The Surgical Critical Care Handbook

Guidelines for
Care of the Surgical Patient in the ICU

The Surgical Critical Care Handbook

Guidelines for Care of the Surgical Patient in the ICU

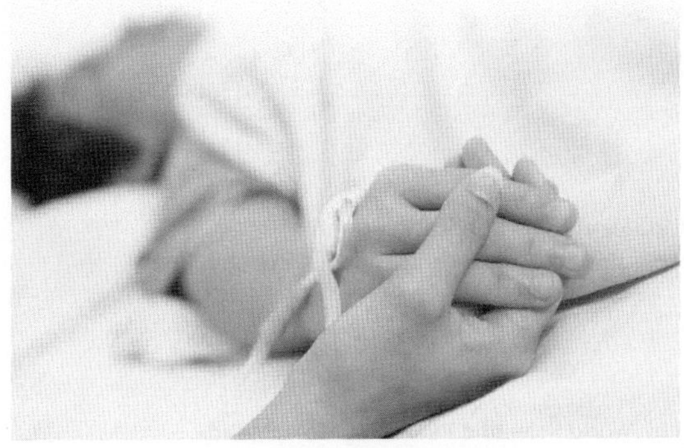

Editor

Jameel Ali

University of Toronto, Canada

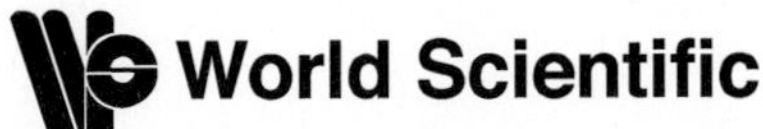

NEW JERSEY · LONDON · SINGAPORE · BEIJING · SHANGHAI · HONG KONG · TAIPEI · CHENNAI · TOKYO

Published by

World Scientific Publishing Co. Pte. Ltd.
5 Toh Tuck Link, Singapore 596224
USA office: 27 Warren Street, Suite 401-402, Hackensack, NJ 07601
UK office: 57 Shelton Street, Covent Garden, London WC2H 9HE

Library of Congress Cataloging-in-Publication Data
The surgical critical care handbook : guidelines for care of the surgical patient in the ICU / [edited] by Jameel Ali.
p. ; cm.
Includes bibliographical references.
ISBN 978-9814663120
I. Ali, Jameel, editor.
[DNLM: 1. Intensive Care--methods--Handbooks. 2. Intensive Care Units--standards--Handbooks. 3. Monitoring, Physiologic--methods--Handbooks. 4. Surgical Procedures, Operative--methods--Handbooks. 5. Wounds and Injuries--surgery--Handbooks. WX 39]
RC86.7
616.02'8--dc23

2015009060

British Library Cataloguing-in-Publication Data
A catalogue record for this book is available from the British Library.

Desk Editor: Dipasri Sardar

Typeset by Stallion Press
Email: enquiries@stallionpress.com

Printed in Singapore

Contents

Foreword

As care givers we are frequently required to manage patients with life threatening disorders. This is more likely in the ICU environment where surgical patients are treated. These patients not only require management of their surgical disorders but also correction of abnormalities characteristic of the critically ill. The surgical intensivist must therefore be well informed in many disciplines other than the surgical disorders in order to care for these patients appropriately. This frequently requires a team approach which includes input from anesthesiologists, internists, respirologists, nurses, respiratory therapists, social workers, ethicists and frequently members of the clergy.

To address all these issues, this handbook has benefited from input from many sources. The authors and coauthors are experts in their disciplines or have had recent personal exposure to management of the critically ill surgical patient during extensive postgraduate training. The first section of the text discusses pathophysiologic processes common to the critically ill patient and sets the stage for applying these general principles in managing specific surgical disorders, dividing these into two subsections — trauma and no trauma.

The geriatric population continues to increase with our improvements in technology and medical/surgical care in general leading to larger numbers of these patients requiring intensive care. Our chapter on the geriatric critically ill patient focuses on problems unique to this population as well general ICU management issues. Likewise there is great emphasis on the care of the critically ill pediatric patient where special skills are required in dealing with the psychological component as well as unique pathophysiologic response to illness.

Family dynamics, life and death issues, futility of treatment, consent for treatment and cessation of treatment are all very important issues in the ICU requiring sensitivity, empathy and honest open discussion with not only the patient but also with their family members and stakeholders. The chapter on application of biomedical ethical principles is aimed at preparing the intensive care team to deal with these issues.

As physicians we are very privileged to be afforded the precious gift of knowledge and skills to make a difference in the lives of our patients and with this privilege comes a deep sense of responsibility and gratitude for having been the recipients of these special gifts. This gratitude is best expressed by applying our skills to the ultimate benefit of our patients and expressing thanks for these gifts to our teachers and the Giver of all knowledge. We are also very privileged not only as physicians but also as teachers giving to our students and patients the benefits of our knowledge in such a way that when our students touch their patients it should be as if our own hands are touching those patients. This brings a level of solemnity and spirituality to our day-to-day care of our patients and their families.

It is my hope that this handbook will enhance the readers' ability to care for the critically ill patient, not only in a very knowledgeable fashion but also with kindness, sensitivity, and humility.

I am deeply indebted to my coauthors who toiled unceasingly in their efforts to make this handbook a special part of the educational armamentarium of our students at all levels.

This handbook is dedicated to my family, my teachers, my students and especially my patients from whom I continue to learn so much, to whom I am forever grateful and through whom I am able to practice this treasured art with (as mentioned by one of my dear colleagues) heart, humility and humanity.

— Jameel Ali, MD, MMedEd

About the Editor

Jameel Ali

Dr Jameel Ali was born in Trinidad and Tobago where he underwent early education at Roman Catholic Missionary Schools. Dr Ali then moved to Winnipeg, Manitoba for Medical School followed by Residency training and clinical Fellowship in General Surgery with basic research training in respiratory physiology.

From Winnipeg, Manitoba he went on to Critical Care and Trauma fellowships at Boston University Medical Centre and San Francisco General Hospital of the University of California — San Francisco. Dr Ali returned to Winnipeg as Assistant Professor and was later promoted as Full Professor in 1985. During this period Dr. Ali continued doing research in respiratory physiology and established one of the first Surgical Critical Care units in Canada. He became the Director of Trauma and established the Advanced Trauma Life Support (ATLS) training program in Manitoba. He was also the Director for Post graduate Training in Surgery for four years there and Chief of the Region XI of the Committee on Trauma of the American College of Surgeons as well as President of the Manitoba Chapter of the American College of Surgeons, National ATLS faculty and member of the ATLS subcommittee. Dr Ali is a Fellow of the Royal College of Surgeons of Canada and of the American College of Surgeons and has a Master's degree in Medical Education from the University of Dundee.

Dr. Ali moved to the University of Toronto in 1987 as the Head of the Divisions of General Surgery at Sunnybrook and later to the Toronto Western Hospital where he was Medical Director of the Trauma Program.

Dr Ali is also the Director of the University of Toronto Advanced Trauma Life support program and was Chairman of the Postgraduate Surgery Committee of the University for 11 years, during which period the Postgraduate Program underwent two successful Royal College reviews. Under Dr. Ali's tenure the Surgical Scientist Program of the University of Toronto secured Ministry of Health funding, under the leadership of Dr. Ori Rotstein with the foresight of the Chair of the Department, Dr. Bernard Langer. The Surgical Scientist Program has trained PhD and MSc surgeons that have gone on to major academic surgical careers in Canada and world-wide including myself.

Dr. Ali has been a prominent member of the international ATLS educator faculty, which trains educators and ATLS faculty across the world. Dr. Ali was a contributing author of 7 editions of the ATLS Provider and Instructor manuals, the Prehospital Trauma Life support manual, the Advanced Trauma Operative Management course and pioneered the TEAM (Trauma Evaluation and Management) program for training medical students in principles of trauma resuscitation. He has also promulgated the Rural Trauma Team Development program in Canada, the Middle East and the Caribbean. Dr. Ali directed the first ATLS course outside North America, which took place in Trinidad and Tobago in 1986. This course was the start of the international ATLS promulgation program through which more than 2 million physicians have been trained in over 65 countries. Dr. Ali has received numerous awards for undergraduate, postgraduate and international teaching including the W T Aikins Faculty teaching award for course development and coordination for undergraduate teaching as well as the Bruce Tovee award for postgraduate teaching at the University of Toronto, the ATLS Meritorious Service Award, the Trauma Achievement award of the American College of Surgeons and the Prehospital Trauma Life Support Scott Frame Award. A measure of Dr. Ali's compassion and zeal for humanitarian care is his receiving the Dr. Vincent J Hughes Physician humanitarian award through the Medical staff association as well as the award named after him — the Jameel Ali St. Michaels Hospital Award in Continuing Education in Surgery. Dr. Ali has been the Associate Editor for 3 editions of one of the leading Text books in Critical Care, and a member of the editorial Board of the Journal of Trauma and Journal of Surgical Research. He has over 240 publications in the areas of respiratory physiology, critical care, trauma and trauma education. After a five-year experience at the Breast Cancer Center at St. Michaels Hospital in Toronto, Dr. Ali travelled to Trinidad and Tobago where he continues his clinical practice in breast cancer and research in a public free Breast Cancer Clinic. Dr. Ali is part of a funded research program in breast cancer genetics in the Caribbean while maintaining his trauma focused teaching activities at the University of Toronto and overseas. Dr. Ali's wealth of experience in clinical and basic science research and educational aspects of trauma and critical care is quite evident in this handbook which is an excellent guide for those interested in surgical critical care at all levels of training.

Sandro Rizoli MD PhD FRCSC FACS
Professor Surgery & Critical Care Medicine, University of Toronto
Medical Director Trauma & Acute Care Service, St Michael's Hospital
Chair in Trauma Care
Past President Trauma Association of Canada

List of Contributors

EDITOR

Jameel Ali, MD, M. Med. Ed., FRCSC, FACS
Professor of Surgery, University of Toronto,
Division of General Surgery, Trauma Program
St. Michael's Hospital
55 Queen Street E. Suite 402
Toronto, ON M5C 1R6 CANADA
Tel: 416 864-6019
Fax: 416 864-6008
Email: alij@smh.ca

CONTRIBUTORS

Addison K. May, MD, FACS, FCCM
Professor of Surgery and Anesthesiology Director,
Surgical Intensive Care Program Director,
Surgical Critical Care, Acute Care Surgery,
and Burn Fellowship Director,
Critical Care Education 1211, 21st Avenue South
404 Medical Arts Bldg.
Nashville, TN 37212-1750
Tel: (615) 936-0303
Fax: (615) 936-0185
Email: addison.may@vanderbilt.edu

Anand Ghanekar, MD, PhD, FRCSC
Assistant Professor of Surgery,
Abdominal Organ Transplant Surgeon,
Multi Organ Transplant Program,
University of Toronto, University Health Network
190 Elizabeth Street Toronto,
Ontario M5G 2C4, Canada
Email: anand.ghanekar@uhn.ca

Andrew Beckett, MD, FRCSC
Trauma and Acute Care Surgery
McGill University Health Centre Montreal,
Quebec Canada H3G 1A4

Andrew S. Barbas, MD
Transplant Fellow,
University Health Network, Toronto
Duke University Hospital
2301 Erwin Rd
Durham, NC 27705
Tel: (919) 970-4267

Andrew Smith, MD, FRCSC
Department of Surgery
Thunder Bay Regional Health Sciences Centre
Northern Ontario School of Medicine
980 Oliver Road
Thunder Bay, Ontario,
Canada P7B 6V4

Arthur Cooper, MD, MS, FACS, FAAP, FCCM, FAHA
Professor of Surgery, Columbia University College
of Physicians & Surgeons;
Director of Trauma & Pediatric Surgical Services
Harlem Hospital Center
Department of Surgery
506 Lenox Avenue, Suite 11-103
New York, NY 10037
Tel: (212) 939-4003
Email: ac38@columbia.edu

Brad S. Moffat, MD, MSc
501-1460 Beaverbrook Ave
London, ON, N6H 5W7

D. Kagedan, MD
General Surgery Resident,
University of Toronto
1 King's College Circle Medical Sciences Building Room 7358
Toronto, Ontario M5S 1A8 Canada

Daniel Roizblatt, MD
Professor of Surgery
Universidad Andres Bello
Trauma and General Surgery
Hospital del Trabajador,
Providencia, Santiago, Chile

David D. Paskar, MD, MSc
University of Western Ontario
General Surgery Resident,
LHSC University Hospital
Department of General Surgery
Room C8 114,339 Windermere Road
London, ON N6A 5A5

G. Papia, MD, MSc, FRCS(C)
Assistant Professor
Department of Surgery
University of Toronto
Division of Vascular Surgery
Department of Critical Care Medicine
Sunnybrook Health Sciences Centre
2075 Bayview Ave.
Toronto, ON M4N 3M5
Tel: 416-480-6100, ext. 83680
Fax: 416-480-5815
Email: giuseppe.papia@sunnybrook.ca

James Mahoney, MD, FRCS
Chief, Division of Plastic Surgery
Medical Director, Perioperative Services
St. Michael's Hospital
30 Bond St., Rm 4080
Toronto, Ontario M5B 1W8
Tel: (416)-864-5385
Fax: (416)-864-5888
Email: amaralh@smh.toronto.on.ca

Joao B. de Rezende-Neto, MD, PhD, FACS
Associate Professor of Surgery,
University of Toronto
Trauma and Acute Care Surgery,
St. Michaels Hospital, Toronto

Jeremie Larouche, MD, FRCSC
Division of Orthopedics
University of Toronto
27 King's College Circle
Toronto, Ontario M5S 1A1 Canada
Tel: 416-978-2011

Jeremy Hall, MD, FRCSC
Assistant Professor of Surgery, Dept of Orhopedics,
University of Toronto,
St. Michael's Hospital
30 Bond St.
Toronto, ON M5B 1W8 Canada
Tel: 416-864-6006
Email: tungl@smh.ca

Joel S. Fish, MD, MSc, FRCSC
Associate Professor of Surgery,
University of Toronto
Medical Director
Burn Program

Plastic and Reconstructive Surgery Sick Kids
555 University Avenue
Toronto, Ontario
Canada M5G 1X8
Phone: 416-813-7654 Ext. 228198
Fax: 416-813-8569
Email: joel.fish@sickkids.ca

John B. Kortbeek, MD, MMedSC, FRCSC FACS
Professor and Chairman,
Dept of Surgery,
University of Calgary, Alberta
Alberta Health Services
10301 Southport Lane SW
Calgary, Alberta T2W 1S7 Canada

John Weigelt, DVM, MD, MMA, FACS
Professor of Surgery
Medical College of Wisconsin
9200 W Wisconsin Ave
Milwaukee, WI 53226

Jonathan Hong, MBBS, MS, FRACS
St. Michael's Hospital
30 Bond Street
Toronto, Ontario
M5B 1W8, Canada
Tel: 416-360-4000

Karen M. Cross, MD, FRCSC
Assistant Professor, Dept of Surgery,
St. Michaels Hospital,
Division of Plastic Surgery,
University of Toronto
30, Bond St. Toronto M5B1W8
Email: Crossk@smh.ca

Katerina Pavenski, BSc, MD, FRCPC
Assistant Professor
Laboratory Medicine and Pathobiology,
University of Toronto
St. Michael's Hospital
30 Bond St. Rm 2-035 CC Wing
Toronto
Ontario
M5B 1W8
Tel: 416-864-5058
Fax: 416-864-3060
Email: pavenskik@smh.ca

Logeswary Rajagopalan, MD
Newark Beth Israel Medical Center
201 Lyons Ave
Newark, NJ 07112
Tel: (973) 926-4000

Lyne Noël de Tilly, MD, FRCPC
Assistant Professor of Radiology,
University of Toronto,
Neuro Radiologist St. Michaels Hospital,
30, Bond St. Toronto
Ontario
M5B1W8
Tel: (416) 864-5674

Marcus Burnstein, MD, MSc, FRCSC
Associate Professor of Surgery,
University of Toronto
Colon and Rectal Surgeon
St. Michael's Hospital
55 Queen Street E. Suite 402
Toronto, ON M5C 1R6
CANADA
Tel: 416 864-6019
Fax: 416 864-6008

Mark W. Bowyer, MD, FACS, DMCC
Professor of Surgery
Chief, Division of Trauma and Combat Surgery
The Norman M. Rich Department of Surgery
Uniformed Services University
Bethesda, Maryland
Attending Surgeon, Trauma and Acute Care Surgery
Washington Hospital Center
Washington, DC

Marshall Beckman, MD, MA, FACS
Assist Professor of Surgery,
Medical College of Wisconsin
9200 W Wisconsin Ave
Trauma And Critical Care Surgery
Milwaukee, WI 53226
Phone: (414) 805-8623
Fax: (414) 805-8641

Mary Joan Marron-Corwin, MD
Clinical Professor of Pediatrics,
Columbia University, New York
Harlem Hospital Center
506 Malcolm X Blvd Ste 4419
New York, NY 10037

Mohammed Bawazeer, MB, ChB, FRCSC
Consultant General Surgery, Trauma, Critical Care Medicine
King Abdulaziz Medical City
Riyadh

Nawaf Al-Otaibi, MBBS
Division of Plastic Surgery, Department of Surgery
St. Michael's Hospital
30 Bond St., Rm. 4080
Toronto, Ontario
M5B 1W8

Neil G. Parry, MD, FRCSC, FACS
Associate Professor of Surgery,
University of Western Ontario
Chair Povincial Committee on Trauma, Ontario
Director Trauma Program,
London Health Science Centre
General and Trauma Surgeon
800 Commissioners Rd East.
London, Ontario N6A 5W9

Priti Dhar, MD
Surgical Oncology Fellow,
University of Toronto
190, Elizabeth St. Toronto
Ontario
M5G2C4
Tel: (989) 790-1001

Pamela Feuer, MD
Pediatric Critical Care
Rhode Island Hosp Crtcl Cr Medc
593 Eddy St # Potter
Providence, RI 02903
Tel: (401) 444-4201

R. Loch Macdonald, MD, PhD, FRCSC, FAANS, FACS
Professor of Surgery,
University of Toronto
Division of Neurosurgery
Head, Division of Neurosurgery
St. Michael's Hospital
Old Administration Building
263 McCaul, Room 120
Toronto, ON. M5T1W7
Phone: (416) 864-5452
Fax: (416) 864-5634
Email: macdonaldlo@smh.ca

Ranjith Kamity, MD
259 First Street
Department of Pediatrics-Neonatology
Mineola, NY 11501
Phone: (516) 663-8453
Fax: (516) 663-8955

Richard M. Bell, MD, FACS
Distinguished Emeritus Professor of Surgery,
University of South Carolina, USA
(503) 224-1371

Robert Chen, MD, FRCP
Department of Clinical Neurological Sciences
University of Western Ontario
Victoria Hospital, London, Ontario, Canada

Safraz Mohammed, MBBS, FRCSC
Neurosurgical Spine Fellow,
University of Toronto
Chief Neurosurgical Resident
University of Toronto
27 King's College Circle
Toronto, Ontario M5S 1A1 Canada

Sami Alissa, MBBS
Security Forces Hospital
Riyadh, Saudi Arabia

Sandro Rizoli, MD, PhD, FRCSC, FACS
Professor of Surgery, University of Toronto
Director Trauma Program,
St. Michael's Hospital
3-074 Donnelly Wing
30 Bond Street
Toronto, ON M5B 1W8
Phone: 416-480-5255
Fax: 416-480-4599
Email: sandro.rizoli@sunnybrook.ca

Sarah Knowles, MD, MSc
London Health Sciences Centre
Human Resources — Perth Drive Complex
339 Windermere Road
London, Ontario
N6A 5A5

Shelly Wang, MD
Neurosurgical Resident
Department of Neurosurgery
University of Toronto
Toronto, Ontario, Canada

Shuyin Liang, MD
General Surgery Resident,
University of Toronto
Dept of Surgery
University of Toronto, Stewart Building
149 College Street, Suite 503
Toronto, ON M5T 1P5

Timothy D. Jackson, BSc, MD, MPH, FRCSC
Assistant Professor of Surgery,
University of Toronto
Department of Surgery
University Health Network
University of Toronto
Toronto, Ontario, Canada
Email: Timothy.Jackson@uhn.ca

Victor Hurth, MD, MHA, CMD, FACP, AGSF
Professor of Medicine and Chief of Geriatrics
University of South Carolina
1600 Hampton Street Suite 738
Columbia, South Carolina 29208
United States

Zoheir Bshouty, MD, PhD, FRCPC
Assistant Professor of Medicine,
Section of Respiratory Diseases,
Director of Pulmonary Function Laboratory,
Health Sciences Centre,
Department of Medicine
University of Manitoba
Winnipeg, Manitoba R3A 1R8, Canada

SECTION 1
General Considerations

Chapter 1

Preoperative Assessment of the High-Risk Surgical Patient

Robert Chen and Jameel Ali

Key Points

1. Perioperative risk assessment by careful history, physical examination, and selective investigation is essential for directing therapy in the high-risk surgical patient.
2. To decrease mortality and morbidity, major medical illnesses must be identified and appropriately managed.
3. Delirium is a common postoperative complication that can be anticipated given risk factors.
4. Perioperative cardiac morbidity can be minimized with preoperative medical evaluation which includes appropriate perioperative testing. Routine beta-blockade is likely harmful.
5. Postoperative pulmonary complications can be reduced by aggressive pre- and postoperative care.
6. Diabetes mellitus and steroid dependence must be completely managed to significantly influence perioperative morbidity and mortality.

Chapter Overview

Anesthesiologists have described elective surgery as "planned trauma". Thus they prepare for all the traumatic sequelae that will occur such as blood loss and fluid shifts, increased myocardial oxygen demands, respiratory changes caused by intubation and ventilation with supplemental oxygen, increased plasma cortisol of the stress response and coagulopathy to name a few. In the average otherwise healthy patient these responses result in no major untoward postoperative events. However, in the medically compromised patient, the additional burden of surgical stress can prove to be very challenging and sometimes insurmountable. Such patients frequently require detailed evaluation and monitoring in the preoperative as well as postoperative periods in the intensive care unit (ICU). Careful planning, preoperative assessment and management of identified abnormalities in these patients are crucial to optimize chances of a good postoperative outcome. A major component of this planning involves the assessment of risks for intraoperative and post-operative morbidity. Patients with cardiac, respiratory, and renal abnormalities pose special risks for postoperative complications. In this chapter, we present guidelines for identifying and managing patients at risk of developing postoperative morbidity.

Preoperative Screening

Appendix 1 is the perioperative screening tool for surgical patients at St. Michael's Hospital in Toronto, Canada. Patients identified preoperatively with severe disease or gravid patients for non-obstetric surgery should be seen by an anesthesiologist in an outpatient clinic where there is time for preoperative risk stratification and disease optimization if possible. If conditions are found that warrant a delay in surgery, early identification minimizes the impact of other scheduled surgeries. At that juncture, additional advice from Internal Medicine or medical subspecialties is sought as necessary for postoperative management.

Codifying or classification leads to more rapid and precise communication among clinicians: Shock classification, solid organ injury grading, and subarachnoid hemorrhage classification are such examples. The American Society of Anesthesiologists (ASA) physical status classification was created with a similar goal (Appendix 2) and is still commonly used as an index of surgical risk.[1] The Dripps American Surgical Association classification is essentially identical.[2] Not surprisingly, for a non-parametric scale, morbidity and mortality does not rise regularly with increasing score. The risk for anesthesia and surgery for ASA 1–2 patients is thought to be better than 1:50,000. The risk rises acutely for ASA 4 but is not 100% for ASA 5.[3] Additionally, statistics are made more difficult to interpret as the score is assigned by a clinician who is free to interpret "constant threat to life". A patient critically dependent on dialysis may logically be called ASA 4 but such patients have competed in triathlons.[4] Therefore, clinicians should not depend entirely on such scales for risk assessment but critically assess the individual.

Assessment of Preoperative CNS risk

Delirium is common postoperative, particularly in elderly patients who are thought to have a 50% occurrence.[5] Longitudinal studies have demonstrated long term cognitive dysfunction in patients who have suffered delirium as inpatients.[6]

The risk factors for delirium are numerous and include surgery and anesthesia (Appendix 3). Patients who have received regional anesthetics, thus likely exposed to less opiates, have the same rate of delirium as those who have undergone general anesthetics.[7] Other factors common to our aging population such as structural (stroke, brain injury) and non-structural (psychiatric) brain disease increase the risk for delirium. A recognized risk of delirium allows early treatment.

Postoperative pain is an important risk factor for delirium. Patients may enter a terrible feedback loop of suffering from delirium only to have opiates removed from their postoperative regime to then experience more pain and more delirium. Inadequate pain control is even more frequent in the critical care units with reliance on PL sedation without concomitant analgesia. Many ICU's do not have a formal sedation and analgesia protocol and, patients risk being sedated without analgesia,[8] increasing risk for postoperative delirium.

Postoperative delirium requires a multimodal treatment strategy. While haloperidol is sometimes considered, the evidence for improved outcomes is lacking. Pre-treating patients at risk for delirium has had limited success.[10]

Identifying risk of delirium allows preventive treatment. This is done by ensuring that environmental, medical and pharmacological factors favor recovery. Examples of such measures include: Ensuring the patient has appropriate vision and hearing aids in place, controlling noise and lighting that affect sleep-wake cycles, ensuring adequate pain control, treatment of dehydration, appropriate nutrition and avoiding polypharmacy.

Assessment of Cardiac Morbidity for Non-Cardiac Surgery

Our aging population, rising rates of obesity and Type II diabetes suggest that more patients presenting for non-cardiac surgery will have diagnosed or clinically suspected ischemic heart disease and thus increased risk for perioperative complications. Using multivariate analysis of 1,001 consecutive patients presenting for non-cardiac surgery, Goldman and associates developed an index for perioperative risk (Cardiac Risk Index; CRI) based on clinical, electrocardiographic (ECG), and routine biochemical parameters.[9] The strongest predictors of cardiac morbidity were the severity of CAD, a recent myocardial infarction (MI) and perioperative heart failure. Detsky and coworkers reworked the scoring system to allow for broader applicability and less dependence on clinical exam findings. At present, the standard for perioperative cardiac risk assessment combines surgery specific risk, the Eagle criteria, (Appendix 4) and medical risk (Revised Lee CRI).[4] The Lee index also includes surgical risks as one of the variables however only considers supra-inguinal vascular surgery to be high risk as opposed to Eagle who considers all vascular surgery risky. Low risk is defined as less than 1% possibility of perioperative cardiac complications. High-risk patients have a predicted risk of greater than 10%. Modern vascular surgery techniques such as endovascular aortic aneursysm repair (EVAR) compared to open surgery, demonstrate reduced perioperative risk thus calling into question Eagle's definition.

In 2007, the American College of Cardiology and the American Heart Association published their guidelines for preoperative assessment. The guidelines were updated only two years later to reflect new perioperative beta blockade information.[12]

Their conclusion was that patients in the low-risk category may proceed directly to surgery with an expectation of a low rate of cardiac complications. Clearly, patients who require emergent surgery should proceed immediately to the operating theatre without delay for cardiac testing. Patients deemed to be in the high-risk group (those who suffer from unstable coronary artery disease (CAD), decompensated congestive heart failure (CHF), severe valvular disease and unstable arrhythmias) should have their non-cardiac surgery delayed for full cardiac evaluation and treatment.

Patients in the intermediate-risk category will benefit most from the investigations, in an effort to further elucidate the extent of their underlying cardiac disease and to attempt to quantify and possibly reduce the perioperative risks before the commencement of the surgical procedure.

Testing becomes more important as patients face intermediate or high risk surgery without good preoperative functional capacity. Patients who suffer from functional limitation due to surgical disease may mask important cardio-respiratory disease. In addition, North America and many other

Western countries are in the midst of an obesity epidemic with associated sedentary lives .The lack of symptoms in this large segment of the population results from "auto Beta blockade." The patients never achieve, in their day-to-day activities, enough physiologic challenge to reveal their disease.

Without symptoms of CHF, the possibility of complete left ventricle (LV) systolic decompensation is low. Routine LV function studies by echocardiography are not indicated. In analyzing patients for low-risk surgery, the addition of a routine echocardiogram to the preoperative evaluation increased mortality. Still, the availability of echocardiography has allowed the diagnosis of valvular disease at a rate much higher than in the era of Goldman and Detsky where clinical exam findings alone defined risk. An increasingly mobile global population results in the presentation of diseases such as rheumatic mitral stenosis, considered uncommon to Western born patients. Recent publications on perioperative antibiotic coverage have addressed the evolving science of endocarditis prevention. In 2006, the enigma of "mitral valve prolapse without mitral valve regurgitation" was a Class III recommendation for antibiotics. The update that followed two years later concluded even more strongly that there were no Class I indications for endocarditis prophylaxis. The committee did recognize that in certain very high-risk populations (previous endocarditis, prosthetic heart valves, valvulopathy following cardiac transplantation and certain congenital heart disease patients) antibiotic prophylaxis "would be reasonable" but with a weaker II a recommendation. The highest risk of bacteremia is attributed to dental surgery or surgery with gingival manipulation. Endoscopy was considered low risk.

The clinical question is: "Does this patient have ischemic risk? Or will the patient infarct perioperatively". In patients who cannot exercise or cannot perform exercise stress testing, the 2007 ACC/AHA guidelines suggest nuclear medicine perfusion studies or stress echocardiography. Both studies also offer the clinician insight into LV function.

Risk Modification

Preoperative coronary revascularization

It is anticipated that in patients having high risk non-cardiac surgery, revascularization should improve outcome. Early recommendations for preoperative coronary artery bypass grafting (CABG) based on retrospective data or historical controls did not include the mortality associated with CABG itself.

Recently, several trials have examined revascularization through percutaneous procedures as well as sternotomy. The CARP trial randomized over 500 patients to have coronary revascularization or not prior to elective surgery. There were no differences between groups in terms of short term or long term outcome. Other trials which addressed relative weakness of CARP reported similar results. It is difficult to dispute that if the patient has an independent reason for urgent coronary revascularization such as left main CAD or continued ischemia following myocardial infarction coronary revascularization should precede elective non-cardiac surgery. Present evidence would suggest that if important but non critical CAD is identified, preoperative revascularization will delay access to non-cardiac surgery without definite benefit. In the setting of oncologic surgery and major vascular surgery, delays may result in important progression of disease or death.

Perioperative beta blockade

Mangano's important and heavily cited[14] trial randomized patients for major surgery including vascular surgery to be beta blocked with atenolol. He demonstrated a decrease in cardiac mortality as well as cause mortality. Studies that followed supported his conclusions and led to enthusiastic embrace of perioperative beta blockade.

The POISE study,[15] a multicentre placebo control trial of fixed metoprolol dosing for patients facing intermediate and high risk surgery with at least one clinical risk factor for CAD echoed Mangano's findings *vis-à-vis* cardiac morbidity. However, the cause mortality for patients who received metoprolol was higher due to the increased rate of stroke. Concluded differently, the beta blockade of intermediate risk patients may cause harm.

Since POISE, an analysis of beta blocker data with only the most secure studies included suggest that beta blockers increase perioperative mortality The authors believe that beta blocking medications should not be discontinued if already initiated by the patients caring physician. Initiation of beta blockers should only be used to treat active ischemia and not as a preventative measure.

Intensive perioperative management

The rationale for using aggressive perioperative medical intervention to reduce cardiac risk is compelling. Many of the major cardiac risk factors such as congestive heart failure, myocardial ischemia, and dysrhythmias are detectable and amenable to therapy. Factors contributing to oxygen supply and demand balance beyond beta blockade would include appropriate treatment of hypertension, diagnosis and treatment of anemia and appropriate treatment of pulmonary disease. Inpatient optimization and resuscitation have not led to changes in outcome. A multicenter randomized trial of the use of the pulmonary catheter derived hemodynamic goals in almost 2,000 high-risk patients undergoing elective abdominal, thoracic, vascular, and major orthopedic surgery, showed no benefit over standard care.[16]

Pulmonary artery catheter

There is no indication for routine use of the pulmonary artery catheter (PAC) to aid decision making for the high-risk surgical patient. Dr. Swan, in an elegantly written review in 2005 stated quite strongly "the PAC is a diagnostic device only and has ***no therapeutic role***" (emphasis the authors').[17] The PAC-man trial,[18] a large prospective cohort study of mixed medical and surgical patients in the ICU showed no improvement in outcome in those patients with pulmonary artery catheterization. Meta-analysis published in JAMA and the Cochrane Database echo these findings. Even more damning, clinicians may be misinterpreting catheter derived data at a high rate. Worse yet, clinicians may be subjecting their patients to the risk of catheter insertion and not using all the information available. The authors do not question the value of identifying right heart failure or pulmonary hypertension in surgical patients. Important changes to anesthesia and surgical care can be made to favor hemodynamics in that setting. Still, given the paucity of data supporting its use and given a known rate of serious complications, Swan's catheter should be reserved for very, very few patients.

Transesophageal echocardiography (TEE)

TEE is a sensitive marker of myocardial ischemia, often revealing segmental wall motion abnormalities before other signs of ischemia become obvious. TEE has been advocated to detect intraoperative ischemia, and has been shown to have superior sensitivity and specificity (sensitivity 75%, specificity 100%) in comparison to two-lead ECG (sensitivity 56%, specificity 98%) and pulmonary capillary wedge pressure (sensitivity 25%, specificity 93%). A larger study (224 patients) confirms that TEE is frequently influential in guiding clinical decision-making.[19] In comparison to two-lead ECG and PAC, intraoperative TEE was the most important intraoperative guiding factor in decision making for anti-ischemic therapy, fluid administration, and vasopressor or inotrope administration. The technique itself requires expensive equipment and specialized training. Even at centers where TEE is standard of care for cardiac anesthesia, the resource is not routinely available for non-cardiac surgery patients. New miniature, disposable technology may allow greater utilization. No guidelines have suggested class 1 indications for TEE in the non-cardiac surgery population.

Resource Allocation

Application of aggressive hemodynamic monitoring in the ICU to achieve the improved survival of patients with ischemic heart disease following non-cardiac surgery is very costly. In Rao's study, more than 1,300 ICU days of care were required to bring about a 2.4% reduction in the re-infarction rate. However, if admission criteria were restricted to congestive heart failure, angina plus congestive heart failure, or angina plus hypertension, this would account for almost 80% of the perioperative infarctions, and reduce ICU days to <300. Studies have suggested that most perioperative myocardial infarctions occur within the first two postoperative days suggesting a shorter period of monitoring may be sufficient.

Type of Surgery: Type of Anesthetic

As discussed previously, Eagle recognized that non-cardiac operations may be divided into those that are likely to provoke perioperative ischemia and those that do not increase the risk of ischemia above normal. Major vascular procedures involving aortic cross-clamping and infra-inguinal arterial bypass carry a high risk of postoperative ischemia, as do major abdominal and thoracic procedures. Orthopedic procedures such as total hip arthroplasty have a lower incidence of cardiac morbidity, and are deemed intermediate risk. Peripheral nonvascular procedures such as transurethral resection of the prostate, an operation frequently performed in patients with coexisting CAD, are associated with a low incidence of perioperative MI.

Major surgery is associated with an intense sympathetic and procoagulant response, which may be implicated in the development of myocardial ischemia. These neurohumoral responses to surgery may be diminished with the use of epidural anesthesia and analgesia (EAA) extending into the postoperative period. Stress-mediated release of hormones such as cortisol, antidiuretic hormone, and catecholamines is blunted by epidural anesthesia.

In addition, postoperative pain may contribute to tachycardia and resultant subendocardial ischemia. Early studies showed a dramatic reduction in cardiac complications in patients treated with EAA in comparison to general anesthesia (GA) alone. This opinion was further upheld by a large systematic review of relevant trials of epidural or spinal anesthesia versus GA over the past 30 years, which showed a statistically and clinically significant reduction in mortality and morbidity after surgery. This retrospective work was prospectively tested by a large (915 patients) randomized controlled trial of high-risk surgical patients who either received EAA (intraoperatively and up to 72 hours postoperatively) with GA or GA alone with intraoperative and postoperative opioids as the mainstay of the analgesic regimen. The group observed no reduction in mortality or cardiac morbidity between groups. The only clinical benefit documented was a reduction in postoperative respiratory failure. However, the authors commented that 15 epidurals were required to prevent one episode of respiratory failure. They also commented that in no cases were there any serious complications with catheter placement or postoperative problems directly attributable to the placement of the epidural.

Recommendations

Evaluation and treatment of patients presenting for non-cardiac surgery requires careful attention to history, functional status, and assessment of clinical evidence of reversible cardiac failure or dysrhythmias, in addition to consideration of the timing and indications for the proposed surgery. There is no doubt that clinical risk factors such as known ischemic heart disease, cardiac failure, diabetes and renal insufficiency are all independently documented to be associated with an increase in perioperative cardiac morbidity.

Following published guidelines and analysis of the literature, it can be recommended that non-invasive cardiac testing will not add to the clinicians' knowledge or improve risk stratification in patients without the above risk factors. Similarly, patients who present a significant clinical risk may have independent cardiac reasons for revascularization prior to proposed non-cardiac surgery. This high-risk group should be intensively monitored in the perioperative period, including a stay in the ICU for approximately 48 hours postoperatively. It is the intermediate-risk group of patients, presenting with one to two clinical risk factors, who will benefit most from non-invasive stress testing. Beta blockers should not be discontinued for patients already receiving them. There is poor evidence supporting their routine use, even in higher risk patients. Due to negative reports regarding the use of the pulmonary artery catheter its routine use for high-risk patients following non-cardiac surgery cannot be supported. Finally, there may be a role for TEE in non-cardiac surgery. Resources, both financial and manpower will dictate its use.

Assessment of Risk of Postoperative Pulmonary Complications

Clinical assessment of pulmonary risk

Postoperative alterations in pulmonary physiology predispose to the development of atelectasis. Marked decreases in forced expiratory volume in 1 second (FEV1) and forced vital capacity (FVC) have been documented with serial postoperative pulmonary function tests (PFT). A reduction in functional residual capacity (FRC) of approximately 70% of basal values may occur by about 18 hours after surgery, resulting in closure of small airways as FRC approximates closing volume. Progressive loss of functional lung tissue and intrapulmonary shunting leads to worsening hypoxemia.

Many risk factors for the development of postoperative atelectasis have been highlighted. Each of the following has been shown to predict postoperative atelectasis: Preoperative severe bronchitis, FEV1 of more than two standard deviations less than predicted, obesity, malnutrition, abdominal surgery, and age. Analysis of risk factors in a group of 272 patients referred for preoperative assessment concluded that statistically significant predictors of postoperative pulmonary complications were: partial pressure of arterial carbon dioxide ($PaCO_2$) ≥45 mm Hg (OR = 61.0), FVC ≤1.5 L/min (OR = 11.1), maximum laryngeal height ≤4 cm (OR = 6.9), forced expiratory time ≥9 seconds (OR = 5.7), smoking ≥40 pack-years (OR = 5.7), and body mass index (BMI) ≥30 kg/m^2 (OR = 4.1).

PFTs such as spirometry have been used to identify patients at risk of developing postoperative pulmonary complications, but lack of randomization, selection bias, and retrospective or unblended analysis of outcome invalidate conclusions. Spirometry as a screening procedure for high-risk patients remains unproven and its routine use has been discouraged. The American College of Physicians recommends preoperative PFT in the following groups: Patients with unexplained dyspnea, patients undergoing high risk surgery (cardiac, thoracic, and upper abdominal), cigarette smokers, symptoms of dyspnea on exertion, and patients undergoing head and neck or orthopedic surgery with uncharacterized lung disease. All patients undergoing lung resection should have PFTs.

The inability to improve pulmonary function despite adequate therapy may be a more sensitive predictor of postoperative respiratory failure. In a prospective study, those at risk of developing postoperative respiratory failure (defined as ventilator dependent >2 postoperative days) were best identified by the failure of 48–72 hours of intensive preoperative preparation to improve FVC, forced expiratory flow over 25% to 75% of the expiratory cycle (FEF25–75), and maximal voluntary ventilation measured over 1 minute (MVV). Five percent of the study group developed postoperative respiratory failure, and all of these patients had an FEF25–75 and MVV less than 50% of predicted values, which had not improved with preoperative therapy. The perioperative mortality in this subgroup was 60%.

Evaluation of risk prior to pulmonary resection surgery

Approximately 80% of patients presenting for lung cancer surgery have concomitant chronic obstructive pulmonary disease (COPD) and 20–30% have severe pulmonary dysfunction. Pulmonary resection for lung cancer has been associated with morbidity of 12–50% and mortality of 2–12%. A more recent retrospective analysis confirms that these figures have not been markedly improved (morbidity 20%, mortality 3%). In addition to the general preoperative preparation of the surgical patient, those patients who will require pulmonary resection must have a preoperative estimation of postoperative pulmonary reserve.

A multifactorial risk index was proposed for patients undergoing thoracic surgery consisting of the Cardiac Risk Index (CRI) and a pulmonary risk index (PRI), known as the cardiopulmonary risk-factor index (CPRI). These pulmonary risk factors had previously been validated as independent risk factors in univariate analysis. The CPRI assesses obesity, cigarette smoking within eight weeks of surgery, productive cough within five days of surgery, FEV1/FVC <70%, and $PaCO_2$ >45 mm Hg. Each of these factors was assigned one point. By combining the CRI (0–4) and the PRI (0–6), patients classified as having a CPRI of 4 or greater were 17 times more likely to develop a postoperative pulmonary complication than patients with a CPRI less than 4.[23]

Guidelines for prediction of outcome following lung resection are generally based on preoperative whole lung function tests. MVV (% of predicted), FEV1 (liters), and FEV1 (% of predicted) have been most commonly used. Guideline values for proceeding with pneumonectomy, lobectomy, or wedge/segmental resection are:

— For pneumonectomy MVV >55%, FEV1 >2 L, FEV1% >55%;
— For lobectomy MVV >40%, FEV1 >1L, FEV1% 40% to 50%; and
— For wedge/segmental resection MVV >35%, FEV1 >0.6 L, FEV1% >40%.

Predicted postoperative FEV1 has been suggested as a sensitive predictor of postoperative pulmonary complications. For this measurement, FEV1 and CT calculation of the number of preoperative functioning lung segments are required. Predicted postoperative FEV1 (ppoFEV1) may then be calculated using the formula:

$$\text{ppo FEV1} = \text{preoperative FEV1}/(\text{No. of pre-op. functioning segments} \times \text{No. of postop functioning segments}).$$

Studies have suggested that if ppoFEV1 is <40% of predicted, this may be a sensitive predictor of prohibitive operative risk and that resection should not be considered. More recent work suggests that a low ppoFEV1 may indeed be a sensitive predictor of postoperative pulmonary complications in lung cancer resection patients, but only in the group without pre-existing COPD. PpoFEV1 was not a significant predictor of postoperative pulmonary complications in patients with a preoperative diagnosis of COPD. This may be due to the fact that while these patients may have been losing lung tissue, a proportionally greater part of it was emphysematous and therefore less involved in gas exchange.[24]

In addition to these standard bedside tests, diffusion capacity of the lung for carbon monoxide (DLCO) may be helpful. If there is evidence of interstitial lung disease on chest X-ray or undue dyspnea on exertion, even if FEV1 and FVC are normal, a DLCO should be obtained. If preoperative FEV1 or DLCO is <40% of predicted, these are independent predictors of postoperative pulmonary complications. These patients may benefit from cardiopulmonary exercise testing. This is a sophisticated assessment of cardiopulmonary reserve and allows calculation of maximal oxygen consumption (VO_2max). Risk of perioperative pulmonary complications can be stratified according the VO_2max measured. Patients with a preoperative VO_2max of >20 mL/kg are not at increased risk of complications; however, patients with VO_2max of <15 mL/kg and <10 mL/kg are at intermediate and high-risk, respectively, for perioperative pulmonary complications.

Risk Modification

Perioperative preparation

Standard preoperative preparation, including the use of intensive chest physiotherapy, bronchodilators, and appropriate use of antibiotics are considered routine practice in an effort to reduce the risks of postoperative pulmonary complications. High-risk patients who were assigned to receive a protocol of intensive pre- and postoperative therapy (including delay of surgery if indicated) had a 22% incidence of postoperative complications, compared to 60% in a group in whom the preoperative preparation was at the discretion of the admitting physician. Aggressive pulmonary therapy resulted in shorter hospital stay despite frequent delays of surgery in the treatment group to improve pulmonary function.

Despite the clinical application of deep breathing exercises, intermittent positive-pressure breathing (IPPB), and incentive spirometry, these treatments have not been shown to be independently successful in the prevention of postoperative pulmonary complications. Incentive spirometry has been shown to be of benefit, but only in high-risk patients. Pre- and postoperative chest physiotherapy ***per se*** is of value only in the treatment of established pulmonary atelectasis. However, high-risk morbidly obese (BMI >40 kg/m^2) patients may benefit significantly from the application of biphasic positive end-expiratory pressure noninvasively and prior to signs of respiratory distress.

Cessation of cigarette smoking

Continued smoking up to the time of surgery is associated with a significant increase in mortality. Cessation of smoking has been shown to result in a significant increase in FRC and reduced postoperative pulmonary complications. For maximum risk reduction, the patient should stop smoking at least eight weeks prior to surgery. Brief interventions during the preoperative visit or even mailed information can make an important difference in preoperative smoking cessation.[25]

Site of surgical incision

Extremity surgical intervention leads to little alteration in lung volume. However, lower abdominal incision results in a 25–30% decrease in FVC and a mild decrease in oxygenation. Upper abdominal and thoracic surgery produces significant impairment of pulmonary ventilation and defense systems independent of the effect of anesthesia. Maintenance of FVC is essential for effective secretion clearance and is reduced by 50–60% immediately following upper abdominal surgery. Gradual restoration of FVC over the next 5–7 days is usual. During the first 24 hours after upper abdominal or thoracic surgery, reductions occur in tidal volume (20%) and FRC (70–80%) as a result of incision pain and reflex diaphragmatic splinting, resulting in rapid shallow breathing, absence of spontaneous sigh, and chest wall splinting.

Laparoscopic surgery has revolutionized the postoperative care of patients undergoing common surgical procedures such as cholecystectomy and fundoplication. Comparing the open subcostal cholecystectomy to the laparoscopic approach, significant improvements in FVC (52% versus 73% baseline), FEV1 (53% versus 72% baseline), and FEF (53% versus 81% baseline) were documented. A similar comparison of the laparoscopic versus open approach resulted in quicker return of postoperative respiratory mechanics towards but not quite to normal compared to open cholecystectomy.[27] A review of over 300 patients following laparoscopic cholecystectomy showed no major postoperative pulmonary morbidity in the entire group, despite the fact that 45 were deemed to be obese, including 18 who were morbidly obese (BMI >45 kg/m^2).[28]

Type of anesthesia and analgesia

Repeated attempts to demonstrate a consistent decrease in postoperative pulmonary complications with the use of regional anesthesia alone or in combination with GA have failed. Anesthetic technique *per se* is not a significant determinant of postoperative respiratory complications.[29] All forms of regional anesthesia such as epidural local anesthetic, epidural narcotic, intercostal nerve blocks, and paravertebral nerve blocks have beneficial effects on postoperative FEV1, FVC, and partial pressure of arterial oxygen (PaO_2). However, these beneficial effects have not proved to alter outcome in terms of pneumonia, respiratory failure, or death. Perhaps this is because the delayed reduction in FRC, resulting in atelectasis and hypoxemia, remains largely unaffected by the intra- and immediate postoperative analgesic regimens.

Repeated studies of intraoperative positive end-expiratory pressure (PEEP) have failed to show benefit in normal patients; however, the intraoperative application of PEEP 10 cm H_2O to morbidly obese patients (BMI >40 kg/m^2) resulted in an improvement in perioperative oxygenation (110–130 mm Hg). However, these patients were studied in the early postoperative period and this improvement may not have been maintained.

Recommendations

Although several questions concerning accurate preoperative assessment for prevention of clinically significant pulmonary complications remain unanswered, from available data a few guidelines may be generated. Likely to benefit the patient preoperatively are: Cessation of smoking (at least four weeks, preferably >eight weeks abstinence), weight loss, and optimization of airway obstruction using bronchodilators. Intraoperative management options that may benefit the patient include: Peripheral incision, limiting duration of surgery, endoscopic procedures, and the use of intraoperative PEEP. Postoperatively, good analgesia by the use of regional analgesia and patient-controlled analgesia delivery devices has shown to be equally effective in reducing morbidity. Postoperative chest physiotherapy has proven value only for the treatment of atelectasis, but is useful as part of a program to encourage deep breathing exercises.

Diabetes Mellitus

Diabetes mellitus is the most common endocrine disorder encountered in the perioperative period, since it occurs in almost 5% of the general population. Traditionally, diabetics presented for surgery for limb amputation and wound debridement, but owing to surgical advances in vitrectomy, cataract extraction, renal transplantation, and peripheral vascular repairs, diabetic patients are frequently presenting for preoperative assessment. Type I (Insulin-dependent diabetes mellitus) comprises approximately 25% of the diabetic population, and affects a relatively younger population who are ketosis prone. They have no endogenous insulin production and thus insulin is an absolute need. Type II (often and incorrectly called Non-insulin-dependent diabetes mellitus) patients are older and often obese and have a decrease in the number and responsiveness of insulin receptors, together with impaired insulin secretion, features which are accentuated in the perioperative period. The stresses of surgery that have already been discussed also include increases in endogenous glucocorticoids predisposing to postoperative hyperglycemia.

Perioperative management problems also arise when Type II diabetic patients who have now transitioned to high dose insulin are labeled "insulin requiring" and are managed as if they were ketosis prone. Type II diabetics often require several times the daily physiologic requirement for insulin. If they are hypoglycemic, insulin is contraindicated. The ketosis prone Type I requires continuous access to physiologic insulin.

The aim of therapy is to avoid excess morbidity and mortality, which may be caused or exacerbated by extremes in blood glucose levels, undue protein catabolism, and fluid and electrolyte disturbances.

Risk Assessment

As discussed previously, diabetes is an important cardiac risk indicator and it is accepted that diabetics encounter increased perioperative morbidity and mortality.

A perioperative myocardial infarction rate of 5.2% is reported in diabetics undergoing abdominal aortic reconstruction compared to 2.1% of non-diabetic patients. Inadequate control of blood glucose can lead to ketosis and acidemia in Type I patients and dehydration in Types I and II diabetics. Decreased wound healing occurs at glucose levels greater than 200 mg/dL. Glucose concentrations greater than 250 mg/dL have been shown to impair leukocyte function and exacerbate ischemic brain damage. In addition to the effects of abnormal blood glucose levels, diabetics are at particular risk of atherosclerotic disease in cerebral, coronary, and renal vasculature. Peripheral vasculopathy is an important complication of diabetes.

Preoperative clinical markers for increased perioperative complications have been introduced previously. The important risk factors of CAD, congestive heart failure, renal failure, and vascular disease could all be considered simply sequelae of diabetes. Autonomic neuropathy is found in over 40% of patients presenting for surgery and may alter hemodynamic responses to intubation and surgery.

Apart from anesthesia for cataract extraction, choice of anesthetic technique has not been associated with altered outcome. Thoracic epidural and spinal anesthesia techniques are associated with reduced intraoperative catecholamine release. However, to date, no study focusing entirely on diabetic patients has compared outcome between regional and GA techniques.

Risk Reduction

Preoperative evaluation should include thorough clinical assessment for cardiac, neurologic, and peripheral vascular abnormalities. A careful history for the presence of ischemic heart disease or prior myocardial infarction should be supported by cardiac investigations where appropriate. Glycosylated hemoglobin (HbA1c) levels less than 10% suggest satisfactory glycemic control. Some past evidence suggested that intensive insulin therapy to achieve strict control of blood sugar (80–110 mg/dL) improved outcome in non-diabetic surgical ICU patients and that the typical practice (to maintain a blood sugar <200 mg/dL) may be inadequate in the postoperative diabetic.[30] Logically, an intensive regime adds hypoglycemia risks which may mitigate any benefit. The NICE SUGAR research group studied over 6,000 critically ill patients randomly assigned to strict or more liberal blood glucose control. A small but significant mortality signal was associated with strict control.

Non-diabetic patients recovering from surgery commonly show transient hyperglycemia with diminished insulin secretion and end-organ responsiveness secondary to increased circulating catecholamines.[31] However, these patients secrete sufficient insulin to suppress lipolysis and ketogenesis. Diabetics present with decreased or absent preoperative insulin secretion and a pre-existing insulin resistance, which serves to worsen the hyperglycemic response to surgery. Decreased peripheral use of glucose results in lipolysis, ketogenesis, possible acidemia, glycosuria, and dehydration.[32] A variety of insulin regimens have been suggested for the routine perioperative management of diabetics undergoing surgery. No single regimen has proved markedly superior. Currently, perioperative intravenous glucose infusions are recommended, and insulin may be administered via a variety of dosages and routes. Subcutaneous administration of half the regular daily dose before surgery, using a variable-rate glucose infusion to maintain normoglycemia, has proved successful. Mixing insulin, potassium, and 5% or 10% glucose has also been suggested. Most authors suggest a variable-rate insulin infusion using an automated syringe device with a simultaneous glucose infusion through an alternative intravenous access.

Insulin requirements vary widely in the perioperative patient. The normal state (approximately 0.25 unit of insulin per gram of glucose) is influenced by many factors such as obesity, concomitant glucocorticoid administration, and the septic state, which may increase insulin requirements to as high as 0.4–0.8 unit of insulin per gram of glucose. The highest insulin requirements have been observed in patients undergoing CABG (0.8–1.2 U/g of glucose).[33]

Recommendations for glucose infusion to prevent catabolism suggest between 5 and 10 g of glucose per hour,[34] although the optimal dose of glucose necessary for prevention of fat and protein catabolism has not been clearly determined. However, clinical experience suggests that most surgical diabetics can be maintained within the normal blood glucose range with an insulin infusion set between 1 and 2 U/hour.

Patients receiving total parenteral nutrition, which is generally up to 25% dextrose, usually require an additional 2–3 units of insulin per hour. Apart from careful monitoring of blood glucose levels, the patient's overall clinical status (particularly neurologic and hemodynamic) should be closely observed.

Avoidance of hypoglycemic episodes while allowing mild hyperglycemia without ketosis is prudent in the diabetic whose blood sugar is extremely difficult to control.

What emerges from all the studies dealing with perioperative diabetes management is that the most important factor in optimal perioperative glycemic control is frequent measurement of blood sugar and appropriate therapeutic interventions by trained staff. Perioperative metabolic management should be planned and coordinated by surgeons, anesthetists, and diabetic care teams in conjunction with the patient when possible. With the exception of type II diabetic patients presenting for minor surgery, all diabetic patients should receive intravenous infusions of glucose with appropriate insulin to achieve normoglycemia until the preoperative regimen is resumed.

Glucocorticoid Supplementation in Chronic Glucocorticoid Users

Perioperative glucocorticoid supplementation for patients receiving steroid therapy is common. The rationale for its use is the avoidance of hypoadrenalism, resulting in a variety of clinical signs including fever, nausea, dehydration, abdominal pain, hypotension, and shock. Other evidence of hypoadrenalism includes low-voltage complexes on the ECG, hypoglycemia, and eosinophilia. Despite many patients presenting with chronic steroid use, the incidence of perioperative adrenal insufficiency is low (0.01–0.1%).[23]

Retrospective and prospective data suggest that routine steroid supplementation for all glucocorticoid-treated patients may not be necessary. Well-known adverse effects of exogenous glucocorticoids include immunosuppression, exacerbation of osteoporosis, avascular necrosis of the femur, diabetes, peptic ulcer disease, diminished wound healing, and neuropsychiatric disorders.

Daily endogenous cortisol release in normal adults approximates 25–30 mg per day at rest. Stressors such as major surgery or critical illness increase endogenous production to five to ten times that amount because of increased secretion of adrenocorticotropic hormone (ACTH) from the anterior pituitary gland. Increased cortisol secretion returns to normal within 24 hours of skin incision in uncomplicated minor surgery.[36]

The clinical rationale for steroid supplementation in the perioperative period is based on the known protracted recovery of the hypothalamus-pituitary-adrenal (HPA) axis following prolonged glucocorticoid administration.[37] The stress response observed in typical perioperative patients results in

ACTH levels far in excess of that required for maximal adrenocortical stimulation. A number of studies have suggested that patients on chronic steroid therapy undergoing elective major surgery may not require perioperative steroid supplementation in addition to their regular steroid regimen. In a study of 40 renal transplant recipients on chronic prednisone therapy, none of the patients received more than baseline glucocorticoid therapy during admission for moderately stressful surgery or critical illness. Despite biochemical evidence of decreased adrenal response to exogenous ACTH in 67% of the patients, none of the patients exhibited clinically overt hypoadrenalism, and 97% of all patients excreted normal or increased urinary cortisol concentrations during their hospital stay. This suggested that cortisol concentrations were sufficient to meet requirements during the time of stress.

Since endogenous cortisol secretion in normal individuals rarely exceeds 200 mg/day, exogenous steroid supplementation should be similar. To date, no data suggest that supplemental glucocorticoid therapy exceeding this amount is beneficial. Patients on chronic steroid therapy undergoing minor surgery should have their regular steroid dose on the morning of surgery and no additional doses if surgery is uncomplicated. Candidates for major surgery should receive no more than physiologic doses of glucocorticoid. A regime might consist of 25 mg hydrocortisone intravenously on induction of anesthesia, and 100–150 mg per day over the following 24–72 hours. If a patient presenting for surgery is already receiving a maintenance steroid dose greater than the estimated requirement, additional steroid coverage is not necessary.

Clinical and biochemical preoperative assessment of patients on chronic steroid therapy is invaluable in the identification of patients at risk for adrenal insufficiency in the perioperative period. Published recommendations for supplemental steroid coverage should be followed by dosing to physiologic levels.

References

1. Keats AS. The ASA classification of physical status: A recapitulation (editorial). *Anesthesiology* 1978; 49: 233.
2. Dripps RD, Lamont A, Eckenhoff JE. The role of anesthesia in surgical mortality. *JAMA* 1961; 178: 261–266.
3. Lagasse RS. Anesthesia safety: Model or myth? A review of the published literature and analysis of current original data. *Anesthesiology* 2002; 97(6): 1609–1617.

4. http://www.ironshad.com/home/ (accessed on July 1, 2014).
5. Milbrandt EB, Deppen S, Harrison PL *et al.* Costs associated with delirium in mechanically ventilated patients. *Crit Care Med* 2004; 32(4): 955–962.
6. Jackson JC, Gordon SM, Hart RP, Hopkins RO, Ely EW. The association between delirium and cognitive decline: A review of the empirical literature. *Neuropsychol Rev* 2004; 14(2): 87–98.
7. Bryson GL, Wyand A. Evidence-based clinical update: General anesthesia and the risk of delirium and post-soperative cognitive dysfunction. *Can J Anaesth* 2006; 53(7): 669.
8. Mehta S, Burry L, Fischer S *et al.* Canadian survey of the use of sedatives, analgesics, and neuromuscular blocking agents in critically ill patients. *Crit Care Med* 2006; 34(2): 374–380.
9. Inouye SK, Bogardus ST Jr, Charpentier PA *et al.* A multicomponent intervention to prevent delirium in hospitalized older patients. *N Engl J Med* 1999; 340(9): 669–676.
10. Kalisvaart KJ, de Jonghe JF, Bogaards MJ *et al.* Haloperidol prophylaxis for elderly hip-surgery patients at risk for delirium: A randomized placebo-controlled study. *J Am Geriatr Soc* 2005; 53(10): 1658–1666.
11. Goldman L, Caldera DL, Nussbaum SR *et al.* Multifactorial index of cardiac index in noncardiac surgical procedures. *N Engl J Med* 1977; 297: 845.
12. Fleisher LA, Beckman JA, Brown KA *et al.* 2009 ACCF/AHA focused update on perioperative beta blockade incorporated into the ACC/AHA 2007 guidelines on perioperative cardiovascular evaluation and care for noncardiac surgery. *J Am Coll Cardiol* 2009; 54(22): e13–e118.
13. McFalls EO, Ward HB, Moritz TE *et al.* Coronary-artery revascularization before elective major vascular surgery. *N Engl J Med* 2004; 351(27): 2795–2804.
14. Mangano DT, Layug EL, Wallace A, Tateo I. Effect of atenolol on mortality after non-cardiac surgery. Multicenter Study of Perioperative Ischemia Research Group. *N Engl J Med* 1996; 335: 1713.
15. Devereaux PJ, Yang H, Yusuf S *et al.* Effects of extended-release metoprolol succinate in patients undergoing non-cardiac surgery (POISE trial): A randomised controlled trial. *Lancet* 2008; 371(9627): 1839–1847.
16. Sandham JD, Hull RD, Brant RF *et al.* A randomised, controlled trial of the use of pulmonary-artery catheters in high-risk surgical patients. *N Engl J Med* 2003; 348: 5
17. Swan HJ. The pulmonary artery catheter in anesthesia practice. *Anesthesiology* 2005; 103(4): 890–893.
18. Harvey S, Harrison DA, Singer M *et al.* PAC-Man study collaboration. Assessment of the clinical effectiveness of pulmonary artery catheters in management of patients in intensive care (PAC-Man): A randomised controlled trial. *Lancet* 2005; 366(9484): 472–477.

19. Kolev N, Brase R, Swanevelder J *et al.* The influence of transoesophageal echocardiography on intra-operative decision making. A European multicentre study. European Perioperative TOE Research Group. *Anaesthesia* 1998; 53: 767.
20. Rao TLK, Jacobs KH, El-Etr AA. Reinfarction following anesthesia in patients with myocardial infarction. *Anesthesiology* 1983; 59: 499.
21. De Nino LA, Lawrence VA, Averyt EC *et al.* Preoperative spirometry and laparotomy — blowing away dollars. *Chest* 1997; 111: 1536.
22. Marshall M, Olsen GN. The physiologic evaluation of the lung resection candidate. *Clin Chest Med* 1993; 14: 305.
23. Brunelli A, Al Refai M, Monteverde M *et al.* Predictors of early mortality after major lung resection in patients with and without airflow limitation. *Ann Thorac Surg* 2002; 74: 999.
24. Epstein SK, Faling J, Daly BDT *et al.* Predicting complications after pulmonary resection. *Chest* 1993; 104: 694.
25 Lee SM, Landry J, Jones PM, Buhrmann O, Morley-Forster P. The effectiveness of a perioperative smoking cessation program: A randomized clinical trial. *Anesth Analg* 2013; 117(3): 605–613.
26. Ford GT, Whitelaw WA, Rosenal TW *et al.* Diaphragm function after upper abdominal surgery in humans. *Am Rev Respir Dis* 1983; 127: 43.
27. Ali J, Gana T. Lung volumes after laparoscopic cholecystectomy — justification for early discharge. *Can Respir J* 1998; 5: 109.
28. Sperlongano P, Pisaniello D, Parmeggiani D *et al.* Laparoscopic cholecystectomy in the morbidly obese. *Chir Ital* 2002; 54: 363.
29. Peyton P, Myles PS, Silbert BS *et al.* Perioperative epidural analgesia and outcome after major abdominal surgery in high-risk patients. *Anesth Analg* 2003; 96: 548.
30. Van den Bergh G, Wouters P, Weekers F *et al.* Intensive insulin therapy in the critically ill patient. *N Engl J Med* 2001; 345: 1359.
31. NICE-SUGAR Study Investigators, Finfer S, Chittock DR, Su SY *et al.* Intensive versus conventional glucose control in critically ill patients. *N Engl J Med* 2009; 360(13): 1283–1297.
32. Gavin LA. Perioperative management of the diabetic patient. *Endocrinol Clin North Am* 1992; 21: 457.
33. Gill GV, Sherif IH, Alberti KG. Management of diabetes during open-heart surgery. *Br J Surg* 1981; 68: 171.
34. Rosenstock J, Raskin P. Surgery: Practical guidelines for diabetes management. *Clin Diabetes* 1987; 5: 49.
35. Alford WC, Meador CK, Mihalevich J *et al.* Acute adrenal insufficiency following cardiac surgical procedures. *J Thorac Cardiovasc Surg* 1979; 78: 489.
36. Snow K, Jiang NS, Kao PC, Scheithauer BW. Biochemical evaluation of adrenal dysfunction: The laboratory perspective. *Mayo Clin Proc* 1992; 67: 1055.
37. Livanou T, Ferriman D, James VHT. Recovery of hypothalamo-pituitary-adrenal function after corticosteroid therapy. *Lancet* 1967; 2: 856.

Appendix 1. Considerations for preoperative Anesthesia assessment

1. Request for Consultation — either patient- or surgeon-initiated request for preoperative anesthetic care discussion, particularly if EOL decisions have been formalized.
2. Anesthetic Considerations
   - Patient has personal history of anesthesia-related serious adverse event
   - Patient or family history of Malignant Hyperthermia
   - Anticipated or past history of difficult intubation
   - Chronic pain requiring medication or other treatments
3. Surgical Considerations
   - Major cardiac, vascular, or intrathoracic procedures
   - Cervical spinal procedures
   - Implantable cardiac defibrillator procedures
   - Percutaneous procedures to repair aneurysms (aortic or cerebral) or cardiac valves
4. Patient Considerations
   a. General
   - Gravid patient for non-obstetric surgery
   - Poor functional capacity (unable to walk one block or climb one flight of stairs)
   - Recent deterioration of chronic medical problem
   - Admission to hospital in last two months for acute (or exacerbation of a chronic medical) problem
   - Unusual or complicated medical problem

   b. Cardiovascular
   - CAD (history of angina or myocardial infarction)
   - Congestive heart failure
   - Valvular heart disease or other structural cardiac abnormality (e.g., congenital VSD)
   - History of CABG/PTCA, valvular repair, structural cardiac repair, or cardiac defibrillator implantation
   - Diffuse vasculopathy
   - Diastolic blood pressure >100 mmHg
   - Symptomatic arrhythmia, particularly new or undiagnosed atrial fibrillation

c. Respiratory

- Asthma or COPD
- Obstructive sleep apnea (including symptomatic patients who have not had a sleep study)
- Pulmonary hypertension
- Other serious lung diseases e.g., cystic fibrosis, sarcoidosis, idiopathic pulmonary fibrosis
- Upper or lower airway tumor tumors or obstructions
- Any chronic respiratory disease requiring home oxygen, ventilatory assistance or monitoring

d. Neurologic

- Neuromuscular diseases e.g., myasthenia gravis, muscular dystrophy, myotonic dystrophy
- Quadri-, hemi- or paraplegia
- Cervical spine instability, myelopathy or radiculopathy
- Other serious neurologic disease e.g., poorly-controlled seizures, cerebral palsy
- Perioperative delirium risk (see Appendix 3)

e. Metabolic

- Morbid obesity — >1.5*x* ideal body weight or BMI >40
- Diabetics on insulin
- Diabetics on oral agents only if co-morbidities are present

f. Hematologic

- Anemia
- Sickle cell disease
- Coagulopathy e.g., hemophila, von Willebrand's disease, thrombocytopenias
- Patients on anticoagulant (Coumadin, heparins, thrombin inhibitor, Factor X*a* inhibitor) therapy or prophylaxis

g. Other

- Severe latex allergy
- Significant renal dysfunction or dialysis-dependent
- HIV
- Chronic hepatitis or known hepatic dysfunction
- History of ongoing drug or alcohol abuse

Appendix 2. ASA classification

1. Healthy
2. Illness which does not impede activities of daily living
3. Illness which impedes activities of daily living
4. Illness which represents a constant threat to life
5. Not expected to survive 24 hours (with our without surgery)
6. Patient declared dead for purposes of organ donation

The suffix "E" denotes emergency surgery.

Appendix 3. Partial list of risk factors for delirium

1. Patient factors:

- Advanced age
- Dementia
- CNS and psychiatric disease
- Severe medical disease
- Drug or alcohol addiction
- Vision or hearing loss

2. Postoperative factors:

- Anesthesia
- Surgery/Trauma
- Pain
- Severe illness
- sleep deprivation/Noisy environment
- Polypharmacy
- Psychotropic Rx (including opiates)

Appendix 4. Eagle criteria: Surgery specific risk for cardiac complications

1. High Risk (>5%)

- Emergency surgery
- Vascular surgery
- Prolonged operation
- Large fluid shifts or blood loss

2. Intermediate Risk (1–5%)

- Carotid endarterectomy
- Head and neck surgery
- Intraperitoneal or intrathoracic surgery
- Orthopedic surgery
- Prostate surgery

3. Low risk (<1%)

- Endoscopic procedures
- Superficial procedures
- Cataract surgery
- Breast surgery

Chapter 2

Shock: Cardiovascular Dynamics, Endpoints of Resuscitation, Monitoring, and Management

Jameel Ali

Chapter Overview

Shock is the commonest indication for ICU admission of the surgical patient. It is therefore essential that the intensivist has a clear understanding of the definition, pathophysiology, classification, and principles of management of shock in order to guide therapy.

In this chapter, these topics will be presented with a major surgical focus.

Definition of Shock

Although shock has been defined differently by many clinicians and physiologists, the underlying abnormality and its sequelae arise from decreased tissue perfusion.

Shock may be defined, therefore as a generalized state of cellular hypoperfusion.

Tissue perfusion is responsible for the delivery of oxygen and other substrates to the cells. Decrease in this perfusion therefore leads to cellular hypoxia, anaerobic metabolism, activation of a myriad of systemic responses including initiation of an inflammatory process, endocrine, microvascular, hemodynamic, and organ dysfunction resulting in eventual death if left unabated.

Classification of Shock

Although shock may be categorized in many ways the most commonly used classification is based on the mechanism responsible for the hypoperfused state as this mechanism affects the pumping function of the heart, circulating volume and the state of the conduits transporting the blood volume i.e., the blood vessels. Shock may thus be classified as:

(a) Hypovolemic: Related to inadequate circulating volume as seen in blood loss.
(b) Obstructive: Due to extracardiac obstruction to blood flow e.g., cardiac tamponade.
(c) Cardiogenic: Due to pump failure secondary to decreased myocardial contractility, dysrhythmia, etc.
(d) Distributive: Due to maldistribution of blood flow and volume e.g., septic or neurogenic.

Conceptually, decreased tissue perfusion may be considered to arise from abnormality in one or all of the determinants of cardiac output or blood flow viz blood volume (preload), cardiac contractility or systemic vascular resistance (afterload). Cardiac output or blood flow is the product of stroke volume and heart rate. As preload decreases such as in hypovolemia the stroke volume decreases because of the decreased ventricular volume and stretch of the myocardial muscle (Starling's Law). Cardiac output is then maintained by an increase in heart rate. This compensatory response is limited by the maximum heart rate attainable and the limitation of stroke volume as heart rate increases limiting time for cardiac filling. Systemic blood pressure which is the product of cardiac output and systemic vascular resistance (determined by the tone of the peripheral vasculature) is maintained and may even be elevated in early hypovolemic states due to the increase in peripheral vascular resistance secondary to the vasoconstrictive effect of catecholamine release. This blood pressure is however maintained at the expense of a decrease in systemic blood flow to the tissues.

Hypovolemic shock

Decreased circulating blood volume is the *sine qua non* of hypovolemic shock and although it may arise from loss of fluids from third spacing, as in ileus, peritonitis, bowel obstruction, burns, other gastrointestinal disorders and pancreatitis, the commonest cause in the surgical patient is hemorrhage. The prime goal then is to identify the source of hemorrhage, stop it, and replace the volume loss. The source is identified by external examination (extrinsic source) when control is affected by direct pressure or in some instances the application of tourniquets. Internal sources are identified by a systematic assessment of the chest (by physical examination and chest X-ray, occasionally a chest tube insertion); abdominal examination including ultrasound; Pelvic X-ray with examination and assessment of the retroperitoneum (the extremities are included in the search for an external or extrinsic source). When the source of the bleeding is in the abdomen, chest, pelvis or retroperitoneum surgical intervention is frequently required (see chapters on chest trauma, abdominal trauma and pelvic and extremity injuries). Initially, volume replacement is by crystalloid but when major blood loss is obvious or anticipated massive transfusion protocol is initiated which includes early red blood cell, plasma, platelets, cryoprecipitate, and fibrinogen infusion (see chapter on massive transfusion).

Obstructive shock

The underlying mechanism is mechanical obstruction to cardiac output resulting in decreased tissue perfusion. Cardiac tamponade, tension pneumothorax massive pulmonary thromboembolus, air embolism are causes of this type of shock and are described elsewhere in the text.

Cardiogenic shock

This results from primary pump failure which may be secondary to myocardial infarction, dysrhythmias, cardiomyopathy, ventricular outflow obstruction (aortic dissection or valvular stenosis), ventricular septal defect, etc. In the absence of a surgically correctable lesion which should be sought, treatment is guided by response to volume infusion, inotropes and vasoactive drugs to modify cardiac contractility, afterload and preload as described below.

Distributive shock

This type of shock is usually ascribed to a septic etiology but many other entities (spinal cord injury, anaphylaxis, and liver dysfunction) may manifest signs of distributive shock in which there are the following signs: decreased systemic vascular resistance, normal to low cardiac filling pressures and increased cardiac output. In spite of increased cardiac output, signs of diminished oxygen extraction are present and many theories have been put forward to explain this including the notion that in early septic shock there is cellular inability to utilize oxygen in face of supernormal to normal oxygen delivery which may be related to an effect of endotoxin on the cells. Depression of myocardial contractility has also been demonstrated in these patients frequently ascribed to the endotoxin as well. Neurogenic shock, another form of distributive shock is described elsewhere in this text.

In this conundrum, it is important to utilize parameters of endpoints of resuscitation to guide therapy as described below. In septic shock, however, the main goals are to identify the septic focus, administer specific antimicrobial therapy, and eradicate the septic focus which frequently requires surgical or image guided drainage while managing the hypoperfused state.

Responses to the Shock State

Recognizing the responses to the shock state is not only important in diagnosing its presence but also its response to treatment. Reversal of the parameters manifested in the shock state is a sign of effectiveness of treatment measures.

Endocrine and catecholamine release

Baro and chemo receptors in response to the shock state stimulate activation of the hypothalamic — pituitary — adrenal axis resulting in release of catecholamines.

The effects of the released catecholamine are many, including:

Tachycardia maintains cardiac output which is the product of stroke volume and heart rate. The increased heart rate compensates temporarily to maintain cardiac output in spite of the decreased preload, but there is a point of diminishing return when the heart rate is so high that the decreased cardiac filling time decreases stroke volume and cardiac output. Volume loading to increase preload should be instituted early in hypovolemic states in order to reverse this process.

Vasoconstriction maintains blood pressure by increasing peripheral vascular resistance, blood pressure being the product of stroke volume and peripheral vascular resistance. Note that blood pressure is maintained at the expense of hypoperfusion resulting from the vasoconstriction, so that hypotension is a late sign of hypovolemic shock. Both pre and post capillary sphincters initially constrict decreasing capillary hydrostatic pressure with movement of fluid into the capillaries (plasma refill). Later, under acidotic conditions the pre capillary sphincters relax but the post capillary sphincters remain constricted leading to pooling in the capillaries and "stagnant" circulation.

Cold clammy extremities with pallor and decreased capillary refill are due to the vasoconstriction and stimulation of secretory glands at the base of hair follicles.

Regional differences in perfusion are because of differences in vasoreactivity in vascular beds — vascular beds such as cardiac and cerebral preferentially perfused versus splanchnic, skin and muscle with relative decreased perfusion.

ADH and aldosterone release preserves sodium and water, maintaining vascular volume.

Anaerobic metabolism

Anaerobic metabolism leads to lactic acidosis with compensatory hyperventilation. Optimum pH for cellular enzyme function is disrupted with cellular dysfunction. Lower ATP generation under anaerobic conditions leads to lower energy availability for cellular function. Energy requiring mechanism such as the 'sodium pump' for maintaining higher sodium to potassium ratio extracellularly is disrupted leading to movement of sodium (with water) intracellularly with cellular edema, further diminishing extracellular circulating volume exacerbating the hypovolemic state and hyperkalemia. Intracellular lysozymes are released and auto digest cells leading to cell death, tissue death, organ death, and finally organism death unless the cycle is broken by therapeutic intervention.

Reperfusion Injury

Cellular hypoxia predisposes to reperfusion injury, with local vasoconstriction, thrombosis, regional perfusion maldistribution, release of superoxide radicals with direct cellular damage with activation of neutrophils and proinflammatory cytokine release such as tumor necrosis factor (TNF), interleukin-1 (IL-1), platelet activating factor all resulting in cellular injury, organ dysfunction, organ failure, interference with gut mucosal permeability, and bacterial translocation frequently leading to multiorgan failure and death.

End Points of Resuscitation

As indicated above, shock is a state of generalized hypoperfusion associated with a decrease in oxygen delivery and other substrates to the cells resulting in cellular dysfunction. The aim of resuscitation is to return perfusion to normal. Our endpoints of resuscitation in shock should be to monitor the effect of our therapy with the goal of achieving perfusion normalcy. To identify the normalcy endpoint, normalcy itself needs to be defined in terms of the parameters which we monitor. To date, there is no consensus of what monitoring parameters should reflect normalcy in perfusion and cell function.

One of the problems is related to the lack of uniformity of perfusion particularly in the shock state where there is preferential perfusion of some vascular beds e.g., brain and heart with maintained high perfusion as opposed to splanchnic and cutaneous beds. Endpoints may thus be categorized as: clinical, organ specific, or global.

Clinical parameters: Heart rate, blood pressure, temperature, urine output, and pulse oximetry are good indices of the presence of shock but their return to normal values does not constitute reversal of the shock state especially in complex cases. Age premorbid physiology and drug history may make interpretation of these parameters difficult. However, these parameters are attractive because of their simplicity and ease of application and generally suffice as good indicators of the presence of shock and its resolution or response to therapy in uncomplicated cases. A blood pressure which falls and then rises to the patient's normal level, a heart rate which rises in shock or falls drastically and comes back to normal with treatment, a urine output which falls and then rises to normal with treatment and O_2 saturation value which falls in shock and then rises to normal values after treatment ordinarily are good indicators of resolution or improvement of the shock state. However, blood pressure, heart rate, and urine output could be problematic as endpoints of resuscitation.

Blood pressure may be normal or even elevated in early shock because of compensatory vasoconstriction. Blood pressure in hypovolemic shock does not fall until at least Class II–III hemorrhage — 15–30% blood volume loss.[1] In a study of 81,000 patients[2] from the National trauma Database of the American College of Surgeons, the traditional definition of hypotension as 90 mmHg systolic was questioned because at 110 mmHg blood pressure the slope of the mortality curve increased 4.8% for every 10 mmHg drop in pressure. The change in base deficit as an index of hypoperfusion increased at 118 mmHg. Based on change in base deficit and mortality, it was suggested that a systolic blood pressure of 110 mmHg was a more clinically relevant definition of hypotension.

Urine output — generally, good quality and volume of urine represent normal perfusion and a good index of adequate tissue perfusion. However, surgery, stress, trauma, ADH, and aldosterone release may result in low urine output in spite of normovolemia. Volume infusion alone may not result in reversing this endocrine effect on urine output with attendant risk of pulmonary edema. Furthermore, confounding factors such as diabetes insipidus, ketoacidosis, diuretic therapy, and renal tubular disorders limit the use of urine output as an index of adequate perfusion.

Pulse oximetry is convenient and an easily applicable technique of measuring tissue oxygenation and may be used as an index of adequate perfusion. Its unreliability in face of vasoconstriction which accompanies shock is however problematic.

Aerobic to anaerobic metabolism accompanying hypoperfusion states and its return to the aerobic state results in changes in serum lactate and base deficit which generally reflect changes in perfusion. Lactate and base deficit are superior to changes in hemodynamics and pH in assessing hypotensive states and clearance of acidosis.[3,4] However, in large series these have failed to represent a uniform index of perfusion and its relation to mortality.

Oxygen delivery, consumption, and oxygen debt in hypoperfusion states have been utilized to monitor adequacy of shock resuscitation. Tissue oxygen extraction is generally constant in spite of variation in oxygen delivery accompanying variation in perfusion until the critical delivery level when oxygen extraction varies with delivery leading to the state of 'oxygen debt'. This concept led to the supranormal oxygen delivery model to avoid critical oxygen delivery.[5] Although encouraging initial results were reported, recent large clinical trials have yielded inconclusive results.

Mixed venous oximetry through a centrally placed catheter allows determination of oxygen delivery and extraction. A low mixed venous O_2 saturation always indicates increased extraction suggesting inadequacy of oxygen delivery whereas normal or high values are more difficult to interpret.[6–8]

Intramucosal pH monitoring is an indirect measure of splanchnic perfusion. Because perfusion differs in vascular beds for the same degree of shock and the splanchnic circulation is one of the first to be deprived of oxygenated blood leading to local anaerobic metabolism and acidosis, gastric pH monitoring has been used to monitor the degree of hypoperfusion and response to therapy. Several studies have demonstrated that a gastric mucosal pH of less than 7.32[9] is correlated with mortality and the development of multisystem organ failure. This is gaining wider usage but is not universally adopted.

Invasive Hemodynamic Monitoring

Indwelling arterial catheters, monitoring of ventilatory gases, in combination with specially designed flow directed catheters have allowed not only monitoring of gas exchange but also cardiac output, mixed venous blood sampling, pulmonary artery dynamics as well as left heart hemodynamics. The pressures measured through these catheters allow assessment of right heart dynamics as well as left sided dynamics. The resistance or afterload of the right and left ventricles could be measured and alterations resulting from therapeutic manipulations can be used to guide changes in therapy. The measured variables include mixed venous O_2 saturation which can be used to measure oxygen delivery and extraction, systolic blood pressure, diastolic blood pressure, pulmonary systolic and diastolic pressure, central venous pressure, heart rate and cardiac output as well as right ventricular ejection fraction (Table 1). Derived variables (Table 1) from these which are computer generated based on standard derivation formulas include mean arterial and pulmonary arterial pressure, cardiac index, stroke volume, stroke volume index, systemic vascular resistance index, pulmonary vascular resistance index, left ventricular, and right ventricular stroke work index. These measured and derived variables which are continuously and instantaneously available in most ICUs guide choice of therapy, the monitoring of response to therapy as well as the need to alter therapy in the continuously changing and dynamic process characteristic of shock states.

Monitoring Principles that Govern Treatment

The goals of therapy in shock are: to diagnose and establish the etiology of shock, to restore adequacy of systemic and regional perfusion, and prevent death and multiorgan failure from the shock.

Utilizing the above hemodynamic parameters allows determination of the degree of preload, myocardial contractility, and afterload, deviations from normal, indications for specific interventions to normalize these parameters and modify these interventions based on the response to specific interventions.

Table 1. Hemodynamic measured and derived variables.

Measured variables			Derived variables		
Variable	**Normal**	**Unit**	**Variable**	**Normal**	**Unit**
SBP	90–140	Torr	MAP	70–105	Torr
DBP	60–90	Torr	MPAP	9–16	Torr
PAS	15–30	Torr	CI	2.8–4.2	L/min/m^2
PAD	4–12	Torr	SV	varies	mL/beat
PAOP	2–12	Torr	SVI	30–65	ML/beat/m^2
CVP	0–8	Torr	SRVI	1600–2400	dyne-s-cm^{-5}
HR	varies	beats/min	PVRI	250–340	dyne-s-cm^{-5}
CO	varies	L/min	LVSWI	43–62	gm·m/m^2
RVEF	0.40–0.60	Fraction	RVSW	I7–12	gm·m/m^2
			Coronary	PP>60	Torr
			RVEDVI	60–100	mL/m^2

Note: I: Indexed to body surface area, SBP: Systolic Blood Pressure, DBP: Diastolic Blood Pressure, PAS: Systolic Pulmonary Artery Pressure, PAD: Diastolic Pulmonary Artery Pressure, PAOP: Pulmonary Artery Occlusion Pressure, CVP: Central Venous Pressure, HR: Heart Rate, CO: Cardiac Output, RVEF: Right, Ventricular Ejection Fraction, MAP: Mean Arterial Pressure, MPAP: Mean Pulmonary Artery Pressure, CI: Cardiac Index, SV: Stroke Volume, SVI: Stroke Volume Index, SVRI: Systemic Vascular Resistance Index, PVRI: Pulmonary Vascular Resistance Index, LVSWI: Left Ventricular Stroke Work Index, RVSWI: Right Ventricular Stroke Work Index, Coronary PP: Coronary Perfusion Pressure, RVEDVI: Right Ventricular End-Diastolic Volume Index.

Frequently, the abnormality is many fold and not only in one of the parameters of preload, contractility or afterload and the response or lack of response to one intervention based on these parameters may dictate changes in these interventions. As shock is a dynamic process its therapy must be altered to match these dynamic changes.

Preload

In almost all types of shock an initial diminished preload exists and the first maneuver through reliable large bore intravenous access is the administration of crystalloid although in situations where massive blood loss has occurred, massive blood transfusion protocols are immediately initiated (see chapter on massive transfusion protocol). Although there is much controversy over the choice between crystalloid and colloid, meta-analysis[10,11] have shown a survival advantage with crystalloid recognizing that larger volumes are required for the same circulating blood volume result. Because of this, in addition to the increased cost of colloids, crystalloid is preferred. The fluid bolus must result in increased stroke volume otherwise it serves no useful purpose and may indeed be harmful. According to the Frank Starling principle as preload increases, stroke volume increases until the optimum preload after which there is no further increase in stroke volume (Fig. 1). This optimum preload is related to the maximum overlap of the actin–myosin fibrils and is different for different patients and different hemodynamic events in the same patient. Traditionally, CVP central venous pressures has been used as an indirect measure of preload responsiveness in terms of changing stroke volume. There are many reasons why this is a false notion (changes in venous tone and intrathoracic pressures, right and left ventricular compliance and geometry in the critically ill). Based on this information, CVP should no longer be routinely used for guiding fluid management in the ICU, OR, or ER.

A key element in determining the need for increasing preload is the volume responsiveness to fluid infusion. Recently, many dynamic tests of

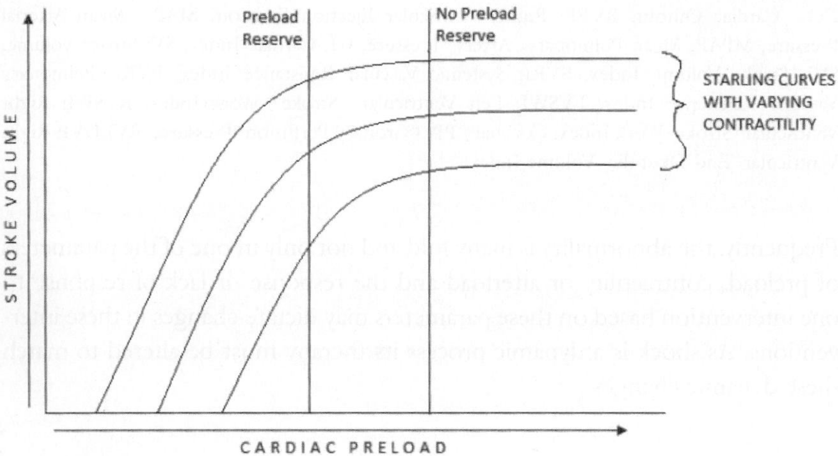

Fig. 1. Variations in stroke volume with changes in preload reflect varying myocardial contractility

Note: On the steep part of the curves, there is preload reserve and volume expansion produces increased stroke volume (PLR, EEO are positive: PPV and SVV variations are marked). Near flat part of the curves, there is no preload reserve and volume expansion has little effect on stroke volume. *Source*: Adapted from Ref. 12.

volume responsiveness have been described. These tests dynamically monitor the change in stroke volume in response to increasing or decreasing preload. These tests include: pulse pressure variation (PPV) derived from analysis of the arterial waveform, the stroke volume variation (SVV) derived from pulse contour analysis and variation of the amplitude of the pulse oximetry plethysmographic wave form, dynamic changes in aortic flow velocity/stroke volume assessed by Doppler methods, positive pressure ventilation induced changes in vena caval diameter, the end-expiratory occlusion test, passive leg raising test.[12] The ideal management of fluid therapy should also include the response or lack thereof of volume expansion on cardiac output and tissue oxygen consumption — all of which could be measured by monitoring the above described parameters in the ICU patient.

Myocardial contractility

Optimization of the heart rate is important in monitoring changes in contractility in response to therapy. Also, contractility agents should be applied only after optimization of preload and afterload.

Commonly used contractility agents are: dopamine, dobutamine, norepinephrine, and amrinone.

Dopamine is a precursor of norepinephrine with dosing related variability. Low doses ('renal doses') of 0–3 μg/kgm increases GFR and renal blood flow. However, the benefit of the renal dosing in critically ill patients has been questioned.[13] In modest doses (5–10 μg/kgm), cardiac contractility and heart rate increase through cardiac beta receptor stimulation. In higher doses (>10 μg/kgm), alpha adrenergic receptor stimulation occurs with elevation of systemic blood pressure. Caution should be exercised in the use of dopamine for improving myocardial contractility in patients with coronary artery stenosis because of the potential deleterious effects of tachycardia and increase in myocardial oxygen demand.

Dobutamine also acts on beta-1 receptors but unlike dopamine, does not directly release norepinephrine. When there is minimal chronotropic effect, there is little effect on myocardial oxygen demand probably because of accompanying systemic vasodilatation which could lead to decreased blood pressure and overall decrease in systemic perfusion. Caution should therefore be exercised in using dobutamine in hypovolemic vasodilated patients.

Norepinephrine possesses both alpha and beta adrenergic activity and is a potent vasoconstrictor. This latter effect could result in decreased mesenteric and renal blood flow. Its main use is in maintaining blood pressure in acute situations associated with hypotension when the improved blood pressure may result in improved renal function. As soon as a sustained blood pressure response is achieved cessation of norepinephrine therapy and replacement by alternative inotropic agents should be considered because of the deleterious effect of prolonged norepinephrine use on splanchnic and renal blood flow.

Amrinone is a non-catecholamine phosphodiesterase III inhibitor which raises cyclic AMP. In congestive heart failure it increases stroke volume without increasing heart rate. Because of its vasodilatory effect it may be contraindicated in some patients because of profound hypotension.

Many other agents are used in the ICU for modifying myocardial contractility and the intensivist needs to be familiar with the therapeutic profiles of these agents in order to use them effectively.

Afterload

After optimizing preload and myocardial contractility if perfusion goals are not met, afterload reduction should be considered provided the patient is not persistently hypotensive. In patients with decreased contractility, afterload reduction should improve cardiac output by improving ventricular ejection fraction and stroke volume. Agents commonly used are sodium nitroprusside, nitroglycerine and angiotensin converting enzyme inhibitors.

Sodium nitroprusside is both a venous and arterial vasodilator with rapid onset and short duration making it ideal for testing the patient for response and quickly stopping if there are deleterious side effects. It should be used with caution in patients with coronary artery disease who are at risk for coronary artery steal and resulting myocardial ischemia.

Nitroglycerine primarily affects venous capacitance but also decreases arterial resistance which may improve cardiac output.

Ace inhibitors are of significant value in reducing afterload in normovolemic patients with poor cardiac function.

Afterload may also be reduced mechanically through a percutaneously placed intra-aortic balloon pump for couterpulsation. This is commonly used in the immediate postoperative period after coronary bypass to allow the newly perfused myocardium to recover from the acute insult of the surgery. Afterload reduction is effected mechanically with improved coronary artery perfusion by augmenting diastolic perfusion pressure while decreasing resistance to ventricular ejection during systole. This is particularly effective in myocardial infarction with reversible pathology.

The patient with aortic stenosis is not a good candidate for afterload reduction because of the resulting reduced coronary perfusion pressure.

Summary

Shock is commonly seen in the ICU patient. A clear understanding of its etiology is required to focus therapy at correcting the underlying disturbance in physiology. The approach to management is to improve and maintain cellular perfusion and oxygenation. Understanding the interrelationships of the heart, blood vessels and blood volume, their behavior in shock and the ability to modify and monitor them through various therapeutic approaches is essential for successful outcome and survival.

References

1. Advanced Trauma Life Support for Doctors. American College of Surgeons Committee on Trauma. Chapter 4. *Shock.* 9th ed. Chicago: American College of Surgeons.
2. Eastridge BJ, Salinas J, McManus JG, Blackburn L *et al.* Hypotension begins at 110 mmHg: Redefining "hypotension" with data. *J Trauma* 2007; 63(2): 291–297.
3. Davis JW, Shackford SR, Mackersie RC, Hoyt DB. Base deficit as a guide to volume resuscitation. *J Trauma* 1988; 28: 1464–1467.
4. Rutherford EJ, Morris JA, Reed G, Hall KS. Base deficit stratifies mortality and determines therapy. *J Trauma* 1992; 33: 417–423.
5. Bland RD, Shoemaker WC, Abraham E, Cobo JC. Hemodynamic and oxygen transport patterns in surviving and nonsurviving postoperative patients. *Crit Care Med* 1985; 13: 85–90.
6. Burchell SA,Yu M, Takiguchi SA *et al.* Evaluation of a continuous cardiac output and mixed venous oxygen saturation catheter in critically ill surgical patients. *Crit Care Med* 1997; 25: 388–391.
7. Nelson LD. Continuous venous oximetry in surgical patients. *Ann Surg* 1986; 203: 329–333.
8. Orlando R. Continuous mixed venous oximetry in critically ill surgical patients. *Arch Surg* 1986; 121: 470–471.
9. Ivatury RR, Simon RJ, Havriliak D *et al.* Gastric mucosal pH and oxygen delivery and oxygen consumption indices in the assessment of resuscitation after trauma: A prospective randomized study. *J Trauma* 1995; 39: 128–136.
10. Schierhout G, Roberts I. Fluid resuscitation with colloid or crystalloid solutions in critically ill patients: A systematic review of randomized trials. *BMJ* 1998; 316: 961–964.

11. Choi PTL, Yip G, Quinonez LG *et al.* Crystalloid vs Colloid in fluid resuscitation. A systematic review. *Crit Care Med* 1999; 27: 200–210.
12. Marik PE, Monnet X, Teboul JL. Hemodynamic parameters to guide fluid therapy. *Ann Intensive Care* 2011; 1: 1–9.
13. Kellum JA, Decker J. Use of Dopamine in acute renal failure: Ameta analysis. *Crit Care Med* 2001; 29: 1526–1531.

Chapter 3

Gas Exchange

Zoheir Bshouty

Chapter Overview

Gas exchange involves the exchange of gases between the lung and the blood. The gases of interest are oxygen and carbon dioxide. The general objectives behind this chapter are to leave you with enough basic physiological knowledge that would enable you to identify derangements in gas exchange based on the interpretation of arterial blood gases and to try to identify the mechanism(s) leading to these derangements.

Although pH plays a certain role in interpreting arterial blood gases, when dealing with gas exchange, emphasis is on interpreting derangements in the partial pressure of arterial oxygen (P_aO_2) and the partial pressure of arterial carbon dioxide (P_aCO_2).

To help with these, some key equations will be used. The derivation of these equations is beyond the scope of this chapter but the principles used in deriving these equations will be mentioned. Equations that are useful in clinical practice are boxed.

The chapter will start with derangements in carbon dioxide followed by derangements in oxygen. The reason for this order, as you will see later, is that derangements in carbon dioxide can directly lead to derangements in oxygen, while derangements in oxygen do not affect carbon dioxide. The goal is to keep the topic as simple as possible and at the same time clinically relevant. Often, learners fail to understand the link between theory and clinical applicability; therefore, the chapter starts with two clinical scenarios that will be referred to occasionally to help maintain this link.

Many surgical patients in the intensive care unit (ICU) will have problems related to gas exchange. The concepts in this chapter will allow understanding of the basic mechanisms involved in these gas exchange abnormalities and guide therapeutic interventions.

In this chapter and in pulmonary physiology in general, V indicates volume. Subscripts are used to identify the various types of volumes (e.g., V_D for dead space). When written with a diacritic period such as V it indicates volume measured over a period of one minute (e.g., V_E for minute ventilation).

The Problem

Case 1. An elderly man is brought to the Emergency Department by his daughter. He tells the resident that his chronic cough and shortness of breath have become worse in the last few days, during which time he has had periods of drowsiness and confusion. The patient is drowsy and uncooperative, blue and in obvious respiratory distress. The resident decides to take an arterial blood gas sample on room air.

P_aO_2	33 mmHg
S_aO_2	45%
P_aCO_2	80 mmHg
pH	7.15

Case 2. An elderly woman presents to the outpatient clinic complaining of increased fatigue and shortness of breath on exertion that were insidious in nature and have gradually progressed over the past five years. As part of her investigation an arterial blood gas on room air is drawn with the following results:

P_aO_2	60 mmHg
S_aO_2	90%
P_aCO_2	32 mmHg
pH	7.45

Analyzing P_aO_2 and P_aCO_2 and identifying the mechanism(s) for the gas exchange disturbances in the earlier context is the topic of this chapter.

Normal values for arterial blood gases

Textbooks often reference the following normal ranges for arterial blood gases,

P_aO_2	80–100 mmHg
P_aCO_2	35–45 mmHg
pH	7.36–7.44
HCO_3^-	23–27 mEq/L

In some ways, however, it is difficult to define **"normality"** particularly for P_aO_2, which may vary with body position, age, and smoking history, to mention the more important factors. Also, as you will see later, the three variables are linked physiologically. A normal P_aO_2 of 80 mmHg at a normal P_aCO_2 of 45 mmHg will be abnormal at a P_aCO_2 of 35 mmHg. Similarly, a normal P_aCO_2 of 45 mmHg at a HCO_3^- of 24 mEq/L will be abnormal at a HCO_3^- of 15 mEq/L.

The lungs are the first link in the O_2 transport chain to the tissues (for metabolism) and the last link in the CO_2 transport chain (by-product of metabolism). There is no doubt that both patients have a problem getting O_2 into their blood. In addition, the first patient has a problem getting rid of CO_2.

As mentioned earlier, we will refer back to these two cases as new concepts are learned to maintain the link between theory and clinical practice.

Anatomic dead space (V_{Danat}) is the volume of all non-gas-exchanging airways from the nose (or mouth, during mouth-breathing) down to the respiratory bronchioles Fig. 1.

Alveolar dead space (V_{Dalv}) is the volume of inspired air that is <u>delivered to alveoli</u> in which there is no gas exchange or gas exchange is incomplete. V_{Dalv} is primarily the result of under perfusion of the affected alveoli Fig 1. V_{Dalv} is too small to be measured in healthy subjects, particularly young people, but can become large enough to interfere with alveolar ventilation (V_A) in patients who have certain lung diseases, in spite high V_E.

Physiologic dead space (V_D) is the <u>sum</u> of V_{Danat} and V_{Dalv}. V_D defines the portion of each inspiration that <u>does not</u> equilibrate with gas pressures of the pulmonary capillary blood Fig. 1.

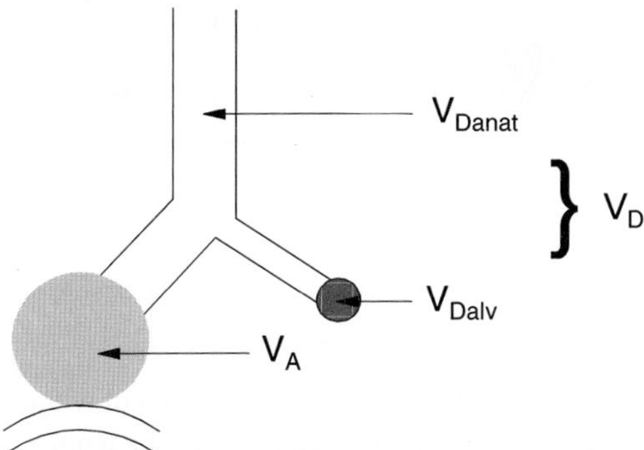

Fig. 1. Dead space (V_D). In this figure, the white area represents anatomic dead space (V_{Danat}), the grayed circle represents alveolar dead space (V_{Dalv}), and V_D represents physiologic dead space which is the sum of V_{Danat} and V_{Dalv}.

In the lungs, not all alveoli are ventilated and perfused at ideal proportions. For a given perfusion rate, some alveoli are underventilated (or hypoventilated), while others are overventilated (or hyperventilated) with respect to the ventilation required to accomplish adequate gas exchange. The same is true for blood perfusion (i.e., for a given V_A some areas are underperfused, while others are overperfused). The ratio between ventilation (V) and perfusion (V) is referred to as the ventilation to perfusion ratio (V/Q). This concept and the concept of V/Q mismatch will be discussed in detail at the end of the chapter. Despite the existence of a wide spectrum of V/Q ratios, dead space and shunt (see later) are calculated under the assumption that the lung consists of:

1. Alveoli that are optimally and equally ventilated and perfused (with complete equilibration of gas pressures between alveoli and capillary blood, V/Q = 1, Fig. 2 compartment 1).
2. Alveoli that are optimally ventilated but not perfused at all ("V_{Danat}", V/Q Fig. 2 compartment 2 = ∞)
3. Alveoli that are optimally perfused but not ventilated at all (contributing to "shunt", V/Q Fig. 2 compartment 3 = 0)

Thus, V_D is a theoretical rather than an actual volume.

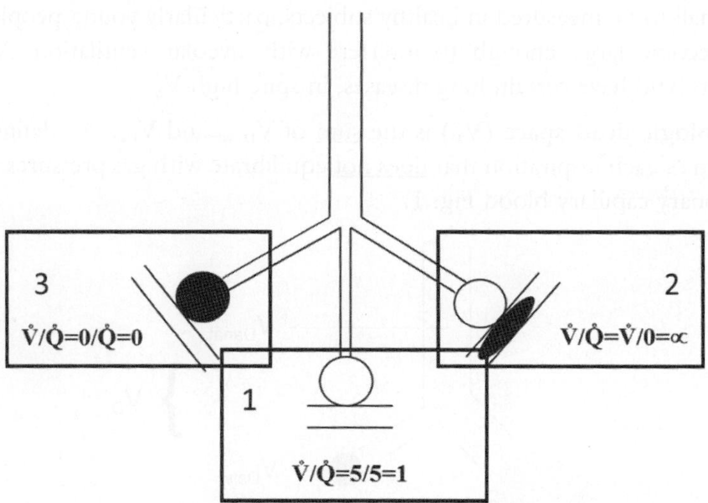

Fig. 2. This figure represents the three main compartment within the lung based on the ventilation to perfusion ratio. Clear circles represent adequately ventilated alveoli (compartments 1 and 2) whereas the black filled circle represents non-ventilated alveoli (compartment 3). Similarly, the clear parallel lines represent capillaries that are perfused (compartments 1 and 3) and the parallel lines with the black ellipse (compartment 2) represents capillaries that are not perfused.

Factors affecting V_{Danat}

Size of subject. V_{Danat} is highly dependent on body size. A good estimate is based on ***body height*** (rather than body weight), a relationship that holds true for both children and adults.

Age. V_{Danat} increases slightly with age. This increase is probably due to loss of elasticity (i.e., increased compliance) of airways.

Breathing pattern. V_{Danat} increases with increasing tidal volume (V_T). This is due to the increase in distending pressure that parallels the increase in V_T which stretches the elastic airways as well as the lungs.

Factors affecting V_{Dalv}

Pulmonary embolism. Occlusion of pulmonary vessels creates a situation where alveoli continue to be ventilated yet unperfused, hence contributing to an increase in V_{Dalv}.

Mechanical ventilation with high Positive End-Expiratory Pressure (PEEP). Similar situation to pulmonary embolism except that pulmonary vessels are occluded by the high alveolar pressure.

The increase in V_{Danat} is usually not enough to cause a disturbance in gas exchange. Diseases that affect gas exchange through their effect on dead space do so by increasing V_{Dalv} which, in turn, leads to an increase in V_D. So, it suffices to calculate V_D in order to determine whether it is contributing to a gas exchange derangement.

Calculation of V_D

Why is it important to calculate V_D? The answer is very simple, Dead Space ventilation (V_D) is considered wasted ventilation. The larger the dead space volume, V_D (or ventilation, V_D) the less volume is available for adequate gas exchange (termed alveolar volume, V_A, or ventilation, V_A, Eq. 3.3). And, as you will see later, V_A, and in turn V_A, have a large impact on carbon dioxide elimination.

V_E. The total amount of gas that is moved in and out of the lung per minute and is equal to the product of V_T and respiratory frequency (f):

$$\dot{V}_E = V_T \cdot f \tag{3.1}$$

V_D. The amount of gas that moves in and out of the <u>dead space</u> of the lung per minute and is equal to the product of V_D and f:

$$\dot{V}_D = V_D \cdot f \tag{3.2}$$

V_A. The volume of gas that is introduced into the gas-exchanging regions of the lung per minute. It is equal to V_E minus V_D,

$$\dot{V}_A = \dot{V}_E - \dot{V}_D = (V_T - V_D)\cdot f \tag{3.3}$$

Bohr equation. The Bohr Equation enables us to estimate V_D (as a proportion of V_T) using a sample of CO_2 in mixed expired gas ($P_{ME}CO_2$) and P_aCO_2. The derivation of this relationship is based on the laws of conservation of mass for CO_2,[1]

$$\frac{V_D}{V_T} = \frac{(P_aCO_2 - P_{ME}CO_2)}{P_aCO_2} \tag{3.4}$$

Going back to *Case 1*, if the patient's $P_{ME}CO_2$ was 36 mmHg, given a P_aCO_2 of 80 mmHg, the proportion of the total ventilation that is being wasted in dead space is (applying Eq. (3.4)):

$$V_D/V_T = (80 - 36)/80$$
$$= 0.55$$

Indicating that over half of his V_T is wasted on dead space. Under normal condition, at rest, V_D/V_T is approximately 0.3 (30%).

One of the factors that has a large impact on the distribution of ventilation between dead space and gas exchanging alveoli is breathing pattern. Consider the patient in *Case 1*, when assessed he was noted to having rapid shallow breathing. His respiratory frequency was 40 per minute and his estimated V_T was approximately 200 mL. As his V_D/V_T was 0.55, his V_D would have been $200 \cdot 0.55 = 110$ mL. The subject's V_E was $40 \cdot 0.2 = 8$ L/minute, $V_D = 40 \cdot 0.11 = 4.4$ L/minute, and $V_A = 8 - 4.4 = 3.6$ L/minute. If V_E were to remain the same (8 L/minute) and his breathing pattern were to change to slower and deeper, for example $f = 20$ and $V_T = 400$ mL. In this latter case V_D would be $20 \cdot 0.11 = 2.2$ L/minute and compartment V_A would be $8 - 2.2 = 5.8$ L/minute. What impact will this have on his gas exchange? This is the topic of the next section.

V_A and CO_2

Relation between V_A and P_aCO_2

During steady state conditions of ventilation and perfusion, the rate of CO_2 production (V_{CO_2}), at the tissue level, is constant and equals the rate of CO_2 elimination at the lung. Alveolar CO_2 concentration is directly related to

CO_2 production (V_{CO_2}) and inversely related to CO_2 elimination which is controlled by V_A. This relationship is also derived using the laws of conservation of mass for carbon dioxide,[2]:

$$P_ACO_2 = \frac{\dot{V}_{CO_2} \cdot (P_B - 47)}{\dot{V}_A} \tag{3.5}$$

where P_B is barometric pressure and 47 is water vapor pressure at 37°C.

Conventionally, P_ACO_2 is expressed in mmHg, V_A in L/minute at BTPS (Body Temperature Pressure Saturated) and V_{CO_2} is expressed in mL/minute at STPD (Standard Temperature Pressure Dry). To account for P_B, the difference in units between V_A (L/minute) and V_{CO_2} (mL/minute), and to standardize BTPS conditions with STPD one needs to multiply the right-hand side of the equation by a correction factor ***k*** (equals 0.863). Also, since CO_2 is a very diffusible molecule across biologic membranes P_aCO_2 can be substituted for P_ACO_2 and the equation can be written in the following form:

$$P_aCO_2 = \frac{\dot{V}_{CO_2} \cdot k}{\dot{V}_A} \tag{3.6}$$

This equation expresses a very important core concept as it relates effective breathing (as represented by V_A) to the metabolic rate of CO_2 production (V_{CO_2}). Thus, the measurement of P_aCO_2 expresses whether V_A is adequate for the metabolic needs of the body without measuring either V_A or V_{CO_2}. If normally P_aCO_2 is 40 mmHg, then a doubling to 80 mmHg means that V_A is only half of what is normally required for the body's CO_2 output. In other words, at a given metabolic rate, P_aCO_2 is inversely proportional to V_A.

Going back to *Case 1*, at the end of the last section, we wondered what would happen to the patient's gas exchange if he were to change his breathing pattern.

From Eq. (3.6), substituting 80 for P_aCO_2, 0.863 for ***k***, and 3.6 for V_A, gives a V_{CO_2} of 333 mL/minute. Using the same equation, by changing V_A from 3.6 to 5.8 L/minute, and assuming that V_{CO_2} remains the same, the subject's P_aCO_2 would drop to $333 \cdot 0.863/5.4 = 53$ mmHg. This is achieved by simply changing the breathing pattern without changing V_E.

The "steady-state"

P_aCO_2 has just been considered as an indication of the balance between ventilation and the metabolic production of CO_2. This is a valid concept which holds only if the output of CO_2 by the lungs and the production of CO_2 by body tissues are equal. This is known as a **"respiratory steady-state"**. In some situations this may not apply. For example, when a patient is hyperventilating because of anxiety, perhaps occasioned by the approach of a nervous student about to take his first arterial blood sample, pulmonary output of CO_2 becomes temporarily higher than the body's metabolic production of CO_2. Similarly, at the onset of exercise, changes in P_ACO_2 will occur if ventilation does not increase in parallel with the increase in body metabolism. As long as one is reasonably careful, the assumption of a "steady-state" in most clinical situations will hold true, but learn to question the assumption, so that you are not caught out in the occasional instance where circumstances have led to changing conditions in gas exchange and an unsteady state.

The V_a graph

Figure 3 shows the relationship between V_A and P_aCO_2 (as expressed by Eq. 3.6). It is an easy graph to draw, and once you have drawn it you will understand the implications of the V_A equation for carbon dioxide. Also, the message to be obtained from the equation is easier to appreciate graphically.

Starting with a normal V_A of 4.3 L/minute and a P_aCO_2 of 40 mmHg, when V_A is halved (to 2.15 L/minute), P_aCO_2 doubles to 80 mmHg. Now when V_A is doubled to 8.6 L/minute and again to 17.2 L/minute, P_aCO_2 is halved to 20 mmHg and 10 mmHg, respectively. The solid line curve describes a resting level of CO_2 production of about 200 mL/minute. Similar curves could be drawn for other values of CO_2 output. The dotted line in Fig. 3, for example, is for a CO_2 output twice the resting value (400 mL/minute).

Notice that the lines are **hyperbolic**. This follows from the equation $P_aCO_2 \cdot V_A = k$, where k is constant. Notice also that once ventilation has fallen by more than one liter from the normal point, a small drop in V_A will lead to a big rise in P_aCO_2. This accounts for the behavior of some patients with respiratory disease who manage to exist well with moderately elevated P_aCO_2, say at 60 mmHg, and then, with only a slight fall in their ventilatory capacity, perhaps due to an infection, their P_aCO_2 rapidly rises to 70 or 80 mmHg.

Looking at the other end of the scale, notice that a modest increase in V_A will produce quite a dramatic fall in P_aCO_2, initially. However, it requires a greater and greater increase in V_A to produce an equivalent fall in P_aCO_2 once P_aCO_2 becomes low. This may be clinically important in states of metabolic acidosis. Increasing ventilation to lower P_aCO_2 is one way to

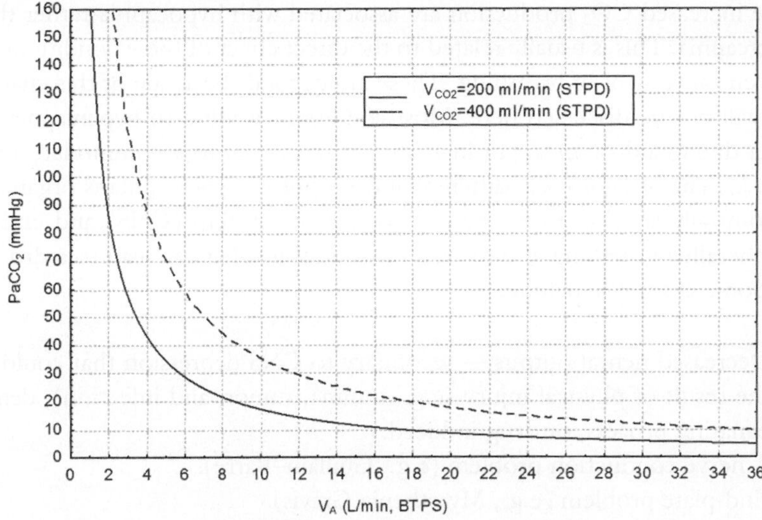

Fig. 3. Relationship between Alveolar volume and P_aCO_2.

minimize the changes in pH due to metabolic acidosis. Early in the process, achieving a large drop in P_aCO_2 by increasing ventilation is relatively easy, but as acidosis becomes more severe it becomes more difficult to lower P_aCO_2, particularly as patients in this situation tend to become fatigued.

When assessing the ventilation state of a patient, the ability to place the subject on this hyperbolic relationship indicates their ability (or lack thereof) to compensate for various metabolic insults. The closer the subject is to P_aCO_2 40 mmHg and V_A of 4 L/minute, the more stable they are and the more capable they are to compensate for metabolic insults. As they deviate away from this central point, in either way, the more unstable they become and their ability to compensate for metabolic insults rapidly diminishes.

Causes of hypercapnia

From Eq. (3.7) it is quite apparent that hypercapnia occurs as a result of either an increase in V_{CO_2}, a drop in V_A, or a combination of both. An increase in V_{CO_2} usually occurs under conditions in which metabolic rate is increased (such as fever and hyperthyroidism) or because of an increase in caloric intake (e.g., hyper alimentation). Interestingly though, many conditions that cause increased CO_2 production are associated with hypocapnia rather than hypercapnia. This is usually related to the direct effect of these conditions on the central control of breathing. These are beyond the scope of this chapter and will not be discussed here. Most conditions leading to hypercapnia are either due to a drop in V_A, or inability to increase V_A to accommodate a rise in V_{CO_2}. The physiological differential diagnosis of hypercapnia is organized anatomically starting from the central nervous system (CNS) and ending peripherally in the lung and focuses on conditions that can lead to a drop in V_A. Some examples include,

1. Decreased neural output — secondary to CNS depression that could be the result of physical injury (e.g., trauma, tumor, and infection), demyelinating process, or drug induced.
2. A nerve conduction problem (e.g., Guillain–Barre).
3. End-plate problem (e.g., Myasthenia Gravis).
4. A muscle problem (e.g., muscle fatigue or myopathy).
5. A pulmonary problem in which all lung volumes are decreased (e.g., restriction secondary to chest wall deformities or lung parenchymal processes), secondary to alveolar destruction (e.g., severe chronic obstructive pulmonary disease — COPD); or is increased V_D/V_T as occurs in rapid shallow breathing.

As mentioned in the introduction though, normocapnia is not an absolute term with a normal range of 35–45 mmHg. Each level of HCO_3^- is associated with its normal range. Several prediction equations for normal P_aCO_2 for a given level of HCO_3^- exist in the literature. The one I like to use is[3]:

$$P_aCO_2 = 1.5 \cdot HCO_3^- + 8 \pm 5. \qquad (3.7)$$

A patient with a HCO_3^- of 10 and a P_aCO_2 of 30 is relatively hypercapnic as his predicted P_aCO_2 is $1.5 \cdot 10 + 8 = 23$. Waiting for the patient's P_aCO_2 to rise above 45 to identify hypercapnia is physiologically unsound and potentially dangerous.

Alveolar Oxygen Pressure (P_AO_2)

The simplified alveolar air equation for oxygen

The alveolar air equation for oxygen is a bit more complicated than the relationship between P_AO_2 or P_aCO_2 and V_A. This is due to several facts including the dilution of inspired oxygen by the dead space, the continuous dumping of CO_2 into the alveoli, and the continuous transfer of oxygen from the alveoli into the blood. The principles used in deriving this equation are based on the laws of conservation of mass for oxygen. Oxygen consumption, V_{O_2}, under steady-state conditions, at the tissue level, is assumed equal to the amount of oxygen take-up by the hemoglobin (Hgb) in the lung. The equation in its simplified form is[4]:

$$P_AO_2 = P_IO_2 - \frac{P_aCO_2}{R}, \tag{3.8}$$

where P_IO_2 is the partial pressure of inspired oxygen and is calculated by multiplying F_IO_2 (the fractional concentration of inspired oxygen, 0.21 for air) by barometric pressure (P_B) minus water vapor pressure (47 mmHg at 37°C) as follows,

$$P_IO_2 = F_IO_2 \cdot (P_B - 47). \tag{3.9}$$

And R is the respiratory quotient (V_{CO_2}/V_{O_2}) and is often assumed equal to 0.8.

Breathing room air (F_IO_2 = 20.9%) at sea level (P_B = 760 mmHg), with a normal respiratory exchange ratio R = 0.8) and V_A (P_aCO_2 = 40 mmHg),

$$\begin{aligned} P_AO_2 &= 0.209 \cdot (760 - 47) - (40/0.8) \\ &= 0.209 \cdot (713) - 50 \\ &= 149 - 50 \\ &= 99 \text{ mmHg.} \end{aligned}$$

Notice that by calculating P_AO_2 one also defines the highest possible value for arterial P_{O_2} (P_aO_2). Given the conditions just defined, one cannot have a P_aO_2 higher than 99 mmHg (unless supplemental oxygen is being administered), even if gas exchange in the lungs is perfect.

Hypoxemia in the presence of a normal alveolar–arterial O_2 gradient

As mentioned earlier, P_AO_2 represents the ceiling for P_aO_2 and hence, any mechanism that causes a drop in P_AO_2 will cause a parallel drop in P_aO_2. From Eq. (3.8) it is apparent that a drop in P_IO_2 or a rise in P_aCO_2 (hypercapnia) will both cause such an effect. The former occurs most frequently upon ascent to high altitude. At an altitude of 2,400 meters above sea level, barometric pressure is approximately 585 mmHg (cabin pressure at most commercial airlines). Hence, P_IO_2 while flying on a commercial airline is 112.4 mmHg rather than 149 mmHg and a subject with a normal P_aCO_2 of 40 mmHg will have a P_AO_2 of 62.4 mmHg.

Going back to *Case 1* at the beginning of the chapter whose arterial sample was obtained while breathing room air, P_aCO_2 was 80 mmHg. This patient's P_AO_2 is (assuming a P_B of 760),

$$P_AO_2 = 149 - (80/0.8)$$
$$= 49 \text{ mmHg}$$

Notice that the patient's P_aO_2 was 33 mmHg while his calculated P_AO_2 is 49 mmHg. That is, there is a step down between alveolar oxygen and arterial blood oxygen. This step down is termed the alveolar–arterial oxygen gradient ($P_{A-a}O_2$).[5] In other words, his $P_{A-a}O_2$ is 16 mmHg. A normal $P_{A-a}O_2$ is considered less or equal to 12 mmHg. As many parameters, especially when using estimate equations, there is a gray zone between 12 and 18 mmHg. Most references would consider a $P_{A-a}O_2$ greater than 18 mmHg as large.

In clinical practice, a normal $P_{A-a}O_2$ indicates that the lung is able to transfer oxygen adequately from the alveoli into the blood. When faced with a patient who is hypoxemic ($P_aO_2 < 60$ mmHg) while breathing room air, the first step in attempting to identify the cause of the hypoxemia would be to calculate $P_{A-a}O_2$. If $P_{A-a}O_2$ is less than 12 mmHg, the cause of the hypoxemia is either a low barometric pressure or hypercapnia. If low barometric pressure is not a logical option then hypercapnia is the only possible cause. When examining the blood gas, if hypercapnia is not present then there is an error in the calculations.

The question remains, what clinical implications do all these calculations have? Determining the physiological cause of the hypoxemia determines the intervention, for example in *Case* 1, where $P_{A-a}O_2$ was 16 mmHg, the first intervention should focus on treating the hypercapnia. Treating the hypercapnia in this case will most likely resolve the hypoxemia.

Shunt and V/Q Mismatch and their Contribution to Hypoxemia

The reader is referred back to Fig. 2 where shunt was described as a compartment in which venous blood passes through unchanged. If deoxygenated (i.e., systemic venous) blood bypasses ventilated alveoli and mixes with well

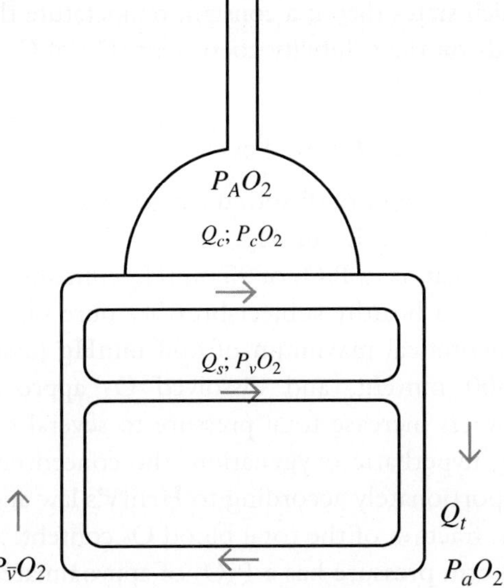

Fig. 4. The concept of shunt.

oxygenated blood that has passed through ventilated alveoli, the oxygen content of blood finally leaving the lungs will be less than that leaving the ventilated areas (Fig. 4). This is the concept of "shunt".[6]

The derivation of the shunt equation is also based on the laws of conservation of mass for oxygen as blood passes through the lung. The shunt equation is described by the following relationship:

$$\frac{Q_s}{Q_t} = \frac{C_cO_2 - C_2O_2}{C_cO_2 - C_{\bar{v}}O_2}, \tag{3.10}$$

where Q_s is blood flow (in L/minute) that is bypassing oxygenated alveoli, Q_t is total blood flow (i.e., cardiac output), C_cO_2, C_aO_2, and C_vO_2 are oxygen content in capillary, arterial, and mixed venous blood, respectively.

Blood carries O_2 in two ways: (1) in physical solution as dissolved O_2, and (2) in a loose reversible chemical combination with Hgb, as oxyhemoglobin. ***In both cases the amount of*** O_2 ***depends on the partial pressure of*** $O_2(P_{O_2})$ ***to which the blood is exposed.***

Dissolved oxygen. Dissolved O_2, also termed O_2 in physical solution, comprises little more than 1% of total blood O_2 content under ordinary physiologic conditions. The amount of dissolved oxygen is determined by

Henry's law which states that at a constant temperature the amount of dissolved O_2 depends on the solubility coefficient (C_s) of O_2 in blood and is a linear function of P_{O_2}:

$$C_{diss}O_2 = C_s \cdot P_{O_2} \tag{3.11}$$

where, $C_{diss}O_2$ is the amount of dissolved oxygen in one liter of blood and C_s for O_2 at 38°C is 0.03 mL/L/mmHg.

Arterial blood that has a P_aO_2 of 95 mmHg contains about 2.85 mL/L dissolved O_2. When a healthy subject breathes pure O_2 at sea level, P_AO_2 rises toward a theoretical maximum of 663 mmHg (assuming R = 0.8), P_aO_2 exceeds 600 mmHg, and dissolved O_2 approaches 20 mL/L. Hyperbaric chambers increase total pressure to several times atmospheric pressure. During hyperbaric oxygenation, the concentration of dissolved O_2 increases proportionately according to Henry's law and may then comprise a significant fraction of the total blood O_2 content. A subject breathing pure O_2 at 3-atm pressure has a P_AO_2 of approximately 2,000 mmHg, and arterial blood content of about 60 mL/L of dissolved O_2. This amount of dissolved O_2 would theoretically satisfy the O_2 requirements of a subject at rest. However, the toxicity of O_2 at high pressures limits the medical use of hyperbaric oxygenation to treatment of only certain conditions by experts.

Hgb combined oxygen. It is clear that the amount of O_2 dissolved in blood or plasma is insufficient for tissue needs even at rest. At rest, more than 95% of the O_2 delivered to the tissues is transported in combination with Hgb, and during exercise this value may exceed 99%.

Each gram of Hgb can combine chemically with a maximum (i.e., when fully saturated) of about 1.36 mL [STPD] of O_2. One liter of blood containing 150 g of Hgb can combine with 150 × 1.36 = 204 mL [STPD] of O_2. The amount of O_2 actually combined with Hgb depends on oxygen saturation (S_{O_2}) which is in turn dependent on blood P_{O_2} (Fig. 5). The relationship between saturation and P_{O_2} is sigmoid in shape and the position of the curve is dependent on multiple factors including temperature, pH, and P_{CO_2} to mention a few.[7] The curve slopes steeply between 10 and 50 mmHg and has a nearly flat portion above 70 mmHg. The unique shape of this oxyhemoglobin dissociation curve is an important example of physiologic adaptation. The relatively flat portion above 70 mmHg ensures the oxygenation of most Hgb despite wide variations in P_AO_2. On the other hand, the steep portion of the curve between 10 and 50 mmHg assures unloading of large amounts of O_2 in the systemic capillaries in response to small tissue P_{O_2} (P_tO_2) decrements.

Equation (3.12) describes the relationship between the amount of oxygen that is combined with Hgb ($C_{comb}O_2$) per liter of blood and S_{O_2}:

$$C_{comb}O_2 = 1.36 \cdot Hgb \cdot S_{O_2} \tag{3.12}$$

When calculating shunt, both components of oxygen (dissolved and attached to Hgb) must be included in Eq. (3.10). For arterial blood, C_aO_2 is the sum of $C_{a(diss)}O_2$ (derived from Eq. (3.11) and P_aO_2 obtained from an arterial blood sample) and $C_{a(comb)}$ O_2 (derived from Eq. (3.12) and S_aO_2 which can be either measured directly or derived from P_aO_2 utilizing the appropriate oxygen saturation curve from various available nomograms). Similarly, C_vO_2 is calculated from a sample of mixed venous blood (usually obtained from the distal port of a pulmonary artery catheter). Since capillary blood cannot be sampled, in practice C_cO_2 is calculated from P_AO_2 and S_AO_2

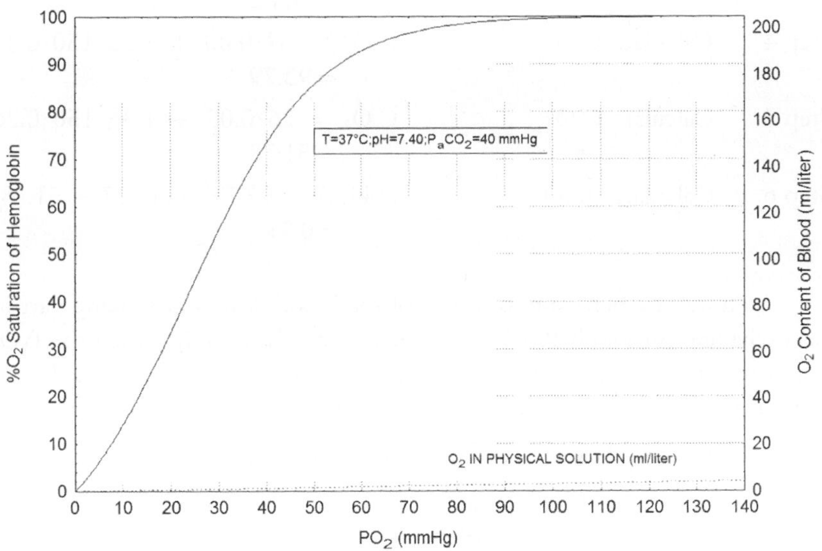

Fig. 5. Relationship between O_2 saturation and arterial PO_2

(using the same approach as for arterial blood) by assuming they are equal to P_cO_2 and S_cO_2, respectively.

Going back to *Case 1*, a mixed venous blood sample had the following results,

P_vO_2	26 mmHg
S_vO_2	25%
P_vCO_2	85 mmHg
pH	7.12

Assuming a Hgb of 150 g/L, and a barometric pressure of 760 mmHg, to calculate shunt one would have to go through the following steps:

Step 1	Calculation of P_AO_2	$P_AO_2 = 149 - 80/0.8 = 49$ mmHg
Step 2	Derive S_AO_2 from P_AO_2	At a P_AO_2 of 49 mmHg and pH 7.15, S_AO_2 is approximately 70%
Step 3	Calculate C_cO_2	$C_cO_2 = 49 \cdot 0.03 + 1.36 \cdot 150 \cdot 0.70 = 144.27$
Step 4	Calculate C_aO_2	$C_aO_2 = 33 \cdot 0.03 + 1.36 \cdot 150 \cdot 0.45 = 92.79$
Step 5	Calculate C_vO_2	$C_vO_2 = 26 \cdot 0.03 + 1.36 \cdot 150 \cdot 0.26 = 51.78$
Step 6	Calculate shunt	$(144.27 - 92.79)/(144.27 - 51.78) = 0.55$

The lungs are behaving as if 55% of the blood flow is not taking part in gas exchange. Although $P_{A\text{-}a}O_2$ difference is only 16 mmHg, when the P_aO_2 values are on the steep part of the O_2 dissociation curve even a small $P_{A\text{-}a}O_2$ difference could indicate a gross degree of shunt.

For *Case 2*, P_AO_2 and $P_{A\text{-}a}O_2$ are calculated as follows:

$$P_AO_2 = 149 - (32/0.8) = 109 \text{ mmHg}$$

$$P_{A\text{-}a}O_2 = 109 - 60 = 49 \text{ mmHg}$$

Calculating Q_s/Q_t for *Case 2* illustrates that, at times, the shunt fraction is not as severe as one would expect in the presence of a large A–a gradient. A mixed venous blood in this case had the following results:

P_vO_2	38 mmHg
S_vO_2	72%
P_vCO_2	45 mmHg
pH	7.40

Again assuming a Hgb of 150 g/L, and a barometric pressure of 760 mmHg, to calculate shunt one would have to go through the same steps:

Step 1	Calculation of P_AO_2	$P_AO_2 = 149 - 32/0.8 = 109$ mm Hg
Step 2	Derive S_AO_2 from P_AO_2	At a P_AO_2 of 109 mmHg and pH 7.45, S_AO_2 is approximately 99%
Step 3	Calculate C_cO_2	$C_cO_2 = 109 \cdot 0.03 + 1.36 \cdot 150 \cdot 0.99 = 205.23$
Step 4	Calculate C_aO_2	$C_aO_2 = 60 \cdot 0.03 + 1.36 \cdot 150 \cdot 0.90 = 185.40$
Step 5	Calculate C_vO_2	$C_vO_2 = 38 \cdot 0.03 + 1.36 \cdot 150 \cdot 0.72 = 148.02$
Step 6	Calculate shunt	$(205.23 - 185.40)/(205.23 - 148.02) = 0.34$

The calculated shunt fraction is not as severe as the one obtained for *Case 1* in spite of a very large $P_{A-a}O_2$.

From the earlier calculations it is quite evident that the shunt can be a major contributor to hypoxemia. The mechanism of this hypoxemia is through the mixing of deoxygenated blood with well-oxygenated blood. The shunt fraction is not always apparent from the blood gas results and an attempt to calculate it should always be made (especially when $P_{A-a}O_2$ is greater than 12 mmHg). The pathophysiology underlying shunt is not necessarily the result of a congenital or acquired cardiac disease with right-to-left shunt or an intrapulmonary shunt secondary to atelectasis or pneumonia. In fact, neither patient had any of these conditions. This brings us back to the last physiological cause of hypoxemia, namely, ventilation–perfusion (V/Q) mismatch.

V/Q mismatch as a cause of hypoxemia

To help one understand the concept of V/Q mismatch we will proceed with the management of *Case 1*. The patient was intubated and mechanically ventilated. He was initially ventilated with 100% oxygen. After approximately 30 minutes new samples of arterial and mixed venous blood were obtained with the following results:

P_aO_2	450 mmHg	P_vO_2	40 mmHg
S_aO_2	100%	S_vO_2	75%
P_aCO_2	40 mmHg	P_aCO_2	45 mmHg
pH	7.45	pH	7.42

With these results, and by following the previous steps for calculating Q_s/Q_t, the following results were obtained (Remember F_IO_2 in this case is 100% and therefore P_IO_2 is 713 mmHg):

Step 1	Calculation of P_AO_2	$P_AO_2 = 713 - 40/0.8 = 663$ mmHg
Step 2	Derive S_AO_2 from P_AO_2	At a P_AO_2 of 663 mmHg and pH 7.45, S_AO_2 is approximately 100%
Step 3	Calculate C_cO_2	$C_cO_2 = 663 \cdot 0.03 + 1.36 \cdot 150 \cdot 1.00 = 223.89$
Step 4	Calculate C_aO_2	$C_aO_2 = 450 \cdot 0.03 + 1.36 \cdot 150 \cdot 1.00 = 217.50$
Step 5	Calculate C_vO_2	$C_vO_2 = 45 \cdot 0.03 + 1.36 \cdot 150 \cdot 0.75 = 154.35$
Step 6	Calculate shunt	$(223.89 - 217.50)/(223.89 - 154.35) = 0.09$

One may wonder how the shunt fraction dropped from 55% to 9% by merely intubating the patient and administering 100% oxygen. It is quite possible that the patient had areas of atelectasis (due to mucous plugging for example) and/or pneumonia both of which could have easily contributed to the shunt. But these were not present on the chest X-ray or CT scan of the chest. This brings us back to the concept of V/Q mismatch.

In the presence of unequal distribution of V_A and perfusion, there will be units with low V/Q ratios that will cause hypoxemia and hypercapnia (shunt-like effect) and units with high V/Q ratios that will cause an increase in P_aO_2 and a drop in P_aCO_2 (dead-space-like effect). What impact do these low and high V/Q units have on gas exchange?

Similar to the oxygen dissociation curve, CO_2 has its own dissociation curve. In the physiologic range, the relationship between CO_2 content and P_{CO_2} is linear. Because of this linear relationship, the high P_aCO_2 coming out of low V/Q units when mixed with the low P_aCO_2 coming out of high V/Q units will tend to normalize the final P_aCO_2. Hence, the presence of V/Q mismatch is not a contributor to either hypercapnia or hypocapnia. The situation with respect to P_aO_2 is quite different. The O_2 dissociation curve is not linear but rather sigmoid in shape with the Hgb being almost completely saturated at a P_aO_2 of 80 mmHg. Although P_aO_2 coming out of units with high V/Q ratios may be very high, saturation, and hence, content is only marginally increased. Thus when this blood is mixed with blood coming out of low V/Q units the mean content drops precipitously and P_aO_2 will fall accordingly. In summary, the high V/Q units can compensate for the increased P_aCO_2 coming out of low V/Q units but cannot do so for oxygen because of the peculiar shapes of the O_2 and CO_2 dissociation curves.

Notice that with administration of 100% O_2, all the units with low V/Q mismatch are eliminated through better oxygenation of alveolar units that are receiving minimal ventilation. This is well illustrated in our last example in which the calculated shunt following the administration of higher levels of oxygen had eliminated part of the low V/Q units that were contributing to shunt. Units that are not ventilated at all (i.e., V/Q = 0) are not corrected with this maneuver and continue to contribute to the shunt fraction. These units are often referred to as "true shunt".

To summarize, when applying the shunt equation at any F_IO_2 other than 100% oxygen, the calculated shunt includes the contribution of V/Q mismatch. Calculation of shunt at 100% oxygen determines "true shunt". "True shunt" contributing to hypoxemia cannot be fixed by the administration of oxygen (as evidenced by its existence even with 100% oxygen). Calculating shunt at any F_IO_2 (*Case 1*, 55% on room air) is "true shunt" plus the contribution of V/Q mismatch. If one subtracts "true shunt" (in *Case 1*, 9%) from the calculated shunt on room air or any F_IO_2 other than 100% oxygen, one can derive the contribution of V/Q mismatch to the calculated shunt (in this case 46%). From the intervention point of view, hypoxemia that is due to V/Q mismatch can be treated by the administration of oxygen, whereas, hypoxemia that is due to "true shunt" requires the reversal of the primary disorder causing the "true shunt".

Summary

In summary, one can identify gas exchange problems through a sample of arterial blood gas. This should be obtained, when possible, while breathing room air. The most significant gas exchange problem related to CO_2 is hypercapnia. From Eq. (3.6), it is evident that hypercapnia can result from either an increase in V_{CO_2}, a decrease in V_A or a combination of both. However, most clinical causes of hypercapnia result from either a drop in V_A or inability to increase V_A in response to an increase in V_{CO_2}. The differential diagnosis to hypercapnia is approached anatomically starting from CNS, through the conduction system, end plate, muscular, thoracic cage, lung, peripheral airways and ending up in the central airways.

With regards to Q_2, the most significant gas exchange problem is hypoxemia. The approach to hypoxemia is physiological (i.e., trying to identify the physiological cause) as the physiological cause determines the intervention. The first two steps in trying to identify the physiological cause are to calculate P_AQ_2 and $P_{A\text{–}a}Q_2$. If the $P_{A\text{–}a}Q_2$ is less than 12 mmHg (normal A–a gradient), then the cause of hypoxemia can either be a drop in barometric pressure (as occurs with accent to altitude) or hypercapnia. If the cause of the hypoxemia is hypercapnia, then the treatment should focus on treating the hypercapnia, as treating the hypercapnia will resolve the hypoxemia. If the A–a gradient is greater than 18 mmHg, then shunt and V/Q mismatch should be considered. One can estimate the degree of shunt and V/Q mismatch by applying Eq. (3.10). Shunt that is calculated at any F_IO_2 other than 100% includes V/Q mismatch. Shunt that is calculated at a 100% F_IO_2 is termed "true shunt". This component of the shunt cannot be reversed by the administration of oxygen and requires treatment of the primary cause.

References

1. Anthonisen NR, Fleetham JA. Ventilation: Total, alveolar, and dead space. *Am Physiol Soc* 1987; IV: 113–129.

2. Mithoefer JC, Bossman OG, Thibeault DW *et al.* The clinical estimation of alveolar ventilation. *Am Rev Respir Dis* 1968; 98: 868–871.
3. Fulop M. A guide for predicting arterial CO_2 tension in metabolic acidosis. *Am J Nephrol* 1997; 17: 421–424.
4. Raymond LW. The alveolar air equation abbreviated. *Chest* 1978; 74: 675–676.
5. Mellemgaard K. The alveolar–arterial oxygen difference: Its size and components in normal man. *Acta Physiol Scand.* 1966; 67: 10.
6. Glenny RW. Teaching ventilation/perfusion relationships in the lung. *Adv Physiol Educ* 2008; 32: 192–195.
7. Roughton FJW. Transport of oxygen and carbon dioxide. *Amer Physiol Soc* 1964; I: 767–825.

Chapter 4

Perioperative Respiratory Dysfunction

Jameel Ali

Chapter Overview

One of the main reasons for surgical patients being admitted to the intensive care unit (ICU) is the necessity for respiratory support. Increasingly elderly patients require surgical procedures and age carries increased risk for respiratory compromise. The metabolic stress of the surgery and the need for nutritional support may require administration of supplemental nutrition which itself could increase the demand on the respiratory system contributing to respiratory dysfunction. Positioning of patients during operative procedures predispose them to specific alterations in lung volumes leading to respiratory dysfunction. Pain from peritonitis or incisions restrict lung volumes leading to abnormalities in gas exchange. Injudicious volume resuscitation in the perioperative period combined with borderline cardiac reserve in elderly patients and those with coronary artery disease could lead to elevated pulmonary capillary hydrostatic pressure with the elaboration of extravascular lung water and deleterious respiratory consequences. Also, there are many conditions in the surgical patients particularly sepsis which could lead to increase in pulmonary capillary permeability resulting in pulmonary edema and hypoxemia. Surgical procedures could also lead to abnormal function of the diaphragm itself resulting in respiratory compromise. In this chapter, these factors are discussed in greater detail setting the framework for understanding their role in perioperative respiratory dysfunction and guiding therapy to prevent and manage these abnormalities.

One major cause of morbidity and mortality affecting surgical patients in general and specifically in the ICU is thromboembolic disease. This topic is discussed in a separate chapter in the book.

Effect of Metabolic Stress, Fluid Volume, Oxygen Requirement, and Nutritional Support on Respiratory Function

Release of antidiuretc hormone (ADH) and aldosterone is a well-known response to surgical stress and fasting.[1,2] These hormones result in sodium and water retention as well as decreasing urine output. The decrease in urine output may persist in spite of normovolemia. These changes, combined with unmeasurable third space loss secondary to surgical procedures and peritonitis make estimation of circulating volume status very difficult. Traditional estimate of volume requirements based on urine output[3] is therefore likely to be very inaccurate and frequently leads to fluid overload and pulmonary edema related hypoxemia in the presence of "inadequate" urine output. In these circumstances, clinical indices other than urine output must be used to assess adequacy of fluid volume status, such as level of consciousness, capillary return, skin warmth, pulse rate, and character as well as blood pressure. In situations where these clinical indices also prove imprecise especially in the elderly surgical patient with poor cardiopulmonary reserve, central hemodynamic monitoring in the ICU environment is required. In addition, the syndrome of inappropriate ADH release (SIADH) is relatively common in the postoperative period resulting in water intoxication and severe hyponatremia[4] even when water in modest volume is administered. In these circumstances treatment should be guided by frequent monitoring of electrolytes and central hemodynamics.

The early phase of negative nitrogen balance following surgical stress can be shortened or even aborted by appropriate nutritional support before and after surgery. Early institution of enteric feeding has been reported to decrease postoperative complications including septic sequelae after abdominal surgery.[5] If daily caloric goals could not be achieved entirely by enteric feeds before day 8 of ICU stay then parenteral nutrition should be instituted to meet the estimated caloric needs and to prevent further loss of muscle mass.[6] Loss of muscle mass affects the ability to maintain normal respiratory function and results in dependence on ventilatory support as well as prolongation of the time to weaning off the respirator. The increased metabolic rate after surgery is associated with an increase in oxygen requirement and utilization, and a fall in muscle protein synthesis.[7,8] While this increased oxygen demand is easily met without untoward sequelae in patients with normal cardiorespiratory reserve, nutritionally depleted patients and those with already compromised cardiorespiratory function may be unable to meet these increased oxygen demands leading to decompensation, muscle fatigue, and respiratory failure. Such patients may require intubation and mechanical ventilatory support until the acute insult has abated and the oxygen demand can be met.

Apart from loading oxygen onto the red cell for delivery to the tissues, the respiratory apparatus is responsible for providing the necessary ventilation for carbon dioxide elimination. Excessive caloric delivery particularly in the form of carbohydrates,[8] can lead to production of Carbon dioxide (CO_2) in amounts that exceeds the ventilatory capacity of the lung to excrete the CO_2 thus leading to respiratory failure, the requirement for respirator support and prolongation of weaning.[9] Thus, in providing nutritional support not only should one try to provide the necessary calories, but also prevent overburdening of the respiratory system. If the caloric requirements are such that they cannot be provided without overwhelming the respiratory capability then the choice is between limiting caloric delivery and adding mechanical ventilator support to the treatment regime.

Generally, since the magnitude and duration of the surgical procedure affect the intensity of the metabolic response, the aim should be to decrease the duration and extent as well as frequency of surgical procedures in critically ill patients particularly in those with poor nutritional or cardiopulmonary reserve. This aim, however, should be considered in the context of the patient's underlying problem. The surgical procedure should not be minimized at the expense of incomplete eradication of a surgical lesion such as a source of sepsis since failure to eradicate the septic focus would result in further complications including respiratory failure. In the setting of the multiple injured patient requiring massive blood transfusion, who is hypocoagulable, hypothermic, and/or acidotic, abbreviated laparotomy ('damage control laparotomy') should be considered in which the patient's bleeding is stopped by techniques such as packing, control of sources of contamination by such procedures as irrigating, suctioning, and stapling without resection or anastomosis and taking the patient to the ICU for monitoring, warming, blood replacement, correction of hypothermia, and metabolic derangements including acidosis with mechanical ventilatory support which is followed as soon as possible by return to the Operating Room (OR) for completion of definitive care as the patient's condition in the ICU allows.[10]

Elaboration of Extravascular Lung Water in Surgical Patients

All three of the forces in Starling's equation governing transcapillary fluid flux i.e., capillary hydrostatic pressure, oncotic pressure, and capillary permeability are implicated in the generation of lung water (pulmonary edema) in the surgical patient.

Hydrostatic pressure

As aforementioned, the metabolic response to surgery and stress involves release of ADH, aldosterone, and catecholamines. We have discussed how water and sodium retention combined with low urine output in response to ADH and aldosterone release could lead the clinician who uses urine output as an endpoint of fluid resuscitation, to unintentionally fluid overload the surgical patient leading to increased capillary hydrostatic pressure particularly in the patient with poor cardiopulmonary reserve thus generating pulmonary edema and hypoxemia. The increase in afterload that accompanies the effect of catecholamine release on the systemic arteriolar bed can result in a decrease in left ventricular systolic stoke volume. This could result in a relative increase in end diastolic ventricular volume and thus ventricular end diastolic pressure which will be reflected in an increase in pulmonary capillary hydrostatic pressure predisposing to the elaboration of extra vascular lung water and hypoxemia particularly in the patient with diminished cardiorespiratory reserve. This may not only occur secondary to the response to stress and surgery, but has been implicated as one of the mechanisms in neurogenic pulmonary edema in the head injured patient although there is suggestion that some degree of increased capillary permeability may also play a role in the pathogenesis of neurogenic pulmonary edema.[11] Because of these factors consideration should be given to central hemodynamic monitoring in the ICU using a pulmonary artery catheter in these patients during fluid administration.

Oncotic pressure

The nutritionally depleted surgical patient with an underlying hypoalbuminemia or the patient with decreased intravascular protein concentration from non-colloid fluid infusion could also be at risk for pulmonary edema because of this decrease in capillary oncotic pressure. However, attempts to attenuate this effect by protein infusion has not been uniformly successful.

Capillary permeability

Increased pulmonary capillary permeability occurs in many settings in the surgical patient with the systemic release of cytokines and other vasoactive agents[12,13] but the most common cause is unrecognized sepsis which commonly arises in the abdomen as a result of complications of such inflammatory conditions as appendicitis, diverticulitis, perforated ulcer, or other perforations which could be secondary to abdominal trauma which is a frequent source of unrecognized sepsis and death. Increased capillary permeability is also implicated in reperfusion injury after restoration of perfusion after a period of ischemia in vascular occlusive disorders, or after shock resuscitation, after decompression of fascial compartments in compartment syndromes, early and late phases of multiple organ dysfunction syndrome etc. Intra-abdominal sepsis is frequently secondary to an undrained intra-abdominal abscess requiring a surgical or percutaneous radiologic approach.

Although both increased microvascular hydrostatic pressure and capillary permeability are important in the generation of extravascular lung water, manipulation of the microvascular hydrostatic pressure (by the use of vasoactive agents and regulation of the state of hydration) is the most direct means of altering pulmonary edema in the surgical patient. A search for a septic focus is crucial when increased capillary permeability is suspected. Control of capillary permeability can then be achieved, though indirectly, by treating the septic focus which may require a surgical approach. The link between sepsis and permeability is thus broken and the capillary permeability lesion is allowed to resolve with time. The resolution of the increased capillary permeability is accompanied by improvement in perioperative respiratory failure. An undrained septic focus should be suspected in patients who continue to have worsening of respiratory function including failure to wean off the respirator and until that septic focus is eradicated, dependence on ventilatory support and inability to wean will continue. Aggressive investigation for a septic source followed by appropriate eradication of this source is of paramount importance in managing these patients. Until the permeability is corrected, though indirectly, reduction of pulmonary artery wedge pressure to the lowest level compatible with adequate peripheral perfusion should be the goal.

Differentiation between pulmonary edema due to increased pulmonary capillary hydrostatic pressure and that due to capillary permeability is very important because the treatment may need to be modified based on which one of these entities may be considered responsible for the pulmonary edema. Treatment based on hemodynamic and fluid volume endpoints such as the use of diuretics, inotropes, vasodilators guided by central hemodynamic monitoring are the main focus in treating the high hydrostatic pressure pulmonary edema whereas pulmonary edema secondary to capillary leak requires a focus on trying to identify and treat the cause of the capillary leak such as identification and eradication of a septic focus. Usually, identification of a high measured capillary hydrostatic pressure with a central catheter such as SwanGanz catheter in the presence of radiologic and clinical evidence of pulmonary edema is considered evidence of high hydrostatic pressure pulmonary edema. However, caution must be exercised because of the recognized lag phase between the normalization of central hemodynamics and the radiologic clearance of signs of pulmonary edema.[14] In these settings, the presence of normal capillary hydrostatic pressure with radiologic signs of pulmonary edema could be falsely considered to be due to capillary leak edema not recognizing that the pulmonary edema occurred initially under high pulmonary capillary hydrostatic pressure conditions and with diuresis and other maneuvers the hydrostatic pressure is normalized, but the radiologic signs of pulmonary edema persists for a variable period.

Atelectasis and Hypoventilation

Ventilation and perfusion are not equally matched in the normal lung, because the shape of the thoracic cavity and the descent of the diaphragm result in greater expansion of the dependent areas of the lobes. Also blood flow is greater in dependent areas of the lung during spontaneous ventilation and changes with body position. The normal lung has an average ventilation perfusion ratio of approximately 0.8. In the surgical patient, many factors cause a reduction in these ratios to very low values, causing severe ventilation/perfusion mismatch and hypoxemia. Similar factors result in resorption of alveolar gas behind closed airways (compression atelectasis). This resorption atelectasis can occur as early as five minutes after induction of anesthesia.[15,16]

In surgical patients, hypoventilation is characteristically caused by impairment of ventilation due to the restrictive effect of painful incisions or peritonitis. It may also result from Central Nervous System (CNS) depression secondary to poorly titrated narcotic analgesia, anesthesia, or CNS injury.

The respiratory system is protected from sepsis and atelectasis by a respiratory mechanism that responds to hypoxemia, hypercapnia, acidosis, and the presence of irritating or noxious stimuli in the airway. These defense mechanisms can be significantly depressed by excessive postoperative narcotic analgesia or anesthesia. Inhalational anesthetics are noted for their respiratory depressive effect resulting in hypoventilation and a reduced to carbon dioxide as well as blunted response to hypoxemia and acidosis. Whereas in optimal doses narcotic analgesics decrease abdominal pain and increase the ability to clear secretions and ambulate, in larger doses they may depress the respiratory center leading to hypoventilation, hypercapnia, and hypoxemia.

The cough reflex is the main mechanism whereby particles are cleared from the upper airway, this reflex may be blunted by narcotic analgesics. Clearance of particles from the lower airway is effected through the action of the mucociliary system. Mucociliary activity as well as mucus production are altered by anesthetics leading to the production of mucus plugs which plug the lower airway leading to hypoxemia. In addition cellular defense mechanisms of the respiratory system are altered by anesthetic agents predisposing to respiratory compromise.

Shunting results from continued perfusion of non-ventilated lung units. In the surgical patient this frequently occurs as a result of perfusion of areas of postoperative atelectasis, although it can also occur with continued perfusion of edema filled alveolar units from capillary leak or increased pulmonary capillary hydrostatic pressure.

Age, Position, and Lower Airway Closure

Body position, age, and incisional pain all affect the relationship between the functional residual capacity (FRC) of the lung and the closing volume of the lung.[17,18] The FRC which is the volume of gas in the lung at the end of normal expiration represents the balance of opposing forces on the rib cage at resting lung volume and is considered the most important index of mechanical abnormality in the lung.[19] The closing volume is that volume of the lung at which small peripheral airways close. When FRC exceeds closing volume, lower airway patency is maintained and when FRC falls below closing volume lower airway closure begins. FRC falls with age and in all patients it is lower in the supine position which is the usual position for most surgical procedures. The lithotomy position results in a greater decrease in FRC predisposing to lower airway closure. As shown in Table 1, in the seated position 80% of patients (all below 35 years of age) maintain FRC above closing volume; in the supine position this percent falls from the 80% to 60% ; in the lithotomy position FRC is above closing volume in only 40% of patients all in the less than 30 year age group.

Table 1. FRC relative to closing volume with age and position.

Position	% FRC above closing volume (with Age)	% FRC below closing volume (with Age)
Seated	80% (all below age 35)	20% (age ≥ 35 yrs)
Supine	60% (all below age 35)	40% (age ≥ 35 yrs)
Lithotomy	40% (all below age 30)	60% (≥ 30 yrs)

Legend: Age and position affect degree of airway closure
Source: Modified from Ref. 26.

When the difference between FRC and closing volume is plotted against the alveolar–arterial oxygen tension gradient,[20] the gradient increases as FRC falls below closing volume. The most dependent areas of the lung are the first to undergo airway closure and in the supine position which is the commonest patient position for surgical procedures, more of the lung is dependent thus predisposing to airway closure and hypoxemia in these patients. General anesthesia itself, as mentioned earlier, could predispose the patient to compression atelectasis in dependent areas of the lung leading to hypoxemia. In both normal individuals and smokers, increasing age is associated with increasing closing volumes, predisposing the patient to airway closure at higher lung volumes.[21]

As a group, smokers have higher closing volumes so that the combination of smoking with increasing age predisposes to perioperative hypoxemia. Chronic cigarette smoking is generally considered to be associated with an increase in postoperative respiratory complications which may result from alteration in respiratory defense mechanisms, as well as increase in airway resistance and work of breathing. Cessation of smoking for a period of over eight weeks is associated with a decrease in postoperative respiratory complications.[22] Although abstinence too soon prior to surgery has been suggested to increase the risk of postoperative respiratory complications. Aggressive counseling for smoking cessation prior to any elective surgical procedure still appears to be the best approach.

The lack of cartilage support in the periphery of the lung makes these peripheral airways very susceptible to pleural pressures. The negative intrapleural pressures tend to maintain patency of these peripheral airways through the preservation of a positive transpulmonary pressure gradient. However, breathing at low FRC, that occurs with abdominal pain from incisions in patients in the supine position — all contribute to the development of positive pleural pressures predisposing to alveolar collapse.

Continued perfusion of these collapsed lung units lead to hypoxemia from shunting. Even when the airways are not completely collapsed but merely narrowed, this leads to hypoxemia from decreased ventilation–perfusion ratios.

Multiple fractures increase the risk of pulmonary complications not only from the restrictive effect of chest wall pain from rib fractures but pulmonary fat embolism from other fractures and the prolonged period of bed rest in the supine position, leading to atelectasis and secondary pneumonia from decreased clearance of lung secretions from inhibition of effective coughing. Early operative stabilization of fractures allowing early ambulation and physiotherapy as well as frequent changes in body position all minimize dependent alveolar collapse and resulting hypoxemia.[23]

Loss of use of the intercostal muscles in traumatic quadriplegia is a major cause of respiratory dysfunction in these patients. This can be minimized by maintaining these patients in the horizontal to 35° head-up bed position and maximum FRC is achieved in the 60°–90° head-up position.[24,25]

Diaphragm Dysfunction and Abdominal Surgery

Although the factors discussed in the preceding paragraphs are present in patients undergoing most surgical procedures, the most serious sequelae are found in patients undergoing upper abdominal surgery. Within the first 4 hours of surgery in these patients there is an immediate significant decrease in Vital Capacity (VC). There is a slower but definite fall in FRC which peaks at about 24 hours (see Figs. 1 and 2) and is associated with hypoxemia.[26]

The depression in VC and FRC is more pronounced in upper abdominal incision compared to lower abdominal incision. Perhaps the decrease in vital capacity represents restriction due to pain leading to breathing at lower lung volumes, an inability to cough effectively and with time a fall in the FRC with alveolar collapse and hypoxemia. Healthy patients with no pre-existing cardiorespiratory comorbidities are able to tolerate and recover from these disturbances in lung mechanics without significant respiratory complications. However, in elderly patients and those with pre-existing cardiopulmonary disorders these alterations in respiratory mechanics can result in severe hypoxemia and respiratory failure. The postoperative decrease in VC is primarily a restrictive rather than obstructive phenomenon, as evidenced by the maintenance of a normal ratio between the forced expired volume in one second and the forced vital capacity (FEV1/FVC). This restriction may be related to incisional pain with inability to cough vigorously and clear

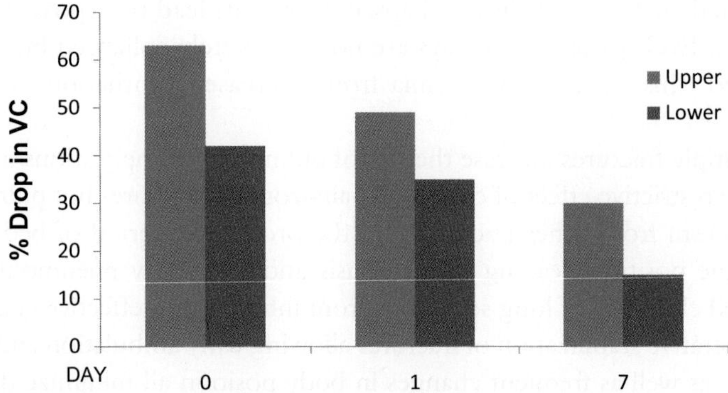

Fig. 1. % drop in VC in upper and lower abdominal incisions.

Legend: Immediate drop in VC occurs within four hours with significant improvement by Day 7. Depression of VC is greater with upper compared to lower incision.
Source: See Ref. 17.

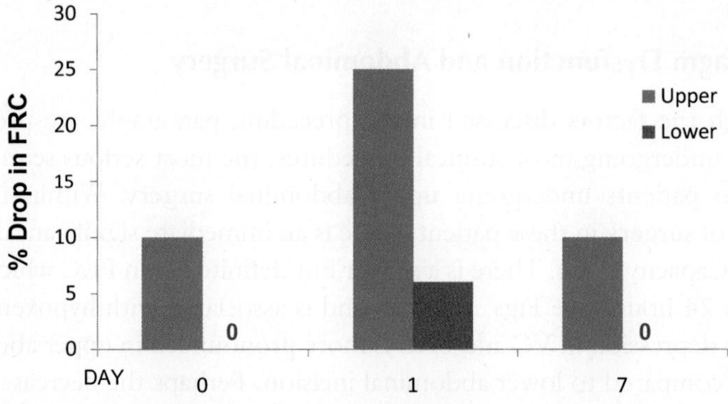

Fig. 2. % drop in FRC in upper and lower abdominal incisions.

Legend: The drop in FRC is delayed compared to VC with maximum depression in 16–24 hours. FRC is back to normal by seven days in lower abdominal incision.

pulmonary secretions leading to an increase in closing volumes and decrease in FRC — if not corrected hypoxemia from atelectasis results. Pain control using such techniques as transcutaneous electric nerve stimulation, epidural, and intercostal blockade[27] have been used to counteract these changes in lung mechanics. Although all of these techniques have improved VC and FRC, none have been successful in immediately achieving preoperative FRC and VC levels. This suggests that these techniques either do not completely control the pain or that the pain is not the only cause of the postoperative respiratory dysfunction.

One of the responsible factors may be diaphragmatic dysfunction as suggested by the finding that patients undergoing upper abdominal surgery have a significant decrease in maximal transdiaphragmatic pressure at FRC which is not altered by epidural analgesia.[28] There may be a primary or secondary effect of the surgical procedure on diaphragmatic function. A switch from predominantly abdominal breathing to rib cage breathing has been identified in patients undergoing upper abdominal surgery[29,30] and similarly in animal models undergoing cholecystectomy[31] Mere traction on the gall bladder has produced similar effects on diaphragmatic function in animals.[31] The ratio of measured abdominal wall motion to chest wall motion is an index of the degree of diaphragmatic movement during respiration, the lower ratio representing more rib cage than diaphragmatic contribution to respiration. As depicted in Fig. 3, immediately after upper abdominal surgery the diaphragmatic contribution to respiration is diminished as reflected in a decrease in the ratio of abdominal to rib cage excursion. These studies suggest that there may be factors other than pain and general anesthesia such as endogenous agents which are responsible for the respiratory dysfunction related to changes in diaphragmatic function following upper abdominal surgical procedures.

Laparoscopic cholecystectomy has been demonstrated to be associated with postoperative changes in VC and FRC as well but the depression in

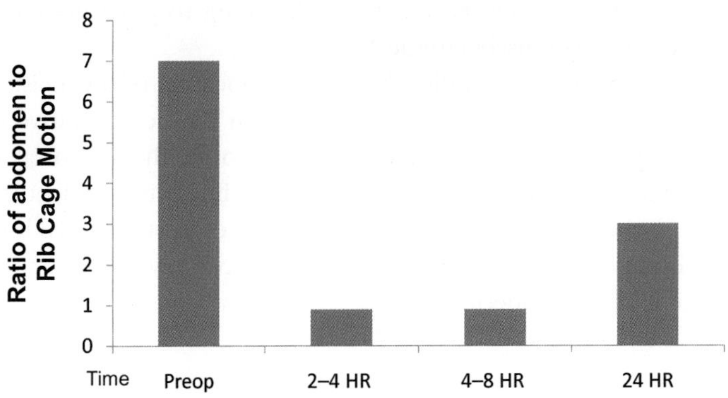

Fig. 3. Ratio of abdomen to rib cage motion versus time.

Legend: Diaphragm motion is decreased post-op and still depressed at 24 hours compared to pre-op.

FRC and VC is less and returns to preoperative levels within 24 hours when compared to open cholecystectomy which demonstrates longer time to recovery of these parameters.[32–34] From the respiratory standpoint, therefore, the laparoscopic procedure should be chosen wherever possible over the open technique particularly in patients with compromised cardiorespiratory status as is so often the case in the ICU patient. The increase in intra-abdominal pressure with pneumoperitoneum during laparoscopic cholecystectomy has a minimal hemodynamic effect[35] but in patients with borderline cardiopulmonary reserve this could be significant warranting close hemodynamic monitoring in the operating room. Shock and cardiac failure also affect diaphragmatic function as demonstrated by changes in diaphragmatic force as well as glycogen depletion in diaphragmatic muscle.[36]

Apart from the factors mentioned in earlier paragraphs, aging has been associated with reduced elastic recoil of the lung, decreased expiratory flow rate and diminished airway protective reflexes all of which would increase the risk of postoperative pulmonary complications.

The obese patient

There are many risks for postoperative pulmonary complications in the obese patient. These patients breathe at lower lung volumes so that closing volume often exceeds FRC leading to atelectasis and hypoxemia. The increased mass, especially in the supine position, increases the work of breathing and places major stress on the respiratory system predisposing to pulmonary dysfunction from respiratory muscle fatigue.[37]

Not only the type of operation but also the location of the incision tend to affect the degree of respiratory impairment in the postoperative period. There is a suggestion that in open cholecystectomy, the subcostal muscle transecting incision may be associated with less impairment of pulmonary function than the midline incision.[38] The severity of postoperative lung dysfunction decreases in the following order: thoracotomy, upper abdominal, lower abdominal, and superficial.[26]

Aspiration

The combination of depression of normal respiratory protective reflexes during anesthesia[39] and the supine position of many surgical patients predisposes to aspiration of gastric contents into the respiratory tract. This is more likely to occur with a full stomach and the patient under general anesthesia or recovering from general anesthesia with retching and coughing soon after or during endotracheal extubation as well as during intubation. The sequence is first obstruction from aspiration of debris and chemically induced bronchoconstriction, then a chemical burn of the airway with fluid loss into the injured area, followed by an intense inflammatory response and finally lung infection. The clinical presentation is quite variable, with mild cases showing transient coughing and minimal bronchospasm all the way to a progressive downhill course including hypovolemic shock, hypoxemia, and finally fulminant bacterial pneumonia.[40,41]

The management of acid aspiration is mainly supportive, including: (1) rapid suctioning of debris — fiber optic bronchoscopy facilitates rapid suction and lavage of gross debris; (2) gastric intubation to aspirate the stomach and prevent further aspiration into the airway; (3) oxygen administration — mechanical ventilation may be required as determined by the severity of respiratory compromise; (4) bronchodilator for severe bronchospasm (5) maintenance of normovolemia and perfusion by monitoring and replacement of fluid — vasoactive drugs including inotropes may be required to temporarily support the circulation. Antibiotics are not recommended unless there is fulminant bacterial pneumonia which occurs later or if there are grossly contaminated contents from the stomach. Steroids have not been proven of benefit. Preventive measures to consider in high risk patients are: gastric decompression, placing intubated patients in the semirecumbent position unless contraindicated, continuous drainage of subglottic secretions,[42] and consideration of inhibitors of gastric secretions.

Prevention of Perioperative Lung Dysfunction

Many techniques have been used to improve postoperative lung function such as incentive spirometry, Intermittent positive pressure breathing (IPPB) and nasal continuous positive airway pressure (CPAP). Although incentive spirometry has been reported to be ineffective in decreasing postoperative pulmonary complications following cardiac and upper abdominal surgery,[43] IPPB, incentive spirometry, CPAP, and physiotherapy generally improve postoperative pulmonary function.[44,45] IPPB offers no advantage over physiotherapy when the latter is maximized in the postoperative period. Non-yielding abdominal binders provide comfort by decreasing incisional pain but this is outweighed by the restrictive effect on lung volumes postoperatively. However, elastic binders may not only improve comfort but also allow coughing without unduly restricting lung volume.[46] None of these measures completely reverses the postoperative respiratory dysfunction.

Predicting postoperative respiratory risk by preoperatively assessing respiratory mechanics as well as identifying risk factors such as age, obesity, smoking, and strategic location of incisions is useful in planning therapeutic approaches. Although no individual respiratory parameter precisely predicts postoperative respiratory compromise or morbidity and mortality, it is recognized that the poorer the measured preoperative respiratory function, the more likely the patient is to develop severe postoperative respiratory dysfunction. Based on cumulative experience, the following have been recommended: If the FEV1 is < 1 L, the FEVC < 1.5 L, FEV1/FVC <30% or the forced expiratory flow rate (FEF 25%–75%) is < 0.6 L/sec and if the maximum minute ventilation is <50% of the predicted value for that patient, then the risk of postoperative respiratory complications is very high.[47–49] In patients whose parameters are below these thresholds, the strategy is to implement measures aimed at improving function to levels above these thresholds by such factors as cessation of smoking, diaphragm muscle conditioning, weight loss, treatment of heart failure, fine tuning the fluid status, to avoid fluid overload, and correcting any identifiable reactive airway disease where possible.

The patient undergoing lung resection is at even greater risk of developing postoperative pulmonary complications, particularly if functional lung tissue needs to be removed. In these patients, the effect of the excised functioning lung tissue must be considered in addition to the above factors.[48,49] A quantitative lung perfusion scan[49] can be used to predict the lung function postoperatively by determining how much lung tissue will remain after the planned procedure. The postoperative FEV1 is then calculated as the product of the preoperative FEV1 and the fractional perfusion of the remaining lung as determined by the preoperative lung perfusion scan. The usual guideline for an adult patient is that if the predicted postoperative FEV1 is < 0.8 L, the operative risk is prohibitive. The preoperative measured diffusing capacity[48] is also an accurate predictor of major morbidity and mortality after lung resection. A useful guide is to exclude from major resection all patients with diffusing capacity <60% of predicted, even if other spirometric parameters appear satisfactory. It is recommended that patients with only slightly impaired function (FEV1 and diffusing capacity >80% predicted) with acceptable cardiovascular risk factors can safely undergo pulmonary resection including pneumonectomy. For others, exercise testing as well as pulmonary split-function test studies are recommended. The symptom limited cardiopulmonary exercise testing measures the maximum volume of oxygen utilization (VO_2 max) as an index of pulmonary and cardiovascular reserve. A VO_2 max <10ml/kg/min is generally considered a contraindication to any pulmonary resection whereas a value >20 ml/kg/min or >75% of predicted is considered safe for major resections. Resections that involve no more than one lobe usually result in early functional deficit during which temporary ventilatory support may be necessary followed by recovery and permanent loss in pulmonary function is usually <10%. Generally, pulmonary function tests tend to overestimate the functional loss after lung resection but this is not necessarily a bad thing except when patients requiring important surgery may be denied such procedures based on these test results. Arterial blood gas criteria may also be used to exclude patients from major lung resection. Patients with a room air PO_2 of <50 mmHg or PCO_2> 45 mmHg at rest are considered at very high risk for pulmonary complications and prohibitive operative risk. Surgical intervention may need to be considered in spite of these prohibitive risks but only for lifesaving mandatory operations in urgent situations where patient and physician are fully aware of the risks involved and are prepared to accept these risks and the possibility of an unfavorable outcome.

Treatment Principles for Perioperative Respiratory Dysfunction

(1) Maximization of the patient's preoperative status when time allows (cessation of smoking, diaphragmatic conditioning exercises, weight loss, nutrition, aggressive treatment of reversible cardiorespiratory disorders — including congestive heart failure, bronchopneumonia, or bronchospasm);
(2) Early ambulation and physiotherapy to overcome the effects of the supine position on lung volumes and early operative stabilization in patients with fractures to allow ambulation and physiotherapy;
(3) Early identification and treatment of sepsis and shock including surgery and interventional radiology to minimize pulmonary capillary leak;
(4) Judicious fluid administration to maintain normal perfusion and hydration and avoid fluid overload;
(5) Optimal use of analgesics without producing respiratory depression;
(6) Specific treatment of identifiable causes of hypoxemia (bronchodilator for bronchospasm, antimicrobials directed against specific microorganisms in pneumonia);
(7) Preoperative pulmonary assessment especially in those with poor pulmonary reserve and those undergoing lung resection; and

(8) Institution of mechanical ventilation when the above measures are not sufficient. Frequently mechanical ventilation can be avoided with appropriate preventive measures which can also shorten the duration of mechanical ventilatory support when this becomes necessary.

References

1. Wilmore DW. Metabolic response to severe surgical illness — overview. *World J Surg* 2000; 24: 705–720.
2. Bessey PQ, Walters JM, Aoki TJ, Wilmore DW. Combined hormonal infusion simulates the metabolic response to surgery. *Ann Surg* 1984; 200: 264–270.
3. Giesecke AH Jr, Egbert LD. Perioperative fluid therapy, in Miller RD (ed). Crystalloids in Anesthesia, 2nd ed. New York, Churchill Livingstone, 1986, 3132–3146.
4. Chung HM, Rudiger K, Schrier RW, Anderson RJ. Postoperative hyponatremia: A prospective study. *Arch Intern Med* 1986; 146: 333–345.
5. Moore FA, Feliciano DV, Andrassy RJ *et al.* Early enteral feeding, compared with parenteral, reduces postoperative septic complications: The results of a meta-analysis. *Ann Surg* 1992; 216: 172–180.
6. Casaer MP, Mesotten D, Hermans G *et al.* Early versus late parenteral nutrition in critically ill adults. *New Engl J Med* 2011; 365: 506–515.
7. Hammarqvist F, Wennerman J, Ali R *et al.* Addition of glutamine total parenteral nutrition after elective surgery spares free glutamine in muscle, counteracts the fall in muscle protein synthesis and improvement in nitrogen balance. *Ann Surg* 1989; 209: 455–460.
8. Herve P, Simmoneau G, Girard P *et al.* Hypercapneic acidosis induced by nutrition in mechanically ventilated patients. Glucose versus fat. *Crit Care Med* 1985; 13: 537–542.
9. Hall JB, Wood LDH. Liberation of the patient from mechanical ventilation. *JAMA* 1987; 257: 1621–1632.
10. Burch JM, Ortiz VB, Richardson RJ *et al.* Abbreviated laparotomy and planned reoperation for critically injured patients. *Ann Surg* 1991; 215: 476–488.
11. Colice GL, Mathay MA, Bass E, Mathay RA. Neurogenic pulmonary edema. *Am Rev Respir Dis* 1984; 130: 941–946.
12. Cinat M, Waxman K, Vaziri ND *et al.* Soluble cytokine receptors and receptor antagonists are sequentially released after trauma. *J Trauma* 1995; 39: 112–117.
13. Michie HR, Eberline TJ, Spriggs DR *et al.* Interleukin-2 initiates metabolic responses associated with critical illness in humans. *Ann Surg* 1988; 208: 493–501.
14. Ali J, Duke K. Decreasing hydrostatic pressure does not uniformly decrease high pressure pulmonary edema. *Chest* 1987; 91: 588–592.

15. Brismar B, Hedenstierna G, Lindquist H *et al.* Pulmonary densities during anesthesia with muscular relaxation — a proposal of atelectasis. *Anesthesiology* 1985; 62: 422–430.
16. Tokics L, Hedenstierna G, Brismar B *et al.* Thoracoabdominal restriction in supine men: CT and lung function measurements. *J Appl Physiol* 1988; 64: 599–604.
17. Craig Db, Wahba WM, Don HF *et al.* "Closing Volume" and its relationship to gas exchange in seated and supine positions. *J Appl Physiol* 1971; 31: 717–731.
18. Alexander JI, Horton PW, Millar PW *et al.* The effect of upper abdominal surgery on the relationship of airway closing point to end tidal position. *Clin Sci* 1972; 43: 137–143.
19. Hoeppner VH, Cooper DM, Zamel N *et al.* Relationship between elastic recoil and closing volume in smokers and non-smokers. *Am Rev Respir Dis* 1974; 109: 81–92.
20. Hedenstierna G. Mechanisms of postoperative pulmonary dysfunction. *Acta Chir Scand* 1989; 550 (Supplement): 152–163.
21. Moores LK. Smoking and postoperative pulmonary complications. An evidence-based review of the recent literature. *Clin Chest Med* 2000; 21: 139–150.
22. Warner MA, Divertie M, Tinker JH. Preoperative cessation of smoking and pulmonary complications in coronary artery bypass patients. *Anesthesiology* 1984; 60: 380–388.
23. Johnson KD, Cadambi A, Seibert AB. Incidence of adult respiratory distress syndrome in patients with multiple musculoskeletal injuries: Effect of early operative stabilization of fractures. *J Trauma* 1985; 25: 375–388.
24. Reines HD, Harris RC. Pulmonary complications of acute spinal cord injuries. *Neurosurgery* 1987; 21: 193–199.
25. Ali J, Qi W. Pulmonary function and posture in traumatic quadriplegia. *J Trauma* 1995; 39: 334–338.
26. Ali J, Weisel RD, Layug AB *et al.* Consequences of post-operative alterations in respiratory mechanics. *Am J Surg* 1974; 128: 376–382.
27. Ali J, Yaffe C, Serrette C. The effect of transcutaneous electric nerve stimulation on postoperative pain and pulmonary function. *Surgery* 1981; 89: 507–512.
28. Simonneau G, Vivien A, Sartener R *et al.* Diaphragm dysfunction induced by upper abdominal surgery. *Am Rev Respir Dis* 1983; 128: 899–905.
29. Ford GT, Whitelaw WA, Rosenal TW *et al.* Diaphragm function after upper abdominal surgery in humans. *Am Rev Repir Dis* 1983; 127: 431–437.
30. Road JD, Burges KR, Whitelaw WA, Ford GT. Diaphragm function and respiratory response after upper abdominal surgery in dogs. *J Appl Physiol* 1984; 57: 576–582.
31. Ford GT, Grant DA, Rideout KS *et al.* Inhibition of breathing associated with gall bladder (GB) stimulation in dogs. *J Appl Physiol* 1988; 65: 72–79.
32. Erice F, Fox GS, Salib YM *et al.* Diaphragmtic function before and after laparoscopic cholecystectomy. *Anesthesiology* 1993; 79: 966–971.

33. Schulze S, Thorup F. Pulmonary function, pain and fatigue after laparoscopic cholecystectomy. *Eur J Surg* 1993; 159: 361–369.
34. Ali J, Gana T. Lung volumes at 24 hours after laparoscopic cholecystectomy — justification for early discharge. *Can Respir J* 1998; 5: 109–113.
35. Obeid F, Saba A, Fatah J *et al.* Increasing intra-abdominal pressure affects pulmonary compliance. *Arch Surg* 1995; 130: 544–549.
36. Roussos C. The failing ventilatory pump. *Lung* 1982; 160: 59–64.
37. vonUngera-Sternberg BS, Regli A, Schneider MC *et al.* Effect of obesity and site of surgery on perioperative lung volumes. *Br J Anaesth* 2004; 92: 202–208.
38. Ali J, Khan TA. The comparative effects of muscle transecting and median upper abdominal incisions on postoperative pulmonary function. *Surg Gynecol Obstet* 1979; 148: 863–868.
39. Brain JD. Anesthesia and respiratory defense mechanisms. *Int Anesthesiol Clin* 1977; 15: 169–180.
40. Wynne JW, Modell JH. Respiratory aspiration of stomach contents. *Ann Intern Med* 1977; 87: 466–472.
41. Torres A, Serra-Battles J, Ros E *et al.* Pulmonary aspiration of gastric contents in patients receiving mechanical ventilation: The effect of body position. *Ann Intern Med* 1992; 166(7): 540–545.
42. Dezfulian C, Shojania K, Collard HR *et al.* Subglottic secretion drainage for preventing ventilator-associated pneumonia: A meta-analysis. *Am J Med* 2005; 1118(1): 11–18.
43. Overend TJ, Anderson CM, Lucy SD *et al.* The effect of incentive spirometry on postoperative pulmonary complications — a systematic review. *Chest* 2001; 120: 971–982.
44. Celli BR, Rodriguez KS, Snider GL. A controlled trial of intermittent positive pressure breathing, incentive spirometry and deep breathing exercises in preventing pulmonary complications after abdominal surgery. *Am Rev Respir Dis* 1984; 130: 12–28.
45. Ali J, Serrette C, Wood LDH, Anthonisen NR. Effect of postoperative intermittent positive pressure breathing on lung function. *Chest* 1980; 77: 337–343.
46. Ali J, Serrette C, Khan TA. The effect of abdominal binders on postoperative pulmonary function. *Infect Surg* 1983; 2: 875–881.
47. Ali MK, Mountain CF, Ewer MS *et al.* Predicting loss of pulmonary function after pulmonary resection for bronchogenic carcinoma. *Chest* 1980; 77: 337–348.
48. Ferguson MK, Little L, Rizzo L *et al.* Diffusing capacity predicts morbidity and mortality after pulmonary resection. *J Thorac Cardiovasc Surg* 1988; 96: 894–901.
49. Schuurmans MM, Diacon AH, Bolliger CT. Functional evaluation before lung resection. *Clin Chest Med* 2002; 23: 159–169.

Chapter 5

Mechanical Ventilation in the ICU

Robert Chen and Jameel Ali

Chapter Overview

Mechanical ventilation is a frequent and very important part of management of the ICU patient. It is therefore essential that doctors working in this environment are familiar with the basics of mechanical ventilation. In this chapter, we discuss the function of the respiratory system and its relation to abnormalities requiring mechanical ventilatory support, the indications for mechanical ventilation, the setting up of the ventilator, monitoring the ventilated patient and the process of liberation from the ventilator.

Functions of the respiratory system and its malfunction leading to respiratory failure

The two main functions of the respiratory system are to eliminate carbon dioxide (ventilation) and to provide oxygenation. Respiratory failure may thus be classified into (1) Ventilatory or Hypercapnic Respiratory Failure and (2) Hypoxemic Respiratory failure.

Hypercapnic Respiratory failure results from: reduced respiratory drive from a variety of causes including drugs, chest wall abnormalities, neuromuscular disorders including muscular fatigue and other causes of increased work of breathing. The resulting increased alveolar pCO_2 also leads to decreased alveolar pO_2 and secondary hypoxemia.

Hypoxemic Respiratory failure results from (1) continued perfusion of non-ventilated lung units (shunt hypoxemia which is relatively resistant to increasing inspired oxygen concentration) (2) ventilation–perfusion mismatch hypoxemia which is responsive to increasing inspired oxygen concentration and (3) increased pulmonary capillary permeability leading to increase in the elaboration of extravascular lung water.

Goals of Mechanical Ventilation

Based on the categorization of Respiratory failure, following are the goals of mechanical ventilation:

1. Decrease work of breathing
2. Improve gas exchange
3. Alleviate muscle fatigue
4. Allow time for lung healing in acute lung injury
5. Provide Hyperventilation — e.g., in head trauma

In overall management of the Respiratory failure the approach involves consideration of patient factors and those related to the ventilator.

Patient factors

The work of breathing should be decreased to the extent possible by:

1. Decreasing ventilatory demand-decrease CO_2 production by decreasing carbohydrate and caloric load, decreasing dead space and maintaining oxygen supply, correcting metabolic acidosis and decreasing respiratory drive by reducing psychologic stress (including use of sedation);
2. Improving secretion clearance;
3. Reverse broncho spasm;
4. Optimize fluid balance by assessing for fluid overload, treating congestive heart failure including the use of diuretics where appropriate;
5. Reversing any correctible neuroendocrine-musculoskeletal abnormality, which may interfere with the mechanics of respiration;
6. Identifying and treating causes of increased pulmonary capillary permeability e.g., eradicating a septic focus.

Ventilator factors

This involves identifying factors that require ventilator assistance:

Mechanical ventilator assistance is required when the respiratory system can no longer maintain its normal function of providing adequate oxygen uptake and carbon dioxide clearance and this is manifested by:

1. Inability to maintain PaO_2, $PaCO_2$ and pH at acceptable levels ($PaO_2 <$ 70 on FiO_2 of 60%; PaO_2/FiO_2 <200, $PaCO_2$ >55 torr and rising; pH 7.25 and lower.
2. Abnormal chest wall and/or lung compliance.
3. Inability to generate an adequate mechanical inspiratory force to sustain respiratory function (negative inspiratory force <15 cm H_2O).

Clinical correlates of the above indications for institution of mechanical ventilation include: tachypnea, dyspnea, central cyanosis, hypertension, headache, sweating, tachycardia, irritability, confusion, loss of consciousness.

The Alveolar Gas Equation (Age) And Modes of Ventilation

Reviewing the AGE will facilitate understanding of the modes of ventilation and types of ventilators used:

$P_AO_2 = (P_{Atm} - P_{H2O}) \times Fi_{O2} - (P_{CO2}/RQ)$,
P_AO_2 = alveolar oxygent tension
P_{Atm} = atmospheric pressure
P_{H2O} = pressure of water vapor (often assumed as 100% humidified)
Fi_{O2} = fraction of inspired oxygen
P_{CO2} = pressure of alveolar carbon dioxide (CO_2)
RQ = respiratory quotient (often assumed as 0.8).

Whereas the pressure inside the circuit of a mechanically ventilated patient is often measured in centimetres of water (cm H_2O), partial pressures of gasses are expressed in millimetres of mercury (mm Hg). Atmospheric pressure at sea level is considered to be 760 mmHg. As a standard, this also equals "zero" airway pressure as measured in cm H_2O. Inspired air saturated with water vapour represents 47 mmHg of partial pressure displaced. By the time inspired air reaches the alveolus, it shares that volume (and thus partial pressure) with the CO_2 continually transported by the alveolar capillaries. The

RQ represents a "fudge factor" that allows peripherally measured arterial CO_2 to better represent conditions within the lung. By substituting 0.21, or the fraction of atmospheric oxygen, the equation produces results nearing 100 mmHg for typical P_{CO2} values.

Recognizing that an airway pressure of zero refers to the pressure of 760 mmHg in the AGE opens up a new understanding of oxygenation. Increasing mean airway pressure (MAP) (i.e., 760 mmHg plus MAP) will result in increased P_AO_2. Increasing tidal volume delivered by a ventilator (thus airway pressure) increases MAP. Adding and increasing positive end expiratory pressure (PEEP) substantially increases MAP. Using pressure controlled (or pressure limited) ventilation (PCV) changes the shape of the inspiratory pressure curve such that a maximum pressure is maintained during the entire inspiratory phase. This further incrementally increases MAP. Changing the ratio of time spent in inspiration versus exhalation (I:E ratio) also significantly affects MAP. "Inverse ratio" ventilation, where more time is spent in the inhalation phase versus the exhalation phase further increases MAP. The ultimate version of prioritizing the inspiratory phase is airway pressure release ventilation (APRV). High airway pressures are maintained with only a brief moment where airway pressure is allowed to fall to allow for ventilation. Theoretically, if the patient never exhales such as the case with high frequency oscillation (HFO) or jet ventilation, the MAP is maximized.

Carbon dioxide removal from the alveolus serves as the other half of mechanical ventilation. pCO_2 control can be summarized as related directly to minute ventilation.

Minute ventilation ($V = V_t * RR$),
V_t = tidal volume,
RR= respiratory rate.

Historically set tidal volumes and ventilation rates of 10–12 mL/kg × 10 breaths/minute in anaesthesia led to physiologic minute volumes but were found to be harmful in patients with lung injury.[1] Such volumes may even have contributed to lung injury through mechanisms beyond barotraumas (i.e., pneumothorax).[2] Current lung protective strategies in critical care suggest 6 mL/kg of ideal body weight as a starting point. Respiratory rates are increased as a consequence.

In the sickest patients, reducing the volume or pressure within the alveolus results in reduced lung injury through barotrauma and the volutrauma of surfactant insult with repeated alveolar collapse and distension.[3] Prioritizing lower peak airway pressure and thus lower ventilating volume results in some hypoventilation. This strategy of permissive hypercapnia leads to a respiratory acidosis that is well tolerated.

In certain patients, pCO_2 control will be more important. Avoidance of hypoventilation is the key in brain injury care. Many trauma patients present with concomitant CNS injury. Brain injury through congenital or acquired disease must be considered similarly. Other patients may tolerate acidosis poorly such as renal failure who might not tolerate pH related potassium shifts. Patients with sickle cell anaemia or pulmonary hypertension will also need to have good pCO_2 control.

Related to pCO_2 control is the titration of exhalation. As discussed earlier, oxygenation could be prioritized by increasing the percentage of the respiratory cycle spent in inhalation. Chronic lung disease, particularly of the obstructive variety is defined by elevated pCO_2. Asthma, and other reversible reactive airways diseases are also marked by pCO_2 elevation when in exacerbation. Those patients, by definition, have exhalation disease. Longer time spent in exhalation results in improved ventilation. Decreasing respiratory rate in special patients also increases time spent in exhalation.

Whereas the AGE predicts the theoretical pO_2 generated by a ventilation strategy, the difference between the calculated pO_2 and the measured pO_2 is the alveolar–arterial gradient (A–a gradient). The normal gradient is in the 10–20 mmHg range. The PF ratio is calculated as $PF = P_aO_2\,(mmHg)/FiO_2$ (as decimal). The PF ratio is a relative shortcut compared to the A–a gradient where a ratio of ≤200 defines adult respiratory distress syndrome (ARDS).[4] Oxygenation failure is defined by an increased A–a gradient or abnormal PF rather than peripheral oxygen saturation while ventilated without consideration of FiO_2.

Modes of Ventilation

There are two major categories of commonly used ventilators. Many modern ventilators are capable of delivering ventilation in both modes.

Volume Control (VC) ventilation is where rigidly timed mechanical breaths of set tidal volumes are delivered irrespective of the patient's effort or respiratory phase. With obstructive processes or compliance changes, the set volume is still delivered but changes in airway pressure will result unless there is a feedback cut off maximum pressure alarm which inhibits further pressure increase and prompts intervention to protect from barotrauma.

Pressure Control (PC). In PC ventilation the same rigidly timed mechanical breaths are pressure limited rather than volume limited. With changes in lung/chest wall compliance or obstructive processes the volume delivered will be affected i.e., with obstruction from secretions lower volumes will be delivered unless there is a feedback low volume alarm that will prompt intervention such as suctioning or searching for the presence of a pneumothorax which will require prompt decompression.

Based on the theoretical concept that surfactant synthesis is stimulated by fluctuation in degree of alveolar wall stretch with varying alveolar volume, 'sighs' or larger volumes are programmed to be delivered by the ventilator at set intervals in both VC and PC ventilators.

The "ASSIST" mode both for VC and PC ventilators allows the patient to trigger each breath before the set volume or pressure is delivered. The sensitivity setting on the ventilator allows the set inspiratory effort of the patient to initiate the delivery of the tidal volume. The PC and VC modes are kept in the initial settings for the patient and then later changed determined by the patient condition e.g., initially when the patient is still sedated after anesthesia and unable to spontaneously initiate a breath, the control mode is used and later switched to 'assist' as the patient becomes more alert. AC (Assist control) allows the patient to receive PC or VC breath triggered by their own inspiratory effort in addition to the set respiratory rate.

Synchronized Intermittent Mandatory Ventilation (SIMV) describes a ventilation evolution where the ventilator would allow the patient to breathe between mandatory (set) breaths in addition to mandatory inhalations that were timed with the patients own inspiratory efforts if those efforts fell within a timed "trigger" zone. This has virtually replaced the earlier intermittent mandatory ventilation mode in which the 'mandatory' breath is delivered without regard to the patient's own phase of respiration. Both assist control and synchronized IMV are preferred when possible because they allow use of the patient's respiratory efforts and thus facilitate the weaning process off the ventilator by maintaining tone and use of the respiratory muscle during ventilator support.

Like home therapy received by patients with sleep apnea, chronic lung disease or heart failure CPAP (continuous positive airway pressure) and BiPAP (Bi level Positive Airway Pressure) augment a patient's spontaneous respiratory effort by maintaining sufficient gas flow to the patient to keep airway pressure constant (CPAP) throughout the respiratory cycle, or augment airway pressure particularly during inhalation (BiPAP). Pressure support (PS) ventilation in the ICU does the same. Inhaled pressure above baseline (PEEP) triggered only by the patient's spontaneous inhalation can augment the patient's weakened respiratory muscles or compensate for decreased respiratory compliance.

Modern ventilators, even those on anaesthesia machines make use of all the above modes simultaneously, each with different proprietary names. Pressure Regulated Volume Control (PRVC) by Maquet Servo, Pressure Control Volume Guarantee (PCVG) by GE, Pressure Control Ventilation Volume Guarantee (PCVVG) by Datex Omeda and Volume Control Auto Flow (VCAF) all use software controlled ventilation to vary airway pressure during inhalation titrated to achieve desired minute ventilation. The ability to provide simultaneous pressure support in addition to the above modes is near universal in ICU ventilators.

Initial Ventilator Settings

1. Mode

Full ventilatory support is provided initially assuming all the work of breathing, with a switch to Assist Control after initial ABG measurement and clinical assessment

Initial FiO_2 is at 80–100% and adjusted after ABG in about 20 minutes.

The aim should be to use the lowest FiO_2 to achieve PaO_2 of 60–70 torr (O_2Sat of over 90%).

PEEP may be required to decrease FiO_2.

FiO_2 of 1.0 for up to 24 hours does not result in significant toxicity but caution is practised to limit the time on FiO_2 of 1.0.

It is ideal to maintain FiO_2 at below 60% to avoid oxygen toxicity and absorption atelectasis.

It is important to consider the effect of PEEP in depressing cardiac output[5] while improving PaO_2.

Optimum PEEP is the one with highest O_2 delivery (O_2 content × CO) and usually coincides with the maximum chest wall/lung compliance.[6]

2. Tidal Volume

Spontaneous Tidal volume for adults is 5–7 mL/Kg ideal body weight. For ventilated patients a range of 6–12 mL/kg for adults is used: 10–12 mL/kg in normal lungs, 8–10 mL/kg in obstructive lung disease 6–8 mL/kg in ARDS-sometimes as low as 4 mL/kg.

Ideally a plateau pressure <30 cm H_2O should be achieved with the chosen tidal volume.

3. Respiratory rate

Respiratory rate is chosen with tidal volume to achieve adequate minute ventilation which is normally 5–10 L/min.

Use ABG to adjust minute ventilation

— if $PaCO_2 > 45$, increase minute ventilation via rate and/or tidal volume.
— if $PaCO_2 < 35$, decrease minute ventilation via rate and/or tidal volume.

4. Inspiratory flow rate

Flow is normally set to deliver inspiration in about 1 sec (0.8–1.2 sec), yielding an I:E ratio of 1:2 or less (usually 1:4).

Flow is set to meet the patient's inspiratory demand.

This can be met with an initial peak flow of about 60 L/min (range of 40–80 L/min).

Other Methods of Mechanical Ventilation

1. Inverse Ratio Ventilation

This is based on the notion that sustained elevation in airway pressure may recruit collapsed alveoli more effectively than conventional ventilation with lower peak alveolar pressure and lower PEEP. These patients require sedation and/or paralysis because of the associated discomfort. There is marked gas trapping and tidal volume may decrease with increased pCO_2.

Indications and methodology for this technique is not well defined.[7]

2. Permissive Hypercapnia

This is based on the theory that high tidal volumes produce lung injury. It utilizes tidal volumes as low as 5 mL/kg allowing pCO_2 to rise above the 60's with pH in the range of 7.02–7.38 with decreased mortality.[8]

Other techniques of ventilator support reported with variable success and not used in most ICU's are not discussed in detail here. These include: (1) High frequency ventilation — where very low tidal volumes at high frequency are delivered to minimize barotrauma and maintain oxygenation while lung healing occurs in severe ARDS unresponsive to conventional ventilator modes[9]; (2) Extracorporeal membrane oxygenator (ECMO) where veno-venous connection to a membrane oxygenator allows oxygenation and elimination of carbon dioxide in anticoagulated patients with severe ARDS[10]; (3) The use of nitric oxide inhalation to maximize vaso dilation and perfusion to ventilated lung units thus improving oxygenation at lower FiO_2[11]; (4) Prone position ventilation in which the patient is ventilated for variable periods in the prone position with reported success[12]; (5) Non-invasive nasal ventilation[13]; and (6) Tracheal insufflation of Oxygen (TRIO).[8,14] As a last resort, in appropriately equipped centers, the use of lung transplant.

Monitoring the Ventilated Patient

Apart from maintaining oxygenation and ventilation, the period of ventilatory support should be viewed as a time during which the patient is being prepared for separation from the ventilator. This involves monitoring the patient for signs of initiating the weaning process. The patient's nutritional and fluid volume status, identification of and eradicating any source of sepsis which will perpetuate the elaboration of extravascular lung water on the basis of increased pulmonary capillary permeability, correcting abnormalities that require sedation or, narcotics, establishing normality of the hemodynamic status ideally without the continued need for extensive pharmacologic support of the circulatory system all require close attention.

Although the patient's initial ventilator setting may require varying degrees of control of the ventilator apparatus and even total control, the aim should be to initiate preparation for separation from the ventilator by having the patient do more and more of the respiratory work and the ventilator doing progressively less. This is accomplished by modifying ventilator settings to encourage use of the patients own respiratory apparatus through techniques such as SIMV, decreasing pressure support and PEEP as well as decreasing FiO_2.

Monitoring of the patient on the ventilator, therefore requires continuous assessment of the hemodynamic status, gas exchange and the patient's ability to generate enough muscular force to spontaneously breathe.

There is a fine line between decreasing the work of breathing and challenging the patient to generate intrinsic mechanical force to maintain breathing. The patient–ventilator interaction should not excessively increase the patient's work of breathing.[15] Synchrony between patient and ventilator should be maintained throughout all phases of the respiratory cycle-breath initiation, delivery, termination and exhalation. Ineffective triggering is a common asynchrony. Others are flow and cycling asynchrony. These can be identified and should be promptly corrected. Their identification can be based not only on assessing built-in ventilator wave forms but also examination of the patient, looking for changes in facial expression, mouth breathing, use of accessory muscles, active exhalation and contraction of the abdominal muscles.

Liberation from Mechanical Ventilation

The questions to be posed and answered in the process of liberation from the ventilator are:

1. Is the patient ready?
2. What is the optimum mode of liberation?

Is the patient ready?
The following steps should be taken before initiating the weaning process:
Patient factors

— Re-examine the patient factors that prompted the decision to institute mechanical ventilatory support.
— Has the patient's hemodynamic status, neurologic status, nutritional status and dependence on narcotics and sedation changed?
— Has a septic process been corrected?
— Is the patient's ability to generate an adequate inspiratory force improved?
— Have causes for increased work of breathing asynchrony been corrected?

Ventilator and Gas Exchange Factors

Trial at spontaneous breathing

If the patient factors have been corrected and were the prime indications for institution of mechanical ventilation, then the patient could be liberated from the ventilator very quickly by a trial of spontaneous ventilation off the respirator with supplemental humidified oxygen through a T-piece, monitoring gas exchange and clinical signs of respiratory distress. A successful spontaneous breathing trial allows extubation followed by humidified oxygen by rebreathe mask then quickly to nasal oxygen and finally room air while monitoring adequacy of oxygenation and ventilation. This is the method that is commonly applied in most acute situations in surgical patients e.g., following a surgical procedure, with no underlying respiratory disorder, adequate control of pain and no need for high dose sedation or narcoltic analgesics in respiratory depressing dosages.

The slower stepwise liberation process

The patient who fails at spontaneous breathing is a candidate for a slower process. The process is individualized and many techniques have been described and published. Our abilities to determine the need and method of weaning are surprisingly diverse.[16] Daily assessments of hemodynamically normal patients who oxygenate and ventilate adequately based on recognized parameters, and can initiate an adequate spontaneous breath as well as successfully pass a spontaneous breathing trial can be weaned over a very brief period of time.[17,18] Otherwise, intervals where the patient breathes on minimal CPAP/PS or even T-piece are gradually lengthened. An intermediary style is that of a patient ventilated with gradually reducing pressure support until able to ventilate and oxygenate adequately on CPAP alone (zero PS). An entirely software driven ventilator wean based on ventilator settings alone has also been described.

Mindful of the wide variabilty in weaning techniques, we describe broad general principles of liberation from ventilatory support in the patient who requires a slower wean rather than present detailed specific recipes for weaning these patients:

1. Consider mechanical ventilation and weaning of the patient a team effort including, physicians, respiratory therapists, nurses, physiotherapist, speech and swallowing therapist all with specific designated roles and responsibilities.
2. Consider weaning strategies and prepare for weaning at the onset of mechanical ventilation, preparing the patient for weaning through implementation of measures such as SIMV with decreasing frequency of mandatory breaths and degree of pressure support as well as providing emotional support and encouragement to the patient.
3. Make weaning plans a priority during ICU team morning rounds by preparing measured parameters to be discussed in the context of weaning and formulate a team strategy for the day.
4. Until weaning for the entire day is possible, keep the night time as a period of rest so that a well-rested patient is ready for the day's weaning strategy.
5. After determining patient factors to be acceptable for weaning use a step wise process for weaning, beginning with decreasing FiO_2 to 0.4–0.5.
6. Measure ABG and other parameters and if satisfactory, gradually decrease PEEP to less than 5 cm H_2O, while decreasing support such as the SIMV rate, implementing one change at a time and checking for the impact of each change on gas exchange and other parameters.
7. If after 3 minutes of decreasing PEEP there is a greater than 20% decrease in PaO_2, then replace the same level of PEEP.
8. Place on increasing short periods of spontaneous ventilation as tolerated aiming eventually for full spontaneous breathing.

9. Obtain input from all members of the team to formulate a team approach to the weaning efforts.
10. Follow standardized criteria for switching from endotracheal tube to tracheostomy and standardized care of the tracheotomized patient to the point of removal of the tracheostomy tube, involving the expertise of members familiar with testing of swallowing and for signs of aspiration before initiating oral feedings.

Summary

1. Large percentage of patients in the ICU require mechanical ventilatory support.
2. Most surgical ICU patients do not require prolonged mechanical ventilation.
3. Early recognition of the indications for and prompt initiation of mechanical ventilatory support are important.
4. Knowledge of the different modes of ventilation, establishing and adhering to protocols agreed upon by attending staff in collaboration with respiratory therapist, nurses, physiotherapists and careful monitoring of the ventilated patient are essential.
5. Identifying readiness for liberation from the ventilator and prompt initiation of a weaning protocol are critical for successful management of the mechanically ventilated patient.
6. The type of ventilatory assistance, the process of monitoring and method of liberation from the ventilator are quite variable but common principles based on accumulated experience in the field provide a good framework for successful management of these patients.

References

1. The Acute Respiratory Distress Syndrome Network: Ventilation with lower tidal volumes as compared with traditional tidal volumes for acute lung injury and the acute respiratory distress syndrome. *N Engl J Med* 2000; 342: 1301–1308.
2. Pingleton S. Complications of acute respiratory failure. *Am Rev Respir Dis* 1988; 137: 1463–1493.
3. Bilek A, Dee K, Gaver D. Mechanisms of surface-tension-induced epithelial cell damage in a model of pulmonary airway reopening. *J Appl Physiol* 2003; 94: 770–783.
4. Bernard G, Artigas A, Brigham K. The American-European Consensus Conference on ARDS. Definitions, mechanisms, relevant outcomes, and clinical trial coordination. *Am J Respir Crit Care Med* 1994; 149(3): 818–824.

5. Rouby JJ, Lu Q, Goldstein I. Selecting the right level of positive end expiratory pressure in patients with acute Respiratory distress Syndrome. *Am J Respir Crit Care Med* 2002; 165: 1182–1186
6. Badet M, Bayle F, Richard JC, Guerin C. Comparison of optimal end expiratory pressure and recruitment maneuvers during lung protective mechanical ventilation in patients with acute lung injury/acute respiratory distress syndrome. *Resp Care* 2009; 54(7): 847–8547.
7. Gurevitch MJ, VanDyke J, Young ES, Jackson K. Improved oxygenation and lower peak airway pressure in severe adult respiratory distress syndrome. Treatment with inverse ratio ventilation. *Chest* 1986; 89(2): 211–213.
8. Laffey JG, O'Croinin D, Mcloughlin P, Kavanagh BP. Permissive Hypercapnia-role in protective lung ventilatory strategies. *Intens Care Med* 2004; 30: 347–358.
9. Drazen JM, Kamn RD, Slutsky AS. High frequency ventilation. *Physiol Rev* 1984; 64: 505–542.
10. Brogan TV, Thiagarajan RR, Rycus PJ *et al.* Extracorporeal membrane oxygenation in adults with severe respiratory failure: A multi-centre data base. *Intens Care Med* 2009; 35: 2105–2111.
11. Rossaint R, Gerlach H, Schmidt R *et al.* Efficacy of inhaled nitric oxide in patients with severe ARDS. *Chest* 199; 107: 1107–1115.
12. Guerin C. Prone ventilation in acute respiratory distress syndrome. *Eur Respir Rev* 2014; 23: 249–257.
13. Brott J, Carroll MP, Conway JH *et al.* Randomized control trial of nasal ventilation in acute ventilatory failure due to chronic obstructive airways disease. *The Lancet* 1993; 341: 1555–1557.
14. Kuo PH, Wu HD, Yu CJ, Yang SH *et al.* Efficacy of tracheal gas insufflation in acute respiratory distress syndrome with permissive hypercapnia. *Am J Respir Crit Care Med* 1996; 158: 612–616.
15. deWit M, Monitoring of patient-ventilator interaction at the bedside. *Resp Care* 2011; 56(1): 61–72.
16. Afessa B, Hogans L, Murphy R. Predicting 3-day and 7-day outcomes of weaning from mechanical ventilation. *Chest* 1999; 116(2): 456–461.
17. MacIntyre NR, Cook DJ, Ely EW, Jr, Epstein SK, Fink JB, Heffner JE *et al.* Evidence-based guidelines for weaning and discontinuing ventilatory support: A collective task force facilitated by the American College of Chest Physicians; the American Association for Respiratory Care; and the American College of Critical Care Medicine. *Chest* 2001; 120(6 Suppl): 375S–395S.
18. Robertson T, Sona C, Schallom L, Buckles M, Cracchiolo L, Schuerer D. Improved extubation rates and earlier liberation from mechanical ventilation with implementation of a daily spontaneous- breathing trial protocol. *J Am Coll Surg* 2008; 206(3): 489–496.

Chapter 6

Nutrition in the Surgical ICU Patient

Mohammed Bawazeer and Jameel Ali

Chapter Overview

Many patients will require some form of nutrition during their stay in the intensive care unit (ICU) due to inability to eat, increased metabolic needs, and physiologic stress. In this chapter, we discuss the physiologic response to stress and starvation, assessment of the nutritional status of the patients and the energy requirements, which will determine their nutritional needs. Enteral Nutrition (EN) is the mode of choice where possible, parenteral nutrition being reserved for other patients in whom EN cannot be provided.

Physiologic Adaptation to Fasting States, Stress, and Sepsis

In the Surgical ICU, patients are usually kept nil per OS for a variable duration. For brief period of 2–3 days, nutritional supplements are not a major issue but patients in the ICU for prolonged periods require nutrition support. Restoration of glucose levels for organs dependent on glucose as a fuel (brain, erythrocytes, and kidney) occurs initially by hepatic glycogenolysis which is short lived. As levels of insulin fall and glucagon rises, lipolysis in adipose tissue and proteolysis in skeletal muscle stimulate gluconeogenesis in the liver. At the same time, peripheral tissues switch to utilization of fatty acids and ketones to produce Acute Thrombocytopenic Purpura (ATP).

After about one week of continuous fasting, the brain adapts to use ketones for 50% of its fuel needs. Gluconeogenesis and muscle breakdown then slow down dramatically.[1]

During physiologic stress (e.g., Trauma, Burn, sepsis), catecholamines, glucagon, cortisol, and cytokines (IL-1, IL-6, TNF-α, and Interferon-γ) are released, causing major physiologic changes. In skeletal muscle, protein breakdown continues with decreased protein synthesis. As a result, amino acid pools become depleted. Similar changes occur in intestinal mucosa with glutamine becoming an essential amino acidare. Amino acids are delivered to areas where protein synthesis continues (Lungs, heart, spleen, and liver). In the Liver, alanine is utilized in gluconeogenesis and synthesis of acute phase reactant proteins. This gluconeogenesis is not reversible by hyperglycemia or administration of glucose. A state of insulin resistance results in hyperglycemia. Lipolysis also occurs in this highly catabolic phase. These factors should be considered when assessing the nutritional needs.[1,2]

Nutrition Assessment

Determination of the nutritional status as well as the energy expenditure are important in planning nutritional support. The most commonly used formula for nutritional requirements is weight based and estimates the caloric requirement at 25–35 Kcal/Kg/day.[2] Harris–Benedict Equations are also used as follows:

Male: Basal Energy Expenditure (BEE)
$$= 66.5 + (13.8 \times \text{weight in kg}) + (5 \times \text{height in cm}) - (6.8 \times \text{age})$$

Female: Basal Energy Expenditure (BEE)
$$= 66.5 + (9.6 \times \text{weight in kg}) + (1.7 \times \text{height in cm}) - (4.7 \times \text{age})$$

BEE is then multiplied by activity factors or stress factors.[2]

Indirect Calorimetry measures oxygen consumption and Carbon dioxide production and provides values on measured energy expenditure using the Respiratory Quotient (RQ), which is the ratio of O_2 consumption to CO_2 production. RQ between 0.9–1 indicates Carbohydrates, 0.8–0.9 indicates proteins, 0.7–0.8 indicates fat as the main fuel. Values >1.1 suggest overfeeding, and values <0.7 suggests ketogenesis.[1,2] One pilot randomized trial comparing feeding targeted by indirect calorimetry to the weight-based formula showed a trend toward improved survival with indirect calorimetry.[3] However, achieving a target dose of enteral nutrition, by starting at a target dose, accepting higher threshold of gastric residual volumes, use of prokinetic agents and small bowel feeding, collectively as a bundle may change patient outcome.[4]

Intentional trophic feeding which involves fixed small volumes feeding such as 10ml/hour for the first six days has been studied in two randomized trials in patients with acute lung injury. Trophic feeding did not improve ventilator-free days or 60-day mortality but had fewer episodes of gastrointestinal intolerance.[5,6] Hypocaloric intake has been compared to full caloric intake in one randomized trial, and there was a trend toward improvement in survival. A larger trial (Permit Trial) is ongoing and may answer this clinical question.[7]

Recently, a conceptual model has been described (see Fig. 1) involving several factors affecting the nutritional status of the critically ill. Using these factors, a novel score has been described and validated. The score is described

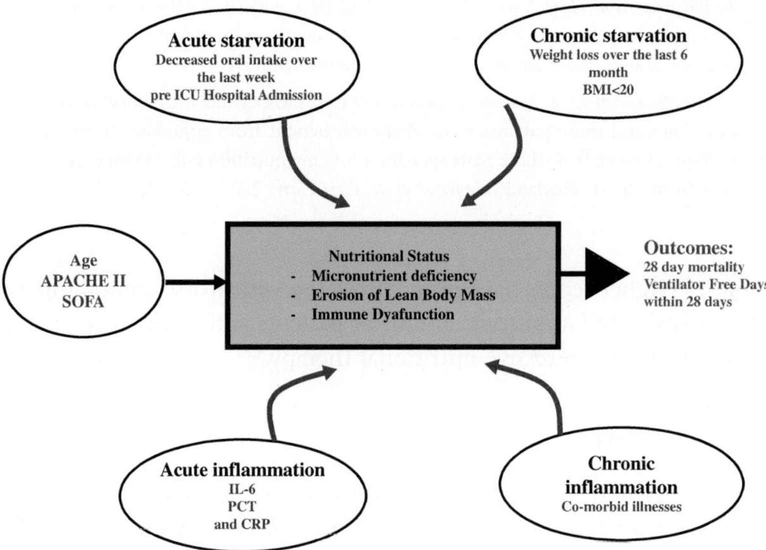

Fig. 1. A conceptual model for nutrition risk assessment in the critically ill.

APACHE, Acute physiology and chronic health evaluation score, BMI, body mass index, CRP, C-reactive protein, IL-6, interleukin 6, PCT, procalcitonin, SOFA, sequential organ failure assessment score. (With permission from Dr. D. Heyland, Heyland *et al. Crit Care* 2011; 15(6)).[8]

Table 1. NUTRIC score.

Variable	Range	Points
Age	<50	0
	50–<75	1
	≥75	2
APACHE II	<15	0
	15–<20	1
	20–28	2
	≥28	3
SOFA	<6	0
	6–<10	1
	≥10	2
Number of co-morbidities	0–1	0
	≥2	1
Days from hospital to ICU admission	0–<1	0
	≥1	1
IL-6	0–<400	0
	≥400	1

In the presence of IL-6: A score between 6 and 10 is associated with worse clinical outcomes and these patients most likely will benefit from aggressive nutrition. A score of 0–5, these patients have a low malnutrition risk.

In the absence of IL-6: A score between 5 and 9 is associated with worse clinical outcomes and these patients most likely will benefit from aggressive nutrition therapy. A score 0–4, these patients have a low malnutrition risk. (With permission from Dr. D. Heyland, Heyland *et al. Crit Care.* 2011; 15(6)).

in Table 1. Higher scores have been correlated with worse clinical outcomes (mortality and ventilation days) and these patients with such scores will most likely benefit from aggressive nutritional therapy.[4,8]

General Principles

Generally, every effort should be made to use the gut and institute enteral nutrition (EN) rather than parenteral (PN). There is strong evidence that EN is associated with significant reduction of infectious complications and is more cost effective.[4] However, there was no difference in mortality or in hospital length of stay. EN feeding should be started early within 24–48 hours following ICU admission. Early EN is associated with lower mortality and lower infectious complications. Although there is no difference in length of stay nutritional goals are better achieved with early EN.[4]

Many patients in the surgical ICU are hemodynamically compromised and some may require vasopressors. Institution of early EN in these patients is controversial. During hypotension blood will be shunted from the gut to more vital organs (heart and brain). Vasopressors increase the blood pressure but increase risk of gut ischemia due to vasconstriction. After volume resuscitation, blood flow to the gut will not be restored immediately because of concomitant increase in endogenous vasoconstrictors (endothelin I, angiotensin II, and vasopressin) and decrease in endogenous vasodilators (nitric oxide). However, EN will increase blood flow to the gut. Two studies in cardiac surgery patients showed that EN is feasible, safe and not associated with major complications. In severely burned patients, early feeding within 48 hours did not increase CO_2 gap and it was well tolerated. A retrospective study in septic patients showed early EN had some delayed gastric emptying. In a large observational study in patients on vasopressors and mechanical ventilation, early EN was associated with lower hospital mortality. This study suffers from selection bias where patients with poor ICU status received delayed nutrition. These studies suggest that early EN is feasible and may not be associated with serious complications but a large randomized trial is warranted.[9]

Enteral Nutrition

A. Routes of Administrations

In the short term, nasoenterirc tubes (gastric, duodenal, or jejunal) may be used for EN. The large tubes (16 or 18-F) that come with the patient from the operating room may be used for feeding as well. They allow measurement of gastric residuals and do not clog easily. They can be uncomfortable and theoretically increase reflux. The small caliber tubes (e.g., stylet-type) allow advancement into the duodenum or jejunum (under fluoroscopic- or endoscopic-guidance) and can be used for feeding in patients with poor gastric emptying (high gastric residuals or with gastroparesis). Usually tubes placed in the small bowel require continuous feeding and those placed in the stomach allow bolus feeding. Complications include malposition in the bronchus with potential feeding into the lung. A chest X-Ray (CXR) showing the tube below the diaphragm is therefore mandatory before institution of EN. Sinusitis due to nasally placed tube can be a cause of fever in the critically ill. Other complications include tube migration, esophageal and gastric mucosal erosions, pulmonary aspiration, pneumothorax, esophageal stricture, esophageal perforation, and fatal dysrrhythmias.[1,10]

For the long-term, gastrostomy or jejunostomy tubes should be used. Gastrostomy tubes can be inserted via a small laparotomy incision (the Stamm Gastrostomy), endoscopically (so-called Percutaneuos Endoscopic Gastrostomy (PEG) tube) or percutaneuosly by interventional radiology. PEG tubes are less expensive with lower complications than conventional Stamm Gastrostomy. In patients with previous upper abdominal surgery, the blind percutaneuos technique is contraindicated because of possible adhesions and inadvertent insertion into the colon. In experienced hands, laparoscopic-assisted PEG tube insertion is a good option, during which the laparoscope guides insertion of the needle into the stomach.[11] Another option is open Stamm Gastrostomy via a left upper quadrant incision.[1,10]

Jejunostomy tube may be inserted surgically via open or laparoscopic techniques. It may also be inserted endoscopically by extension of the existing gastrostomy (called G-J tube) or percutaneuosly by interventional radiology. The G-J tube has a double lumen with an advantage of decompression of the stomach during small bowel feeding. The J tube is often required in patients who are not tolerant of gastric feeding (e.g., Gastroparesis). In the critically ill patient, hypo-osmolar or iso-osmolar feeding should be used in a continuous fashion rather than bolus feeding. Small bowel does not tolerate bolus feeding and hyper-osmolar feeding is associated with pneumatosis and necrosis.[1,10]

Multiple trials compared gastric and small bowel feeding and consistently showed that small bowel feeding is associated with a reduction in pneumonias. Therefore, small bowel feeding should be routinely used especially in patient not tolerating gastric feeding (e.g., on vasopressors, high doses of sedatives or paralytic agents, and high gastric output) or patients at high risk of regurgitation and aspiration (e.g., nursed in supine position).[4]

One small trial compared early PEG tube insertion to nasogastric feeding in patients with stroke and head injury. This trial included only 41 patients and showed lower incidence of ventilator-associated pneumonia with early PEG tube insertion.[12] Because of lack of strong evidence at this time, this approach is not recommended.

EN can be administered in the critically ill either continuously or intermittently. Continuous administration is usually started at a low rate of 20 cc/hr and increased by 20 cc increments every 8–12 hours until the goal rate is achieved. Intermittent administration (or bolus feeding) is given by 100–125 cc bolus by gravity over 15 minutes every 4–8 hours and increased by increments of 100–125 cc every 8–12 hours. Multiple trials compared the two techniques and showed no difference in mortality, infections, length of stay, frequency of interrupted feeds, percent of goal feeds achieved, or diarrhea.[4]

B. Practical Issues

- *Protein versus peptides*

Peptide-based formula has been compared with whole-protein formula in several randomized trials. The hypothesis is that introduction of simple peptides are better absorbed in the critically ill and produce less diarrhea. These studies demonstrated no difference in mortality, infection rate and length of stay with varying effects on diarrhea. Despite the higher cost of peptide-based formula, however, certain groups of patients (e.g., short-bowel syndrome and pancreatitis) may benefit from them.[4]

- *Feeding protocols*

The use of prokinetics is usually reserved for patients who are intolerant of gastric feeding with high gastric residuals. Concomitant prokinetics use with small bowel feeding have shown a trend toward a reduction in hospital mortality and reduction of hospital length of stay but not the ICU length of stay.[13,14] The use of early prokinetics with high gastric residuals has shown a reduction of gastric aspiration and less time to achieve nutritional goals from admission to ICU.[15]

Feeding practices vary widely amongst ICUs. A novel way of feeding patients was recently published based on a proactive strategy. The protocol is based on six elements:

1. Starting at a high-volume rate and giving a certain volume that should be administered over 24 hour period rather than an hourly rate, so-called "volume-based feeding".
2. The use of trophic-feeding (low volume) of concentrated formula for patients who are intolerant of high volume rate.
3. The use of semi-elemental feeding solution to maximize absorption, tolerance and assimilation.
4. Protein supplementation is started early at initiation of EN to prevent negative nitrogen balance.
5. Start metochlopramide early at initiation of EN.
6. Accept higher gastric residuals (between 250–500 mL). If the patient continued to have high residuals, the rate can be decreased by 25 mL/hour and erythromycin is added.

The intervention group in this study received significantly larger amounts of prescribed calories and proteins. There was no difference in the clinical outcomes in terms of mortality and length of stay. The protocol was deemed to be safe and feasible because there was no difference in the complications rate between the groups (vomiting, macro-aspiration, regurgitation, and ICU-acquired pneumonia).[16]

- *Body position*

Semirecumbent position has been compared to supine position in two randomized trials. In one study, body position was an independent risk factor for Ventilator-associated Pneumonia (VAP) and head-of-bed elevation to at least 30° significantly reduced the incidence of VAP.[17] In another study, 45° elevation was compared to standard position. Head-of-bed elevation was never achieved in the majority of patients probably because of feasibility issues. There was no difference in the incidence of pneumonia in this study.[18] Based on these data, all critically ill patients should be fed in the head elevated position, unless contraindicated, to decrease the incidence of VAP.[4] The most common contraindications for head-of-bed elevationare: c-spine instability, hemodynamic compromise, Pelvic fractures, prone positioning, intra-aortic balloon pump and technical issues like obesity.

- *Gastric residuals, checking, threshold, and refeeding*

The issue of checking Gastric Residual Volumes (GRV) is controversial. One study compared checking versus not checking and showed no difference in outcome. Patients without checking for GRV had higher caloric intake but slightly higher vomiting episodes.[19]

The threshold of GRV (500 mL versus 250 mL) was compared in another study. Higher GRV did not worsen outcome or rate of gastrointestinal complication but showed better caloric delivery.[20]

The other controversial issue is refeeding versus discarding GRV. A small RCT showed that refeeding GRV up to a maximum of 250 mLs is safe and not associated with increased gastrointestinal complications.[21]

Composition in Different Disease States

Patients with renal failure generally need low-protein and electrolyte-restricted but high-caloric formula. Patients on dialysis need higher protein requirements which may reach up to 1–1.4 g/kg/day and patients on continuous venovenous hemofiltration up to 1.5–2.5 g/kg/day.[10]

In patients with hepatic failure, there is a decrease in branched-chain amino acids and increase in aromatic amino acids. Formulas provided should have high branched-chain and low aromatic amino acids to prevent encephalopathy.[10]

The aim for patients with Respiratory failure and specifically patients with Acute Respiratory Distress Syndrome (ARDS) is to decrease carbon dioxide production. Generally they should get an enteral formula that is low in carbohydrate and high in fat, containing Omega-3 fatty acids.[10]

Patients with Traumatic Brain injury are usually hypercatabolic. Hyperglycemia, which may complicate ischemic brain injury, should be avoided. Patients with severe burns are severely hypercatabolic and have profound immunosuppression. EN should aim to improve the immune status by using formulas containing Arginine, Omega-3 fatty acids and vitamins E and C. These showed reductions of infectious complications and improved graft survival.[10]

The goal in patients with pancreatitis is to provide EN with minimal exocrine pancreas stimulation. This can be achieved with post-pyloric feeding tubes with the use of elemental EN formulas.[10]

A. Composition of EN

• *Glutamine*

Glutamine is not an essential amino acid, but becomes conditionally essential during trauma and critical illness because its intracellular levels fall. It has been proposed that Glutamine supplementation in enteral nutrition may enhance the immune function of the enterocytes.[1] This clinical question has been addressed in several studies. Overall, there was a significant reduction of hospital length of stay with enteral glutamine in burn and trauma patients. There was no statistically significant reduction in mortality and infectious complication. Enteral glutamine should be considered in burn and trauma patients but not in other critically ill.[4]

• *Fish oils, Borage oils and Antioxidants*

It has been suggested that supplementation with fish oils (Omega-3 fatty acids), Borage oils (γ-Linolenic acid) and antioxidants produce less active metabolites and potentially anti-inflammatory cytokines in patients with acute lung injury but the studies show conflicting results. Supplementation with fish oil, borage oil and antioxidant did not improve mortality or infectious complications but there was reduction in the number of ventilator-free days. With ARDS, continuous supplementation when compared to the standard/high fat formula, there was a significant reduction in mortality, ICU length of stay and duration of mechanical ventilation and should be considered in this patient population.[4]

Fish oil supplementation alone as bolus has also been studied in patients with ARDS. There was no reduction in mortality or infectious complications. There was a trend toward a reduction of the duration of mechanical ventilation.

• *Arginine*

This is a semi-essential amino acid. In sepsis, its levels drop dramatically. It has some immune modulating functions. However, beneficial effects have not been demonstrated in the co-critically ill. Therefore, it cannot be recommended for use in such patients.[4]

• *Probiotics*

The use of probiotics with EN has been evaluated. Several studies used different methodology and different probiotics. The studies showed there was a reduction of the overall infections and a trend toward reduction of VAP. But there was no difference in other important clinical outcomes.[4]

B. Complications with enteral nutrition

Complications related to enteral nutrition can be categorized into tube-related and non-tube-related. Tube-related conditions have already been described. Non-tube-related diarrhea can be caused by acquired lactase-deficiency, which is self-limited and resolves within a few days. Diarrhea can occur also because of lack of absorption of fat, which is dependent on bile and pancreatic enzymes. Surgical procedures that alter their mixing (e.g., Billroth II) may cause fat malabsoprtion. Administration of hyperosmolar enteral formula may also cause diarrhea, dehydration, electrolyte imbalance, and hyperglycemia. Aggressive administration of Hyperosmolar enteral formula through jejunostomy feeding tubes may lead to pneumatosisintestinalis, bowel necrosis, perforation, and potentially death.[1]

Refeeding syndrome is a common condition in critically ill rather than a complication. It is usually manifested by respiratory muscle weakness and hypophosphatemia. Phosphate is primarily intracellular, and with institution of nutrition, the intracellular compartment expands and phosphate steal occurs from the extracellular compartment. Therefore, frequent monitoring and early replacement of depleted electrolytes are very important.[1,10]

Parenteral Nutrition

A. Routes of Administration

Parenteral Nutrition (PN) in the ICU is usually administered when EN is not tolerated or cannot be used as a primary source of nutrition. If the surgical patient cannot be or expected not to be offered EN for period of at least 10 days, PN should be considered. Total Parenteral Nutrition (TPN) is then administered as highly osmolar formula and should be given through a central catheter with the tip in the superior vena cava (central TPN). Less concentrated formula (that do not exceed 5% dextrose) can be given peripherally (peripheral TPN) but this can only be administered for a short period between 5–7 days. It is usually difficult to achieve the daily caloric requirement with peripheral TPN alone. With the addition of lipids (250–500 ml of 20% fat emulsion daily), daily caloric requirement may be achieved. The use of peripherally inserted central lines (PICC) is also an option for administering TPN. PICC lines can be used for 4–6 weeks if they are not infected or thrombosed.[1]

B. Parenteral versus Standard care

EN is always considered the first line of artificial nutrition. In patients with intact GI tract, PN should never be considered ahead of EN. When compared to standard care (IV fluids and oral diet), PN is associated with more infectious complications. In patients who are clearly well nourished, standard therapy should be used and TPN is deferred because of the risks associated with it.[4]

C. Composition of TPN solution

- *Formulation of the TPN solution*

The following is a practical way to formulate the composition of the TPN solution using a 70 kg patient as an example:

1. Determine the caloric requirements: for the above mentioned example, the most commonly used formula is 25–35 kcal/kg/day (= 2100 kcal/day). Take into account when administering propofol as a sedative, it provides 1.1 kcal/ml.
2. Determine the caloric contents of each element: Glucose provides 3.4 kcal/g, amino acids 4 kcal/g and fat 9 kcal/g.

   If using the 3-1 solution, fat usually constitutes 20% of the total calories.

   $(2100 \times 0.2 = 420$ kcal from fat).

   420 kcal $\div$ 9 kcal/g $= 47$ g of lipids.

For amino acids, the usual daily requirements 1.5 g/kg/day

$$(1.5\ \text{g/kg} \times 70\,\text{kg} = 105\ \text{g/day}).$$

Calories from amino acids,

$$105\ \text{g} \times 4\ \text{kcal/g} = 420\ \text{kcal}.$$

Calories from dextrose, is the difference after subtracting calories from lipids and amino acids

$$(2100 - 420 - 420 = 1260\ \text{kcal}),$$

$$1260\ \text{kcal} \div 3.4\ \text{kcal/g} = 370\ \text{g of dextrose}.$$

3. Make up the final solution
   Dextrose 70% solution, (370 g = 528 mL),
   Amino acids 10% solution, (105 g = 1050 mL),
   Fat 20% solution, (47 g = 238 mL),
   Total solution = 1813 mL/day.
4. Other additives
   Electrolytes:
   Sodium: 80 mmol/day as sodium chloride.
   Potassium: Between 40–60 mmol/L of TPN/day (either as K chloride or K phosphate).
   Magnesium: 10 mmol/day as Magnesium sulfate.
   Phosphate: Usually dependent on the carbohydrate load. If high risk of refeeding syndrome, start with 15 mmol/day as potassium phosphate.
   Acetate: Consider if the patient is acidotic or hyperchloremic.
   Multivitamins mixture: (Total 10 mL).

Ascorbic acid 100 mg	Thamine 3 mg	Niacinamide 40 mg	Biotin 60 mcg
Vitamin A 3300 IU	Riboflavin 3.6 mg	d-pantothenol 15mg	Folic acid 400 mcg
Vitamin D 200 IU	Pyridoxine 4 mg	Vitamin E 10 IU	Vitamin B12 5 mcg

• ***The Use of Branched Chain Amino Acids (BCAA)***

The use of BCAA has been studied in patients receiving PN and whether that improves outcome is controversial. A higher amount of BCAA was compared to standard amount. There was a trend toward improvement of mortality especially in septic patients, but it did not reach statistical significance. There was no difference in other clinical outcomes.[4]

- *Type of Lipids*

The use of lipids with the initial PN is controversial. If lipids were to be used, the type of lipids is also controversial. Overall, strategies used to decrease omega 6 fatty acids or Long Chain Triglycerides (LCT, also known as Soybean oil sparing strategy) are associated with decrease in mortality, ICU length of stay and duration of mechanical ventilation.

When combined LCT plus Medium Chain Triglycerides (MCT) compared to LCT alone, there was a significant improvement in nutritional parameters (nitrogen balance and prealbumin) in the combined group but there was no difference in clinical outcomes.

Fish oil emulsions were compared to LCT or combined LCT + MCT. Their use was a trend toward reduction of duration of mechanical ventilation but other clinical parameters were not different. In one study, there was a reduction for the need of surgery due to a subsequent septic episode.

Olive oil containing emulsions were compared to LCT + MCT. There was a significant reduction of duration of mechanical ventilation with the use of olive oils but a trend toward increased infections. There was no difference in mortality, length of stay or ICU length of stay.

- *Zinc*

Zinc is an important trace metal of the human body. It has several functions including being a cofactor for ribonucleic acid (RNA) polymerase and deoxyribonucleic acid (DNA) polymerase. Its levels can be severely depleted in patients with diarrhea or short bowel syndrome and serum levels do not reflect its deficiency.[1]

Multiple studies investigated PN enriched with IV Zinc. One study compared higher to lower Zinc supplementation and other studies compared IV Zinc along with other antioxidants (Selenim, α tocopherol, and copper) to placebo. Data from these studies show a trend toward reduction in mortality but with a wide confidence interval and non-significant p value. Given its low cost, safety and feasibility, patients with GI losses or short bowel syndrome may benefit from Zinc supplementation.[4]

- *Glutamine Supplementation*

PN supplemented with IV Glutamine has been studied in several randomized trials. Although there was a reduction of hospital mortality and both ICU and hospital length of stay, its high cost and lack of availability limits its use.[4]

• *Combined PN and EN Glutamine Supplementation*

REDOX trial used a unique methodology comparing high doses of parenteral and enteral Glutamine supplementation in critically ill patients with two or more organ failure. There was an increase in hospital, 28-day, 3-month and 6 month mortality. There was a trend toward increase in ICU length of stay and duration of mechanical ventilation. Therefore, high dose IV and enteral Glutamine is not recommended.[22]

• *Antioxidants supplementations: combined vitamins and trace elements*

Various types of antioxidants have been studied in critically ill patients, eitheralone (Zinc and Selenium) or in combinations (selenium, copper, zinc, vitamins A, C, E, and N-acetylcystiene). A meta-analysis of these studies, showed that supplementation in various forms (parenterally, enterally, or in combination) reduce overall mortality in critically ill. There was also a significant reduction of the overall infectious complications, while there was no effect on ICU or total hospital length of stay.[23]

D. Practical issues

• *Dose of PN*

There are significant numbers of patients in critical care settings who are enterally fed but they are not getting adequate nutrition for various reasons. In those, a low dose TPN (either by removing lipids or reducing the carbohydrate dose) may be considered for the short term (usually less than 10 days). Studies on this subject showed that low-dose PN is feasible and not harmful. While there was no effect on mortality there was a reduction in infections. Patients who require longer-term PN (more than 10 days), were obese or malnourished were excluded.[4]

• *The Use of Lipids*

As mentioned in a previous section, the use of lipids in controversial. As mentioned, patients who require short term PN (less than 10 days) and are getting inadequate EN, withholding PN high in soybean oil should be considered. This has been shown to decrease the infection rates. The evidence in patients requiring longer-term PN or malnourished is lacking.[4]

• *Mode of Lipid Delivery*

Lipids may be administered separately in a piggyback or mixed with PN solution, which is called Total Nutrient Admixture (TNA). Only one study compared infectious complications between the two modes and showed no difference.[4]

• *Optimal Glucose (insulin therapy)*
Most critically ill patients on PN will require some form of insulin therapies to manage the carbohydrate load delivered. The target blood sugar has been a subject of debate. Intensive insulin therapy to target blood sugar between 4–6 mmol/L or 4–8 mmol/L was compared to the conventional blood sugar between 9–12 mmol/L. Intensive insulin therapy has been associated with a trend toward reduction of mortality and reduction of the ICU length of stay and duration of mechanical ventilation. There was no effect on infections or the hospital length of stay. However, this was associated with significant episodes of hypoglycemia. From this, it is concluded that hyperglycemia (>10 mmol/L) should be avoided in all critically ill patients. As well, probably the safest blood sugar target should be between 7–9 mmol/L.[4]

E. Role of supplemental TPN

Supplemental PN and EN have been compared. Several trials compared combined PN and EN to EN alone either with the same amount of calories or higher calories in the combined group. Analysis of these trials showed no effect on mortality or infectious complications. However, the combined nutrition group had lower hospital length of stay and a trend toward reduction of ICU length of stay. Because of the lack of clear benefit and potential harmful effects of PN, it is probably better to maximize efforts to improve EN tolerability (e.g., the use of small bowel feeding tube and promotility agents). The use of supplemental PN should be reserved for patients not tolerating EN after all efforts have been exhausted.[4]

Early supplemental PN (within three days) together with high IV glucose has been compared to delayed supplemental PN (by day 8) in a large multicenter trial. While there was no difference in mortality, there was a significant increase in infections, longer ICU and hospital length of stay and longer duration of mechanical ventilation. Therefore, early TPN supplementation and high IV glucose should not be used. Delayed supplementation may be used if adequate nutrition cannot be provided by EN alone as mentioned previously.[24]

F. Monitoring During TPN

For the critically ill in whom TPN is planned, baseline (pre-TPN) laboratory investigations are required initially, then twice weekly thereafter. This includes Liver Function tests (LFTs), Total Bilirubin, Total Triglyceride and Cholesterol. This also includes the investigations that are usually done as part of the ICU routine; Complete Blood Count (CBC), Electrolytes, Ca, Mg, and Po4. Blood glucose is usually monitored as per the monogram or every 6 hours if they are diabetic or blood glucose >10 mmol · L. Daily evaluation of the fluid status is also essential. Patients with alcoholic liver disease may require LFTs and Bilirubin more often than twice weekly. Once patients reach a steady state and pass the critical illness phase, the frequency of checking LFTs, Bilirubin, and Lipids may be decreased to once weekly. The frequency of the routine serum lectrolytes maybe decreased even more to three times weekly once the patients receive the appropriate TPN composition and does not require any more adjustments.[25,26]

Micronutrients and trace elements are not routinely checked initially since the results are not available for several days usually and are very costly. However, patients who present to the ICU with significant malnutrition pre-TPN, serum Vitamin B12, Folate and serum Zinc is useful and are often measured. Patients with significant GI losses are at risk of Zinc deficiency and its measurement prior to starting TPN is helpful. The physician and the clinical dietician should keep a high index of suspicion for micronutrient deficiencies and excess which can be of concern in patients on home TPN and present with critical illness.[25,26]

References

1. Sabiston DC, Townsend CM. Sabiston textbook of surgery: The biological basis of modern surgical practice. 18th ed. Philadelphia, PA: Saunders/Elsevier, 2008, 143–190.
2. Asensio JA, Trunkey DD. Current therapy of trauma and surgical critical care. 2008. Philadelphia, PA: Mosby/ELSVIER; 2008 Preoperative and Postoperative Nutritional Support: Strategies For Enteral and Parenteral Therapies, 710–717.
3. Singer P, Anbar R, Cohen J, Shapiro H, Shalita-Chesner M, Lev S *et al.* The tight calorie control study (TICACOS): A prospective, randomized, controlled pilot study of nutritional support in critically ill patients. *Intensive Care Med* 2011 April; 37(4): 601–609.
4. Dhaliwal R, Cahill N, Lemieux M, Heyland DK. The Canadian Critical Care Nutrition Guidelines in 2013: an update on current recommendation and implementation strategies. *Nutr Clin Pract.* 2014 Feb;29(1):29–43. 2013; Available at criticalcarenutrition.com.
5. Rice TW, Mogan S, Hays MA, Bernard GR, Jensen GL, Wheeler AP. Randomized trial of initial trophic versus full-energy enteral nutrition in mechanically ventilated patients with acute respiratory failure. *Crit Care Med* 2011 May; 39(5): 967–974.

6. National Heart, Lung, and Blood Institute Acute Respiratory Distress Syndrome (ARDS) Clinical Trials Network, Rice TW, Wheeler AP, Thompson BT, Steingrub J, Hite RD *et al.* Initial trophic versus full enteral feeding in patients with acute lung injury: The EDEN randomized trial. *JAMA* 2012 Feb 22; 307(8): 795–803.
7. Arabi YM, Tamim HM, Dhar GS, Al-Dawood A, Al-Sultan M, Sakkijha MH *et al.* Permissive underfeeding and intensive insulin therapy in critically ill patients: A randomized controlled trial. *Am J ClinNutr* 2011 March; 93(3): 569–577.
8. Heyland DK, Dhaliwal R, Jiang X, Day AG. Identifying critically ill patients who benefit the most from nutrition therapy: The development and initial validation of a novel risk assessment tool. *Crit Care* 2011; 15(6): R268.
9. Yang S, Wu X, Yu W, Li J. Early enteral nutrition in critically ill patients with hemodynamic instability: An evidence-based review and practical advice. *Nutr Clin Pract* 2014 Feb; 29(1): 90–96.
10. Cameron JL. Current surgical therapy. 10th ed. Philadelphia, Mosby Elsevier, 2010.
11. Lopes G, Salcone M, Neff M. Laparoscopic-assisted percutaneous endoscopic gastrostomy tube placement. *JSLS* 2010 Jan–Mar; 14(1): 66–69.
12. Kostadima E, Kaditis AG, Alexopoulos EI, Zakynthinos E, Sfyras D. Early gastrostomy reduces the rate of ventilator-associated pneumonia in stroke or head injury patients. *Eur Respir J* 2005 Jul; 26(1): 106–111.
13. Martin CM, Doig GS, Heyland DK, Morrison T, Sibbald WJ, Southwestern Ontario Critical Care Research Network. Multicentre, cluster-randomized clinical trial of algorithms for critical-care enteral and parenteral therapy (ACCEPT). *CMAJ* 2004 Jan 20; 170(2): 197–204.
14. Doig GS, Simpson F, Finfer S, Delaney A, Davies AR, Mitchell I *et al.* Effect of evidence-based feeding guidelines on mortality of critically ill adults: A cluster randomized controlled trial. *JAMA* 2008 Dec 17; 300(23): 2731–2741.
15. Pinilla JC, Samphire J, Arnold C, Liu L, Thiessen B. Comparison of gastrointestinal tolerance to two enteral feeding protocols in critically ill patients: A prospective, randomized controlled trial. *JPEN* 2001 Mar–Apr; 25(2): 81–86.
16. Heyland DK, Murch L, Cahill N, McCall M, Muscedere J, Stelfox HT *et al.* Enhanced protein-energy provision via the enteral route feeding protocol in critically ill patients: Results of a cluster randomized trial. *Crit Care Med* 2013 Dec; 41(12): 2743–2753.
17. Drakulovic MB, Torres A, Bauer TT, Nicolas JM, Nogue S, Ferrer M. Supine body position as a risk factor for nosocomial pneumonia in mechanically ventilated patients: A randomised trial. *Lancet* 1999 Nov 27; 354(9193): 1851–1858.
18. van Nieuwenhoven CA, Vandenbroucke-Grauls C, van Tiel FH, Joore HC, van Schijndel RJ, van der Tweel I *et al.* Feasibility and effects of the semirecumbent position to prevent ventilator-associated pneumonia: A randomized study. *Crit Care Med* 2006 Feb; 34(2): 396–402.

19. Reignier J, Mercier E, Le Gouge A, Boulain T, Desachy A, Bellec F *et al.* Effect of not monitoring residual gastric volume on risk of ventilator-associated pneumonia in adults receiving mechanical ventilation and early enteral feeding: A randomized controlled trial. *JAMA* 2013 Jan 16; 309(3): 249–256.
20. Montejo JC, Minambres E, Bordeje L, Mesejo A, Acosta J, Heras A *et al.* Gastric residual volume during enteral nutrition in ICU patients: The REGANE study. Intensive Care Medicine 2010 Aug; 36(8): 1386–1393.
21. Juve-Udina ME, Valls-Miro C, Carreno-Granero A, Martinez-Estalella G, Monterde-Prat D, Domingo-Felici CM *et al.* To return or to discard? Randomised trial on gastric residual volume management. *Intensive Crit Care Nurs* 2009 Oct; 25(5): 258–267.
22. Heyland D, Muscedere J, Wischmeyer PE, Cook D, Jones G, Albert M *et al.* A randomized trial of glutamine and antioxidants in critically ill patients. *N Engl J Med* 2013 Apr 18; 368(16): 1489–1497.
23. Manzanares W, Dhaliwal R, Jiang X, Murch L, Heyland DK. Antioxidant micronutrients in the critically ill: A systematic review and meta-analysis. *Crit Care* 2012 Dec 12; 16(2): R66.
24. Casaer MP, Mesotten D, Hermans G, Wouters PJ, Schetz M, Meyfroidt G *et al.* Early versus late parenteral nutrition in critically ill adults. *N Engl J Med* 2011 Aug 11; 365(6): 506–517.
25. Canada T. *ASPEN Parenteral Nutrition Handbook*, New York, NY, ASPEN Publishers, 2009.
26. Mahan LK, Escott-Stump S, *Krause's Food, Nutrition, and Diet Therapy*, St Loius, MS. Saunders, 2004.

Chapter 7

Management of the Anticoagulated Injured Patient

K. Pavenski

Chapter Overview

With the aging population, the likelihood of injured patients being admitted to hospital including the (intensive care unit) ICU, while on anticoagulant therapy is ever increasing, posing significant therapeutic challenges. The indications for anticoagulant and/or antiplatelet drugs include atrial fibrillation, venous thromboembolism, and cardiovascular diseases including intravascular or cardiac prostheses. These challenges are compounded by the recent addition of new oral anticoagulants, which cannot be easily reversed in the bleeding patient.

The patient's healthcare team needs to be aware of these agents and to recognize the need for a timely consultation with a coagulation or transfusion medicine specialist.

In this chapter, the epidemiology, significance, classification, and differentiating features of these anticoagulant and antiplatelet agents are described as well as general principles of managing the bleeding injured patient who is on such therapy.

Epidemiology and Significance

The exact proportion of injured patients on anticoagulants and/or antiplatelet medications is not known. Retrospective studies have shown that about

4% of trauma patients were on warfarin,[1] while up to 13% were on warfarin, aspirin, clopidogrel, or various combinations of these drugs.[2] The proportion of anticoagulated patients approached 40% in the group of older patients with hemorrhagic brain injury.[3]

Pre-injury warfarin is associated with increased mortality in trauma patients,[2] especially those aged 65 years or older[1] or those with traumatic brain injury.[4] Antiplatelet agents do not seem to confer a higher risk of mortality,[2] while the data on new oral anticoagulants are largely lacking.

General Principles of Managing a Bleeding Patient on Anticoagulant and Antiplatelet Agents

The first step in the management of an injured anticoagulated patient is to obtain a basic past medical history. Use of anticoagulant or antiplatelet medication should be suspected in older patients with a history of atrial fibrillation, cardiovascular disease, valve surgery, or thromboembolism. Information on what co-morbidities the patient has and how these may affect the metabolism of these medications or the bleeding risk should be sought. Patients with chronic liver disease may have an underlying coagulopathy, while patients with renal disease may have impaired clearance of dabigatran. Information on the type of medication, the dose and when these medications were last taken should be obtained. Appropriate laboratory investigations should be ordered to determine the extent of the hemostatic defect as well as to estimate the time to drug clearance. Options for removal or reversal of the drugs and their attendant risks should be considered. For a patient with only a minor hemorrhage or non-urgent surgical indication, and especially if there is a significant thrombotic risk, urgent anticoagulant reversal may not be the best management strategy.

The earlier approach can be summarized in the following five questions:

- What anticoagulant/antiplatelet drug does the patient take? What laboratory tests, if any, may be helpful to determine the degree of hemostatic defect?
- When was the last dose? What is the half-life of the drug?
- Does the patient have relevant co-morbidities affecting the bleeding risk or drug clearance?
- Is there an effective antidote? Can the drug be removed?
- Are the risks of the urgent drug reversal acceptable?

In case of major hemorrhage in anticoagulated patients, if available, antidote should be administered or arrangements made for a drug removal procedure as soon as possible. Unfortunately, not all drugs can be effectively reversed or removed. Attempt should be made to rapidly identify the source of bleeding and, if possible, control it locally with compression, surgery, angiography, or endoscopy. The patient should receive appropriate resuscitation with IV fluids and red blood cells, whereas plasma and platelet transfusions may be used to treat dilutional coagulopathy and thrombocytopenia respectively. Although there is no evidence to support this practice, nonspecific hemostatic agents such as tranexamic acid are also frequently administered. During resuscitation, maintenance of normothermia and normocalcemia is important in order to prevent exacerbation of bleeding due to platelet dysfunction and coagulopathy.

Introduction to Common Anticoagulants

Currently available oral anticoagulants include warfarin, direct thrombin (factor IIa) inhibitors, and factor Xa inhibitors (see Fig. 1).

Warfarin

Warfarin is the oldest and still most commonly used oral anticoagulant. It acts by inhibiting vitamin K_1-2,3 epoxide reductase, preventing vitamin K from being converted to its active form and thus causing deficiency of vitamin K dependent proteins (clotting factors II, VII, IX, and X, and proteins C and S) (refer to Fig. 1). Warfarin is used to prevent as well as treat venous and arterial thromboembolism. The medication is taken once a day and its duration of action is 2 to 4 days. Warfarin predictably prolongs PT and increases INR.

The case fatality rate of major warfarin associated bleeding approaches 10%.[5] Therefore, it is imperative to expeditiously diagnose and treat warfarin related hemorrhage. Fortunately, warfarin does have effective antidotes. Over-anticoagulation without bleeding can be effectively managed by stopping the medication and administering vitamin K. Vitamin K can be administered orally or intravenously and will start to reverse the anticoagulant effect in about 6 hours. For urgent reversal, such as clinically significant bleeding or impending surgical intervention in the next 6 hours, either a four factor prothrombin complex concentrate (PCC) or frozen plasma may be used. Vitamin K should also be administered since the duration of action for both PCC and plasma is about 6 hours. PCC is a pathogen reduced plasma derived product containing all vitamin K dependent clotting factors and proteins. It is usually dosed as per patient INR and weight and administered by a slow IV bolus. The most important risk of PCC is thrombosis and the

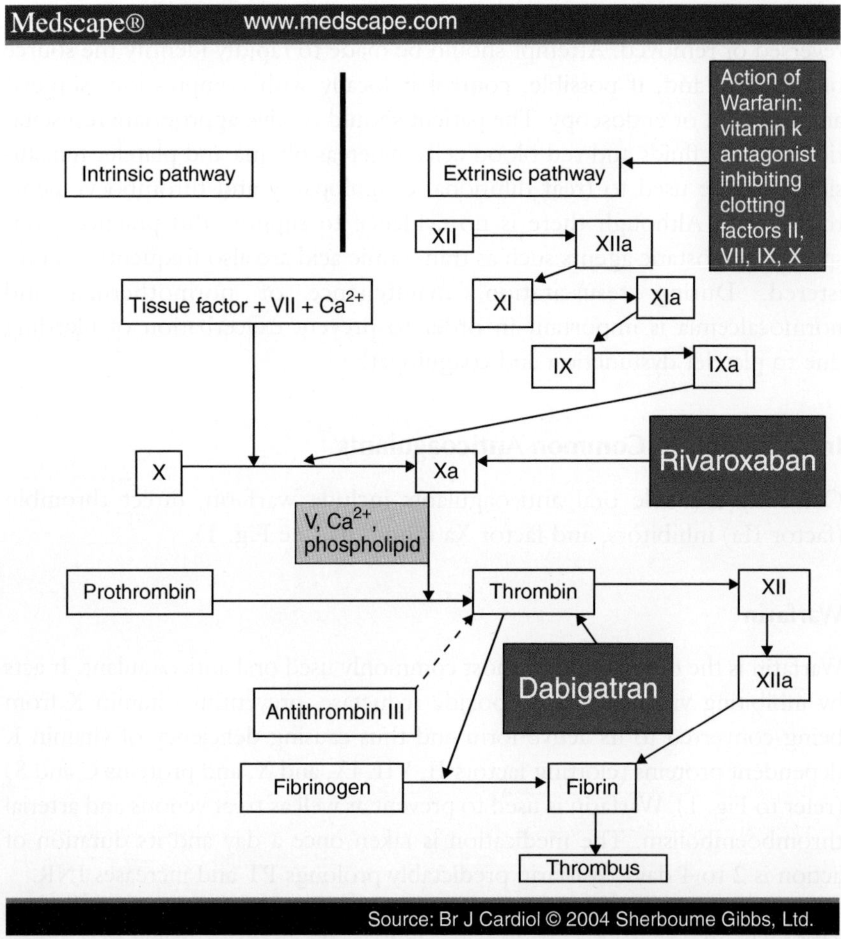

Fig. 1. Coagulation eascade and sites of action of warforin, dabigtran and rivaroxaban.

rate of thrombotic complications ranges from 1.5[6] to 7.8%.[7] The dose of plasma is 15cc/kg and its preparation may take 20 minutes or longer as it requires pre-transfusion testing and thawing. Adverse events related to plasma infusion may include circulatory overload, transfusion related lung injury, allergic reactions and transmission of blood borne pathogens. As compared to plasma, PCC provides more rapid and complete correction of INR.[7] It is important to point out, however, that no study to date has demonstrated that emergent reversal of anticoagulant effect in warfarinized bleeding patients results in improved patient outcomes.

Factor IIa inhibitors (Dabigatran)

Dabigatran is a direct thrombin (Factor IIa) inhibitor. Dabigatran is used to prevent venous or arterial thromboembolism. It is an oral medication that is taken twice a day and its half-life is about 17 hours. Since dabigatran is excreted primarily by the kidneys, renal insufficiency will significantly prolong its half-life. The drug has little effect on prothrombin time (PT) and its effect on activated partial thromboplastin time (aPTT) is not dose-dependent. APTT above 40 seconds suggests that the drug is present in the circulation and causes anticoagulant effect. Thrombin time is significantly prolonged in patients on dabigatran but the extreme sensitivity of this test limits its clinical utility. The best currently available laboratory test to determine the degree of anticoagulation is Hemoclot which is a diluted thrombin time and is reported as a dabigatran level. At present, this test is not available in most laboratories. When evaluating a bleeding patient on dabigatran, a serum creatinine should be ordered since this will give an idea of how long it will take for the drug to clear. Whereas the half-life of dabigatran is 14–17 hours in a patient with creatinine clearance of 50 or more ml/minute, the half-life would be closer to 18 hours in someone with a lower creatinine clearance.[8] It is also important to remember that dabigatran interferes with the assays for fibrinogen and other clotting factors yielding falsely low levels and this may potentially lead to unnecessary treatments with blood products. In clinical studies, dabigatran was associated with less major bleeding, including intracranial hemorrhage.[9] On the other hand, the drug does not have an antidote. The 30-day mortality following the first major bleed was reported to be 9.1% in one study.[10] In case of a major hemorrhage and if the drug was taken within the past two hours, an attempt could be made to remove the drug by activated charcoal.[13] Dabigatran can also be partially removed by hemodialysis or hemofiltration.[12] In reality, performing hemodialysis in a hemodynamically unstable trauma patient for 3–4 hours may prove to be impractical. In animal bleeding studies as well as two human volunteer studies,[11,12] recombinant VIIa or activated PCC (FEIBA) showed some efficacy in reversing the anticoagulant effect of dabigatran. It is important to point out, however, that the optimum doses for these agents have not been established in this clinical context. Anecdotally, administration of these clotting factors does not result in a significant improvement of coagulation tests even though a clinical effect (i.e., hemostasis) may occur. Recent studies have shown that idarucizumab, a humanized antibody fragment, immediately and completely reverses anticoagulation with dabigatran in healthy volunteers.[14] A Phase 3 study evaluating its efficacy as a specific antidote in patients with severe bleeding or emergency surgery has recently begun recruitment.

Factor Xa inhibitors (rivaroxaban, apixaban)

Currently available factor Xa inhibitors are rivaroxaban and apixaban. Rivaroxaban is used to prevent and treat venous thromboembolic events, while apixaban is used to prevent arterial thromboembolic events. Both have rapid onset of action and short half-lives ranging from 8 to 15 hours. Rivaroxaban is taken once a day, while apixaban is taken twice a day. Rivaroxaban, unlike apixaban, is mainly excreted by the kidneys. Both drugs may prolong PT and aPTT but prolongation may be minimal even at therapeutic concentrations. A much more accurate measure of drug effect is a chromogenic assay that measures Xa inhibition and is specifically calibrated for these drugs. Just like Hemoclot, these assays are reported as a drug level and are not widely available.

Factor Xa inhibitors were associated with less bleeding as compared to warfarin in clinical trials. According to one registry, the case fatality rate of rivaroxaban-related bleeding is about 6% at 90 days post-bleeding.[15] There are no antidotes for factor Xa inhibitors. Since these drugs are highly protein bound, plasmapheresis may theoretically be able to remove them. In a few animal bleeding studies and two human volunteer studies[11,12] four factor PCC, recombinant VIIa and activated PCC (FEIBA) were at least partially effective in correcting the hemostatic defect. According to a few published retrospective studies,[15] administration of PCC was associated with cessation of bleeding. However, the optimum dose of PCC has not been determined and dose ranges from 25 to 50 IU/kg. A Phase 2 study of the antibody PRT064445 directed against factor Xa inhibitors, a specific antidote, has been completed and a Phase 3 study is forthcoming.[14]

Antiplatelet agents

Discussion of inhibitors of hemostasis may not be complete without mentioning antiplatelet drugs. These medications are generally prescribed to prevent arterial thromboembolic diseases. The currently available antiplatelet drugs can be divided into four groups: COX-1 inhibitors (ex. Aspirin), ADP receptor inhibitors (ex. Clopidogrel), GPIIb/IIIa inhibitors (ex. Abciximab), and miscellaneous others.[16] For discussion of antiplatelet agents in injured patients only COX-1 inhibitors and ADP receptor inhibitors are relevant. Characteristics of a few commonly used antiplatelet drugs are listed in Table 1.[17] The listed medications do not have specific antidotes and they vary with regards to their mechanisms of action, half-lives and potency of antiplatelet effect. There is no readily available and reliable laboratory test

Table 1. Characteristics of select antiplatelet agents.

	ASA	**Clopidogrel**	**Prasugrel**	**Ticagrelor**
Mechanism of action	Inhibits synthesis of TXA2	Antagonist of platelet receptor $P2Y_{12}$ (irreversible)	Antagonist of platelet receptor $P2Y_{12}$ (irreversible)	Antagonist of platelet receptor $P2Y_{12}$ (reversible)
Route of administration	po	po	po	po
Time to peak effect	20 minutes (650 mg)	6 hours (300 mg)	1 hours	2–4 hours
Drug elimination half-life	ASA < 20 min Salicylate 3–5 hours	7.2–7.6 hours	3.7 hours	12 hours
Duration of action	1–3 days	5–10 days	5–10 days	24 hours

that can accurately determine the degree of platelet dysfunction in a bleeding patient on an antiplatelet agent. In a bleeding patient with a history of recent intake of an antiplatelet agent, a platelet transfusion may be tried. Whereas a single adult platelet dose (one apheresis concentrate or one buffy coat pool of platelets) may be sufficient to reverse the effect of aspirin, reversal of clopidogrel is likely to require at least two adult doses[18] and reversal of ticagrelor even more doses.[19] Other interventions that may be used include desmopressin (DDAVP), a drug frequently used to treat platelet dysfunction; tranexamic acid, an antifibrinolytic agent; and recombinant VIIa. The data on optimum dosing and efficacy of these interventions are lacking.

References

1. Dossett LA[1], Riesel JN, Griffin MR *et al.* Prevalence and implications of preinjury warfarin use: An analysis of the National Trauma Databank. *Arch Surg* 2011; 146(5): 565–570.
2. Bonville DJ[1], Ata A, Jahraus CB, Arnold-Lloyd T *et al.* Impact of preinjury warfarin and antiplatelet agents on outcomes of trauma patients. *Surgery* 2011; 150(4): 861–868.
3. Fortuna GR[1], Mueller EW, James LE *et al.* The impact of preinjury antiplatelet and anticoagulant pharmacotherapy on outcomes in elderly patients with hemorrhagic brain injury. *Surgery* 2008; 144(4): 598–603.
4. Ott MM[1], Eriksson E, Vanderkolk W *et al.* Antiplatelet and anticoagulation therapies do not increase mortality in the absence of traumatic brain injury. *J Trauma* 2010; 68(3): 560–563.
5. Guerrouij M[1], Uppal CS, Alklabi A *et al.* The clinical impact of bleeding during oral anticoagulant therapy: Assessment of morbidity, mortality and post-bleed anticoagulant management. *J Thromb Thrombolysis* 2011; 31(4): 419–423.
6. Dentali F[1], Marchesi C, Pierfranceschi MG *et al.* Safety of prothrombin complex concentrates for rapid anticoagulation reversal of vitamin K antagonists. A meta-analysis. *Thromb Haemost* 2011; 106(3): 429–438.
7. Sarode R[1], Milling TJ Jr, Refaai MA *et al.* Efficacy and safety of a 4-factor prothrombin complex concentrate in patients on vitamin K antagonists presenting with major bleeding: A randomized, plasma-controlled, phase IIIb study. *Circulation* 2013; 128(11): 1234–1243.
8. Schulman S, Crowther MA. How I treat with anticoagulants in 2012: New and old anticoagulants, and when and how to switch. *Blood* 2012; 119: 3016–3023.
9. Ruff CT[1], Giugliano RP[2], Braunwald E[2] *et al.* Comparison of the efficacy and safety of new oral anticoagulants with warfarin in patients with atrial fibrillation: A meta-analysis of randomised trials. *Lancet* 2014; 383(9921): 955–962.

10. Majeed A, Hwang HG, Connolly SJ *et al.* Management and outcomes of major bleeding during treatment with dabigatran or warfarin. *Circulation* 2013; 128(21): 2325–2332.
11. Eerenberg ES[1], Kamphuisen PW, Sijpkens MK *et al.* Reversal of rivaroxaban and dabigatran by prothrombin complex concentrate: A randomized, placebo-controlled, crossover study in healthy subjects. *Circulation* 2011; 124(14): 1573–1579.
12. Marlu R[1], Hodaj E, Paris A *et al.* Effect of non-specific reversal agents on anticoagulant activity of dabigatran and rivaroxaban: A randomised crossover ex vivo study in healthy volunteers. *Thromb Haemost* 2012; 108(2): 217–224; Lauw MN[1], Coppens M[2], Eikelboom JW[3]. Recent advances in antidotes for direct oral anticoagulants: Their arrival is imminent. *Can J Cardiol* 2014; 30(4): 381–384.
13. Alikhan R[1], Rayment R, Keeling D *et al.* The acute management of haemorrhage, surgery and overdose in patients receiving dabigatran. *Emerg Med J* 2014; 31(2): 163–168.
14. Kamphuisen PW. Gaining experience with the NOACs. *Blood* 2014; 124(6): 836.
15. Beyer-Westendorf J, Förster K, Pannach S *et al.* Rates, management, and outcome of rivaroxaban bleeding in daily care: Results from the Dresden NOAC registry. *Blood* 2014; 124(6): 955–962.
16. Sarode R. How do I transfuse platelets (PLTs) to reverse anti-PLT drug effect? Transfusion 2012; 52(4): 695–701.
17. Lopes RD. Antiplatelet agents in cardiovascular disease. *J Thromb Thrombolysis* 2011; 31(3): 306–309.
18. Vilahur G, Choi BG, Zafar MU *et al.* Normalization of platelet reactivity in clopidogrel-treated subjects. *J Thromb Haemost* 2007; 5(1): 82–90.
19. Tanaka KA, Subramaniam K. Looking into the future of platelet transfusion in the presence of $P2Y_{12}$ inhibitors. *British Journal of Anaesthesia* 2014; 112(5): 780–784.

Chapter 8

Pneumonia in the Surgical Intensive Care Unit

Mohammed Bawazeer and Jameel Ali

Chapter Overview

Pneumonias are generally classified as Community Acquired (CAP) or Health Care Associated (HCAP) both of which may be found in Intensive Care Unit (ICU) patients. The most common form of pneumonia in ICU patients is Ventilator-Associated (VAP) which is a subcategory HCAP with which it bears many similarities in microbiology and treatment. Because the most common causes for ICU admission in these patients is not the pneumonia itself but associated hypoxemic respiratory failure and severe sepsis the mortality is quite high and prompt early diagnosis and therapeutic intervention are crucial to survival. Major therapeutic challenges arise because of a higher frequency of resistant organisms associated with previous antibiotic usage and longer hospital stay with exposure to organisms specific to the institution making it difficult to apply therapeutic recommendations from other clinical settings. This chapter discusses the epidemiology, classification, diagnosis of CAP and HCAP. Because VAP is the most common pneumonia in the surgical ICU, special emphasis will be given to this entity to help formulate an approach to this serious disorder in order to improve treatment and outcome.

Introduction

About 10% of CAP patients require ICU admission because of development of hypoxemic respiratory failure or systemic signs of sepsis. In only about 25% of these cases the pathogen is identified on admission to the ICU leading to delayed specific therapy with increased complications and mortality.[1] HCAP runs a worse clinical course because of multi drug resistant (MDR) organisms and coexistent morbidities with an overall mortality of 25% which is even higher if associated with Adult Respiratory Distress Syndrome (ARDS).

Classification

The most common classification is based on the origin of the pneumonia — CAP or HCAP. The pathogens involved in these two are different with different drug susceptibility profiles. CAP is associated with easily identified and treatable pathogens, while HCAP is associated with MDR pathogens especially when hospital stay is prolonged (see Table 1 for identification of the common pathogens in these two categories).

Table 1. Classification of pneumonia by its origin and most common pathogens in each of them.

	CAP	HCAP
Bacterial	*Streptococcus pneumonia* *Haemophilus influenza* *Staphylococcus aureus* *Legionella* species Gram-negative bacilli	*Pseudomonas aeruginosaw* *Acinetobacter* spp. Enterobacteriaceae (*Klebsiella pneumoniae*; *Escherichia coli*; *Enterobacter* spp.) *Staphylococcus aureus*
Viral	Adenovirus, Respiratory syncytial virus Seasonal influenza and parainfluenza Herpes viruses (immunocompromised)	
Fungi	*Aspergillus* species (immunocompromised) *Pneumocystic jiruveci* (immunocompromised) *Cryptococcus neoformans* (immunocompromised)	
Mycobacterial	*Mycobacterium* species	

Source: (De Pascale G *et al. Curr Opin Pulm Med* 2012; 18(3): 213–221).

In one observational study, the most common pathogens associated with CAP admitted to ICU are *Streptococcus pneumoniae*, *Staphylococcus aureus* and *Pseudomanas aeruginosa*.[2] *Legionella pneumophila* is one of the atypical pathogens that can cause severe CAP that is associated with immune-mediated extrapulmonary symptoms.[1] *Staphylococcus aureus* is also a causative organism that can cause severe CAP with a growing number being methicillin-resistant (MRSA).[1]

In immunocompromised patients (e.g., Human immunodeficiency Virus (HIV)), opportunistic pathogens like Herpes viruses, *Aspergillus* species, *Pneumococcus jiroveci* and *Cryptococcus neoformans may* be involved. Antimicrobial therapy should be directed at these organisms when suspected or identified.

In another observational study, the most common pathogens associated with HCAP were MRSA and *Pseudomonas aeroginosa*.[3] Because of their associated morbidity and mortality, every effort should be made to establish an early microbiological diagnosis including drug sensitivity.

Diagnosis and Microbiology

Once the diagnosis of pneumonia is considered, cultures from the blood as well as the sputum should be obtained before starting the antibiotics. The risk of bacteremia is dependent on multiple factors. A prediction score has been suggested and evaluated in a retrospective study involving 1,136 patients. The overall rate of bacteremia was between 12–16%. The score consisted of 6 variables: liver disease, pleuritic pain, tachycardia, tachypnea, systolic hypotension, and absence of prior antibiotic treatment. With a score of 1, the risk of bacteremia was < 8%, while a score of 2, the risk of bacteremia was between 14–63%.[4]

Urine should be sent for Antigen assays for *S. pneumoniae* and *L. pneumophila*. For *Legionella*, urinary antigen assay has a sensitivity of 74% and specificity of 99%, while the pneumococcal antigen assay has a sensitivity of 71% and specificity of 96%.

In non-intubated patients, the reliability of sputum obtained from deep coughing is unknown. In those patients, awake Fiberoptic Bronchoscopy (FOB) and Bronchoalveolar Lavage (BAL) may be employed to obtain sputum samples. In intubated patients, multiple techniques are available including Protected Specimen Brushing (PSB), FOB with BAL and miniBAL (without FOB). Diagnostic accuracy is similar with each of these techniques. Their use is largely dependent on resources and center experience. Quantitative cultures may differentiate true infection from contaminants in the respiratory tract. Most of the literature is extrapolated from studies done on VAP.[5]

Polymerase Chain Reaction (PCR) is being used increasingly as a diagnostic technique. Its advantages include rapidity, sensitivity, and detection of both bacterial and viral pathogens. It has also some limitations including cost and inability to differentiate between colonizations from true infections.[1] In immunocompromised patients, BAL samples should be sent for fungal antigens. PCR assays also may have some role in this patient population.[1]

Treatment

Recommended criteria for ICU admission are shown in Table 2. The presence of one major criterion is an indication for ICU. The presence of ≥3 minor criteria is an indication for admission to high-level monitoring settings (e.g., level II bed).[6]

Once the diagnosis is suspected, early initiation of antimicrobial therapy is very important since it is associated with better outcome. This is especially important in patients with severe sepsis or septic shock. A summary of antibiotic regimens recommended for both severe CAP and HCAP is shown in Table 3. For severe CAP in the ICU, combination therapy is recommended to cover the most common pathogens and is superior to monotherapy.[6] This should consist of a β-lactam plus a macrolide or a fluoroquinolone. Antipseudomonal coverage is only required if there are risk factors for Pseudomonal infections, such as structural lung disease, bronchiectasis, repeated exacerbations of Chronic Obstructive Pulmonary Disease (COPD) with frequent steroid and/or antibiotic administration, and prior antibiotic

Table 2. Major and minor criteria for ICU admission.

Major criteria	1. Mechanical ventilation
	2. Septic shock and the need for vasopressors
Minor criteria	1. Respiratory rate ≥ 30 breaths/min
	2. PaO_2/FiO_2 ratio ≥ 250
	3. Multilobar infiltrates
	4. Confusion/disorientation
	5. Uremia (BUN level ≥ 20 mg/dL)
	6. Leukopeniac (WBC count < 4,000 cells/mm^3)
	7. Thrombocytopenia (platelet count < 100,000 cells/mm^3)
	8. Hypothermia (core temperature < 36°C)
	9. Hypotension requiring aggressive fluid resuscitation

Source: (Mandell *et al. Clin Infect Dis* 2007; 1: 44).

Table 3. Recommended empiric antibiotic therapy.

CAP	HCAP
No risk factors for Pseudomonas and MRS:	Early onset HCAP (no risk factors for MDR pathogens):
Option I: β-lactam (cefotaxime or ceftriaxone) *plus* a macrolide (azithromycin)	Option I: Penicillin plus β-lactamase inhibitor (amoxicillin/clavulanic acid or ampicillin sulbactam)
Option II: Respiratory fluoroquinolone (moxifloxacin, levofloxacin)	Option II: 2nd or 3rd generation cephalosporin (cefuroxime, cefotaxime, ceftriaxone)
	Option III: Ertapenem
Risk factors for Pseudomonas:	Late-onset, high risk of MDR pathogens:
Option: I: An anti-pseudomonal β-lactam (piperacillin-tazobactam, cefepime, imipenem or meropenem) *plus* a fluoroquinilone (ciprofloxacin or leveofloxacin)	Option I: Anti-pseudomonal β-lactam (piperacillin-tazobactam), or cephalosporin (cefepime, ceftazidime) or carbapenem (imipenem or meropenem) *plus* Anti-pseudomonal fluoroquinolone (ciprofloxacin or levofloxacin) or aminoglycoside (amikacin, gentamycin or tobramycin) *plus* Linezolid or vancomycin
Option II: An anti-pseudomonal β-lactam plus an aminoglycoside and a macrolide	
Risk factors for MRSA: Add linezolid or vancomycin	

Source: (Mandell *et al. Clin Infect Dis* 2007; 1: 44).

use.[6] If there are risk factors for MRSA; such as end-stage renal disease, injection drug abuse, and prior antibiotic use, addition of linezolid or vancomycin is recommended.[6]

In HCAP, the antibiotic choice will depend on the risk of MDR pathogens. "Early-onset" HCAP patients (within four days of the index admission) usually have low risk. "Late-onset" HCAP that occurs after five days and early onset with recent hospitalization or coming from a health-care facility (nursing home, dialysis center) usually have a high risk of MDR pathogens.[7] Those should be treated with triple therapy to cover for ***Pseudomonas*** species, MDR gram negatives, and MRSA until cultures are available.[7]

After 48–72 hours, checking the cultures and reassessment of the clinical response are required. If the patient has a good clinical response and a causative pathogen is identified, de-escalation of the antibiotics according to the cultures and sensitivity is recommended. Consideration should be given to stopping the antibiotics if all reliable cultures from the respiratory tract are negative. If the patient is not improving and organisms identified, adjustment of the antibiotics obviously is required. If cultures are still negative by that time, consider complications (e.g., empyema) or other diagnoses. All patients should receive intravenous antibiotics initially. Switching to oral/enteral route is reasonable in patients with good clinical response. Combination therapy is recommended in all patients with high risk of MDR organisms. Monotherapy is acceptable in the absence of resistant organisms. Total duration of directed therapy is 7–8 days and there is no benefit from longer courses.[7]

Management of Organ Failure

The two most common indications for an ICU admission in patients with severe pneumonia are septic shock and respiratory failure. Severe sepsis and septic shock should be managed according to the guidelines in Surviving Sepsis Campaign. The first bundle, which should be completed within three hours, includes measuring serum lactate, obtaining blood cultures, administering broad-spectrum antibiotics, and fluid resuscitation. The second bundle, which should be completed within six hours, includes starting vasopressors (for persistent hypotension), measuring central venous pressure (CVP) and central venous oxygen saturation ($ScvO_2$) and remeasuring lactate if initially elevated. End points of resuscitation are CVP $\geq$ 8 mmHg, central venous oxygen saturation $\geq$ 70% and normalization of lactate.[8]

Hypoxemic and/or hypercapnic respiratory failure can be managed initially by a trial of Non-Invasive Ventilation (NIV). Contraindications for

NIV include decreased level of consciousness, hemodynamic instability, inability to protect the airway or clear secretions, severe gastrointestinal bleeding and inability to fit the mask, or undrained pneumothorax.[1] Failure of NIV and/or clinical criteria of ARDS (acute onset, Partial Pressure of Arterial Oxygen/Fraction of Inspired Oxygen (PaO_2/FiO_2) ratio < 300, bilateral pulmonary infiltrates with normal left ventricular function) are indications for intubation and mechanical ventilation.[1] Management of hypoxemia in ARDS is beyond the scope of this chapter.

VAP

VAP is traditionally defined as a hospital-acquired pneumonia that develops in patients who have been mechanically ventilated for ≥48 hours. It is subclassified into early onset and late onset. Early onset VAP usually develops within four days of mechanical ventilation, while late onset develops after four days. Early onset is usually caused by antibiotic-susceptible organisms and late-onset by MDR organisms.[9]

VAP is the most common nosocomial infection that develops in mechanically ventilated patients. Its incidence has been estimated as 9–27% of mechanically ventilated patients, with about five cases per 1,000 ventilator days. VAP has been a significant hospital burden due to increased ICU and hospital mortality, with an estimated attributable mortality of 9%.[9]

Risk factors and pathophysiology

The main risk factor for developing VAP is the presence of an endotracheal tube. The tube interferes with the normal protective mechanism of the upper airways including an effective cough. It also facilitates microaspiration of contaminated oropharyngeal secretions, which is the main pathophysiolpogic mechanism for VAP. The incidence of VAP is significantly lower with non-invasive ventilation.[9]

Commonly after intubation with an inflated cuff, colonization of the oropharynx rapidly occurs. These contaminated secretions accumulate above the inflated cuff and slowly gain access to the airway via folds in the wall of the cuff. A bacterial biofilm gradually forms on the inner surface of the endotracheal tube. This biofilm serves as a nidus for infection. With each breath, bacteria with its biofilm are propelled into the distal airways.[9]

Immunosuppression associated with critical illness is a key risk factor for the development of VAP. There is also a significant reduction of the phagocytic activity of the neutrophils with critical illness. This finding has been consistent and precedes the development of VAP.[9]

Other risk factors that increase the risk of aspiration and hence the risk of VAP, include nursing in supine position and feeding through gastric feeding tubes. As well, risk factors that prolong the duration of mechanical ventilation also increase the risk of VAP.[9]

Prevention

Prevention of VAP is an important strategy that should be implemented in the critically ill patients who are mechanically ventilated. Many preventive interventions to decrease the incidence of VAP have been described. Some of them are effective more than others. But even those, which are effective in reducing VAP, do not change patient outcome. The Canadian Critical Care Trials Group published clinical practice guidelines for VAP prevention in 2008.[10] The strategies were physical, positional, and pharmacological. All these strategies can be classified into three categories: (A) reducing colonization, (B) prevention of microaspiration, (C) limiting the duration of mechanical ventilation.[9] Using care bundles aimed at reducing the incidence of VAP is probably better than using a single intervention alone.[11]

Reducing colonization

Route of endotracheal intubation has an impact on the incidence of VAP. Nasal intubation has been associated with more sinusitis and increased incidence of VAP. Orotracheal intubation has been associated with a trend towards reduction of VAP but has no effect on patient outcome.[10] In patients who are nasally intubated for various reasons, systematic search for maxillary sinusitis by (computed tomography) CT scan and subsequent treatment was compared to those without this systematic CT scan search and there was a significant reduction in the incidence of VAP and mortality without effect on duration of ICU and mechanical ventilation.[10] Some even advocate prevention of maxillary sinusitis. This is done by xylometazoline nasal drops followed by budesonide spray. This practice has been associated with a decreased incidence of maxillary sinusitis but not the incidence of VAP.[10]

Changing the ventilator circuit has been also studied. Scheduled changing of the circuit every two days has been compared to no change. This failed to show any effect on the incidence of VAP. However, a new circuit should be used for each patient just put on mechanical ventilation. The circuit is changed when clinically indicated.[10]

Airway humidification has been recommended in every patient receiving mechanical ventilation to prevent hypothermia, atelectasis, airway obstruction, and possibly obstruction of the endotracheal tube by inspissated secretions. Two types are available, active humidification by Heated Humidifier (HH) and passive humidification using Heat and Moist Exchanger (HME).[12] The two types have been compared and there was no difference on the incidence of VAP. In those using HME as a humidifier, more frequent (e.g., daily) changing of the humidifier system did not show benefit over less frequent (e.g., every 5–7 days). The panel concluded that less frequent changing may be associated with VAP reduction and might be considered a cost-effective measure.[10]

Prophylactic antibiotics directed toward VAP reduction have been studied using different routes, including aerosolized, nasal, intravenous alone, and topical and intravenous combinations. Two randomized trials studied antibiotics using the nebulized form. One compared ceftazidime against placebo and the other compared tobramycin against no antibiotics. Both studies showed a significant reduction of VAP in the treatment arm.[10] Another randomized trial compared nasal mupirocin ointment to placebo. This showed a significant reduction of VAP due to MRSA but no effect on the overall incidence of VAP.[10] Intravenous antibiotics in the form of IV Cefuroxime (1.5 gm for two doses, 12 hours apart) showed also a significant reduction of VAP but no effect on other outcomes. The use of topical (oropharyngeal gel) alone or in combination with intravenous ones also showed significant reduction of VAP and inconsistent effects on other outcomes.[10] However, despite all these positive effects on the reduction of VAP with different routes, the committee of the Canadian Critical Care Trials raised serious concerns on the emergence of resistance with their widespread use. Therefore, no consistent strong recommendations have been made.[10]

Oral decontamination with different agents has been studied in an effort to decrease oral colonization. 0.2% Chlorhexidne oral rinses of gingival and dental plaque have been compared to placebo. Another compared Chlorihexdine to combined Chlorhexidine/colistin and to placebo. Both studies showed a trend toward reduction of VAP but it did not reach statistical significance. In head injured patients, povidone–iodine in the form of oropharyngeal and nasopharyngeal rinses followed by aspiration has been compared to saline. This was associated with significant reduction of VAP. Oral iseganan failed to show any reduction of VAP when compared to placebo. Taken all these together, Chrohexidine should be considered in all mechanically ventilated patients, and povidone–iodine in head-injured patients in efforts to reduce the incidence of VAP.[10]

A recent meta-analysis included all trials comparing tooth brushing to no-tooth brushing. There was a trend toward reduction of VAP but it did not reach statistical significance with substantial heterogeneity between the studies. Interestingly, in a subgroup analysis, in one study that did not use chlorhexidine as part of the routine oral care, VAP was lower with tooth brushing, while in trials that used chlorhexidine in both groups, there was no difference.[13]

The type of endotracheal tube suctioning system (closed versus open) has been a topic of interest in many trials. This has been raised because open systems might introduce organism and contribute to further contamination of the airways. This type of the system had no effect on the incidence of VAP. However, because of safety concerns (to patients and health-care workers) the closed systems have been favored by many ICUs. As well, the frequency of changing the suctioning system (scheduled daily versus as clinically indicated) has no influence on VAP incidence. Probably, it is more cost-effective to change the system only whenever it is clinically indicated.[10]

Because microbial biofilms form on the inner surface of the endotracheal tube, silver, as a broad-spectrum antimicrobial agent, has been studied in a large multicenter randomized trial. In this trial, silver-coated endotracheal tubes were compared to the conventional ones and there was a significant reduction of VAP with silver-coated tubes as well as delayed occurrence of VAP.[14]

The last method that was studied in an effort to decrease colonization is the use of bacterial filters. In one randomized trial, bacterial filers (99.9% filtration effectiveness) were compared to no filters. There was no effect on the incidence of VAP; as well, there was a trend toward increase in mortality with the use of filters. Therefore, the use of bacterial filters has not been recommended.[10]

Preventing microaspiration

The first method that was studied is the use of rotating beds. Multiple methods were described including a kinetic treatment table, continuous postural oscillation, and continuous lateral rotational therapy. Compared to manual turning, the use of rotating beds was associated with significant reduction of VAP. However, implementation of this method can be a problem for feasibility, safety, and cost reasons.[10]

Another method is head-of-bed (HOB) elevation or semi-recumbent position. This has been studied in two randomized trials. In one study, body position was an independent risk factor for VAP and HOB elevation to at least 30° significantly reduced the incidence of VAP. In another study, 45° elevation was compared to standard but this was never achieved in the majority of patients probably because of feasibility issues. There was no difference in the incidence of pneumonia in this study. Therefore, all critically ill patients, if there is no contraindication, should have enteral feeding with head of bed elevated to at least 30° (if 45° is not feasible) to decrease the incidence of VAP.[10]

The last positional strategy to prevent microaspiration is prone positioning. In one trial, prone positioning for four hours was compared to supine. In another, prone positioning for eight hours was compared to supine with HOB at 30°. Combining the two studies, there was a trend toward reduction of VAP. However, feasibility and safety issues are of concerns here.[10]

As described previously, colonized secretions can accumulate above the cuff of the endotracheal tube. Specially designed endotracheal tubes with subglottic secretion drainage have been compared to conventional tubes. A meta-analysis of five randomized trials showed that these tubes are associated with VAP reduction. Feasibility and cost were reasonable. Therefore, these tubes are recommended in patients expected to be on mechanical ventilation for more than 72 hours.[10]

Another method studied for prevention of microaspiration is the use of ultrathin polyurethrane cuffed endotracheal tubes. Those have narrower longitudinal folds that might limit microaspiration when inflated. In a retrospective study, the use of this kind of tubes was associated with VAP reduction.[15] However, randomized trials are needed.[9]

Limiting the duration of mechanical ventilation

It is well known that, the longer the duration of mechanical ventilation the higher the incidence of VAP. Daily sedation interruption (when appropriate) has been associated with decreased duration of mechanical ventilation.[9] Implementation of a weaning protocol in each ICU also has been associated with a decrease in the duration of mechanical ventilation.[9]

Early tracheostomy has been advocated to decrease the incidence of VAP. Many randomized trials compared early versus late tracheostomy. Early tracheostomy failed to show any benefit.[10]

Microbiology

To choose the appropriate antibiotics, a general understanding of the causative organism is required. VAP is like any hospital-acquired pneumonia and the microbiology of the two conditions are very similar. Table 4 summarizes the organism involved in VAP.[9]

Early VAP (that develops within four days of mechanical ventilation) is usually caused by drug-susceptible organisms, such as *Haemophilus* spp., *Streptococcus* spp., and methicillin-sensitive *Staphylococcus aureus*. Late VAP (that usually develops after four days of mechanical ventilation) is usually caused by MDR organisms, such as *Pseudomonas aeroginosa*, *Acinetobacter* spp., and MRSA. The antibiotic choice also should take into consideration recent hospital admission for ≥ two days in the last 90 days. That includes chronic hemodialysis, patients from nursing homes, patients on Intravenous antibiotics, and on chemotherapy. This patient population has also a high likelihood of MDR organisms.[9]

Nosocomial fungal and viral infections are uncommon in immunocompetent hosts. *Aspergillus* spp. and *Candida* spp. can be found in organ transplant or immunocompromised patients. In immunocompetent patients, *Candida* spp. are commonly found in cultures from tracheal aspirates. But these usually represent a contamination rather than a true infection.[7]

Diagnosis

Making a diagnosis of VAP is quite challenging. This is because of lack of a "gold standard" diagnostic method. The most commonly used clinical criteria are the presence of a new or persistent pulmonary infiltrate in chest radiograph plus two of the three following criteria:

(1) Temperature greater than 38.3°C
(2) Leukocytosis (<12 × 10^9 while blood cell/L) or leucopenia (<4 × 10^9 white blood cell/L)
(3) Purulent tracheal secretions

The use of these clinical criteria alone may put a large number of patients on antibiotics unnecessarily because it is overly sensitive. There is also a

Table 4. The most common pathogens involved in VAP bases on their frequencies.

Pathogen	Frequency
Pseudomonas aeruginosa	24.4
Acinetobacter spp.	7.9
Stenotrophomonas maltophilia	1.7
Enterobacteriaceae:	14.1
Klebsiella spp.	15.6
Escherichia coli	24.1
Proteus spp.	22.3
Enterobacter spp.	18.8
Serratia spp.	12.1
Citrobacter spp.	5.0
Hafnia alvei	2.1
Haemophilus spp.	9.8
Staphylococcus aureus:	20.4
MRSA	55.7
Methicillin-sensistive	44.3
Streptococcus spp.	8.0
Streptococcus pneumoniae	4.1
Coagulase-negative staphylococci	1.4
Neisseria spp.	2.6
Anaerobes	0.9
Fungi	0.9
Other (<1% each):	3.8
Corynebacterium spp., *Moraxella* spp., and *Enterococcus* spp.	

Source: (Hunter *et al.*, *BMJ* 2012; 29: 344).

30–35% false negativity and 20–25% of false positivity. It is not uncommon in critical care settings to have a patient with pulmonary infiltrates on chest X-ray that is not related to infection. This can be caused by pulmonary edema, hemorrhage, and ARDS. Also, purulent tracheal secretions may be related to tracheobronchitis. Fever and leukocytosis is very common in the critical care settings and may be caused by extrapulmonary sources.

Therefore, obtaining microbiological samples is mandatory in all patients with suspected VAP.[7,9]

The two main reasons to obtain microbiological samples are to document a true infection rather than contamination and to identify the organism involved. This should be done ideally before starting antibiotics. Samples can be taken non-invasively (using tracheal aspirates) or invasively (using bronchoscopically obtained "BAL" or "PSB"). An increasingly common technique to obtain samples from the lower respiratory tract using a specially designed catheter that is wedged in the lower airways and called "mini-BAL" or "blind BAL". If endotracheal aspirates are used and cultured quantitatively using a diagnostic threshold of 10^6 CFU/ml, this technique has a sensitivity of 56–69% and specificity of 75–95%.[9] The quantitative culture of BAL usually uses a diagnostic threshold of 10^4 CFU/ml. Reported sensitivity with BAL is 42–93% and specificity is 45–100%.[7] While the quantitative cultures of PSB uses a diagnostic threshold of 10^3 CFU/ml, it has a sensitivity of 33–100% and specificity of 50–100%.[7] When blind sampling is used, the diagnostic threshold varies according to the technique, whether a mini-BAL or mini-PSB. Those have a sensitivity of 63–100% and 58–86% respectively. The specificities of these techniques are 66–96% and 71–100% of mini-BAL and mini-PSB respectively.[7] Because of the multifocality and diffuse nature of VAP, BAL and endotracheal samples can produce more representative samples than PSB and blind-BAL or PSB may be as accurate as bronchoscopically derived samples.[7] When invasive techniques were compared to non-invasive ones in many trials, there was no difference in patient outcomes.[16] A meta-analysis of all the trials showed no difference in hospital mortality, ICU length of stay, and rate of antibiotics usage.[17] A negative tracheal aspirate without a recent change in antibiotics has a negative predictive value of 94% for VAP.[7]

Rarely, the diagnosis can be made from blood cultures or samples from pleural fluids. Therefore, blood cultures should be obtained from any patient with febrile illness in the ICU. Blood cultures have a sensitivity of 25% when positive. As well, organisms may be originating from extrapulmonary source. It is very important to sample pleural fluids to rule out empyema or parapneumonic effusion if the patient has a large pleural effusion especially in the presence of a febrile illness not explained by other causes.[7]

In order to improve the diagnostic accuracy of the clinical criteria, the Clinical Pulmonary Infection Score (CPIS) was developed. This incorporates clinical, radiographic, physiological, and microbiological criteria. Table 5 summarizes the criteria used and the scoring system. A score of more than 6

Table 5. Clinical Pulmonary Infection Score (CPIS).

Criteria	**Score**
Tracheal secretions	Absent = 0 point Presence of non-purulent secretions = 1 point Presence of purulent secretions = 2 points
Chest X-ray	None = 0 point Diffuse (or patchy) = 1 point Localized infiltrate = 2 points
Progression of pulmonary infiltrate	No radiographic progression = 0 Progression (after CHF or ARDS excluded) = 2
Temperature	36.5–38.4°C = 0 points 38.5–38.9°C = 1 point <36 or >39°C = 2 points
White cell count	4,000–11,000 = 0 point <4,000 or >11,000 = 1 point <4,000 or >11,000 + bands ≥50% = 2 points
PaO_2/FiO_2	>240 or ARDS = 0 point ≤240 or no ARDS = 2 points
Culture of tracheal aspirate	Pathogenic bacteria cultured in rare or light quantity = 0 points Pathogenic bacteria cultured in moderate or heavy quantity = 1 point Same pathogens on gram stain — add 1 point

A score > 6 is considered suggestive of pneumonia.
ARDS = Adult Respiratory Distress Syndrome, CHF = Congestive Heart Failure, PaO_2/FiO_2 = Ratio of the arterial oxygen pressure to fraction of inspired oxygen.

Source: (Pugin *et al. Minerva Anesthesiol* 2002; 68(4):261–265).

is suggestive of pneumonia and initiation of antibiotics warranted.[18] A meta-analysis of the studies that used the CPIS score showed that the sensitivity and the specificity were 65% and 64% respectively. Although not very sensitive, it is simple and easy to perform.[19]

Another system commonly used in Europe is Hospitals in Europe Link for Infection Control through Surveillance (HELICS). Table 6 summarizes these criteria for VAP.[9] This system is not very well adapted in North America and its sensitivity and specificity are still unknown.

Table 6. Hospitals in Europe Link for Infection Control through Surveillance (HELICS) criteria for VAP.

Categories	Criteria
Radiography	In patients with underlying cardiac or pulmonary disease: ≥2 serial chest radiograph or CT scan suggestive of pneumonia.
	In patients without underlying cardiac or pulmonary disease: one definitive chest radiograph or CT.
Symptoms	**And atlest one of the following:**
	Fever > 38°C with no other cause.
	Leucopenia (<4 × 10^9 WBC/L) or leukocytosis (>12 × 10^9 WBC/L).
	And at least one of the following (or at least two if clinical pneumonia only = PN4 and PN5):
	New onset of purulent sputum or change in sputum character.
	Cough, dyspnea, or tachypnea.
	Suggestive auscultation (rales or bronchial breathing), wheeze, worsening gas exchange (e.g., oxygen desaturation, increase oxygen demand, or increased ventilator demand).
Microbiology	**And according to the used diagnostic method:**
	PN1: Positive quantitative culture from minimally contaminated lower respiratory tract specimen — BAL ≥ 10^4CFU/ml.
	PN2: Positive quantitative culture from lower respiratory tract (tracheal aspirate) with a threshold of 10^5 CFU/ml.
	PN3: Positive culture related to no other source of infection — Positive pleural fluid culture, pulmonary abscess with Positive needle aspirate, positive histology, or positive exams for pneumonia with virus or particular organism.
	PN4: Positive sputum culture or non-quantitative lower respiratory tract culture.
	PN5: no positive microbiology.

Source: (Hunter *et al.*, *BMJ* 2012; 29: 344).

Treatment

Once clinical suspicion of VAP is present, immediate cultures should be taken followed by immediate administration of antibiotics. Obtaining cultures should not delay administration of antibiotics. In one randomized trial, empiric early administration was compared to delayed and culture-directed administration. In this trial, there was no difference in mortality or duration of mechanical ventilation, but there was a trend toward reduction of costs and hospital length of stay.[16] In another observation study, delay in administration of antibiotics was associated with increased mortality.[7] Given these results, early empiric antibiotic administration is essential.

The factors that influence the choice of antibiotics are as follows: severity of illness, duration of hospital stay, and recent antibiotics use.[9] Patients with severe sepsis should be treated aggressively with broad-spectrum antibiotics according to the Surviving Sepsis Campaign Guidelines.[8] The longer the duration of hospital stay (more than four days), the higher the likelihood of MDR.[7] Finally, recent exposure to antibiotics usually predicts resistant microorganisms. Therefore, patients who have been treated for a different infection and develop a VAP shortly after should be treated empirically with a different antibiotic class.[7] In addition to early administration of antibiotics, appropriate choice (and dose) can influence outcome. Inappropriate selection of initial therapy is a major risk factor for higher mortality, increased length of stay, and emergence of antibiotic-resistant organisms.[7]

No antibiotic regimen has shown superiority in many randomized trials.[16] Apart from the factors mentioned previously, local resistance patterns according to their antibiogram should be considered in the initial choice of antibiotics.[7,16] Generally, antibiotics should have a high degree of activity against aerobic gram-negative bacilli. For early onset VAP, with no risk factors for MDR, ampicillin–sulbactam, 2nd or 3rd generation cephalosporin (cefuroxime, ceftriaxone), a fluoroquinolone (levofloxacin or ciprofloxacin) or ertapenem are appropriate.[7,9] For late onset VAP, antibiotics should have activity against MDR and particularly ***Pseudomonas aeruginosa***. Options include a Cephalosporin (Ceftazidime or Cefepime), Carbapenem (Imipenem or meropenem), piperacillin–tazobactam plus a Fluoroquinolone (ciprofloxacin or levofloxacin), or an Aminoglycoside (amikacin or gentamycin).[7,9] When MRSA is a possibility, vancomycin or linezolid is added. It was thought than linezolid is better than vancomycin because it has better lung penetration. A meta-analysis of all the trials comparing linezolid to glycopeptides antibiotics (vancomycin and teicoplanin) showed no difference between the two. Therefore, the choice between the two depends on local availability and resistance patterns.[20]

Combination therapy is a common practice for the following reasons: to provide synergy in the treatment of ***Pseudomanas***, to prevent emergence of resistance during therapy, and to provide broad-spectrum coverage to ensure activity against MDR organisms.[7] Studies comparing monotherapy to combination therapy failed to show superiority of combination therapy and there was no effect on mortality or clinical response.[16] Monotherapy should be used whenever possible because it is more cost-effective and it avoids unnecessary exposure to antibiotics. Agents that are effective as monotherapy are ciprofloxacin, levofloxacin, imipenem, meropenem, and piperacillin–tazobactam.[7] Combination therapy should be reserved only for situations where high rates of resistance patterns are seen on local antibiogram.[16]

All antibiotics should be administered initially systemically through the intravenous route. Nebulized and local instillation of tobramycin has been studied in two randomized trials. Both routes did not improve outcomes when compared to the systemic routes alone. However, with nebulized tobramycin, there was a trend toward earlier extubation. However, this trial was underpowered because of small numbers.[16] More studies are required to further answer this question. In the meantime, nebulized may be used as an adjunctive therapy to MDR gram-negative organisms in patients not responsive to systemic therapy.[7]

After 48–72 hours of therapy, and when cultures are available, it is very important to de-escalate the broad-spectrum antibiotics to a more culture-directed therapy, switching to oral or enteral route in patients with intact gastrointestinal (GI) tract and showing good clinical response.[7] Most patients can be safely treated for a total of eight days provided they receive adequate initial therapy. One randomized trial compared 8-day to a 15-day course. There was no difference in mortality, length of stay or ventilator-free days between the two groups. The shorter course was associated with decreased antibiotic use and emergence of resistant organisms. There was also a higher rate of relapse without worsening clinical outcome. However, the recurrent VAP due to MDR organism was less with the short course.[7,16] The decision whether to discontinue the antibiotics should be based on clinical criteria (resolution of signs and symptoms of infection) rather than physician discretion. In one randomized trial, this seems to shorten the duration of antibiotic use without worsening clinical outcome.[16]

References

1. De Pascale G, Bello G, Tumbarello M *et al.* Severe pneumonia in intensive care: Cause, diagnosis, treatment and management: A review of the literature. *Curr Opin Pulm Med* 2012; 18(3): 213–221.
2. Restrepo MI, Mortensen EM, Velez JA *et al.* A comparative study of community-acquired pneumonia patients admitted to the ward and the ICU. *Chest* 2008; 133(3): 610–617.
3. Schreiber MP, Chan CM, Shorr AF. Resistant pathogens in nonnosocomial pneumonia and respiratory failure: Is it time to refine the definition of health-care-associated pneumonia? *Chest* 2010; 137(6): 1283–1288.

4. Falguera M, Trujillano J, Caro S *et al.* A prediction rule for estimating the risk of bacteremia in patients with community-acquired pneumonia. *Clin Infect Dis* 2009; 49(3): 409–416.
5. Chastre J, Trouillet JL, Combes A *et al.* Diagnostic techniques and procedures for establishing the microbial etiology of ventilator-associated pneumonia for clinical trials: The pros for quantitative cultures. *Clin Infect Dis* 2010; 51(Suppl 1): S88–92.
6. Mandell LA, Wunderink RG, Anzueto A *et al.* Infectious Diseases Society of America/American Thoracic Society consensus guidelines on the management of Community-acquired pneumonia in adults. *Clin Infect Dis* 2007; 44(Suppl 2): S27–72.
7. American Thoracic Society, Infectious Diseases Society of America. Guidelines for the Management of adults with hospital-acquired, ventilator-associated, and health-care-associated Pneumonia. *Am J Respir Crit Care Med* 2005; 171(4): 388–416.
8. Dellinger RP, Levy MM, Rhodes A *et al.* Surviving sepsis Campaign: International guidelines for management of severe sepsis and septic shock: 2012. *Crit Care Med* 2013; 41(2): 580–637.
9. Hunter JD. Ventilator associated pneumonia. *BMJ* 2012; 29 344: e3325.
10. Muscedere J, Dodek P, Keenan S *et al.* Comprehensive evidence-based clinical practice guidelines for ventilator-associated pneumonia: Prevention. *J Crit Care* 2008; 23(1): 126–137.
11. Morris AC, Hay AW, Swann DG *et al.* Reducing ventilator-associated pneumonia in intensive care: Impact of implementing a care bundle. *Crit Care Med* 2011; 39(10): 2218–2224.
12. American Association for Respiratory Care, Restrepo RD, Walsh BK. Humidification during invasive and noninvasive mechanical ventilation: 2012. *Respir Care* 2012; 57(5): 782–788.
13. Alhazzani W, Smith O, Muscedere J *et al.* Toothbrushing for critically ill mechanically ventilated patients: A systematic review and meta-analysis of randomized trials evaluating ventilator-associated pneumonia. *Crit Care Med* 2013; 41(2): 646–655.
14. Kollef MH, Afessa B, Anzueto A *et al.* Silver-coated endotracheal tubes and incidence of ventilator-associated pneumonia: The NASCENT randomized trial. *JAMA* 2008; 300(7): 805–813.
15. Miller MA, Arndt JL, Konkle MA *et al.* A polyurethane cuffed endotracheal tube is associated with decreased rates of ventilator-associated pneumonia. *J Crit Care* 2011; 26(3): 280–286.
16. Muscedere J, Dodek P, Keenan S *et al.* Comprehensive evidence-based clinical practice guidelines for ventilator-associated pneumonia: Diagnosis and treatment. *J Crit Care* 2008; 23(1): 138–147.
17. Berton DC, Kalil AC, Teixeira PJ. Quantitative versus qualitative cultures of respiratory secretions for clinical outcomes in patients with ventilator-associated pneumonia. *Cochrane Database Syst Rev* 2012; 1: CD006482.

18. Pugin J. Clinical signs and scores for the diagnosis of ventilator-associated pneumonia. *Minerva Anestesiol* 2002; 68(4): 261–265.
19. Shan J, Chen HL, Zhu JH. Diagnostic accuracy of clinical pulmonary infection score for ventilator-associated pneumonia: A meta-analysis. *Respir Care* 2011; 56(8): 1087–1094.
20. Walkey AJ, O'Donnell MR, Wiener RS. Linezolid vs glycopeptide antibiotics for the treatment of suspected methicillin-resistant *Staphylococcus aureus* nosocomial pneumonia: A meta-analysis of randomized controlled trials. *Chest* 2011; 139(5): 1148–1155.

Chapter 9

Hypothermia and Hyperthermia

John B. Kortbeek

Chapter Overview

Patients suffering from hypothermia or hyperthermia of varying degrees are frequently admitted to the ICU. Treatment of these patients presents many challenges, including metabolic, cardiorespiratory, fluid, and electrolyte derangements which often can only be effectively managed in the ICU setting. The classification of hypothermia and hyperthermia will be presented. Definitions, mechanisms, etiology, pathogenesis, clinical presentation, and principles of management of these entities will assist physicians caring for these critically ill patients in understanding and effectively managing these disorders.

Maintenance of Temperature

Temperature homeostasis, maintenance of normothermia is essential for human life. Body temperature is centrally regulated and affected by changes in muscle activity, metabolism, and the cardiovascular system. The hypothalamus is the center of thermoregulation. The optic nuclei in the anterior hypothalamus receive temperature feedback from peripheral nerves in the skin and mucous membranes as well as from perithalamic thermosensors.

Normal temperature is defined as 36.5°C +/− 0.5°C. There is a normal diurnal variation of up to 1°C with peak mid day and nadir around 4 am. Temperature also varies depending on measurement site with core temperatures (rectal > oral > skin).

Temperature is affected by body mass, body habitus, gender, and ovulation. Physical activity, medications, and illness may affect body temperature and regulation. Temperature typically rises with meals and exercise. Environmental exposure to heat and cold produce physiologic responses to maintain normothermia.

Heat and exercise result in peripheral vasodilation and sweating. Tachycardia and hyperventilation may ensue. Exposure to cold results in vasoconstriction, shivering, piloerection, and initially tachycardia as well. Humans are able to maintain thermoregulation across a wide range of temperatures and environments. However, this may be profoundly affected by age, illness, endocrine and metabolic disorders malnutrition, obesity, drugs (including those used in general anesthetic such as muscle relaxants) and alcohol. Muscle mass provides an important mechanism for generating heat. A low relative body surface area to mass ratio conserves heat. Increased insulation with higher adipose ratio serves as an insulator.

Environmental heat gain or loss may occur through several mechanisms:

Conduction: Transfer of heat (energy) through direct contact.
Convection: Transfer of heat through fluids (liquid or gas).
Radiation: Transfer of heat through electromagnetic waves.

Hypothermia and hyperthermia occur when normal adaptive mechanisms are unable to cope with environmental exposure or altered heat production due to changes in metabolic rate or thalamic regulation.

Hypothermia

Etiology and classification

Hypothermia results when body heat loss exceeds the ability to generate or conserve heat. It may also result from loss of central temperature regulation following severe CNS injury affecting the thalamus. Hypothermia should be suspected when patients present following trauma or with diminished level of consciousness. It is common following immersion, near drowning, drowning episodes. Hypothermia often occurs in avalanche victims. It frequently co-exists in patients who have suffered exposure following alcohol or drug intoxication.

Hypothermia may be classified as mild, moderate, or severe. Mild hypothermia (temperature 32–25°C) presents with tachycardia, tachypnea, shivering, and confusion. The most common arrhythmia is atrial fibrillation. J waves may be present on the electrocardiogram (EKG).[1]

Moderate hypothermia (temperature 28–23°C) presents with altered level of consciousness. The Glasgow coma scale is typically less than 12 and the patient may be comatose. In patients with diminished GCS and coma, co-existent traumatic brain injury must be excluded. The respiratory pattern varies. Tachycardia frequently progresses to atrial fibrillation or flutter and PVCs may be present. More profound temperature drops may result in bradyarrythmias. The patient is at risk of progressing to ventricular arrhythmias including ventricular tachycardia and ventricular fibrillation.

Severe hypothermia (temperature <28°C) presents with coma and apnea. These patients frequently progress to ventricular fibrillation and asystole. Correct assessment of core temperature requires use of thermometers capable of recording temperatures less than 28°C. Many standard emergency department thermometers have a low set point of 28°C.

Patients presenting following exposure to cold may also present with characteristic associated soft tissue injuries. These include frostbite, chilblain, and trench foot.

Frostbite, like burns, is classified by depth of injury. Superficial epidermal injury (frostnip) presents with whitish discoloration or simple erythema after rewarming. The wound is typically numb but becomes quite painful on rewarming. Second-degree injury involves the epidermis and dermis and presents with white–yellow discoloration and is accompanied by blister formation. Some tissue sloughing may occur during recovery. Third-degree injury involves subcutaneous tissues and may progress to muscle, tendon, nerve, and bone. Necrosis accompanies the loss of perfusion and the development of ice crystals in the tissues. Tissue loss is universal and debridement or amputation may be required.

Chilblains (or pernio) refer to the development of erythematous patches accompanied by pain and pruritus in response to rapid rewarming after exposure to cold. The extremities, particularly digits are involved. The condition is common with some individuals genetically predisposed. It may also develop following previous cold injury.

Trench foot or immersion injury earned is so named as it occurred frequently in soldiers during World War I, subjected to prolonged exposure and immersion of the feet in cold water and mud. Freezing temperatures are not required. The prolonged exposure to a cold wet environment results in vasoconstriction, tissue hypoxia, and subsequent injury. Pain swelling and erythema progressing to blistering and even necrosis may occur.

Pathophysiology

Hypothermia has significant effects on a number of essential homeostatic mechanisms. Importantly it affects central nervous system metabolism, cardiac conductivity, the vascular system, oxygen transport, platelet aggregation, the coagulation cascade, and the immune response to pathogens.[2]

The brain receives approximately 15% of arterial blood flow and is responsible for approximately 20% of metabolic energy consumption. Hypothermia reduces the metabolic rate dramatically, up to 50% at temperatures of 28°C. Hypothermia has neuroprotective effects in reducing production of lactate through anaerobic metabolism as well as reducing the release of excitatory amino acids such as glutamate. Production of free radicals is reduced, cell membranes are stabilized and cerebral oxygen requirements are lowered. These changes result in resistance to ischemic or hypoxic injury. EEG changes in hypothermia consist of reduced alpha activity with a relative increase in beta and theta activity. Somatosensory evoked potentials are also affected with increased latency. These changes explain the sequential altered level of consciousness observed in hypothermia with progression from confusion to coma.[3]

Mild hypothermia results in shivering and vasoconstriction. Oxygen requirements are increased and there may be compensatory tachycardia and increased cardiac output. As hypothermia progresses impaired cardiac contractility and conduction occurs along with progressive increases in afterload from vasoconstriction which may decrease stroke volume especially in the patient with border line cardiac reserve. This leads to impaired perfusion and lactic acidosis. With severe hypothermia cardiac arrest eventually results.

Mild hypothermia initially results in an intracellular potassium shift. In addition, the hemoglobin oxygen saturation curve shifts to the left resulting in decreased delivery of oxygen to the tissues. As the shock state unfolds and cardiac arrest occurs, hypoxia and necrosis lead to severe acidosis and hyperkalemia.

The coagulation cascade is directly affected by hypothermia resulting in the increased risk of bleeding and associated mortality in trauma. Fibrinolysis is enhanced, platelet aggregation and adhesion is diminished. The enzymatic coagulation cascade is inhibited.

Leukocyte and immunologic effects have been documented with impaired wound healing and increased risk of sepsis, pneumonia, and surgical site infection. Surgical wounds are directly affected through vasoconstriction and relative tissue hypoxia. Systemic effects are many and include reduced leukocyte chemotaxis, aggregation and phagocytosis, altered cytokine production, delayed TNF clearance and impaired monocyte major histocompatibility surface antigen expression.

Diagnosis

Hypothermia should be suspected in patients with a history of prolonged exposure, immersion or near drowning. Mild confusion and delirium may be associated with hypothermia. Patients may exhibit tachycardia, tachypnea and will have cool and possibly mottled extremities.

Current medications should be reviewed to evaluate the confounding effects on cardiovascular response or to suggest contributing metabolic or endocrine conditions. Toxic drug and alcohol ingestion should be excluded. Body habitus will be obvious on inspection and support the history in determining risk of hypothermia particularly in thin, emaciated and malnourished adults. Children are particularly at risk given their large body surface area to mass ratios.

Hypothermia should be excluded in any patient presenting with an altered level of consciousness, major trauma, cardiac arrhythmia/arrest or severe sepsis. Temperature should be measured and documented along with the initial set of vital signs. In severe hypothermia, the thermometer used should be checked to confirm its lowest measurement range. Many thermometers used in the emergency department have a lowest measurement of 28°C and will record this in patients whose core temperature may have fallen significantly lower.

The EKG may exhibit a prolonged PR, QRS, and QT intervals, Osborne waves, sinus tachycardia, and atrial fibrillation. Brady-arrhythmias and ventricular arrhythmias are associated with low moderate to severe hypothermia (Fig. 1, J Wave).

Hypothermia may commonly occur in patients undergoing resuscitation or surgery for trauma or critical illness. It may also occur in patients during prolonged major operative procedures. Close monitoring of core temperature should routinely occur in these circumstances. Increasing operating room temperatures, administration of warmed fluids through warmers or rapid infusion devices, and application of warm air body blankets (e.g., Bair Hugger®) can prevent or correct mild hypothermia.

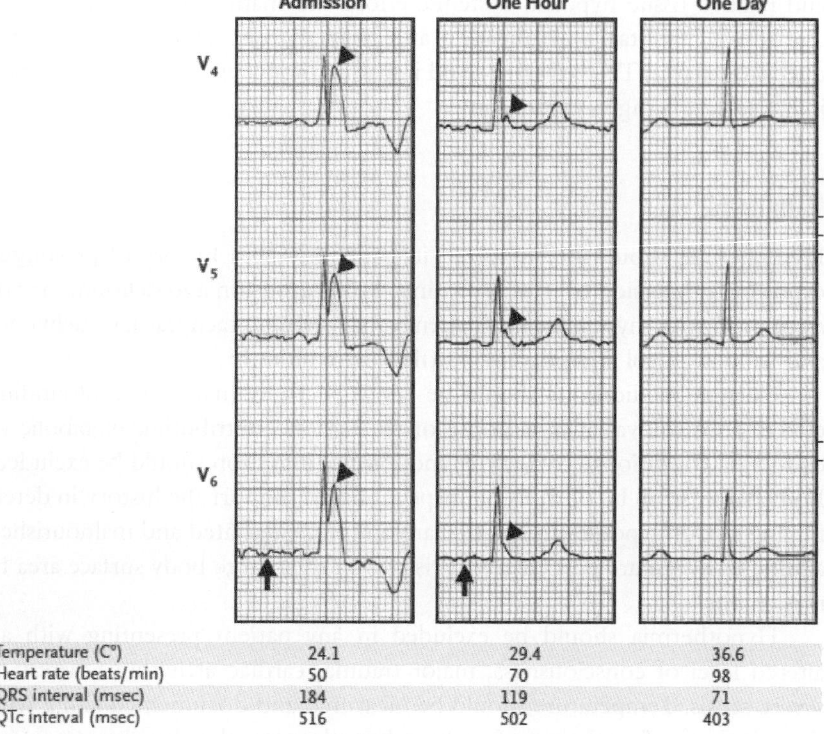

	Admission	One Hour	One Day
Temperature (C°)	24.1	29.4	36.6
Heart rate (beats/min)	50	70	98
QRS interval (msec)	184	119	71
QTc interval (msec)	516	502	403

Fig. 1. Demonstration of J-wave

Source: Krantz MJ, Lowery CM, *N Engl J Med* 2005; 352(2), Available at www.nejm.org.

Management

When hypothermia is recognized steps should be taken to restore normothermia. This may take the form of passive or active rewarming techniques depending on the level of hypothermia and the response to rewarming. The only exception would be when a decision is made to continue moderate hypothermia following cardiac arrest in a patient with suspected hypoxic brain injury and only once oxygenation, ventilation, and adequate perfusion are established.

Passive rewarming is sufficient in most cases of mild hypothermia. Applying warm blankets, clothing, and ambient temperature as well as administering warm fluids and a hot meal if possible, will often suffice.

Active rewarming is required when patients are at risk for ongoing exposure or heat loss (surgery, intoxication, coma, quadriplegia, burns) and when moderate hypothermia is present. Options include a warm humidified ventilator circuit; forced warm air body covers and blankets, IV warmers and massive transfusion high volume IV warmers (40–42°C). Humidified warm air circuits may be provided with endotracheal intubation and mechanical ventilation. Ventilators may have a set maximum temperature of 40°C or 41°C but this can still be very effective. Humidified external nebulizers (41–45°C) may be useful in some cooperative patients. Application of direct heat for conduction and convection warming should be applied to the trunk as a priority to minimize after drop in core temperature associated with select rewarming of the extremities. Gastric, bladder, and peritoneal irrigation with warm fluids (40°C) have all been described. Active rewarming usually result in body temperature elevation of 1–2°C/h.[4]

Severe hypothermia in patients presenting with a perfusing rhythm requires more urgent therapy as cardiac arrest may be imminent. In these cases in addition to the active rewarming measures already described a dialysis circuit may offer rapid rewarming. Consideration may also be given to venovenous bypass and preparation for cardiopulmonary bypass. Placement of cannula or establishing central IV access greatly facilitates bypass access in the event of a cardiac arrest.

Patients who present in cardiac arrest should receive active rewarming with extracorporeal membrane oxygenation (ECMO) if available.[5] Rewarming adult patients with severe hypothermia who have cardiac arrest is extremely difficult if not impossible. In small children active rewarming efforts have been successful but CPB remains the standard for rapid effective rewarming. A cardiac perfusing rhythm is rarely restored before the core temperature is elevated above 30°C and usually returns once the core temperature reaches 32–35°C.

Selection of patients for ECMO requires an assessment for the potential to restore a perfusing rhythm and survive the arrest. Factors that are associated with survival and moderate to good recovery are youth, pH > 7, serum potassium <9. The etiology is also important as patients with isolated exposure hypothermia have better outcomes than those with associated asphyxia (avalanche victims), aspiration and hypoxia (drowning victims) or multiple trauma. A 50 year patient who presents following multiple trauma with a pH of 6, a potassium of 11 and multiple trauma will not survive a hypothermic arrest.[6] These are published criteria for considering cessation of warming techniques.

Prognosis

Survivors of accidental hypothermia have been described after prolonged circulatory arrest. A 57 year old female survived over 300 min of arrest and

CPR and was noted to have only mild cognitive deficits during three months. She had become lost in the Swiss Alps during a snowstorm. Her first documented pH was 7.25 with potassium of 5.8. ECMO using veno-arterial femoral access was established after 307 min.[7] A study from the Netherlands documented 84 patients with accidental hypothermia presenting with temperatures <35°C. There were 60 survivors (71.4%). Indoor exposure and submersion (asphyxia) were associated with higher mortality rates. A total of 42 of the 60 survivors were discharged to home.[8]

A study from Japan evaluated patients with severe hypothermia requiring ECMO. About half were accidental exposures, half were submersion injuries and a small number were avalanche victims. Ten patients (38%) survived with good Glasgow outcome scale recovery. Predictors of mortality included presence of asphyxia (submersion, avalanche) and asystole as the presenting rhythm. Survivors had lower potassium levels. The authors noted that rewarming rates of 8–12°C/h can be achieved by ECMO. Predictors of mortality that have been suggested as relative contraindications to ECMO include serum potassium greater than 9, and pH 6.5. Asphyxia preceding arrest portends a very poor prognosis. Age has been associated with mortality. The statement that a patient is not dead until warm and dead should be taken literally in young adults and children unless they have signs incompatible with survival.[6]

Hyperthermia

Etiology

Hyperthermia is a potentially lethal condition. There are three general classes of hyperthermia. Environmental hyperthermia, exertional hyperthermia and drug induced hyperthermia. Awareness of the typical conditions associated with these types and their presenting characteristics is important in management.

Environmental hyperthermia occurs with exposure to excessive ambient temperatures. Lack of acclimatization in populations subjected to sudden heat waves and resultant increased mortality was described in France. In 2003, record temperatures exceeding the previous 50 years were set. Daily maximum temperatures exceeding 35° lasted for greater than one week. An excess mortality of nearly 15,000 deaths was described over historical norms. The excess mortality was greatest in Paris and central, eastern France where cities typically did not experience high temperatures.[9] Environmental hyperthermia is associated with extremes of age, comorbid illness including skin diseases, cardiovascular disease, endocrine and metabolic disorders, and obesity. Lack of social supports, isolation, and lack of air conditioning have also been described as important factors. The Hajj in Mecca is an event where large populations are suddenly immersed in high ambient temperatures. This has led to the establishment of preventive measures as well as treatment areas including body-cooling units.

Exertional hyperthermia is well described in athletes and military personnel who are subject to extreme physical stress in hot and humid environments. Muscular and mesomorphic build, heavy clothing or sports equipment, heavy carrying loads are all recognized contributing factors. Poor hydration and brief acclimatization periods are also important factors.

Drug induced hyperthermia includes medications which predispose individuals to hyperthermia by impairing normal physiologic mechanisms for dissipating heat loss. Examples are phenothiazines, which antagonize dopamine receptors, impair the thalamic response to rising body temperatures and disrupt thermoregulation. Anticholinergics impair sweating and cardiovascular responses to hyperthermia.

Malignant hyperthermia (MH) refers to an inherited myopathy characterized by an abnormal response to depolarizing neuromuscular blockers (succinylcholine) and volatile halogenated anesthetic agents (e.g., Halothane). Excessive calcium is released by the sarcoplasmic reticulum resulting in muscle rigidity and a cascade of effects including severe hyperthermia. The prevalence is estimated to be as high as 1/5,000.

Hyperthermia presents as a continuum with fever associated with infectious and inflammatory conditions and temperatures of 37.7–39°C. Heat exhaustion is a term that usually describes exertional hyperthermia presenting with temperatures of less than 40°C and muscle cramps, pain, and inability to continue active physical sports or duties. These patients have normal cognition. Heat stroke patients present with hyperthermia, temperatures typically greater than 40°C and altered sensorium progressing to seizures and coma. Initial symptoms include nausea, vomiting, headache, and syncope. They develop progressive multiple organ system failure leading to cardiorespiratory arrest if untreated.

MH patients develop severe hyperthermia and muscle rigidity accompanied by acidosis and hyperkalemia following exposure to a known trigger.[10] Historical rates of death associated with MH events were >60%. A review of the North American Malignant Hyperthermia registry from 1987 to 2006 revealed 291 severe MH events, eight cardiac arrests (2.7%) and four deaths (1.4%).

The registry certainly did not capture all events in North America. The study illustrates that even with great awareness and extensive training severe MH events leading to cardiac arrest and death may still occur.[11]

Pathophysiology

Hyperthermia results from disturbances in the normal thalamic thermo regulation. Normal adaptive responses are impaired or overwhelmed including peripheral vasodilation, sweating, and tachycardia with increased cardiac output. Excessive sweating accompanied by inadequate hydration leads to dehydration. This in turn leads to diminished cardiac output and impaired peripheral circulation diminishing heat loss. Splanchnic circulation is impaired leading to poor organ perfusion and diminished renal and hepatic function. Impaired gut perfusion has been associated with bacterial translocation and exposure to gram-negative lipopolysaccharides. Vasodilation is accompanied by increased endothelial permeability and interstitial fluid loss exacerbating hypovolemia. Inflammatory cytokine release occurs leading to progressive organ dysfunction including ARDS. The response to heat stress is increased production of heat shock proteins. Heat shock proteins help prevent protein denaturation and repair injured proteins. They protect against the effects of endotoxin exposure and attenuate cytokine release. They also reduce apoptosis. Heat acclimatization has been associated with increased levels of heat shock proteins, potentially an important protective adaptation.[12]

Diagnosis

The pathognomonic sign is severe hyperthermia accompanied by an altered sensorium. The definition of severe hyperthermia is greater than 40.5°C. Glasgow coma scale is less than 15. Patients may be experiencing severe headache, nausea, and vomiting. The skin will be hot and frequently dry. Hypoxemia accompanying acute lung injury, oliguria and acute kidney injury, coagulopathy progressing to disseminated intravascular coagulation may follow. Hyperkalemia and acidosis are common. Rhabdomyolysis will accompany hyperthermia and creatinine kinase (CK) will be significantly elevated.

The presenting history and associated medical conditions will establish the diagnosis. Careful documentation of medications is important particularly phenothiazines, anticholinergics as well as medications that affect the cardiovascular response such as beta-blockers. MH should be considered in any patient who develops sudden severe hyperthermia after exposure to a known trigger.

MH should be suspected in patients who present with elevated CK, recurrent myalgias, and in first degree relatives of patients with MH. These patients should be referred for muscle biopsy. The usual site sampled is the vastuslateralis. A 0.5 cm transverse by 1 cm longitudinal specimen of muscle should be submitted fresh to the laboratory for preparation (submit on telfa or gauze moistened with saline in a sterile container, do not immerse in saline or freeze). The procedure should be coordinated with pathology so that they are prepared to receive and process a fresh specimen. The laboratory will examine the specimen for abnormal contracture when exposed to caffeine and halothane. Additional histopathology, immunohistochemistry, and metabolic studies may be performed.

Management

The primary management of hyperthermia is resuscitation, providing airway control, oxygen, ventilation, IV access, fluid therapy, and shock management. Hyperkalemia and acidosis should be treated.

Attempts to reverse hyperthermia and cool the patient should occur immediately.

If MH is suspected dantrolene should be administered.[13]

Cooling techniques include administering cool fluids, surface cooling, and immersion therapy. Invasive techniques involving cooling catheters and the application of limited extracorporeal cooling circuits have also been described. Body cavity lavage techniques have also been used occasionally with success.[14] There are no specific drug therapies to treat exertional or environmental hyperthermia. Dantrolene as noted should be given to MH patients. Associated electrolyte disturbances and seizures should be treated appropriately.

If sepsis is suspected, cultures should be drawn and antibiotics should be immediately administered. The source should be identified and controlled as soon as possible. Other less common conditions that may be associated with severe hyperthermia should be suspected particularly when the history and physical laboratory conditions do not point to a cause. These conditions include thyroid storm, serotonin syndromes, and pheochromocytoma. Intoxication with amphetamines and like substances (ECSTASY) may present with hyperthermia. In the event of cardiac arrest standard advanced cardiac life support measures should be applied while attempts at cooling continue.

Simple cooling measures include exposing the patient and application of ice packs. Immersion in ice water is effective if the patient's condition and hospital clinic infrastructure permit. One study of distance runners with exertional hyperthermia demonstrated that immersion cooled patients in half the time required by air exposure and application of cold towels.[15]

Prognosis

With prompt recognition, diagnosis of the underlying cause and treatment, hyperthermia patients have an excellent prognosis. Greater awareness of MH has resulted in dramatic reductions in mortality. Preventive measures in sports medicine, the military, and in high-risk occupations have proven effective at reducing the risk of severe hyperthermia. The water cooling breaks at the 2014 World Cup in Brazil are an excellent example.

Reduction of environmental hyperthermia mortality associated with warm weather events such as the 2003 French experience will require greater awareness and planning by municipalities. This should be incorporated into regional disaster planning.[16]

Hypothermia and Hyperthermia are important and challenging conditions that commonly affect critically ill patients. Knowledge of the presentation, pathophysiology, and principles of management supports early and effective intervention. Restoration of normothermia reduces morbidity. It provides the critically ill patient with the greatest possibility of survival.

References

1. Rolfast CL, Lust EJ, de Cock CC. Electrocardiographic changes in therapeutic hypothermia. *Crit Care* 2012; 16(3): 1–7. Available at http://ccforum.com/content/16/3/R100.
2. Schubert A. Side effects of mild hypothermia. *J Neurosurg Anesthesiol* 1995; 7(2): 139–147.
3. Parissis H, Hamid U, Soo A, Al-Alao B. Brief review on systematic hypothermia for the protection of central nervous system during aortic arch surgery: A double-sword tool? *J Cardiothorac Surg* 2011; 6(153): 1–5. Available at http://www.pubmedcentral.nih.gov/articlerender.fcgi?artid=3231978&tool=pmcentrez&rendertype=abstract.
4. Soar J, Perkins GD, Abbas G, Alfonzo A, Barelli A, Bierens JJLM *et al.* European Resuscitation Council Guidelines for Resuscitation 2010 Section 8. Cardiac arrest in special circumstances: Electrolyte abnormalities, poisoning, drowning, accidental hypothermia, hyperthermia, asthma, anaphylaxis, cardiac surgery, trauma, pregna. *Resuscitation* 2010; 81(10): 1400–1433. Available at http://www.ncbi.nlm.nih.gov/pubmed/20956045.

5. Walpoth BH, Walpoth-Aslan BN, Mattle HP, Radanov BP, Schroth G, Schaeffler L *et al.* Outcome of survivors of accidental deep hypothermia and circulatory arrest treated with extracorporeal blood warming. *N Engl J Med* 1997; 337(21): 1500–1555. Available at http://www.ncbi.nlm.nih.gov/pubmed/9366581.
6. Sawamoto K, Bird SB, Katayama Y, Maekawa K, Uemura S, Tanno K *et al.* Outcome from severe accidental hypothermia with cardiac arrest resuscitated with extracorporeal cardiopulmonary resuscitation. *Am J Emerg Med* 2014; 32: 320–324. Available at http://www.ncbi.nlm.nih.gov/pubmed/24468125.
7. Boue Y, Lavolaine J, Bouzat P, Matraxia S, Chavanon O, Payen JF. Neurologic recovery from profound accidental hypothermia after 5 hours of cardiopulmonary resuscitation. *Crit Care Med* 2014; 42(2): e167–e170. Available at http://www.ncbi.nlm.nih.gov/pubmed/24158171.
8. Van der Ploeg GJ, Goslings JC, Walpoth BH, Bierens JJLM. Accidental hypothermia: Rewarming treatments, complications and outcomes from one university medical centre. *Resuscitation* 2010; 81(11): 1550–1555. Available at http://www.ncbi.nlm.nih.gov/pubmed/20702016.
9. Vandentorren S, Suzan F, Medina S, Pascal M, Maulpoix A, Cohen JC *et al.* Mortality in 13 French cities during the August 2003 heat wave. *Am J Public Health* 2004; 94(9): 1518–1520. Available at http://www.pubmedcentral.nih.gov/articlerender.fcgi?artid=1448485&tool=pmcentrez&rendertype=abstract.
10. Kim TW, Nemergut ME. Preparation of modern anesthesia workstations for malignant hyperthermia-susceptible patients: A review of past and present practice. *Anesthesiology* 2011; 114(1): 205–212. Available at http://www.ncbi.nlm.nih.gov/pubmed/21169802.
11. Larach MG, Brandom BW, Allen GC, Gronert GA, Lehman EB. Cardiac arrests and deaths associated with malignant hyperthermia in North America from 1987 to 2006. *Anaesthesiology* 2008; 108(4): 603–611.
12. Epstein Y, Roberts WO. The pathopysiology of heat stroke: An integrative view of the final common pathway. *Scand J Med Sci Sports* 2011; 21(6): 742–748. Available at http://www.ncbi.nlm.nih.gov/pubmed/21635561.
13. Wappler F. Anesthesia for patients with a history of malignant hyperthermia. *Curr Opin Anaesthesiol* 2010; 23(3): 417–422. Available at http://www.ncbi.nlm.nih.gov/pubmed/20173632.
14. Hadad E, Rav-acha M, Heled Y, Epstein Y, Moran DS. A review of cooling methods. *Sport Med* 2004; 34(8): 501–511.
15. Armstrong LE, Crago AE, Adams R, Roberts WO, Maresh CM. Whole-body cooling of hyperthermic runners: Comparison of two field therapies. *Am J Emerg Med* 1996; 14(4): 355–358. Available at http://www.ncbi.nlm.nih.gov/pubmed/8768154.
16. Bernard SM, McGeehin MA. Municipal heat wave response plans. *Am J Public Health* 2004; 94(9): 1520–1522. Available at http://www.pubmedcentral.nih.gov/articlerender.fcgi?artid=1448486&tool=pmcentrez&rendertype=abstract.

Chapter 10

Thrombo-Embolism in the ICU patient

Daniel Roizblatt, Andrew Beckett and Jameel Ali

Chapter Overview

In this chapter, we discuss the principles of diagnosis of venous thromboembolism, its prevention and treatment, focusing on factors that guide therapy in the ICU patient.

Risk for Venous Thromboembolism in the ICU

Venous thromboembolism (VTE) is the main cause of pulmonary embolism (PE), which is present in up to 27% of postmortem examinations, contributing to death in up to 12% of ICU patients. Of the deceased patients, there is a clinical suspicion for PE in only 30%.[1]

Virchow's Triad identifies three predisposing factors for VTE. These are hypercoagulability, as in sepsis; vascular stasis as in prolonged major surgery, prolonged bed rest in the supine position, delayed ambulation and vessel injury as in trauma.

The main risks for Deep Vein Thrombosis (DVT) in the general population are well known, including hospital or nursing home confinement, surgery, trauma, malignant neoplasm, chemotherapy, neurologic disease with paresis, central venous catheter or pacemaker, varicose veins, smoking and use of some oral contraceptives. Difficulty in applying screening and the heterogeneity of the ICU population have resulted in few publications on this issue in the ICU population. Ansari *et al.* found that the most common risk factors in medical patients were bed rest >72 hours, age >60 years and age 4,060 years. Among surgical patients the risk factors were major surgery in 80.25%, central venous access and age 40–60 years.[2] When assessing more specifically for ICU acquired risk factors for VTE/DVT, mechanical ventilation (OR 1.56), immobility (OR 2.14), femoral venous catheter (OR 2.24), sedatives (OR 1.52) and paralytic drugs (OR 4.81) were associated with higher risk. On the other hand, VTE heparin prophylaxis (OR 0.08), aspirin use (0.42) and thromboembolic disease stockings (OR 0.63) were associated with a decreased risk for VTE. Warfarin use (OR 0.07 $P = 0.01$) and intravenous heparin (OR 0.04 $P<0.01$) were associated with a significantly decreased risk of VTE.[3]

VTE Prevention

As described by Hyers *et al.* in 1995, oral anticoagulants given after unfractionated heparin, prevents PE in 95% of the patients with proximal DVT.[4]

VTE prophylaxis regimens for non-ICU patients may not necessarily be extrapolated to more critically ill patients, mainly because the risk/benefit ratio in this population for thromboprophylaxis, differs significantly from that of non-ICU patients. [1,5] However, a large meta-analysis of 7,226 patients by Alhazzani *et al.* suggests that any type of heparin thromboprophylaxis decreases deep vein thrombosis and PE in critically ill patients, and low-molecular-weight heparin compared with twice daily unfractionated heparin decreases PE. Major bleeding events and mortality rates did not appear to be significantly influenced by heparin thromboprophylaxis in this study. Therefore the main issue, in the ICU population, is to assess the risk of thromboprophylaxis and the risk of VTE. In 2012, a large multicenter study from Asia, showed that the assessment for high risk for VTE in patients varies among physicians. When using their own clinical judgment, physicians categorized only 8.4% of ICU patients as having high risk for VTE. When applying a stratification objective scale as the Caprini risk stratification, 54.9% of the patients were included in the high risk for VTE group, suggesting that objective parameters should be applied when assessing ICU patients.[6] The assessment of VTE risk and prevention was also described by the ENDORSE study published in 2008. After enrolling 68,183 patients from 32 countries they found 51.8% of the patients being at risk for VTE. In spite of this finding no more than 58.5% of the patients, were receiving adequate prophylaxis as recommended by published guidelines.[7] Similar results were reported by Tapson *et al.* in 2007 after collecting data from 15,156 patients from

12 different countries, finding that only 60% of patients who needed prophylaxis, were actually receiving it.[8] As previously discussed, ICU patients are at high risk of VTE and are prime candidates for prophylaxis. VTE prevention techniques include mechanical, chemical and inferior vena cava filters.

— Mechanical prophylaxis includes:

1. Intermittent pneumatic compression
2. Graduated compression stockings

— Chemical prophylaxis includes:

1. Unfractionated heparin
2. Low-molecular-weight heparin
3. Fondaparinux
4. Warfarin
5. Aspirin
6. Dabigatran, Rivaroxaban
7. Inferior Vena Cava filters (IVC filters)

Megan *et al.* when analyzing 30 public hospital ICU's from Australia and New Zealand, found that of 502 patients, 64% were receiving pharmacological prophylaxis, 80% mechanical prophylaxis and 44% receiving both. Patients who did not receive pharmacological prophylaxis were those having recent neurosurgery, intracranial hemorrhage or coagulopathy as well as other less frequent or not specified causes.[9]

Chemical prophylaxis is suggested in all high risk patients for VTE. ICU patients are all at high risk for VTE so they should receive chemical prophylaxis as soon as possible. The main concern when using chemical prophylaxis is the risk of bleeding, which should be assessed on a case by case basis by considering any possible source of bleeding, recent trauma or surgery etc. As to which chemical prophylactic agent to choose, the literature generally favors low molecular weight heparin while unfractionated heparin is considered as an effective agent, especially in the orthopedic literature.[16]

When chemical prophylaxis is not possible, mechanical prophylaxis should be initiated, most preferably with intermittent pneumatic compression devices (IPC) until chemical prophylaxis is possible and is then added to IPC. Although, using both chemical and mechanical prophylaxis has not been proven in the literature, the combination appears safe.[a]

[a](http://www.guideline.gov/content.aspx?id=39350).

In spite of the strong evidence supporting the use of early thromboprophylaxis in the ICU patient as soon as possible, the literature shows as few as 33% of the patients actually receive adequate prophylaxis.[10] This may be explained by ICU systems where there is no common protocol, with each physician prescribing what he/she considers appropriate. In addition, many patients fail to receive VTE prophylaxis because of the increased risk of bleeding and other complications associated with the surgery or intervention itself. Having strict protocols and quality assurance programs is necessary to ensure that the patients receive the needed prophylaxis. Regarding prevention of DVT/PE in the acutely ill patient, the use of relatively new anticoagulants such as the direct thrombin inhibitors, Rivaroxaban of Dabigatran is not recommended.

Some studies have shown that these drugs are efficient in preventing thromboembolic events in the short and long term, but the risk of bleeding increases when compared to LMWH.[11,12]

Inferior vena cava filters have been very helpful in the prophylaxis of PE disease. First described buy Trousseau in 1865, it was not until 1973 with Greenfield's percutaneous technique, that this device was considered in patients at high risk of PE but in whom anticoagulation was contraindicated. In 1990 with the availability of retrievable IVC filter devices, the use of IVC filters became more widespread in the ICU setting.[13] Decousus *et al.* in 1998, randomized two groups among 400 patients at high risk for PE, one with and the other without IVC filter. At day 12, 1.1% of the filter group had PE, compared to 4.8% in the no filter group (OR 0.22). However, in the filter group, who did not receive anticoagulation, 20.8% had recurrent DVT, compared to 11.6% in those that did not receive an IVC filter but were anticoagulated (OR 1.87). There was no statistical significant difference in mortality between the two groups.[14]

Recommendations in the literature differ on the use of Inferior Vena Cava filters.

In 2006, Kaufman *et al.* of the Society of Interventional Radiology, suggested that any patient with high risk for developing VTE should have an IVC filter inserted.[15] The 9th edition of the American College of Chest Physicians Evidence-Based Clinical Practice Guidelines for Diagnosis, Therapy and Prevention for VTE, with Level 1B recommended against IVC filter in addition to anticoagulants in patients with acute DVT of the leg.[16] However, they did recommend the use of IVC filter in patients with acute DVT of the leg, in whom anticoagulation is contraindicated because of high bleeding risk, as occurs in many ICU patients.

Sarosiek *et al.* assessed more than 900 patients with IVC filter in a level 1 Trauma center and reported that as low as 8.5% of the patients with an IVC filter, had the filter successfully removed. They also reported that 48% of VTE events, occurred in patients with no thromboembolism at time of IVC filter insertion, and that many IVC filters were inserted in patients in whom the risk for bleeding was already low, and anticoagulation could have been initiated.[13] The low retrieval rate of IVC filters have been noted also by the American Association for the Surgery of Trauma in their multicenter study regarding practice patterns of retrievable IVC filters in trauma patients, where they showed that only 22% of the filters were actually retrieved, mainly because of poor follow up of the service that inserted the filter.[13,17] The risks of not retrieving a filter are mainly recurrent in DVT, vena cava thrombosis, organ penetration and mechanical filter complications.[13] The United States Food and Drug Administration, recommends removing the filter as soon as protection from PE is no longer needed.[b]

IVC filters should therefore be used cautiously, with its main indication being the prevention of PE in patients with acute leg DVT in whom anticoagulation is contraindicated, mainly because high risk of bleeding. Patients with a filter, should be carefully monitored and the filter removed as soon as the DVT risk is no longer present. Patients with a filter should be started on anticoagulation as soon as possible (i.e., when the risk of bleeding or need for major surgery is no longer present).

At the University of Toronto, a Best Practice in General Surgery (BPIGS) guideline document has been formulated for many common general surgery issues and includes guidelines for thromboprophylaxis and their rationale based on review of the literature and the opinions of expert practitioners in the field. These guidelines (authored by Drs. Robin Mcleod, Bill Geerts and Darlene Fenech) begin by categorization of patients into (1) Low risk patients (2) General surgery patients having elective or emergency abdominal surgery (3) General surgery patients admitted with acute abdominal conditions treated nonoperatively or for observation prior to surgery. The authors' recommendation from these guidelines are summarized as follows: Low risk patients; includes outpatient surgery, minor procedures such as anorectal procedures, inguinal hernia repairs, laparoscopic cholecystectomy or breast surgery who have no additional thromboembolic risk factors. No prophylaxis is recommended with encouragement of early and frequent ambulation.

---

[b](http://www.fda.gov/MedicalDevices/Safety/AlertsandNotices/ucm396377.htm).

1. General surgery patients having elective or emergency abdominal surgery: Includes all patients having open or laparoscopic procedures regardless of age or other VTE risk factors. When there is no contraindication to anticoagulation it is recommended that these patients should have either of 2 Low molecular weight heparins: Lovenox (enoxaparin) 40 mg scq 24 hours or Fragmin (dalteparin) 5,000 units scq 24 hours starting preoperatively at 'time out' and continuing on the first postoperative day (preferably between 1,000 and 1,200) and daily thereafter until discharge.
2. In patients at high risk for bleeding, bilateral appropriately measured below knee stockings or other compressive device should be applied with daily reassessment and conversion to low molecular weight heparin when bleeding risk is decreased. Early and frequent ambulation is encouraged. Patients having surgery after 6 pm should have half the dose of Low molecular weight heparin preoperatively at "time out" and full dosing daily preferably between 1,000 and 1,200 until discharged, while encouraging early and frequent ambulation.

   Patients with epidural catheters should have the catheter introduced before surgery with the first heparin dose 2–8 hours thereafter and full doses daily. The catheter should be removed 20–24 hours after the dose of heparin and restarted 2 hours after catheter removal, encouraging early and frequent ambulation. Dosage should be adjusted according to weight as follows: <40 kg, 30 mg enoxaparin or 2,500 units dalteparin daily; 40–100 kg, 40 mg enoxaparin or 5,000 units dalteparin daily; 100–125 kg, 40 mg enoxaparin twice daily or 5,000 units dalteparin twice daily; 125–150 kg, 60 mg enoxaparin twice daily or 7,500 units dalteparin twice daily; 150–200 kg, 80 mg enoxaparin twice daily or 10,000 units dalteparin twice daily. The American Society of Regional Anesthesia guidelines recommend that epidural catheters should not be used twice daily, in the presence of, dosing of low molecular weight heparins. This should be considered and discussed with patients on an individualized basis.

   Patients with renal dysfunction: No dosage modification of Fragmin (dalteparin) is required but Lovenox (enoxaparin) should be decreased to 30 mg /day in patients with a creatinine clearance of less than 30 cc/hour.
3. Patients at very high risk of VTE e.g., those undergoing major cancer operations or with multiple risk factors should be considered for receiving low molecular weight heparin for 28 days after discharge while encouraging early and frequent ambulation.

4. General surgery patients admitted with acute abdominal conditions treated nonoperatively or for observation prior to surgery, should have Lovenox (enoxaparin) 40 mg or Fragmin (dalteparin) 500 units scq 24 hours until discharged, while encouraging early and frequent ambulation.

The above recommendations are best implemented with standardized order sheets and regular auditing of prophylaxis regimes.

Apart from General surgery, orthopedic surgery patients and neurosurgery patients constitute large population for VTE prophylaxis in the ICU.

Antithrombotic therapy and prevention of Thrombosis, 9th edition, produced by American College of Chest Physicians Evidence based clinical Practice guidelines provide recommendations based on specific procedures and patient characteristics for these and other patients.[16]

Diagnosis

Diagnosis of VTE in the general population may be facilitated by beginning with a clinical pre-test probability score. This combines risk factors that the patient has with clinical findings to determine when to perform an ultrasound and how to interpret the ultrasound result to guide further treatment or whether having a D-dimer is enough.[18,19]

However, in critical care patients the pre-test probability score lacks specificity and sensitivity because clinical findings are not reliable and risk factors are always high. Common clinical findings in the non-critical population include unilateral calf or thigh pain, leg swelling or redness. However, only 10–20% of patients investigated for DVT actually have the disease.[19]

D-dimer is a degradation product of a cross-linked fibrin blood clot that is typically elevated in patients with acute VTE, but also in the presence of non-thrombotic disorders such as recent surgeries, hemorrhage, trauma or cancer. The D-dimer level is, therefore, not suitable for critical care patients, most of whom will have at least one cause for elevation of the D-dimer level. A negative D-dimer is however useful in excluding DVT in the absence of other findings.

Imaging tests, therefore rule out VTE in the critical care setting, with Doppler ultrasound being the first choice. For PE, there are many possible tests such as conventional contrast angiography and magnetic resonance angiography, but the gold standard is the computerized tomographic pulmonary angiography (CTPA).[19]

Pretest probability of deep vein thrombosis (Wells score) is a widely used scoring system which places patients in high, moderate and low probability groups based on clinical factors such as active cancer, quadriplegia etc. The pretest probability of DVT is determined from the Wells score (calculator 1) and a D-dimer test is performed in the outpatient.

For those with a "low probability" score and a negative D-dimer, DVT is effectively ruled out. If the D-dimer test is positive, ultrasound is performed to rule out DVT.

For those in whom DVT is likely (i.e., Wells score ≥1) ultrasound is performed in all patients to rule out DVT. Diagnosis of suspected deep vein thrombosis of the lower extremity.[20]

Treatment

In 2012, the American College of Chest Physicians published the 9th edition of guidelines regarding the treatment of thromboembolic disease.[16] These guidelines were recommended for the general population, and not specifically for the ICU patient. Nevertheless, these should be applied in the ICU patient.

It is important to consider that when treating below the knee DVT, if the patient has no severe symptoms or risk factor, one of the possibilities is to do serial imaging of the lower extremities for two weeks, as in many cases the DVT will resolve without the need for anticoagulation, with a low threshold for PE. Non-ICU patients can be treated with serial imaging and no anticoagulation. Even if the patient has no severe symptoms at all ICU patients are considered as having high risk factors, so all of them should be started on anticoagulation as soon as possible, and when the risk of bleeding is controlled For acute DVT or PE parenteral anti-coagulant therapy should be started as soon as possible, as well as in the presence of above the knee DVT or below the knee DVT with severe symptoms or high risk patients for PE. All ICU patients are considered as high risk patients. Most heparin anticoagulation protocols start with 80 units/kg bolus, then increase the infusion rate by 4 units/kg per hour in most patients being treated for PE, a heparin infusion should be adjusted to a therapeutic a PTT of 1.5–2.5 times the control aPTT (aPTT range of 46–70 seconds).[16]

— Low molecular weight heparin (LMWH) or Fondaparinux is suggested over intravenous or subcutaneous unfractionated heparin.

— When possible vitamin K antagonists should be started at the same time as parenteral LMWH. LMWH should be maintained at least for five days, or until the international normalized ratio (INR) is 2 or above for at least 24 hours.

—Thrombolytic therapy may be used in patients with PE and hypotension (systolic blood pressure <90 mm Hg). The most studied agent is tissue plasminogen activator (tPA), used at dosage of 100 mg intravenously over two hours. Fibrinolytics should be administered through a peripheral vein. A clear diagnosis of a PE should be made and then confirmed with imaging before attempting thrombolysis. As thrombolysis increases the risk of bleeding, patients with absolute or major contraindications to systemic thrombolytic therapy must be excluded. These conditions include an intracranial neoplasm, recent (i.e., <2 months) intracranial or spinal surgery or trauma, history of a hemorrhagic stroke, active bleeding or a coagulopathy. Relative contraindications include; severe hypertension >200 mmHg, and recent trauma or surgery.
—Ongoing supportive care must be provided including ventilatory and inotropic support, in the ICU setting. Severe hypoxemia not responsive to supplemental oxygen or respiratory failure should prompt intubation and mechanical ventilation. Patients with coexistent right ventricular failure may develop hypotension for which the first line therapy is cautious IV fluid administration recognizing that increased right ventricular wall stress leading to ischemia and right ventricular failure may result. If the blood pressure and hemodynamic status do not improve with fluid administration, consideration should be given to initiating vasopressor therapy. The optimal vasopressor has not been identified by randomized trials. Norepinephrine, dopamine, epinephrine and dobutamine have all been used and titration of type of drug and dosage based on hemodynamic response is required. Using a combination of dobutamine and norepinephrine increases myocardial contractility while minimizing the vasodilatory effects and tendency to hypotension from dobutamine. As the dose of dobutamine is increased, the increased myocardial contractility may exceed the effects of the vasodilation allowing weaning off the norepinephrine.

Other modalities include catheter directed thrombolysis which may be used after failure of systemic use of fibrinolytics. In patients with severe enough acute PE (persistent hypotension) in whom fibrinolytic therapy is contraindicated or unsuccessful, embolectomy should be considered which may be catheter embolectomy (rheolytic, rotational, suction, thrombus fragmentation, ultrasound) or surgical embolectomy depending on availability of resources and expertise. Surgical embolectomy is a treatment of last resort with very high mortality but worth considering in spite of this because of the expected very poor outcome otherwise.[21]

Follow up therapy:

1. Treatment using oral vitamin K antagonists should be extended for 3 months for patients with proximal DVT or PE that is provoked by surgery or by a non-surgical transient risk factor.
2. For unprovoked PE extended therapy is suggested if the bleeding risk is low or moderate. This should be at least six months followed by reevaluation with Doppler ultra sound. However, ICU patients are not considered under this category, as they have at least one factor that explains their DVT, such as immobilization, ongoing sepsis or trauma, which precipitated their ICU admission.
3. In patients with active cancer extended therapy is also recommended. In this group of patients LMWH is suggested over vitamin K antagonists.

When treating DVT or PE in the ICU patient, it is important to consider patients who will be at high risk of bleeding and/or will need further surgical procedures. These patients also usually cannot receive enteral treatment. In that sense treating them with LMWH is recommended over vitamin K antagonists. LMWH has the benefit that it can be stopped only two hours before the procedure and restarted as soon as the risk of bleeding has stopped. On the other hand, for patients receiving vitamin K antagonists, anticoagulation reversal has to be made using drugs such as fresh frozen plasma or prothrombin complex concentrate, which can be more time consuming and costly, than when reversing LMWH in which case only stoppage of the drug administration is required.

It is important to consider that the ICU patients change from day to day, and that risk for VTE, as well as bleeding risk should be evaluated daily.

The surgical ICU patient presents special challenges such as the need for major surgery and risk of postoperative hemorrhage requiring consideration of more options both for therapy and prophylaxis.

1. Generally, prevention is a cornerstone of this disease, preventing as high as 95% of PE in patients with deep vein thrombosis.
2. Primary treatment is, usually with anticoagulation, which should be carefully selected and closely monitored using methods that have proven more efficacious and safe.
3. Inferior vena cava filters play an important role in the prevention of PE in ICU patients that are not candidates for anticoagulants primarily because of the risk of bleeding.

4. Patients with filters should be followed up closely and anticoagulation started as soon as the risk of bleeding permits it, with monitoring and removal of the filter as soon as possible.
5. Surgical embolectomy in its various forms as well as fibrinolytic therapy should be considered when less invasive treatment fails in the severely hemodynamically compromised patient with appropriate pharmacologic and fluid support recognizing the high mortality with these therapeutic options.

References

1. Geerts W, Selby R. Prevention of venous thromboembolism in the ICU. *Chest* 2003; 124: 357S–363S.
2. Ansari K, Dalal K, Patel M. Risk stratification and utilisation of thromboembolism prophylaxis in a medical-surgical ICU: A hospital-based study. *J Indian Med Assoc* 2007; 105: 536–540.
3. Cook D, Attia J, Weaver B *et al.* Venous thromboembolic disease: An observational study in medical-surgical intensive care unit patients. *J Crit Care* 2000; 15: 127–132.
4. Hyers TM. Antithrombotic therapy for venous thromboembolic disease. *Chest* 1995; 1–17.
5. Chan CM, Shorr AF. Venous thromboembolic disease in the intensive care unit. *Semin Respir Crit Care Med* 2010; 31: 39–46.
6. Parikh KC, Oh D, Sittipunt C *et al.* Venous thromboembolism prophylaxis in medical ICU patients in Asia (VOICE Asia): A multicenter, observational, cross-sectional study. *Thromb Res* 2012; 129: e152–e158.
7. Cohen AT, Tapson VF, Bergmann JF *et al.* Venous thromboembolism risk and prophylaxis in the acute hospital care setting: A multinational cross-sectional study. *The Lancet* 2008; 371: 387–394.
8. Tapson VF, Decousus H, Pini M *et al.* Venous thromboembolism prophylaxis in acutely ill hospitalized medical patients: Findings from the International Medical Prevention Registry on Venous Thromboembolism. *Chest* 2007; 132: 936–945.
9. Robertson MS, Nichol AD, Higgins AM *et al.* Venous thromboembolism prophylaxis in the critically ill: A point prevalence survey of current practice in Australian and New Zealand intensive care units. *Crit Care Resusc* 2010; 12: 9–15.
10. Ryskamp RP, Trottier SJ. Utilization of venous thromboembolism prophylaxis in a medical-surgical ICU. *Chest* 1998; 113: 162–164.
11. Albertsen IE, Larsen TB, Rasmussen LH *et al.* Prevention of venous thromboembolism with new oral anticoagulants versus standard pharmocological treatment in acutely ill patients: A systemic review and meta-analysis. *Drugs* 2012; 72: 1755–1764.

12. Cohen AT, Spiro TE, Büller HR *et al.* Rivaroxaban for thromboprophylaxis in acutely ill medical patients. *N Engl J Med* 2013; 368: 513–523.
13. Sarosiek S, Crowther M, Sloan JM. Indications, complications, and management of inferior vena cava filters. *JAMA Intern Med* 2013; 173: 513.
14. Decousus H, Leizorovicz A, Parent F *et al.* A clinical trial of vena caval filters in the prevention of pulmonary embolism in patients with proximal deep-vein thrombosis. Prévention du Risque d'Embolie Pulmonaire par Interruption Cave Study Group. *N Engl J Med* 1998; 338: 409–415.
15. Kaufman JA, Kinney TB, Streiff MB *et al.* Guidelines for the use of retrievable and convertible vena cava filters: Report from the Society of Interventional Radiology multidisciplinary consensus conference. 2006; 200–212.
16. Bates SM, Jaeschke R, Stevens SM *et al.* Diagnosis of DVT: Antithrombotic therapy and prevention of thrombosis, 9th ed.: American College of Chest Physicians Evidence-Based Clinical Practice Guidelines. *Chest* 2012; 141: e351S–418S.
17. Karmy-Jones R, Jurkovich GJ. Practice patterns and outcomes of retrievable vena cava filters in trauma patients: An AAST multicenter study. *J Trauma-Injury Infec and Crit Care* 2007; 62: 17–24.
18. Paramo JA, de Gaona ER, Garcia R *et al.* Diagnosis and management of deep venous thrombosis. *Rev Med Univ Navarra* 2007; 51: 13–17.
19. Wells P, Anderson D. The diagnosis and treatment of venous thromboembolism. *Hematology Am Soc Hematol Educ Program* 2013; 2013: 457–463.
20. Brydon JG. Diagnosis of suspected deep vein thrombosis of the lower extremity. *Forthcoming* 2015; 17 [cited 2015 Jan 9].
21. Victor FT. Fibrinolytic (thrombolytic) therapy in acute pulmonary embolism and lower extremity deep vein thrombosis. *Forthcoming* 2015; 1–3 [cited 2015 Jan 9].

Chapter 11

Broad Principles of Antibiotic Usage and Surgical Antimicrobial Prophylaxis

Jameel Ali and Addison K. May

Chapter Overview

Antibiotic usage is very common in the surgical intensive care unit (ICU) both for management of infection as well as prevention of anticipated infection. Rational use of antibiotics requires an understanding of their role and limitations in preventing infections, antibacterial spectrum of the various antibiotics, and their potential risks, particularly their contribution to the development of resistant infectious complications. In this chapter, we discuss some broad general principles of antibiotic usage, followed by principles of surgical antimicrobial prophylaxis to guide the intensivist in the rational effective use of these agents.

A Listing And Brief Considerations of Broad General Principles of Antibiotic Usage

A. Rational use of antibiotics is important not only for treating and preventing infection but also to avoid complications, including antibiotic resistance.

B. Generally, broad spectrum antibiotics should be avoided when a narrower spectrum more specific agent is available.

The selective influence of exposure to broad spectrum antibiotics on subsequent resistant pathogens is demonstrated in a study by May *et al.* Prior to 2002, Vanderbilt University Medical Centre, a Level 1 Trauma Centre with over 3,000 adult trauma admissions per year, utilized broad spectrum antibiotics (ceftriaxone plus vancomycin plus/minus metronidazole) for intracranial pressure monitor prophylaxis during the course of monitor placement. In April 2002, this practice was changed to narrow spectrum antibiotic prophylaxis with cefazolin at the time of insertion. The overall broad spectrum utilization decreased from 100% in 2002 to less than 20% in 2003. No significant change in the rate of CNS infections occurred as result, although the absolute percent was lower in the narrow prophylaxis group (1.8% with narrow spectrum coverage and 4.0% with broad spectrum coverage, $p > 0.05$).[1] However, patients receiving broad spectrum antibiotics are more likely to be associated with subsequent infections with resistant pathogens. Patients receiving broad versus narrow prophylaxis had a significant increase in the frequency of infections with *Acinetobacter species* (21% versus 13% of pathogens), an increase in resistance of gram-negative pathogens (average resistance to gram-negative classes — 47% in the broad group versus 20% in the narrow group, $p < 0.01$), and a very significant increase in multidrug resistant pathogens (72% versus 23%, $p < 0.01$).

Recent systematic reviews and meta-analyses[2] have allowed examination of important questions regarding combination versus monotherapy. These reviews have clarified the following issues:

(1) In patients who have sepsis, beta-lactam-aminoglycoside combination therapy does not improve patient outcome including mortality, when compared with beta-lactam monotherapy.
(2) In patients with sepsis, broad spectrum beta-lactam monotherapy is associated with improved outcomes when compared with similar spectrum beta-lactam-aminoglycoside combination therapy.
(3) Clinical evidence is lacking for patients who have serious gram-negative and Pseudomonas aeruginosa infections; currently there is no evidence to show that combination therapy improves patient related outcomes in these infections.
(4) Beta-lactam aminoglycoside combination therapy has not been shown to prevent the development of resistance that will have clinical implications for the individual patient.

(5) Among patients with cystic fibrosis, combination therapy might have some microbiological benefit but does not translate to improved patient-related outcomes.
(6) Combination therapy for gram-positive infections and endocarditis is unsupported currently by evidence from randomized trials or prospective studies. The few existing data do not point to an advantage for combination therapy.

Mechanisms of antimicrobial resistance for gram-negative bacteria include:

- Beta-lactamase production;
- Outer membrane impermeability and changes in porins;
- Efflux pumps;
- Degrading and antibiotic-altering enzymes;
- DNA gyrase mutations.

Antibiotic exposure is, however, the single strongest risk factor for subsequent antibiotic-resistant bacterial infection as indicated in the following table:

Author	Year	Study setting	Findings and odds ratio
Trouillet	1998	Risk factors for drug resistant VAP	Prior AB exposure: OR 13.46 Broad AB exposure: OR 4.12
Kollef	1999	Resistant pathogens in nosocomial MICU and SICU	Prior AB exposure: OR 3.39
Harbarth	2000	Surgical prophylaxis following CABG	AB>48 hours increases gram negative resistance: OR 1.6
Velmahos	2002	Severely injured trauma patients	AB>24 hours: OR 2.13
Chastre	2003	Randomized trial of eight days versus 15 days Rx VAP	Significant increase in subsequent resistant infections
May	2006	ICP monitor prophylaxis in trauma	Broad, extended prophylaxis: 3X increase in subsequent MDR infections

Certain classes of antibiotics have a greater likelihood of selecting for resistance as follows:

Broad spectrum cephalosporins:
Methicillin-resistant Staphylococcus aureus (MRSA), Vancomycin-resistant Enterococcus (VRE), C. difficile, ESBLs, *Acinetobacter*

Quinolones:
MRSA, multiply resistant gram-negatives

Vancomycin:
MRSA, VRE

Clindamycin:
C. difficile

C. Timing of initiation and duration of antibiotics are important factors.

Kumar *et al.*[3] demonstrated in 2,731 patients with septic shock and a mortality rate of 56% that time to antibiotic treatment was strongly associated with outcome. With each half hour delay there was a 12% increase in risk of death.

In a prospective, randomized, double blind clinical trial including 401 patients with VAP, Chastre *et al.*[4] compared 197 patients assigned to eight days and 204 to 15 days of antibiotic treatment. There was no difference in mortality (18.8% versus 12.2%) or recurrent infections (28.9% versus 26.0%) but the eight day group had more antibiotic free days (13.1 versus 8.7). Among patients who developed recurrent infections multi resistant pathogens emerged less frequently in the eight day treated group.

In intra-abdominal infection, risk of therapeutic failure is increased when there is:

- Inadequate source control;
- Low albumin;
- High severity of illness (APACHE 11–15);
- Need for vasopressors;
- Diffuse peritonitis;
- Nosocomial origin;
- Comorbidity;
- Advanced age.

The Surgical Infection Society (SIS) guidelines for duration of antimicrobial therapy[5,6] are:

- Antibiotic should be limited to no more than 5–7 days with the decision based on operative findings or upon resolution of fever or leukocytosis.
- Continued clinical evidence of infection at the end of antibiotic treatment should prompt a search for residual infection rather than prolonged therapy.
- In the absence of adequate source control, prolonged antibiotic therapy is warranted.

At the Vanderbilt University Medical Centre Critical Surgical Care Unit our approach to antibiotic therapy is as follows:

- Prophylaxis should only be instituted if there is proven efficacy.
- Broad empiric coverage when necessary should be based on unit specific criteria.
- The narrowest spectrum agent with proven efficacy (de-escalation) should be used.
- The least number of agents and least number of doses with equal efficacy, and dosed aggressively should be used.
- The shortest course with equal efficacy should be used.

If there are signs of infection, search aggressively for site and culture with 'gold standard' techniques.

- If empirical treatment is required before cultures, treat suspected infected site based on most common pathogens for that site.
- If the signs/symptoms are inadequate to suggest the site of infection, do not treat.

In an attempt to promote rational use of antibiotics in the ICU and prevent complications such as the development of antibiotic resistance, Antibiotic Stewardship programs such as those at Vanderbilt University Centre have been initiated. The Stewardship protocols include components on:

- Antibiotic prophylaxis regimes;
- Diagnosis and treatment of pneumonia utilizing quantitative broncho alveolar lavage;

- Diagnosis and treatment of sepsis;
- Antibiotic de-escalation and defined antibiotic courses;
- Hand hygiene program;
- Transfusion guidelines;
- Intensive insulin control;
- Critical care nutrition guidelines;
- VAP bundle (head of bed elevated, oral hygiene, daily spontaneous breathing trials, ICU;
- Sedation/analgesia-scale);
- Stress ulcer/DVT prevention;
- Central line insertion and management;
- Lung protective ventilator protocol.

The antibiotic rotation strategies taught in the Stewardship program have been shown to contribute to a reduction in gram-negative resistant pathogens[7] with a relative change in infection rate from 67–90%. These stewardship programs can be associated with reduced use of broad spectrum antibiotics and a decline in resistant infections over time with significant impact on patient care and outcome.

D. When there is a choice between a bacteriostatic and bacteriocidal agent, the choice should be bacteriocidal unless issues such as toxicity dictate otherwise.
E. One of the first questions that should be answered early in the decision to initiate antibiotic therapy is whether antibiotics are required. Fever may be due to non-infectious causes and when present the infection is frequently non-bacterial and antibiotics could prove harmful.[8] In the presence of a drainable source of infection such as an abscess, prompt drainage would usually avoid antibiotic treatment.
F. Choice of antibiotics is important and depends primarily on etiology of the infection but other patient factors and even cost may influence the choice. The etiology is frequently suggested by clinical presentation including site of the infection even before availability of laboratory culture results. Laboratory reports must be interpreted cautiously to rule out normal flora or contaminants. A positive clinical response is more important in deciding to continue the antibiotics than reliance on sensitivity results. The antibiotic's ability to be absorbed orally, its ability to be concentrated in specific tissue and to cross the blood brain barrier are all

important features to be considered. For instance, an antibiotic with a high urinary concentration would be more appropriately used to treat a urinary tract infection than one which has a lower urinary concentration.

G. The route of administration is determined by the Gastrointestinal (GI) absorption of the drug and the ability to use the gut. Frequently, even when oral absorption is possible, initial doses should be given parenterally for rapidity of onset and reliability of blood levels especially in urgent cases with findings such as hyper or hypothermia tachycardia and hypotension suggesting systemic sepsis. Drug–drug interaction with non-antibacterials may alter the blood level of antibiotics and drug dosage adjustment may be required.
H. Cost also is an important determining factor when not only cost per dose but for the entire duration of treatment should be considered.
I. Antibiotics all have variable toxicity profiles which are dose related. Choice of antibiotics and manner of administration must be taken into account in relation to toxicity particularly in patients with comorbidities most notably renal and hepatic disorders. Close monitoring of drug levels is essential to limit toxicity.
J. Patient factors must also be considered when administering antibiotics e.g., age and genetic abnormalities such as the administration of sulfonamides in patients with glucose-6-phosphate dehydrogenase deficiency.
K. In approaching patient factors, two concepts, among others, are worth considering: pharmacokinetics and pharmacodynamics.[9,10]

Pharmacokinetics relates to the time course of drug absorption, distribution, metabolism and excretion and its principles are applied to optimize drug therapy in an individual patient. Pharmacodynamics refers to the relationship between drug concentration and effect or toxicity. Each antibiotic has its own pharmacokinetic profile. Each class of antimicrobials has its own unique kill or inhibitory characteristics on bacteria. Dosing regimens should use these characteristics to optimize outcomes and minimize antimicrobial resistance recognizing that these profiles change over time particularly in critically ill patients warranting frequent reassessment of dosing regimens. Although these pharmacokinetic changes are highly variable in the ICU patient they may be more predictable if basic antibiotic characteristics (e.g., lipophilic or hydrophilic) are known and changes in patient characteristics such as volume status, end organ perfusion or function and pathophysiologic characteristics related to systemic inflammation and change in hemodynamics are considered. For instance, hydrophilic antibiotics such as beta-lactams, aminoglycosides, vancomycin, linezolid, and colistin have a low volume of distribution with predominantly renal clearance with associated low intracellular penetration, whereas lipophilic antibiotics such as fluoroquinolones, macrolides, clindamycin, and tigecycline have high volume of distribution, with predominantly hepatic clearance and good intracellular concentration. In critically ill patients the variability in pharmacokinetics leads to variability in antimicrobial concentration making it less likely to reach pharmacodynamics targets with resultant risk of treatment failure and increased risk of antimicrobial resistance. This is compounded by the effect of critical illness on volume of distribution and clearance of antibiotics. The septic patient is particularly vulnerable to changes in volume of distribution. For example, aggressive fluid resuscitation, the increased extravascular volume from systemic inflammation and associated capillary leak, third spacing of albumin and high output fistulas through postsurgical drains can result in an increase in volume of distribution with associated decreasing antibiotic serum concentration particularly with hydrophilic drugs such as aminoglycosides and beta-lactams. Other characteristics of the septic patient may also affect drug clearance. For example the hyper dynamic state can increase both creatinine clearance and hepatic perfusion leading to increased drug clearance. End organ dysfunction can reduce metabolism and elimination of drugs leading to decreased clearance. In addition, adaptive mechanisms in MOF can increase clearance in the presence of renal failure e.g., gastrointestinal clearance of ciprofloxacin is increased in renal failure. Also, biliary clearance of piperacillin increases in renal failure.

The relationship between half-life of the drug ($T½$), volume of distribution (V_d) and drug clearance (Cl) is $T1/2 = 0.693 \times V_d / \mathrm{Cl}$. From this equation there is the expected prolonged half-life accompanying decreased clearance but unexpected prolongation of half-life also results from increased volume of distribution.

Protein binding is also a potential source of variability in both clearance and volume of distribution. However, this is only relevant for highly protein bound drugs. Most antibiotics have low protein binding. Notable exceptions are: ceftriaxone (95% bound), ertapenem, teicoplainin, aztreonam, and daptomycin.

The above discussion emphasizes that there are huge inter patient and intrapatient variability in pharmacokinetics which is exaggerated in the ICU patient making our dosing strategy frequently unreliable with frequent failure to reach pharmacodynamic targets. A strategic approach to these problems includes: recognizing their presence; monitoring patients' clinical response and changes in pathophysiologic status that would prompt changes in antibiotic dosing strategies; frequent reevaluation of antimicrobial dosing as clinical changes result in changes in volume of distribution and clearance over time.

L. As pointed out above, duration of treatment is an important factor and a good principle is to limit duration to the period by which the signs and symptoms of infection have resolved and avoid prolonged administration in order to limit the emergence of resistant organisms or super infection. Certain infections require longer duration e.g., endocarditis — 4 weeks, tuberculosis — 4–6 weeks, and osteomyelitis — 4 weeks.
M. Monitoring response to treatment allows determining whether to (a) increase the level by changing routes from oral to intravenous, increasing dosage or spectrum, (b) continue with the chosen regime, (c) decreasing level of treatment-intravenous to oral, decreasing dose or spectrum, and (d) stop antibiotics when the infection has resolved, or the diagnosis has changed.
N. Causes of non-response to antibiotics include:
   (1) Resistant organism;
   (2) Incorrect diagnosis;
   (3) Dose, choice or route is inappropriate;
   (4) Inability to reach the infection site;
   (5) Undrained pus;
   (6) Foreign body or devitalized tissue that requires removal;
   (7) Secondary infection;
   (8) Non-compliance.

These causes should all be pursued by appropriate laboratory and clinical assessment in order to guide therapy.

Surgical Antimicrobial Prophylaxis

Postsurgical wound infection increases morbidity, length of stay and mortality in patients including those in the ICU. Effective antimicrobial prophylaxis is aimed at decreasing these sequelae and is a proven strategy for preventing postsurgical infection rates when there is adherence to clinically proven guidelines. The most recent published guidelines for antimicrobial prophylaxis in surgery was published in 2013[11] having been developed jointly by the American Society of Health-System Pharmacists (AHSP), the

Infectious Diseases Society of America (IDSA), SIS and the Society for Healthcare Epidemiology of America (SHEA). These guidelines are an update of the 1999 guidelines[12] and provide a standardized approach to the use of antimicrobials for the prevention of surgical site infections. The discussion of surgical antimicrobial prophylaxis in this chapter is based on these recently published guidelines and includes: identification of the topics updated, level of evidence used, common principles of surgical prophylaxis and common pathogens. The chapter concludes with two tables reprinted, with permission, exactly as they appear online or in print (the hyperlink to the guidelines is: http://www.ashp.org/DocLibrary/Best Practices/TGSurgery.aspx).

The guidelines document classifies prophylaxis or the prevention of an infection as: Primary — the prevention of an initial infection; Secondary — prevention of recurrence or reactivation of a previous infection; and Eradication–elimination of a colonized organism to prevent the development of an infection. The document focuses on primary perioperative prophylaxis. The level of evidence used for formulating the guidelines are categorized as:

Level 1 (evidence from large, well-conducted, randomized, and controlled trials or a meta-analysis);
Level 11 (evidence from small well-conducted, randomized controlled clinical trials);
Level 111 (evidence from well-conducted cohort studies);
Level 1V (evidence from well-conducted case-control studies);
Level V (evidence from uncontrolled studies that were not well-conducted);
Level V1 (conflicting evidence that tends to favor the recommendation), or
Level V11 (expert opinion or data extrapolated from evidence for general principles and other procedures).

The guidelines state that this system has been used by the Agency for Healthcare Research and Quality, and ASHP, IDSA, SIS, and SHEA support it as an acceptable method for organizing strength of evidence for a variety of therapeutic or diagnostic recommendations.[13] Each recommendation was categorized according to the strength of evidence that supports the use or non-use of antimicrobial prophylaxis as category 'A' for Levels 1–111, 'B' for Levels 1V–V1, 'C' for Level V11.

The guidelines further state that when higher level data are not available, a category C recommendation represents a consensus of expert panel members based on their experience, extrapolation from other procedures with similar microbial or other clinical features, and available published literature.

In these cases, the expert panel also extrapolated general principles and evidence from other procedures. Some recommendations include alternative approaches in situations in which panel members were divided.

In some cases, prophylaxis is recommended on the basis of severity of the potential complications of postoperative infection despite the lack of statistical support e.g., an infected artificial device that is not easily removable.

Classification of Wounds

Wounds are classified using the National Healthcare Safety Network Criteria[14] and included as a separate appendix in the guidelines document. As in the 1999 guidelines, four classes of wounds are described:

(1) Clean — an uninfected operative wound with no inflammation and the respiratory, alimentary, genital or urinary tracts are not entered. These are primarily closed wounds or those with closed drainage. Incisional wounds for blunt trauma are including in this category if the other criteria are met.
(2) Clean-contaminated — operative wounds in which the respiratory, alimentary, genital or urinary tracts are entered under controlled conditions, without unusual contamination. Biliary, tract, appendix, vagina, oropharynx operations without evidence of infection or major break in technique are included in this category.
(3) Contaminated — open, fresh, accidental wounds or those with major breaks in sterile techniques or gross spillage from the gastrointestinal tract and incisions with acute, non-purulent inflammation.
(4) Dirty or Infected — old traumatic wounds with retained devitalized tissue and those with existing clinical infection or perforated viscera. This suggests that the organisms causing the infection were in the operative field before the operation.

In a separate Appendix, the guidelines document includes National Healthcare Safety Network Criteria for defining a Surgical-Site Infection (SSI)[15] as follows:

Superficial incisional SSI — occurs within 30 days postoperatively involving skin or subcutaneous tissue of the incision and at least one of: purulent drainage from the superficial incision; organisms isolated from aseptically obtained culture of fluid or tissue from the superficial incision; at least one of the following signs or symptoms of infection: pain, tenderness, localized swelling, redness, heat, and superficial incision is deliberately opened by the surgeon and is culture positive or not cultured and diagnosis of a superficial incisional SSI by the surgeon or attending physician.

Deep incisional SSI — occurs within 30 days after the operative procedure if no implant is left in place or within one year if implant is in place and the infection appears to be related, involves deep soft tissues (e.g., fascia, muscle) of the incision and the patient has at least one of the following: purulent drainage from the deep incision but not from the organ/space component of the surgical site; a deep incision spontaneously dehisces or is deliberately opened by a surgeon and is culture positive or not cultured and the patient has at least one of: fever > 38°C, or localized pain or tenderness; an abscess or other evidence of infection of the deep incision found in direct examination, during re-operation or by histopathologic or radiologic examination: diagnosis of a deep incisional SSI by a surgeon or attending physician.

Organ/Space SSI — involves any part of the body excluding the skin incision, fascia or muscle layers that is opened or manipulated during the operative procedure. Specific sites are assigned to organ/space SSI to further identify the location of the infection e.g., endocarditis, endometritis, mediastinitis, vaginal cuff, and osteomyelitis.

Organ/space SSI must meet the following criteria: infection occurs within 30 days of procedure if no implant is in place or within one year if implant is in place and the infection appears to be related to the operative procedure; infection affects any part of the body excluding the skin incision, fascia, muscle, that is opened or manipulated during the operative procedure and the patient has at least one of: purulent drainage from a drain placed through a stab wound into the organ/space; organisms isolated from an aseptically obtained culture of fluid or tissue in the organ/space; an abscess or other evidence of infection involving the organ/space that is found on direct examination, during operation or by histopathologic or radiologic examination; and diagnosis of an organ/space SSI by a surgeon cum attending physician.

Generally, prophylaxis is reserved for clean-contaminated, contaminated or dirty wound operations. In clean operations, prophylaxis is justified when consequences of infection could be serious e.g., cardiac operations or orthopedic implants. Patient factors may also dictate prophylaxis e.g., old age, malignancy, malnutrition, steroid use, and immune suppression.

The Key Updates in the Revised Guidelines are

(1) Preoperative Dose Timing — the present time frame is more specific than the previous "at induction". The recommended optimal time is now within 60 minutes before the incision. Some agents like fluoroquinolones and vancomycin require one to two hours of administration and should therefore begin within 120 minutes before the incision.

(2) Selection and Dosing — the need for repeat dosing for prolonged operations is emphasized based on the half-life of the agent used. If the procedure lasts twice the half-life or longer, of the drug, repeat dosing is recommended. This requires knowledge of the half-life of the drugs used in prophylaxis. Intraoperative re-dosing is essential to maintain adequate serum and tissue levels of the drug which may also be required in major blood loss or massive fluid shifts or other circumstances affecting drug levels.

The influence of patient's weight on dosing is discussed[16] because of the link between obesity and SSI's. As mentioned in the guidelines document a non-randomized study comparing gastroplasty morbidly obese patients with control patients undergoing general surgery, both groups receiving 1 gm of cefazolin preoperatively, demonstrated consistently lower blood and tissue levels of the drug, below the MIC's needed for prophylaxis. In the second phase of the study, a preoperative dose of 2 gm cefazolin was associated with adequate blood and tissue levels for prophylaxis with a decreased rate of SSI's compared to the group receiving 1 gm preoperative dosing. Although the optimum preoperative prophylactic dose of cefazolin has not been established, it seems justified to administer 2 gm for patients greater than 80 kg and 3 gm for patients weighing over 120 kg because of the low cost and low toxicity profile of the drug.[17,18] similar prophylactic dose adjustments for the obese patients should be considered for other agents.

(3) Duration of Prophylaxis —a shortened postoperative course of prophylactic antibiotic with one dose or continuation for less than 24 hours is recommended. The need for continuing prophylaxis in the presence of indwelling drains and intravascular catheters is not supported in the new guidelines.

(4) Common Principles —there is a section devoted to principles common to all procedures in the guidelines document and new recommendations for plastic surgery, urology, cardiac, and thoracic procedures are added.

Clinical Applications of the Guidelines

As mentioned in the guidelines, patients with renal or hepatic dysfunction are not specifically singled out but, in general, single dose prophylaxis should not require adjustment based on the presence of these disorders. Local resources, clinician experience, availability or non-availability of agents, institutional patterns of sepsis, and resistance are just a few conditions that would dictate prophylaxis regimes that are different from the guidelines. The dynamic nature of scientific information and technology requires periodic review of the guidelines to be consistent with the changing state of medical knowledge in the field.

Although the guidelines focus on antimicrobial prophylaxis, they recognize that many other factors impact on SSI rate such as basic infection control strategies, surgical experience and technique, duration, the physical environment, sterilization issues, preoperative preparation, perioperative management and the underlying condition of the patient such as extremes of age, nutritional status, obesity, diabetes mellitus, tobacco use, remote infections, altered immune status, corticosteroid use, preoperative length of hospitalization, and colonization with microorganisms.

Regarding colonization, roughly 30% of SSI's in the USA are due to *S. aureus* and colonization particularly in the nares occurs in roughly 25% with increased risk of SSI by 2–14 fold.[19] Preoperative screening for *S. aureus* carriers followed by decolonization is practiced frequently but the data supporting uniform screening in the surgical population are controversial.[20, 21] *S. aureus* decolonization is practised in many centers following positive colonization results particularly for MRSA and prompting addition of antimicrobials such as vancomycin to the prophylactic regime to decrease SSI.

The FDA has approved intranasal mupirocin to eradicate MRSA nasal colonization in adult patients and health care workers.[22] Recent studies have demonstrated a decrease in SSI with *S. aureus* decolonization of the anterior nares.[23] Cardiac and orthopedic patients have seen the greatest use of mupirocin, most commonly administered for five days preoperatively, (although other regimens are used) as an adjunct to other prophylactic preoperative antimicrobials.

Common Principles

The following principles common to surgical prophylaxis are identified in the guidelines. The agent should: (1) prevent SSI, (2) prevent SSI related morbidity and mortality, (3) reduce the duration and cost of health care, (4) produce no adverse effects, and (5) have no adverse consequences for the microbial flora of the patient or hospital.

To achieve these goals, as mentioned in the guidelines the antimicrobial agent should be (1) active against the pathogens most likely to contaminate the surgical site, (2) given in an appropriate dosage and at a time that ensures adequate serum and tissue concentrations during the period of potential contamination, (3) Safe, and (4) administered for the shortest effective period to minimize adverse effects, the development of resistance and costs.

Common Surgical Pathogens

As described in the guidelines document, the predominant organisms in clean procedures are skin flora, including *S. aureus* and coagulase negative staphylococci e.g., *Staphylococcus epidermidis*. In clean contaminated procedures including abdominal procedures and heart, kidney and liver transplantations the predominant organisms include gram negative rods and enterococci in addition to skin flora.

Agents that are FDA approved for surgical antimicrobial prophylaxis are mentioned in the guidelines and include cefazolin, cefuroxime, cefoxitin, cefotetan, ertapenem and vancomycin. However, in order to control vancomycin resistance, this agent is not recommended for routine prophylaxis for any procedure. Each institution is encouraged to develop specific guidelines for vancomycin prophylaxis. When used, it can certainly be administered as a single dose because of its long half-life.

Allergy to beta-lactam antimicrobials is given special emphasis in the guidelines for antimicrobial prophylaxis because these agents, including cephalosporins are the mainstay of surgical antimicrobial prophylaxis as well as the most commonly implicated when allergic reactions occur. Because the predominant organisms in SSI's after clean procedures are gram positive, the guidelines suggest that the inclusion of vancomycin may be appropriate for a patient with a life threatening allergy to beta-lactam antimicrobials.

Although true Type 1 (immunoglobulin E) cross allergy between penicillins, cephalosporins and carbapenems are uncommon, the guidelines suggest that cephalosporins and carbapenems should not be used for surgical antimicrobial prophylaxis in patients with documented or presumed Immunoglobulin E (IgE) mediated penicillin allergy.

Surgical antimicrobial prophylaxis can alter individual and institutional bacterial flora leading to changes in colonization rates and increased bacterial

Table 1. Recommended Doses and Redosing Intervals for Commonly Used Antimicrobiais for Surgical Prophylaxis

	Recommended Dose			
Antimicrobial	**Adults**[a]	**Pediatrics**[b]	**Half-life in Adults with Normal Renal Function, hr**[19]	**Recommended Redosing Interval (From Initiation of Preoperative Dose), hr**[c]
Ampicillin–sulbactam	3g (ampicillin 2 g/sulbactam 1 g)	50 mg/kg of the ampicillin component	0.8–1.3	2
Ampicillin	2 g	50 mg/kg	1–1.9	2
Aztreonam	2 g	30 mg/kg	1.3–2.4	4
Cefazolin	2 g, 3 g for pts weighing ≥ 120 kg	30 mg/kg	1.2–2.2	4
Cefuroxime	1.5 g	50 mg/kg	1–2	4
Cefotaxime	1 g[d]	50 mg/kg	0.9–1.7	3
Cefoxitin	2 g	40 mg/kg	0.7–1.1	2
Cefotetan	2 g	40 mg/kg	2.8–4.6	6
Ceftriazone	2 g[e]	50–75 mg/kg	5.4–10.9	NA
Ciprofloxacin[f]	400 mg	10 mg/kg	3–7	NA
Clindamycin	900 mg	10 mg/kg	2–4	6
Ertapenem	1 g	15 mg/kg	3–5	NA
Fluconazole	400 mg	6 mg/kg	30	NA

Gentamicin[g]	5 mg/kg based on dosing weight (single dose)	2.5 mg/kg based on dosing weight	2–3	NA
Levofloxacin[f]	500 mg	10 mg/kg	6–8	NA
Metronidazole	500 mg	15 mg/kg Neonates weighing <1200 g should receive a single 7.5 mg/kg dose	6–8	NA
Moxifloxacin[f]	400 mg	10 mg/kg	8–15	NA
Piperacillin–tazobactam	3.375 g	Infants 2–9 mo: 80 mg/kg of the piperacillin component Children >9 mo and ≤40 kg: 100 mg/kg of the piperacillin component	0.7–1.2	2
Vancomycin	15 mg/kg	15 mg/kg	4–8	NA
Oral antibiotics for colorectal surgery prophyi axis (used in conjuction with a mechanical bowel preparation)				

(*Continued*)

Table 1. (*Continued*)

Antimicrobial	Recommended Dose		Half-life in Adults with Normal Renal Function, hr[19]	Recommended Redosing Interval (From Initiation of Preoperative Dose), hr[c]
	Adults[a]	Pediatrics[b]		
Erythromycin base	1 g	20 mg/kg	0.8–3	NA
Metronidazole	1 g	15 mg/kg	6–10	NA
Neomycin	1 g	15 mg/kg	2–3 (3% absorbed under normal gastrointestinal conditions)	NA

[a] Adult doses are obtained from the studies cited in each section. When doses differed between studies, expert opinion used the most-often recommended dose.

[b] The maximum pediatric dose should not exceed the usual adult dose.

[c] For antimicrobials with a short half-life (e.g., cefazolin, cefoxitin) used before long procedures, redosing in the operating room is recommended at an interval of approximately two times the half-life of the agent in patients with normal renal function. Recommended redosing intervals marked as "not applicable" (NA) are based on typical case length; for unusually long procedures, redosing may be needed.

[d] Although FDA-approved package insert labeling indicates 1 g, 14 experts recommend 2 g for obese patients.

[e] When used as a single dose in combination with metronidazole for colorectal procedures.

[f] While fluoroquinolones have been associated with an increased risk of tendinitis/tendon repture in all ages, use of these agents for single-dose prophylaxis is generally safe.

[g] In general, gentamicin for surgical antibiotic prophylaxis should be limited to a single dose given preoperatively. Dosing is based on the patient's actual body weight. If the patient's actual weight is more than 20% above ideal body weight (IBW), the dosing weight (DW) can be determined as follows: DW = IBW + 0.4(actual weight – IBW).

Originally published in American Society of Health-System Pharmacists. Clinical practice guidelines for antimicrobial prophylaxiz in surgery. *Am J Health-syst. Pharm.* 2013; 70:195–283

Table 2. Recommendations for Surgical Antimicrobial Prophylaxis

Type of Procedure	Recommended Agents[a,b]	Alternative Agents in Patients with β-Lactam Allergy	Strength of Evidence[c]
Cardiac			
Cardiac device insertion procedures	Cefazolin, cefuroxime	Clindamycin,[d] vancomycin[d]	A
(e.g., pacemaker implantation)	Cefazolin, cefuroxime	Clindamycin, vancomycin	A
Ventricular assist devices	Cefazolin, cefuroxime	Clindamycin, vancomycin	C
Thoracic			
Noncardiac procedures, including lobectomy, pneumonectomy, lung resection, and thoracotomy	Cefazolin, ampicillin–sulbactam	Clindamycin,[d] vancomycin[d]	A
Video-assisted thoracoscopic surgery	Cefazolin, ampicillin–sulbactam	Clindamycin,[d] vancomycin[d]	C
Gastroduodenale			
Procedures involving entry into lumen of gastrointestinal tract (bariatric, pancreaticoduodenectomy[f])	Cefazolin	Clindamycin or vancomycin + aminoglycoside[g] or aztreonam or fluoroquinolone[h–j]	A
Procedures without entry into gastrointestinal tract (antireflux, highly selective vagotomy) for high-risk patients	Cefazolin	Clindamycin or vancomycin + aminoglycoside[g] or aztreonam or fluoroquinolone[h–j]	A
Biliary tract			
Open procedure	Cefazolin, cefoxitin, cefotetan, ceftriaxone,[k] ampicillin–sulbactam[h]	Clindamycin or vancomycin + aminoglycoside[g] or aztreonam or fluoroquinolone[h–j]	A

(*Continued*)

Table 2. (*Continued*)

Type of Procedure	Recommended Agents[a,b]	Alternative Agents in Patients with b-Lactam Allergy	Strength of Evidence[c]
		Metronidazole + aminoglycoside[g] or fluoroquinolone[h–j]	A
Laparoscopic procedure			
Elective, low-risk[l]	None	None	A
Elective, high-risk[l]	Cefazolin, cefoxitin, cefotetan, ceftriaxone,[k] ampicillin–sulbactam[h]	Clindamycin or vancomycin + aminoglycoside[g] or aztreonam or fluoroquinolone[h–j]	A
		Metronidazole + aminoglycoside[g] or fluoroquinolone[h–j]	
Appendectomy for uncomplicated appendicitis	Cefoxitin, cefotetan, cefazolin + metronidazole	Clindamycin + aminoglycoside[g] or aztreonam or fluoroquinolone[h–j]	A
		Metronidazole + aminoglycoside[g] or fluoroquinolone[h–j]	
Small intestine			
Nonobstructed	Cefazolin	Clindamycin + aminoglycoside[g] or aztreonam or fluoroquinolone[h–j]	C
Obstructed	Cefazolin + metronidazole, cefoxitin, cefotetan,	Metronidazole + aminoglycoside[g] or fluoroquinolone[h–j]	C
Hernia repair (hernicoplasty and herniorrhaphy)	Cefazolin	Clindamycin, vancomycin	A

Colorectal[m]	Cefazolin + metronidazole, cefoxitin, cefotetan, ampicillin–sulbactam,[h] ceftriaxone + metronidazole,[n] ertapenem	Clindamycin + aminoglycoside[g] or aztreonam or fluoroquinolone[h–j] metronidazole + aminoglycoside[g] or fluororoquinolone[h–j]	A
Head and neck			
Clean	None	None	B
Clean with placement or prosthesis (excludes tympanostomy tubes	Cefazolin, cefuroxime	Clindamycin[d]	C
Clean-contaminated cancer surgery	Cefazolin + metronidazole, cefuroxime + metronidazole, ampicillin–sulbactam	Clindamycin[d]	A
Other clean-contaminated procedures with the exception of tonsillectomy and functional endoscopic sinus procedures	Cefazolin + metronidazole, cefuroxime + metronidazole, ampicillin–sulbactam	Clindamycin[d]	B
Neurosurgery			
Elective craniotomy and cerebrospinal fluid-shunting procedures	Cefazolin	Clindamycin,[d] vancomycin[d]	A
Implantation of intrathecal pumps	Cefazolin	Clindamycin,[d] Cancomycin[d]	C
Cesarean delivery	Cefazolin	Clindamycin + aminoglycoside[g]	A
Hysterectomy (vaginal or abdominal)	Cefazolin, cefotetan, cefoxitin, ampicillin–sulbactam[h]	Clindamycin or vancomycin + aminoglycoside[g] or aztreonam or fluoroquinolone[h–j] Metronidazole + aminoglycoside[g] or fluoroquinolone[h–j]	A

(*Continued*)

Table 2. (*Continued*)

Type of Procedure	Recommended Agents[a,b]	Alternative Agents in Patients with β-Lactam Allergy	Strength of Evidence[c]
Ophthalmic	Topical neomycin–polymyxinB–gramicidin or fourth-generation topical fluoroquinolones (gatifloxacin or moxifloxacin) given as 1 drop every 5–15 min for 5 doses[o] Addition of cefazolin 100 mg by subconjunctival injection or intracameral cefazolin 1–2.5 mg or cefuroxime 1 mg at the end of procedure is optional	None	B
Orthopedic			
Clean operations involving hand, knee, or foot and not involving implantation of foreign materials	None	None	C
Spinal procedures with and without instrumentation	Cefazolin	Clindamycin,[d] vancomycin[d]	A
Hip fracture repair	Cefazolin	Clindamycin,[d] vancomycin[d]	A
Implantation of internal fixation devices (e.g., nails, screws, plates, wires)	Cefazolin	Clindamycin,[d] vancomycin[d]	C
Total joint replacement	Cefazolin	Clindamycin,[d] vancomycin[d]	A

Urologic			
Lower tract instrumentation with risk factors for infection (includes transrectal prostate biopsy)	Fluoroquinolone,[h–j] trimethoprim–sulfamethoxazole, cefazolin	Aminoglycoside[g] with or without clindamycin	A
Clean without entry into urinary tract	Cefazolin (the addition of a single dose of an aminoglycoside may be recommended for placement of prosthetic material [e.g., penile prosthesis])	Clindamycin,[d] vancomycin[d]	A
Involving implanted prosthesis	Cefazolin ± aminoglycoside, cefazoline ± aztreonam, ampicillin–sulbactam	Clindamycin ± aminoglycoside or aztreonam, vancomycin ± aminoglycoside or aztreonam	A
Clean with entry into urinary tract	Cefazolin (the addition of a single dose of an aminoglycoside may be recommended for placement of prosthetic material [e.g., Penile prosthesis])	Fluoroquinolone,[h–j] aminoglycoside[g] with or without clindamycin	A
Clean-contaminated	Cefazolin + metronidazole, cefoxitin	Fluoroquinolone,[h–j] aminoglycoside[g] + metronidazole or clindamycin	A
Vascular[p]	Cefazolin	Clindamycin,[d] vancomycin[d]	A
Heart, lung, heart–lung transplantation[q]			

(*Continued*)

Table 2. (*Continued*)

Type of Procedure	Recommended Agents[a,b]	Alternative Agents in Patients with b-Lactam Allergy	Strength of Evidence[c]
Heart transplantaion[r]	Cefazolin	Clindamycin,[d] vancomycin[d]	A (based on cardiac procedures)
Lung and heart–lung transplantaion[r,s]	Cefazolin	Clindamycin,[d] vancomycin[d]	A (based on cardiac procedures)
Liver transplantation[q,t]	Piperacillin–tazobactam, cefotaxime + ampicillin	Clindamycin or vancomycin + aminoglycoside[g] or aztreonam or fluoroquinolone[h–j]	B
Pancreas and pancreas–kidney tansplantation[t]	Cefazolin, fluconazole (for patients at high risk of fungal infection [e.g., those with enteric drainage of the pancrease])	Clindamycin or vancomycin + aminoglycoside[g] or aztreonam or fluoroquinolone[h–j]	A
Plastic surgery	Cefazolin	Clindamycin or vancomycin + aminoglycoside[g] or aztreonam or fluoroquinolone[h–j]	A
Clean with risk factors or clean-contaminated	Cefazolin, ampicillin–sulbactam	Clindamycin,[d] vancomycin[d]	C

[a] The antimicrobial agent should be started within 60 minutes before surgical incision (120 minutes for vancomycin or fluoroquinolones). While single-dose prophylaxis is usually sufficient, the duration of prophylaxis for all procedures should be less than 24 hours. If an agent with a short half-life is used (e.g., cefazolin, cefoxitin), it should be readministered if the procedure duration exceeds the recommended redosing interval (from the time of initiation of preoperative dose [see Table 1]). Readministration may also be warranted if prolonged or excessive bleeding occurs or if there

are other factors that may shorten the half-life of the prophylactic agent (e.g., extensive burns). Readministration may not be warranted in patients in whom the half-life of the agent may be prolonged (e.g., patients with renal insufficiency of failure).

[b] For patients known to be colonized with methicillin-resistant *Staphylococcus aureus*, it is reasonable, to add a single preoperative dose of vacomycin to the recommended agent(s).

[c] Strenth of evidence that supports the use or nonuse of prophylaxis is classified as A (levelsI–III), B (levelsIV–VI), or C (level VII). Level I evidence is from large well-conducted, randomized controlled clinical trials. Level II evidence is from small, well-conducted, randomized controlled clinical trials. Level III evidence is from well-conducted cohort studies. Level IV evidence is from well-conducted case-control studies. Level V evidence is from uncontrolled studies that were not well conducted. Level VI evidence is conflicting evidence that tends to favor the recommendation. Level VII evidence is expert opinion.

[d] For procedures in which pathogens other than staphylococci and streptococci are likely, an additional agent with activity against those pathogens could be considered. For example, if there are surveillance data showing that gram-negative organisms are a cause of surgical-site infections (SSIs) for the procedure, practitioners may consider combining clindamycin or vancomycin with another agent (cefazolin if the patient is not β-lactam allergic; aztreonam, gentamicin, or single-dose fluoroquinolone if the patient is β-lactam allergic).

[e] Prophylaxis should be considered for patients at highest risk for postoperative gastroduodenal infections, such as those with increased gastric pH (e.g., those receiving histamine H_2-receptor antagonists or proton-pump inhibitors), gastroduodental perforation, decreased gastric motility, gastric outlet obstruction, gastric bleeding, morbid obesity, or cancer. Antimicrobial prophylaxis is may not be needed when the lumen of the intestinal tract is not entered.

[f] Consider additional antimicrobial coverage with infected biliary tract. See the biliary tract procedures section of this article.

[g] Gentamicin or tobramycin.

[h] Due to increasing resistance of *Escherichia coli* to fluoroquinolones and ampicillin–sulbactam, local population susceptibility profiles should be reviewed prior to use.

[i] Ciprofloxacin or levofloxacin.

[j] Fluoroquinolones are associated with an increased risk of tendonitis and tendon rupture in all ages. However, this risk would be expected to be quite small with single-dose antibiotic prophylaxis. Although the use of fluoroguinolones may be necessary for surgical antibiotic prophylaxis in some children, they are not drugs of first choice in the pediatric population due to an increased incidence of adverse events as compared with controls in some clinical trials.

[k] Ceftriaxone use should be limited to patients requiring antimicrobial treatment for acute cholecystitis or acute biliary tract infections which may not be determined prior to incision, not patients undergoing cholecystectomy for noninfected biliary conditions, including biliary colic or dyskinesia without infection.

(*Continued*)

Table 2. (*Continued*)

[l] Factors that indicate a high risk of infectious complications in laparoscopic cholecystectomy include emergency procedures, diabetes, long procedure duration, intraoperative gallbladder rupture, age of >70 years, conversion from laparoscopic to open cholecystectomy, American Society of Anesthesiologists classification of 3 or greater, episode of colic within 30 days before the procesure, reintervention in less than one month for noninfectious complication, acute cholecystitis, bile spillage, jaundice, pregnancy, nonfunctioning gallbladder, immunosuppression, and insertion of prosthetic device. Because a number of these risk factors are not possible to determine before surgical intervention, it may be reasonable to give a single dose of antimicrobial prophylaxis to all patients undergoing laparoscopic cholecystectomy.

[m] For most patients, a mechanical bowel preparation combined with oral neomycin sulfate plus oral erythromycin base or with oral neomycin sulfate plus oral metronidazole should be given in addition to i.v. prophylaxis.

[n] Where there is increasing resistance to first- and second-generation cephalosporins among gram-negative isolates from SSIs, a single dose of ceftriaxone plus metronidazole may be preferred over the routine use of carbapenems.

[o] The necessity of continuing topical antimicrobials postoperatively has not been established.

[p] Prophylaxis is not routinely indicated for brachiocephalic procedures. Although there are no data in support, patients undergoing brachiocephalic procedures involving vascular prosthesis or patch implantation (e.g., carotid endarterectomy) may benefit from prophylaxis.

[q] These guidelines reflect recommendations for perioperative antibiotic prophylaxis to prevent SSIs and do not provide recommendations for prevention of opportunistic infections in immunosuppressed transplantation patients (e.g., for antifungal or antiviral medications).

[r] Patients who have left-ventricular assist devices as a bridge and who are chronically infected might also benefit from coverage of the infecting microorganism.

[s] The prophylactic regimen may need to be modified to provide coverage against any potential pathogens, including gram-negative (e.g., *Pseudomonas aeruginosa*) or fungal organisms, isolated from the donor lung or the recipient before transplantation. Patients undergoing lung transplantation with negative pretransplantation cultures should receive antimicrobial prophylaxis as appropriate for other types of cardiothoracic surgeries. Patients undergoing lung transplantation for cystic fibrosis should receive 7–14 days of treatment with antimicrobials selected according to pretransplantation culture and susceptibility results. This treatment may include additional antibacterial or antifungal agents.

[t] The prophylactic regimen may need to be modified to provide coverage against any portential pathogens, including vancomycin-resistant enterococci, isolated from the recipient before transplantation.

resistance. It can also predispose to Clostridium difficile-associated colitis. Risk factors for developing *C. difficile enterocolitis* are longer duration of therapy or prophylaxis and use of multiple antimicrobial agents. Limiting the duration of antimicrobial prophylaxis to a single preoperative dose can reduce the risk of *C. difficile* disease.[24]

In most situations, elective surgery should be postponed if possible when the patient has infection at a remote site. However, if surgery is necessary and the patient is receiving therapeutic antimicrobials for a remote infection before the surgery they should also be given antimicrobial prophylaxis before surgery to ensure adequate serum and tissue levels of antimicrobials with activity against likely pathogens for the duration of the procedure. If the agent being used therapeutically is appropriate for prophylaxis as well, administering an extra dose within 60 minutes of the incision is recommended in the published guidelines. Otherwise the recommended antimicrobial prophylactic agent for the specific planned procedure should be used.

Recommended antimicrobial prophylaxis for specific procedures are included in Table 2 and reprinted exactly, with permission, as they appear in the published guidelines.[11] Details on background, organisms involved and efficacy of antimicrobial therapy for each specific procedure are also included in the guidelines which could be accessed as indicated above.

Summary

Antibiotics are a major part of treatment of the ICU patient

Appropriate selection of antibiotics based on:

- Clinical and laboratory data as well as characteristics of the drug used including side effects are Essential, recognizing that findings suggesting infection may be misleading.
- Timing and duration of treatment are important in determining outcome.
- Pharmacodynamics and pharmacokinetic principles should be used to guide therapy.
- Awareness of the potential for drug resistance and institution of preventive strategies are important.
- Antibiotic stewardship protocols are important in guiding selection of therapy, monitoring and prevention of complications including drug resistance.
- Postsurgical wound infection is a major cause of morbidity and mortality in the ICU.

- Effective surgical antimicrobial prophylaxis requires differentiation among various sites of infection and their association with specific surgical procedures.
- Prophylaxis should be specific and targeted as well as of the shortest effective duration.
- Choices of prophylaxis regimens should be guided by recognized clinical practice guidelines derived from experts in the field and based on appropriate levels of evidence.

References

1. May AK, Fleming SB, Carpenter RO *et al.* Influence of broad-spectrum antibiotic prophylaxis on intracranial pressure monitor infections and subsequent infectious complications in head injured patients. *Surgical Infections* 2006; 7(5): 409–417.
2. Paul M, Lebovic L. Combination antimicrobial treatment versus monotherapy: The contribution of meta-analyses. *Infect Dis Clin North Am* 2009; 23(2): 277–293.
3. Kumar A, Roberts D, Wood KE *et al.* Duration of hypotension before initiation of effective antimicrobial therapy is the critical determinant of survival in human septic shock. *Crit Care Med* 2006; 34(6): 1589–1596.
4. Chastre J, Wolff M, Fagon J-Y *et al.* Comparison of 8 versus 15 days of antibiotic therapy for ventilator associated pneumonia in adults. A randomized trial. *JAMA* 2003; 290(19): 2588–2598.
5. Mazuski JE, Sawyer RG, Nathens AB *et al.* SIS guidelines on antimicrobial therapy for intra-abdominal infections: An executive summary. *Surgical Infections* 2002; 3(3): 161–173.
6. Solomkin JS, Mazuski JE, Bradley JS *et al.* Diagnosis and management of complicated intra-abdominal infection in adults and children: Guidelines by SIS and the infectious disease society of America. *Clin Infect Dis* 2010; 50(2): 133–164.
7. Dortch MJ, Fleming SB, Kaufmann R *et al.* Infection reduction strategies including antibiotic stewardship protocols in surgical and trauma ICUs are associated with reduced resistant gram-negative health care associated infections. *Surg Infect* 2011; 12: 15–25.
8. Rangel-Frausto MS, Pittet D, Costigan M *et al.* The natural history of the systemic inflammatory response syndrome (SIRS): A prospective study. *JAMA* 1995; 273(2): 117–123.
9. Hyatt JM, McKinnon PS, Zimmer GS, Schentag JJ. The importance of pharmacokinetic/pharmacodynamics surrogate markers to outcome. Focus on antimicrobial agents. *Clin Pharmacokinet* 1995; 6(2): 1995.

10. Levison ME, Levison JH. Pharmacokinetics and pharmacodynamics of antimicrobial agents. *Inf Dis Clin North Am* 2009; 23(4): 791–808.
11. Bratzler DW, Dellinger EP, Osen KM *et al.* Clinical practice guidelines for antimicrobial prophylaxis in surgery. *Am J Health Syst Pharm* 2013; 70: 195–283.
12. American Society of Health-System Pharmacists. ASHP therapeutic guidelines on antimicrobial prophylaxis in surgery. *Am J Health-Syst Pharm* 1999; 56: 1839–1888.
13. Dotson LR, Witmer DR. Development of ASHP therapeutic guidelines. *Am J Health-Syst Pharm* 1995; 52: 254–255.
14. National Healthcare Safety Network. Patient safety component manual: Key terms. Available at www.cdc.gov/nhsn/PDFs/pscKey Terms_current.pdf (accessed on 23 October 2012).
15. Horan TC, Andrus M, Dudeck MA. CDC/NHSN surveillance definition of health care-associated infection and criteria for specific types of infections in the acute care setting. *Am J Infect Control* 2008; 36: 309–332.
16. Forse RA, Karam B, and Maclean LD *et al.* Antibiotic prophylaxis for surgery in morbidly obese patients. *Surgery* 1989; 101: 770–774.
17. Falagas ME, Karageorgopoulos DE. Adjustment of dosing of antimicrobial agents for body weight in adults. *Lancet* 2010; 375: 248–251.
18. Bratzler DW, Houck PM, Surgical infection prevention guidelines writers workgroup. Antimicrobial prophylaxis for surgery: An advisory statement from the national surgical infection prevention project. *Clin Infect Dis* 2004; 38: 1706–1715.
19. Perl TM. Prevention of Staphylococcus aureus infections among surgical patients: Beyond traditional perioperative prophylaxis. *Surgery* 2003; 134: S10–7.
20. Jain R, Kralovic SM, Evans ME. Veterans Affairs initiatives to prevent *Staphylococcus aureus* infections. *New Engl J Med.* 2011; 364: 1419–1430.
21. Harbarth S, Frankhauser C, Schrenzel J *et al.* Universal screening for M*ethicillin-resistant Staphylococcus aureus* at hospital admission and nosocomial infection in surgical patients. *JAMA* 2008; 299: 1149–1157.
22. Bactroban (mupirocin calcium ointment, 2%) nasal package insert. Research Triangle Park, NC. *GlaxoSmithKLine*, April 2009.
23. Hebert C, Robicsek A. Decolonization therapy in infection control. *Curr Opin Infect Dis* 2010; 23: 340–345.
24. Cohen SH, Gerding DN, Johnson S *et al.* Clinical practice guidelines for C. *difficile* infection in adults: 2010 update by the Society for Healthcare Epidemiology of America (SHEA) and the Infectious Diseases Society of America (IDSA). *Infect Control Hosp Epidemiol* 2010; 31: 431–455

Chapter 12

The Coagulopathic Trauma Patient and Massive Transfusion Protocol

Jameel Ali, Sandro Rizoli and Katerina Pavenski

Chapter Overview

Management of the patient who suffers major blood loss presents many challenges to the intensivists, trauma surgeon and other members of the trauma care team. In the past, crystalloid administration has been the initial resuscitation fluid followed by blood transfusion. However, many patients require immediate infusion of blood, plasma, coagulation factors including platelets and cryoprecipitate, fibrinogen, and tranexamic acid to improve survival as part of a massive transfusion protocol. Although, there is no universally accepted protocol, general principles of massive transfusion should be adopted for rational use of the massive transfusion protocol. This involves collaboration of the intensivists with the surgeon, hematopathologist, anesthetist and other members of the trauma care team.

Simultaneous with massive blood loss, patients develop coagulopathy because of the trauma itself as well as the result of hypothermia, acidosis, dilution, and consumption of coagulation factors. Resuscitation should therefore involve not only fluid and blood with blood products and coagulation factors but also monitor preventing and controlling the coagulopathy accompanying trauma with hypoperfusion from major blood loss.

In this chapter, we discuss the coagulopathy of trauma and surgery, its etiology and diagnosis with principles of monitoring and management.

We also discuss the definition of massive blood transfusion, its identification and criteria for implementing and applying a massive transfusion protocol.

The Coagulopathy of Trauma

The coagulation system is a balance of two major processes — one is aimed at clotting to prevent or stop bleeding (procoagulant and antifibrinolysis) and the other to promote 'liquidity' and flowing of blood through anticoagulation and fibrinolysis. It has been reported that as many as 25% of trauma patients present to the emergency room in a coagulopathic state[1] with overall 21% of deaths following trauma being due to hemorrhage of which 50% die within 12 hours and 70% in 48 hours. This coagulopathic state is thought to result from a series of factors. Early after tissue injury there is release of tissue factor (thromboplastin) which forms a complex with Factor VIIa with direct activation of Factor Xc and activation of Factor IXa forming a complex with Factor VIIa and phospholipids. Also, Factor Xa complexes with Factor Va and phospholipids to convert prothrombin to thrombin which converts fibrinogen to fibrin and clot formation. With continued hemorrhage there is depletion of fibrinogen and platelets in the process of clot formation leading to consumption of platelets and coagulation factors (consumption coagulopathy) which aggravates the bleeding process. Trauma coagulopathy arises in an environment of a complex mixture of inflammation, and cellular dysfunction with rapid evolution over mins to hours from an anticoagulant to a procoagulant state. Although all mechanisms are not clearly delineated, several key processes have been identified including dysfunction of natural anticoagulation mechanisms, platelet dysfunction, fibrinogen consumption, and hyper fibrinolysis[2] compounded by hypoperfuson, dilution from resuscitation fluids, hypothermia, and acidosis secondary to the hypoperfusion. The thrombin–thrombomodulin–protein C anticoagulation system has also been implicated as a mechanism of anticoagulation. Decrease in protein C levels has been attributed to its activation (aPC) by thrombin bound to thrombomodulin.[3] The anticoagulation properties of aPC derives from its degradation of activated Factors V and VIII leading to decreased concentration of these factors as demonstrated by Rizoli *et al.*[4] who reported consistent reduction in Factor V among 110 trauma patients. Endogenous autoheparinization has also been implicated possibly secondary to shedding of the endothelial glycocalyx as suggested by the ability to reverse the anticoagulation by adding heparinase to the blood of trauma patients with coagulopathy.[5]

Platelet dysfunction

The observation that platelet counts are typically normal in early trauma coagulopathy suggests that platelet dysfunction rather than actual dilution or depletion of platelets is a primary contributing factor to the coagulopathy of trauma. Kutcher *et al.*[6] demonstrated early platelet dysfunction through impedance aggregometry in trauma patients on arrival in the emergency room. These platelet defects have been shown to contribute to increased trauma mortality.[7] Platelet contribution to clot firmness as measured by rotational thromboelastometry (ROTEM) was also diminished in non-survivors of major trauma.[8]

Fibrinogen consumption and fibrinolysis

Fibrinogen after activation by thrombin polymerizes to a fibrin mesh which forms a clot with platelets to stop hemorrhage at sites of vascular injury. This is the primary process for hemostasis in areas of injury. Consumption of fibrinogen and fibrinolysis through the action of plasmin are major components of the coagulopathy of trauma. Admission fibrinogen levels correlate with measurement of clot firmness by ROTEM and is an independent predictor of early and late deaths following trauma as reported by Rourke *et al.*[9] Fibrin clot formation is counterbalanced by fibrinolysis which is due to the binding of tissue plasminogen activator (tPA) to plasminogen which is then converted to plasmin which destroys the scaffold of the clot by lysing the fibrin fibers. Increased fibrinolysis or hyperfibrinolysis is a known accompaniment of hemorrhagic shock as demonstrated by increased levels of tPA and the clot breakdown product, D-dimer in patients with hemorrhagic traumatic shock.[3,10] Using visco-elastic methods, hyperfibrinolysis has been shown to correlate with exceedingly high mortality in trauma patients.[11]

In addition to the above mechanisms implicated in trauma coagulopathy there is evidence for a significant role of pro-inflammatory cytokines, neutrophil activation, histones, extracellular DNA etc. uncovering a host of diverse reaction to shock and hemorrhage following trauma with potential disastrous consequences. The main goal of treatment is, therefore, early control of hemorrhage to stop the continued requirement for clot formation and consumptive coagulopathy with depletion of clotting factors and hyperfibrinolysis. With established trauma induced coagulopathy mortality is increased 3–4 fold and 24 hours mortality is increased 8-fold with resulting increase in transfusion requirement, increased ICU stay, mechanical ventilation days and incidence of multiple organ failure. This coagulopathy is not only due to hemodilution and consumption of clotting factors but also direct tissue injury leading to release of potent mediators of the inflammatory response and hypoperfusion which is compounded by hypothermia and acidosis all resulting in hyperfibrinolysis and bleeding. Identifying and treating these triggers of hyperfibrinolysis by maintaining perfusion thus decreasing the base deficit, preventing hypothermia which affects platelet function and other clotting factors, by active aggressive warming techniques are important treatment strategies. However, the coagulation defect itself also needs to be identified and targeted for successful outcome. Whereas, minimal trauma with hemorrhage that is successfully treated, is traditionally managed by initial crystalloid followed by packed cells as needed, the massively bleeding trauma patient in prolonged shock with a predilection to hypothermia and acidosis has to be managed not only by treating the surgical lesion but by early identification and correction of the associated trauma induced coagulopathy by replacement of depleted coagulation factors and curtailing the vicious cycle resulting from continued hemorrhage.

When the clinical history and presentation suggest major hemorrhage and/or when there is associated acidosis or hypothermia with a continued state of hypoperfusion, the treatment protocol should involve active warming of the patient and prompt initial transfusion of not only packed red blood cells (RBC) but also coagulation factors. Many different "Massive Transfusion Protocols (MTP)" have been described in the literature including different ratios of packed cells, fresh frozen plasma, platelets, cryoprecipitate, fibrinogen, tranexamic acid etc.[12] but there is no universal agreement on any one of these protocols. The usual tests of coagulation such as INR, PT, PTT, platelet counts require time to complete and interpret in order to guide therapy. These tests are also performed at the 37°C temperature level in the laboratory thus not reflecting their true measurement in the bleeding patient.[13] These tests do not provide crucial information on clot strength and stability and because whole cells are removed by centrifugation before completing the tests, their contribution to clotting from platelets, erythrocytes and tissue factor bearing cells are not considered and the key role of fibrinogen and hyperfibrinolysis are neglected. Availability of a rapid measurement of the strength of the clot, platelet function and fibrinogen level and the degree of fibrinolysis at the bedside would allow immediate correction of targeted abnormalities to correct the bleeding without the necessity to adhere to any particular ratio.

Triggers for Massive Transfusion Protocols and the Protocols

It is evident that early identification of predictors of Massive transfusion protocols would result in correction of the above mechanisms of trauma coagulopathy and hopefully stop the vicious cycle leading to increased mortality following hemorrhage and hypoperfusion from trauma. Clinically, a patient's history of injury associated with significant hemorrhage and shock should and often does trigger the massive transfusion protocol. However, in order to standardize triggers in specific circumstances many other triggers have been described:

Replacement of the patient' entire blood volume in a 24 hours period (10–12 units of PRBC), replacement of 50% total blood volume in three hours (5–6 units PRBC), need for at least four units RBC's within four hours with continued major bleeding, blood loss exceeding 150 ml/min.

The Shock index (SI) defined as the ratio of heart rate to systolic blood pressure has been used by Mutscher *et al.*[14] demonstrating that with increasing SI there was increased need for transfusion.

The Individual Transfusion Trigger (Cincinnati ITT or CITT) study,[15] the Trauma Associated severe Hemorhage (TASH) score and the Assessment of Blood Consumption (ABC) score[16] have also been utilized as MT triggers. The CITT triggers are: Systolic blood pressure, 90 mmHg, Hb <11 g/dl, temp <35.5 C, INR >1.5 and base deficit of 6 or greater. The ABC score includes SBP <90 mmHg, Heart rate 120 or greater per min, positive Focused Assessment sonogram for Trauma (FAST) and penetrating mechanism.

Transfusion triggers described by Callcut *et al.*[17] are: INR >1.5, systolic blood pressure, 90 mmHg, Hb, 11 g/dl, base deficit>6, FAST positivity, heart rate 120/min, and penetrating trauma mechanism, combining both CITT and ABC criteria to arrive at a total of eight parameters. From these parameters, a Massive transfusion Score (MTS) was derived by assigning one point to each parameter and obtaining the sum of these points. Using the Prospective Observational Multicentre Major Trauma Transfusion (PROMMITT) model,[18] Callcut *et al.*[17] prospectively recruited 1,245 patients with 297 receiving MT. All triggers except penetrating mechanism and heart rate were valid individual predictors of MT with INR being the most predictive. Patients with an MTS of less than two were unlikely to receive MT (neg predictive value –89%). If any two triggers were present, sensitivity for predicting MT was 85%. The authors concluded that parameters which are obtainable early in the initial emergency department evaluation are valid predictors of the likelihood of Massive transfusion.

In spite of the lack of generally uniform triggers for MT, all described triggers have in common evidence of major blood loss and hypoperfusion.

The protocols

Hemorrhage in Trauma results in loss of whole blood which includes not only RBCs but also plasma, platelets, and other coagulation factors. It seems reasonable that whole blood loss should therefore be treated by replacement with whole blood rather than component therapy consisting of red cells, platelets and coagulation factors. Several studies, particularly in the military setting have demonstrated effectiveness of whole blood transfusion. Cottton *et al.*[19] demonstrated that patients receiving modified whole blood (after use of leukoreduction filter and without native platelet function), required fewer products during a 24 hours period compared to those receiving component therapy. However, there were no differences in 24 hours or 30 day mortality. Before wide spread adoption of whole blood transfusion as replacement for blood loss, several obstacles need to be overcome-possible link between white cell contamination and transfusion complications, adequacy of removal of possible pathogens and the availability and procurement of whole blood itself, to name a few. Until these issues are resolved we are left with using packed RBCs and component therapy.

Blood transfusion itself, though very important, has to be combined with other aspects of resuscitation of the trauma patient in hemorrhagic shock viz: Restoration of circulating blood volume, maintenance of perfusion, and prevention of acidosis and hypothermia.

Regarding the blood transfusion, several protocols have been advocated. They practically all have in common the infusion of packed red cells, platelets and fresh frozen plasma but in different ratios, the most common being 1:1:1, although there is no uniformity. Use of component therapy, generally results in better outcome[12] but the optimum ratio still remains elusive.

The non-uniformity in massive transfusion protocol becomes more complex when it is observed that elements such as cryoprecipitate, fibrinogen, calcium, and tranexamic acid are incorporated into some protocols and not in others. While the roles of the other elements such as fibrinogen and cryoprecipitate in some massive transfusion protocols may be evident, special aspects of tranexamic acid are worth considering.

Tranexamic acid (TA) is a synthetic derivative of the amino acid lysine and acts as an antifibrinolytic, binding to plasminogen to block the interaction of plasminogen with fibrin and preventing the dissolution of the fibrin clot with an expected effect on decreasing hemorrhage from points of injury. It has decreased 28 day all-cause mortality in bleeding trauma patients, (all-cause mortality decreasing from 16.0%–14.5%, reduced death from bleeding from 5.7%–4.9%, early TA–<1 hour from injury — was associated with the greatest decrease — 32% — in death from bleeding, between 1 and 3 hours there was still a decrease in death from bleeding but after three hours of injury there was an increased risk of death from bleeding). Interestingly, there was no increased vascular occlusive events with TA in spite of concern for increased clotting.[20]

Point of care parameters and their measurement to guide massive transfusion

As pointed out above, considering the coagulopathy associated with major trauma, coagulation tests would be expected to be helpful in guiding therapy in the massively transfused trauma patient. The time taken to complete and interpret these tests, the fact that they are conducted at 37°C rather than the actual patient temperature among other factors make these tests impractical for guiding therapy in acute situations. There are thus two choices in guiding therapy — (a) using ratios of products that hopefully would be effective in curtailing the hemorrhage as in the various massive transfusion protocols discussed so far or (b) using immediate available results of coagulation tests at the patient's bed side (in the Emergency room, Operating room or ICU) focusing on identified coagulation defects in the hemorrhaging trauma patient to guide rational use of blood and coagulation products — referred to as point of care (POC) coagulation testing. Appropriately applied, this would be expected, not only to target and correct specific deficiencies in a timely fashion but also avoid unnecessary wastage of blood and coagulation products. It has been demonstrated that in massive bleeders, delay in specific coagulation therapy is associated with poor outcome.[21] Also, the use of high plasma: Red cell ratios in some patient groups do not improve survival but may also increase complication rates.[22] Holcomb *et al.*[23] in the PROPPR Randomized clinical trial, compared transfusion of plasma, platelets, and RBCs in a ratio of 1:1:1 to 1:1:2 in massively bleeding patients and found no significant difference in mortality at 24 hours or at 30 days. However, more patients in the 1:1:1 group achieved hemostasis and fewer experienced death due to exsanguination by 24 hours.

Viscoelastic POC coagulation monitoring tools such as ROTEM (ROTEM- Tem International, Munich, Germany) and thromboelastography

(TEG-Hemonetics, Braintree, Massachusetts) have made it possible to rapidly assess the initiation of clot formation, clot strength, and clot stability at the patient's bedside allowing individualized coagulation therapy. Ideally, these tests and results should be immediately available but in situations where they are not immediately available or "setup time" is required, the traditional "blind" protocol ratio guided transfusion is appropriate, the ultimate goal being to support the circulation and hemostasis as expeditiously as possible in the massively bleeding patient.

Both ROTEM and TEG allow identification of different causes of bleeding by assessing both the intrinsic and extrinsic coagulation pathways. The fibrin dependent component of the clot can be accurately and instantly assessed providing data on the stability and strength of the clot as well as the degree of hyperfibrinolysis, prompting specific goal directed therapy. In retrospective analysis of data at a level 1 trauma center[24] TEG provided real time measure of thrombostatic function with the ability to reduce the need for FFP administration. ROTEM allowed detection of more coagulation abnormalities than PT and aPTT in a prospective analysis of deployed military personnel[25] allowing both monitoring and guiding individualized therapy during massive transfusion.

The maximum clot strength measured by ROTEM is a result of the interaction of activated platelets, fibrin and aFXIII. As such, a maximum strength of the clot can be achieved in severe bleeding by administration of sufficient fibrinogen. Output from the ROTEM generated measurements allows focus on fibrin deficit for which specific dosage of fibrinogen concentrate would be recommended to correct the deficit. Similarly, thrombin generation deficit may be uncovered prompting specific treatment as well as platelet deficit prompting administration of platelet concentrate. Severe clot deficiency may be treated with TA, fibrinogen concentrate, high doses of FFP, or increasing platelet counts as determined by the ROTEM guided algorithm. The apparatus also allows detection of potential heparin exposure prompting reversal with protamine and clot instability not related to hyperfibrinolysis could be treated by Factor XIII administration just to highlight a few of the specific abnormalities detectable with suggested intervention through examining the ROTEM output.

Massive Transfusion Protocol Logistics

Regardless of the chosen formula for administering and monitoring the process of massive blood transfusion, the protocol requires a detailed well planned cohesive team approach involving physicians, laboratory staff, nurses, communication, and transport services. The protocol described here is extracted, with permission and authored primarily by Dr. Katerina Pavensky our hematopathologist and coordinator of the Massive transfusion service at St. Michaels Hospital in Toronto with the assistance of Dr. Sandro Rizoli, the Transfusion Committee and Trauma Care Committee of the hospital. Protocols will differ from institution to institution but the details presented here is used to highlight features of one protocol to demonstrate the necessity for having a well-planned institution wide protocol in which all sections involved will be aware of their respective roles and responsibilities having reviewed the protocol in detail and agreed to participate fully in adherence to the protocol. This ensures that when the protocol has been approved by all it will be applied uniformly. Otherwise chaos to the detriment of patient care could easily result at a time when urgent cohesive efforts are required and there is no time for ad hoc protocol implementation.

In this protocol, massive transfusion is defined as requirement for >6 units of RBCs in a four hours period to replace blood loss from trauma, postpartum hemorrhage, upper GI hemorrhage, postoperative bleeding, ruptured aortic aneurysm etc.

The specific goals of MTP include:

(a) Provision of optimal resuscitation.
(b) Prevent or manage coagulopathy.
(c) Timely and appropriate provision of blood components and other supportive measures in a standardized manner.
(d) Guide expedient definitive management of bleeding.
(e) Avoid unnecessary transfusions and their complications.
(f) Avoid wastage of blood components.

MTP TEAM- Roles and responsibilities

(a) At the bedside — physicians, nurses, respiratory therapists, MTP leads, and MTP Assistants.
(b) Transfusion medicine lab — MTP medical laboratory technologist (MLT).
(c) Core lab — medical laboratory technologist.
(d) Portering service — MTP PORTER.
(e) Central locating — phone, communication, pagers, cellular contact.
(f) Others: Critical Care. OR, Endoscopy, interventional Radiology.

Responsibilities during MTP

1. MTP LEAD is a staff physician or clinical fellow

   — Gives order to initiate and terminate MTP.
   — Leads resuscitation efforts (orders blood components, medications, IV fluids and therapeutic interventions.
   — When necessary, obtains central venous access and secures airway.
   — Reasseses need for ongoing MTP q1h.
   — Monitors patient clinically and with laboratory testing.
   — Mobilizes additional resources as necessary e.g., OR.
   — Signs the emergency blood release form if applicable.
   — Following MTP, charts summary of resuscitation.

2. MTP ASSIST is A Registered nurse

   — Aids in preparing patient monitors and necessary equipment including blood warmer.
   — Monitors patient.
   — Obtains peripheral venous access.
   — Performs phlebotomy for laboratory testing as required.
   — Administers medication, resuscitation fluids and blood components.
   — During MTP, documents interventions and clinical data.
   — Acts as a liaison between bedside team and other areas (laboratory, portering, imaging, OR etc). For example informs Transfusion Medicine of patient's changing blood components needs, a significant change in patient's condition or change in patient's location.
   — Available to assist MTP Lead as necessary.

3. RESPIRATORY Therapist

   — Assists with securing an airway and providing oxygen therapy/ventilation as necessary.
   — Assists with set up of a blood warmer.
   — Administers resuscitating fluids and blood components.
   — Available to assist MTP lead as needed.

4. Perfusionist

   — Administers resuscitating fluids and blood components.
   — Available to assist MTP lead as needed.
   — Sets up and performs cell salvage if needed.

5. TM laboratory

   — One staff designated as MTP Technologist.
   — Coordinates blood component preparation and issue.
   — Communicates with the clinical team.
   — Prioritizes preparation of blood components for MTP over other work.
   — May provide recommendations on transfusion management (e.g., Dosing of a component).
   — Fills out MTP Monitoring Tool (record of components issued).

6. Core Lab

   — Prioritizes MTP blood specimens over other work (SUPER STAT).
   — Conveys critical results to the MTP team.

7. Portering Service

   — One staff is designated as an MTP PORTER for the duration of the MTP.
   — Transports blood samples and blood components during MTP.
   — Returns MTP cooler promptly to TM once blood components are transfused or MTP terminated.

Note: If MTP is initiated in the OR, the blood portering process is outlined in the "Obtaining and Administering Blood/Blood Products within Perioperative Services" policy will be followed. If the patient is transferred to the OR with MTP in progress, portering Services will continue with blood sample and blood component in transport until the patient is admitted to the Perioperative Services. At this point, the hospital porter will report to the OR Patient Care Coordinator/Charge Nurse for transfer of accountability. The charge nurse will then assign a USW or PSA to the case. In rare circumstances (e.g., Insufficient staffing, multiple complex patients' demands), the charge nurse may ask the Porter to continue blood transport for an MTP patient the OR.

8. Anesthesiologist staff on call

   — Is available to assist with obtaining venous access, invasive monitoring, securing airway, and transfusion management.
   — Be prepared to take over the role of MTP Lead if required.

9. Central Locating

— Once MTP is activated, Central Locating will notify the appropriate parties (see MTP activation).

10. Others

Surgery, interventional radiology, endoscopy

— MTP lead may consult an appropriate service as needed to coordinate an urgent intervention to definitively control hemorrhage.

Critical Care

— MTP lead may request transfer of a patient to a critical care unit for further management or monitoring.

MTP Activation criteria

- GENERAL

— A recognized need for uncross matched RBC's.
— Substantial and rapid blood loss (>1,500 cc estimated blood loss or at least six units of RBC transfused with anticipated ongoing uncontrolled hemorrhage in the short term (mins to hours).
— Anticipated massive and rapid blood loss requiring transfusion of ≥6 units of RBC within mins to hours.

- TRAUMA

— Penetrating trauma and persistent hypotension (two measurements of SBP <90 mmHg 5 mins apart in the Emergency Department).
— Blunt trauma AND persistent hypotension AND one of the following:

(a) Massive hemothorax
(b) Positive FAST
(c) Pelvic fracture

- OBSTETRICAL HEMORRHAGE

— Vaginal bleeding and hypotension not responsive to crystalloid.
— Suspected bleeding AND hypotension not responsive to crystalloid.

- HEMORRHAGE IN CARDIOVASCULAR PATIENT
  - — Known/suspected ruptured Abdominal Aortic Aneursym.
  - — Postoperative chest tube drainage >1,000 cc in 30 mins or less.
  - — Cardiac rupture.
    - — Aortic rupture.
    - — Atrial leak.

MTP initiation

MTP may be initiated in the following areas:

- — Emergency Department.
- — Operating Rooms (including 15th floor OR).
- — Intensive Care Units (TNICU, CVICU, MSICU).
- — MTP may also be initiated in areas involved with at-risk patients, such as Interventional Radiology and Endoscopy Unit. In these cases, the patient must be transferred to a more appropriate care area as soon as feasible.

MTP may not be directly initiated in public areas, Out-patient areas (including Dialysis Unit) and in-patient areas other than intensive care units. In these situations, Code Blue should be called. The Code Blue leader shall activate MTP if appropriate.

Patient Clinical Area

1. The patient's physician (or delegate) assesses the patient and makes a decision to initiate MTP. She/he calls Transfusion Medicine Laboratory (ext. 5084) and requests to activate MTP and provides the following information:

   - — Patient location and telephone extension at that location.
   - — Patient's identifying data name and Medical Record Number — for unidentified patients, only include gender and approximate age.
   - — Name of the MTP lead.
   - — Whether uncross matched RBC are required STAT?
   - — Whether patient is pregnant (if yes, consider calling Code OB or urgently consulting Obstetrics.

Note: Patient's identifying data should not be modified until the MTP has been terminated. The intent to change any of the patient's identifiers must be communicated to the Transfusion Medicine Laboratory ASAP.

2. The patient's physician or delegate calls Locating (code line) to activate MTP and provides the following information: Patient location and phone extension at that location.
3. The patient's physician assumes MTP lead role. In some clinical areas this role will be taken over as soon as practically possible by the staff anesthesiologist.

   — In the emergency department MTP lead is either the Trauma Team Leader or Emergency physician.
   — In the Operating Room MTP lead is an anesthesiologist.
   — In the Intensive Care Unit MTP lead is the Critical Care physician or senior physician trainee
   — In all other clinical areas, staff anesthesiologist shall assume the role of MTP lead.

If applicable, the patient's nurse will begin carrying out the duties of an MTP Assist. Additional resources (RNs, respiratory therapists, and perfusionists) may be summoned by activating the Critical Care Response team (CCRT) or Code Blue under appropriate circumstances.

4. MTP TEAM collects and sends to the laboratory the following blood samples as soon as possible:

   Transfusion medicine:

   — A pretransfusion compatibility sample.
   — Patient Blood Transfusion Record stamped with patient's name ID info.
   — Transfusion Medicine paper requisition stamped with patient's ID info.
   — Request for uncrossed match RBC stamped with patient's ID info — if requesting uncross matched RBC.

   Hematology:

   — For trauma patients: MTP panel — CBC, INR, aPTT, fibrinogen, ROTEM.
   — For all other patients: MTP panel — CBC, INR, aPT, fibrinogen.

Biochemistry:

- — Electrolytes, Cr, ionized Ca, lactate, arterial blood gas or venous blood gas.
- — All samples must be labeled STAT and delivered to the appropriate lab by a dedicated porter.
- — All requisitions should be stamped with patient ID with clearly legible identifiers.

5. The MTP team resuscitates and monitors the patient:

- — Obtains IV access.
- — Initiates resuscitation with crystalloid- note only 0.9% NaCl is compatible with blood components.
- — MTP Assist sets up blood tubing and starts blood component transfusion.
- — MTP Assist sets up blood warmer.

Central Locating

1. Operator notifies the following individuals that MTP has been initiated and provides patient location and phone extension:

- — Core lab.
- — Portering Services.
- — Respiratory technologist on call.

2. If specifically requested by MTP lead, the following should be contacted:

- — Anesthesiologist on call.
- — GI/endoscopist.
- — Interventional Radiology.
- — Perfusionist on call.
- — Operating Room.
- — Med SURG ICU, CV ICU, CCU or Trauma ICU.

Portering services

The dedicated porter arrives as soon as possible at the bedside to collect and deliver initial blood samples to Transfusion Medicine and the Core lab.

After delivery of samples the porter returns to the Transfusion Laboratory Medicine Lab to pick up blood components in an MTP cooler and delivers to the clinical area.

3. The porter continues to deliver blood samples and blood components as necessary during the MTP.

Transfusion Medicine Laboratory (TM)

1. Upon initiation of MTP, TM issues the following blood components as soon as possible in MTP cooler:

— 6 units of RBCs.
— If compatibility testing is completed-cross matched RBC.
— If only blood group is available-group specific and uncross matched RBC.
— If none of the testing is done-Group O and uncross matched RBC.
— 4 units FP.
— If group is available, group specific.
— If blood group is unknown- Group AB.

2. TM performs compatibility testing.
3. 30 min after initiation of MTP, TM prepares and issues with the 2nd shipment:

— 4 units RBC.
— 4 units FP.
— 10 units cryoprecipitate.
— 1 adult dose of platelets (one buffy coat poor or one apheresis platelet concentrate).

4. TM prepares four additional units of RBC and four additional units of FP every 30 min until MTP is terminated.
5. Further doses of cryoprecipitate or platelets should be requested if needed.

Notes: Uncross matched RBC are immediately available. RBC which have been cross matched ahead of time are also available immediately. If no current transfusion sample is available, cross matching of RBC may take 45 min or longer depending on the antibody screen. Store RBC in the MTP cooler until ready to transfuse. RBC may be transfused through a blood warmer.

Thawing of plasma takes approximately 20 min. Store plasma in the MTP cooler until ready to transfuse. Plasma may be administered through a cooler.

Thawing and pooling of cryoprecipitate takes about 30 min. Store prepared cryoprecipitate at room temperature. Do not place in the cooler and do not transfuse through a blood warmer. Platelets are available immediately. Store at room temperature. Do not place in the cooler and do not transfuse through a blood warmer. If the patient's blood group has not been determined and urgent RBC transfusion is required, TM will issue the following:

RBC: O Rh-negative RBC will be issued for female patients less than 50 years old: O Rh-positive RBC will be issued for all others.
Plasma: AB plasma.

Patients will be switched to group specific RBC as soon as the group has been determined. RBC currently contain less than 10 cc of plasma per unit.

Patients will be switched to cross matched RBC as soon as the compatibility testing is completed.

For patients who are known to be Rh-negative, Rh-negative RBC and platelets will be issued initially but may be switched to Rh-positive components at the discretion of the TM medical director.

Rh immunoglobulin will be offered to all Rh-negative female patients <50 years old and who have received Rh-positive platelets except if they have also received Rh-positive RBC or have evidence of alloimmunization with anti-D.

Ongoing management during MTP

Patient Monitoring:

1. Monitor vital signs and fluid status
   — Vital signs (continuous blood pressure, heart rate, O2saturation, respiratory rate, Temperature) Total input and output.
2. Laboratory monitoring
   — Monitor for complications such as hyperkalemia, hypocalcemia, acidosis.
   — Lab tests should include: ABG/VBG, ionized calcium, electrolytes q 15–30 min; MT panel — at least q1h; Creatinine, liver enzymes, cardiac enzymes and serum lactate — as dictated by clinical situation.

3. Monitor for signs of massive transfusion complications:

   Transfusion Associated Circulatory overload; Transfusion related acute lung injury; Allergic reactions; Citrate toxicity/hypocalcemia; abdominal compartment syndrome.

Transfusion Management

POC management based on ROTEM and TEG data from the bed side would dictate more specific interventions. Otherwise the following goals may be used as a guide.

These goals which are not supported by high quality evidence but endorsed by many clinicians and should be used as guidelines only and not replace clinical judgement. In a bleeding patient:

— Transfuse plasma to maintain INR <1.5 and/or aPTT <1.5X upper limit of normal.
— Transfuse cryoprecipitate (10 units) to maintain fibrinogen >1.5 g/l.
— Transfuse 1 adult dose of platelets to maintain platelet count >50,000 during any active hemorrhage or >100,000 in case of CNS bleeding or traumatic brain injury.
— Tranfuse RBC to maintain hemoglobin >80g/l.

Note: platelets may be indicated regardless of platelet count if platelet dysfunction is suspected

e.g., post cardiopulmonary bypass or following ingestion of an antiplatelet agent.

The use of recombinant Factor VIIa in refractory bleeding is generally not recommended. It may be considered only in the following circumstances:

Refractory bleeding due to trauma, following cardiovascular surgery or childbirth and all of the following:

— Patient potentially salvageable.
— Surgical hemostasis achieved/attempted.
— Platelet count >50,000 or just received platelet transfusion.
— INR <5, aPTT <1.5X normal or just received frozen plasma.
— Fibrinogen >1.5 g/L or just received cryoprecipitate.
— Correction of hypothermia, acidosis, and hypocalcemia achieved/attempted.

Off label use of rVIIa is associated with increased risk of arterial thromboembolic events and must be used cautiously and only if potential benefits outweigh the risks.

Anesthesiologists involved in the resuscitation may order rVIIa 5.0 mg IV followed by another dose in 20–30 min if no cessation of bleeding is observed. All other physicians are required to contact hematology or Transfusion Medicine for approval to use off label rVIIa and complete the form "Off label use of rVIIa" and return to TM.

Supportive Measures

1. Attempt to achieve local hemostasis (e.g., interventional angiography, surgery).
2. If appropriate contact perfusion services to set up cell salvage. *Note*: Use only if blood loss is from a clean surgical field in patient without underlying malignancy or current systemic infection.
3. Administer tranexamic acid 1 gm in 50 cc 0.9% NaCl solution over 10 min (except if there is evidence of DIC or bleeding from the urinary tract). Maintenance dose of 1 gm should be started right after the loading dose and infused over 8 hours.
4. Prevent hypothermia. Aim for core temperature of >35°C to avoid hypothermia induced coagulopathy and/or platelet dysfunction.

   — Level One rapid infuser(s) with blood warmer or hot line should be used.
   — All intravenous fluids administered should be delivered through blood warming devices.
   — Consider methods of passive or active warming for all massively transfused patients until.
   — Sustained normothermia is achieved (warming mattress, warm blankets, Bair Hugger. Drape and cover head and extremities if possible. Increase ambient temperature).
   — Prevent/correct acidosis by adequate IV fluid resuscitation, blood components and temporary bicarbonate solution if indicated to prevent acidosis induced coagulopathy.
   — Maintain normal serum calcium levels.
   — If the patient is on any anticoagulant or antiplatelet agents, consult Hematology or Transfusion Medicine for assistance with specific management.

Terminating the MTP

- — The MTP lead notifies TM as soon as MTP is terminated (patient is stabilized or has expired).
- — MTP team returns cooler and all unused blood components promptly to TM.
- — Clinical team charts and completes the required documents.

Summary

Early identification of patients needing massive transfusion should prompt immediate activation of massive transfusion protocols which should be part of most institutions' approach to dealing with trauma and critically ill patients.

Although there is no uniformity among protocols, establishment of a workable rational protocol is essential with input from the surgeon, intensivists, transfusion specialist/hematopathologist all working as an integrated team which includes a reliable communication and porter system.

Coagulopathy must be anticipated, identified and treated promptly by correcting and preventing deficiencies that result in massive bleeding and death.

Understanding the factors implicated in the coagulopathy of trauma should provide a rational basis for applying massive transfusion protocols which hopefully would improve outcome from hemorrhagic shock particularly secondary to Trauma.

References

1. Floccard B, Rugeri L, Faure A *et al.* Early coagulopathy in trauma: An on scene and hospital admission study. *Injury* 2012; 43: 26–32.
2. Brohi K, Cohen MJ, Ganter MT, Matthay MA. Acute traumatic coagulopathy: Initiated by hypoperfusion: Modulated through the Protein C pathway? *AnnSurg* 2007; 245(5): 812–818.
3. Brohi K, Cohen MJ, Ganter MT *et al.* Acute coagulopathy of trauma: Hypoperfusion induces systemic anticoagulation and hyperfibrinolysis. *J Trauma* 2008; 64(5): 1211–1217.
4. Rizoli SB, Scarpellini S, Callum J *et al.* Clotting factor deficiency in early trauma-associated coagulopathy. *J Trauma* 2011; 71(5 Suppl): 5427–5434.

5. Ostrowski SR, Johansson PI. Endothelial glycocalyx degradation induces endogenous heparinization in patients with severe injury and early traumatic coagulopathy. *J Trauma* 2012; 73(1): 60–66.
6. Kutcher ME, Redick BJ, McCreery RC *et al.* Characterization of platelet dysfunction after trauma. *J Trauma* 2012; 73(1): 13–18.
7. Stansbury LG, Hess AS, Thompson K, Kramer B, Scalea TM, Hess TR. The clinical significance of platelet counts in the first 24 hrs after severe injury. *Transfusion* 2013; 53(4): 783–789.
8. Solomon C, Trantinger S, Ziegler B *et al.* Platelet function following trauma. A multiple electrode aggregometry study. *Thromb Haemost* 2011; 106(2) 322–330.
9. Rourke C, Curry N, Khan J *et al.* Fibrinogen levels during trauma hemorrhage, response to replacement therapy and association with patient outcome. *J Thromb Haemost* 2012; 10(7): 1342–1357.
10. Raza I, Davenport R, Rourke C *et al.* The incidence and magnitude of fibrinolytic activities in the trauma patient. *J Thromb Haemost* 2013; 11(2): 307–314.
11. Levrat A, Gros A, Rugeri L *et al.* Evaluation of rotation thrombelastography for the diagnosis of hyperfibrinolysis in trauma patient. *Br J Anaesth* 2008; 100 (6): 792–797.
12. Mitra B, O'Reilly G, Cameron PA *et al.* Effectiveness of massive transfusion protocols on mortality in trauma: A systematic review and meta-analysis ANZ. *J Surg* 2013; 83: 918–923.
13. Toulon P, Ozier Y, Ankri A, Fleron MH *et al.* Point of care versus central laboratory coagulation testing during hemorrhagic surgery. A multicenter study. *Thromb Haemost* 2009; 101: 394–401.
14. Mutschler M, Nienaber U, Munzberg M *et al.* The Shock Index revisited — a fast guide to transfusion requirement? A retrospective analysis on 21,853 patients derived from the Trauma Register DGU. *Critical Care* 2013; 17: 172.
15. Cotton BA, Dosset LA, Haut ER *et al.* Multicentre validation of a simplified score to predict massive transfusion in trauma. *J Trauma* 2010; (68 Suppl): S33–S38.
16. Nunez TC, Voskresensky IV, Dosett LA *et al.* Early prediction of massive transfusion in trauma: Simple as ABC (assessment of blood consumption)? *J Trauma* 2009; 64 (2Suppl): S57–S63.
17. Callcut RA, Cotton BA, Muskat P *et al.* Defining when to initiate massive transfusion: A validation study of individual massive transfusion triggers in PROMMITT patients. *J Trauma Acute Care Surg* 2013; 74: 59–68.
18. Rahbar MH, Fox EE, del Junco DJ *et al.* Coordination and management of multicenter clinical studies in trauma: Experience from the Prospective Observation Multicentre Major Trauma Transfusion (PROMMITT) study. *Resuscitation* 2012; 83: 459–464.

19. Cotton BA, Podbielski J, Camp E *et al.* A randomized controlled pilot trial of modified whole blood versus component therapy in severely injured patients requiring large volume transfusion. *Annals of Surgery* 2013; 258: 527–532.
20. Napolitano L, Mitchell JC, Cotton BA, Schrieber A, Moore EE. Tranexamic acid in trauma: How should we use it? *J Trauma Acute Care Surg* 2013; 74 (6): 1575–1585.
21. Murad MH, Stubbs JR, Gandhi MJ *et al.* The effect of plasma transfusion on morbidity and mortality: A systematic review and meta-analyis. *Transfusion* 2010; 50: 370–383.
22. Johnson JL, Moore EE, Kashuk JL *et al.* Effect of blood products transfusion on the development of post injury multiple organ failure. *Arch Surg* 2010; 145: 973–977.
23. Holcomb JB, Tilley BC, Baraniuk S *et al.* Transfusion of plasma, platelets and red blood cells in a 1:1:1 vs 1:1:2 Ratio and mortality in patients with severe trauma The PROPPR Randomized clinical trial. *JAMA* 2015; 313(5): 471–482.
24. Kashuk JL, Moore EE, Le T *et al.* Noncitrated whole blood is optimal for evaluation of post injury coagulopathy with point of care rapid thromboelastography. *J Surg Res* 2009; 156: 133–138.
25. Doran CM, Woolley T, Midwinter MJ. Feasibility of using rotational thrombelastometry to assess coagulation states of combat casualties in a deployed setting. *J Trauma* 2010; 69(Suppl 1): S40–S48.

Chapter 13

Geriatric Issues and the ICU

Richard M. Bell and Victor Hurth

Chapter Overview

Population ageing with growth rate of nearly 4% per year in those over 80 years of age is a global phenomenon.[1] Some studies report that the percentage of patients ≥80-years-old admitted to intensive care unit (ICUs) approaches 15%.[1] The ageing process itself reduces physiologic reserve and is frequently referred to as homeostenosis. Those with multiple comorbidities are at even greater risk making admission to the ICU more likely. Although policies for ICU admission are as diverse as are the healthcare systems.[2] Resources must be rapidly expanded to meet the health care needs. Some observers predict that ICU admissions in those over 80 will double by 2015, increasing by 6% per year.[5] Options for how expensive resources like ICU care will be managed are limited. The solution will probably be some form of rationing of resources, as the expense is unaffordable and unsustainable.

Age with associated comorbidities pose many challenges for the intensivist including risks of major complications, drug-related side effects and interactions, a general decrease in organ function and the ability to metabolize administered pharmacotherapeutic agents, as well as the ability to respond to cardiorespiratory threats, infections, and surgical illness.

In this chapter, we discuss issues specific to the derangements physiology associated with the ageing process and how they impact ICU care, in order to assist the intensivist caring for these patients.

Characteristics of ICU Admissions for the Elderly

The characteristics of elderly patients admitted to ICUs vary widely and so do criteria for admission. These include personal bias, physician perception, resources, patient, and family wishes etc. The decision for admission is influenced by many factors and involves application of many models (Simplified Acute Physiology Score — SAPS, Acute Physiologic and Chronic Health Evaluation — APACHE), concurrent comorbidities (Charlson Index or Elixhauser Index), functional status of the patient (Knaus, McCabe, Karnofsky, EuroScore, Katz scores, or Barthel Index etc.), physician perceptions regarding appropriateness, futility, and societal ethos. Many decisions are based on the doctors' impression that the patient is "too sick" or "too well" to benefit from ICU admission and/or aggressive care. Patients admitted to Intensive Care in the United States have lower severity of illness scores, higher admissions for cardiac illness, more chronic medical conditions and half the percentage of patients admitted requiring Mechanical Ventilation (MV) than in the United Kingdom,[6] Australia, or New Zealand.[1] Origin of admission also varies considerably. In the US more ICU admissions are referred by the Emergency Department, while in other countries more admissions come from hospital wards, transfers from other units, or unplanned surgeries.

Outcome following ICU admission for the elderly

Because of the variability described earlier, it is impossible to make generalizations regarding the outcome of elderly patients following ICU admission. Traditionally, ICU mortality has been the endpoint for judging outcome. More recently, surveys of elderly patients suggest that the return to a previous functional state is a strong patient desire and outcome measure.

Most reviews agree that severity of critical illness and diminished pre-admission functional status, have a negative impact on ICU and hospital mortality, length of stay, long-term survival, functional status after discharge, and discharge destination. The requirement for mechanical ventilation within 24-hours of admission or renal replacement therapy also appears to negatively impact survival. ICU admissions from chronic care facilities and those with longer ICU stays also have lower survival rates.

The impact of age alone on outcomes is conflicting. It appears that age >75-years may independently predict bad outcome. In-hospital mortality figures range from 25–80% with one to two organ system failures respectively.[6]

Bagshaw *et al.*[1] reported that the most common reason for ICU admission was for planned surgery and these patient had an ICU and in-hospital mortality of 12% and 25% respectively. More importantly discharge to home occurred in 72% and 57% of patients who had planned surgery were alive at one year compared to 11% who underwent unplanned surgery.[7] Quality of life was good with 83% having no cognitive impairment and three quarters having no physical impairment, the perceived quality of life assessments equating with age-matched controls.[8]

Physiology of senescence and common organ dysfunctions in the elderly ICU patient and their impact on ICU care

The ageing process can be described simply as the "stiffening" of all organ systems, due to genetics, oxidative free radical, glycation, and other forms of cellular damage that occurs over the lifetime of an individual, including healthy older adults and this is magnified by comorbidities. Understanding these physiologic limitations will improve the intensivist's ability to appropriately care for the elderly ICU patient.

Many of the changes seen are associated with a chronic, often low-grade inflammatory process that has been termed "inflammaging". This has been confirmed by a measured increase in serum markers of inflammatory cytokines and a decrease in serum levels of anabolic hormones and inflammatory suppressor cytokines. Strategies that ameliorate inflammation, improve muscle mass, and nutritional status have been shown to improve outcomes, reduce morbidity and mortality, improve the prospect of a return[3,4] to independent living by reducing hospital deconditioning, and mitigate the need for discharge to intermediate care or rehabilitation facilities. Conditioning activities, appropriately termed "Pre-habilitation", are not always possible for those elderly patients acutely admitted to an ICU setting. In addition, the margin for error in treating the older population is extremely narrow. Even trivial perioperative complications are poorly tolerated by the elderly.

Organ System Changes with Ageing

Cardiovascular[9]

The increasing incidence of Coronary Artery Disease (CAD) and Heart Failure (HF), place the elderly patient at risk for acute cardiac decompensation when in the ICU, Table 1. Response to fluid resuscitation in shock from trauma and other causes and rapid change in fluid dynamics in the perioperative period are quite variable in the elderly and often unpredictable necessitating close central hemodynamic monitoring. Resuscitation often requires inotropes or afterload-reducing agents, unlike their younger counterparts. Many of these patients may have concomitant renal impairment. This, together with the release of ADH and aldosterone in response to stress and surgery make urine output alone an unreliable measure of adequate perfusion. Catecholamine release in response to hypoperfusion states is more likely to result in dysrhythmias leading to poor outcome. Associated coronary artery disease predisposes to acute coronary ischemic events including Myocardial Infarction (MI) and death in response to hypoperfusion states. Patients on β-blockers and antihypertensive agents pose major challenges because the usual blood pressure and heart rate response to hypoperfusion and fluid resuscitation are no longer reliable, again necessitating close central hemodynamic monitoring. In these situations traditional clinical indices of perfusion such as level of consciousness, skin warmth, capillary refill, base deficit, and lack of skin pallor can prove very helpful in addition to central hemodynamic parameters.

Many acute cardiac events may be masked particularly in those over the age of 75. Subtle changes such as clinical decline or failure to wean from mechanical ventilation may be the only indications of ischemic changes. Tachycardia, because of the increase in myocardial oxygen demand versus supply in the face of limited flow due to CAD, may precipitate an acute ischemic event. Withdrawal of chronic β-blockers may result in rebound tachycardia and contribute to reduced coronary blood flow due to a reduction in ventricular filling time during diastole. Diastolic dysfunction (stiffening precluding adequate ventricular filling, common in the elderly) compounds the issue. Tachycardia may also promote coronary arteryplaque rupture leading to infarction. Abrupt discontinuation of statins likewise produces a rebound vascular inflammatory response contributing to reduced coronary blood flow and subsequent thrombosis. Chronic HF may be exacerbated by acute changes in renal function and injudicious fluid administration in the face of the acute inflammatory response as a result of surgical stress or acute illness.

The increase in myocardial fat and collagen associated with ageing results in conduction abnormalities including Atrial Fibrillation (AF) which is the most common. Rate control, usually with β-blockade or a calcium-channel blocker for AF is common. Many elderly patients with chronic AF

Table 1. Physiologic changes/geriatric issues and impact on ICU care.

Organ system	Ageing changes	Clinical significance	Treatment goals	Interventions
Cardiovascular	↑CAD and ischemia	↑Perioperative MI/ischemic events	Avoid tachycardia	Continue β-blockers/statins
		Failure to liberate from MV	↑Cardiac Output	Euvolemia/inotropes/after-load reduction
	↑Myocardial fat/ collagen	Conduction abnormalities		
		Sick Sinus Syndrome	Tachy–brady dysrhythmias	Consider pacemaker
		Atrial dysrhythmia	Euvolemia/rate control/ Adequate CO	Volume status monitoring Strict Intake and Output (I&O)
				Accurate daily weights US determination of euvolemia
		Ventricular dysrhythmia	Rate control	Consider β-blocker, Implantable
	Cardioverter Defibrillator (ICD),			
		Ventricular Tachycardia (VT)	Normal electrolytes/ O_2Sat./ Drug Toxicity?	Ablation
		Ventricular Fibrillation *Torsades de pointes*		*Note*: Short runs of VT may require no treatment *Torsades* usually self-limited

(*Continued*)

Table 1. (*Continued*)

Organ system	Ageing changes	Clinical significance	Treatment goals	Interventions
		Bundle Branch Blocks/ (HF)	Rate control	Consider pacemaker/ Cathode Ray Tube (CRT)?
	↓Sympathetic response	HF/↓CO	Euvolemia/normal CO	Volume status
	Valvular disease	Myocardial hypertrophy	Euvolemia/normal CO	
		↑Afterload	Euvolemia/normal CO	
	Peripheral Vascular Disease	↑Afterload/Myocardial hypertrophy/Hypertension	Volume status/ normal CO	
Pulmonary	↓Respiratory muscle strength	↓Respiratory reserve with stress	Maintain O_2 saturation and delivery	Non-invasive ventilator support
	↓Chest wall compliance	↑Risk of Acute Lung Injury c sepsis	Early liberation from MV	Aggressive pulmonary toilet
	↓Alveolar surface area	↓PaO_2		Spontaneous breathing trials
	↓Vital capacity	↑Atelectasis		
	↓Functional residual capacity	↑Relapse after liberation from MV		
	↑Closing volume	↓ICU discharge		
	↓CNS response to hypoxia	↑ICU and in-hospital mortality		
	↓Alveolar compliance			

	↑Risk and frequency of aspiration		Upright posture	
				Bedside swallowing evaluation
				Removal of tubes
Renal	↓Number of glomeruli	↓GFR	Euvolemia	Volume status monitoring
	↑Glomerulosclerosis	↓Conservation Na^+	Normal electrolytes	Electrolyte monitoring
	↑Dilatation/diverticularzation of tubules and collecting system	↑Hyperkalemia	Preservation renal blood flow	Maintain renal perfusion
		↑Risk of volume overload/ dehydration	Avoidance of nephrotoxic agents	Monitoring GFR
	↓Number of renal tubules	Change in drug excretion	Preservation of renal function	
	↑Vascular atrophy and hyalinization	↑Nephrotoxicity		
	↓Renal blood/plasma flow			
Hepatic	↓Hepatic volume	↑Risk of oxidative damage	Attention to medication use	Medication monitoring and serum drug levels
	↓Hepatic blood flow	↑Risk of hepatic failure	Appropriate nutritional support	

(Continued)

Table 1. (*Continued*)

Organ system	Ageing changes	Clinical significance	Treatment goals	Interventions
	↓Smooth endoplasmic reticulum	↑Abnormalities of lipid/glucose metabolism/glycation	Preservation of hepatic blood flow	Avoid over feeding Euglycemia/Serum lipids
	↓Cytochrome p450 activity			
	↑Telomere shortening	↑Risk of adverse drug reactions ↓Capacity for regeneration ↑Hepatocyte senescence		
Gastrointestinal	Motility changes, especially Esophagus and Colon	Possible ↑risk of aspiration, particularly after instrumentation of aerodigestive track	Prevention of aspiration	Upright posture when feeding Swallowing evaluation
		Constipation	Prevention of super-infections	Selective antibiotic use
	Possibly no clinically significant changes due to ageing, *per se*, in GI track function			
<u>Unique geriatric issues</u>				
Delirium (Acute Brain Failure)	Cognitive decline	Negative impact on all outcome measures	Prevention	Provision of sensory aids Family at bedside Pain control Identification and Rx of source of infection or other triggers Medication review Pharmacologic prevention?

Polypharmacy	Multiple medication use	↑ADEs	Avoidance	Discontinue non-essential meds Frequent medication reviews Pharmacist on multidisciplinary team
Frailty	Weakness, anorexia, weight loss, falling or fear of falling, fatigue, sarcopenia	Leads to deconditioning and disability	Recognition	Metabolic support Avoidance of iatrogenic injury
		Negative impact on all outcome measures		Early mobilization PT/OT involvement Delirium avoidance/management Geriatric team involvement
Nutrition (Metabolic support)	High prevalence of malnutrition	Inflammaging	Early and appropriate metabolic support	Early enteric feedings
	Anorexia of ageing Low BMI Hypoalbuminemia	Increase in mortality		Pro- and prebiotics? (Impact unknown)
Expectations	Expectations and values are different in the elderly.	Decisions may be contrary to what others might decide	Patient autonomy, beneficence, and non-malfeasance. Shared decision making	Advanced care planning, Limitations of care, palliative withholding and withdrawing care.

are anticoagulated with warfarin and more recently with direct thrombin inhibitors and consideration must be given to bridging therapy depending on other treatment considerations and acute medical or surgical issues. Short runs of Ventricular Tachycardia (VT) are usually insignificant and require no treatment. Prolonged VT may prompt the insertion of internal defibrillators. *Torsades de points*, more common in the elderly, is usually self-limiting, but may precipitate ventricular fibrillation and careful monitoring is mandatory. Bundle branch block, in particular sick sinus syndrome, may require cardiac pacing. Chronic valvular disease such as aortic stenosis most common in the elderly, requires meticulous attention to volume status and occasionally cautious afterload reduction.

Pulmonary[10]

Ageing results in a decline in all respiratory parameters posing major respiratory challenges in the ICU. Collagen cross-linking results in stiffening of pulmonary parenchyma, increasing the work of breathing, which may necessitate mechanical ventilatory assistance. Frequently this is exacerbated by chronic obstructive and restrictive disease. The tachypneic response to low tidal volume to maintain minute ventilation is frequently misinterpreted as a sign for ventilator dependence.

The known decrease in functional residual capacity and increase in closing volume (see chapter on Perioperative Respiratory Dysfunction) in the elderly which is worse in the supine position leads to alveolar collapse and hypoxemia. Alveolar fibrosis also impairs gas exchange because of ventilation perfusion mismatch. A decrease in responsiveness to hypoxia by the central nervous system results in carbon dioxide (CO_2) retention and secondary worsening of the hypoxemia frequently requiring mechanical ventilator support. The risk of acute lung injury also increases in these patients. Relapse after recovery necessitating resumption of mechanical ventilation is also common in these patients.

The elderly also presents many challenges in securing a definitive airway. Bag valve mask ventilation is impeded by inability to obtain a good seal in the edentulous patient, necessitating temporary placement of the patient's dentures in the mouth to facilitate ventilation. The fragile nasal and oral mucosa may predispose to bleeding during intubation necessitating gentleness. Neck immobility due to kyphoscoliosis and spinal stenosis make visualization of the vocal cords difficult and ancillary airway techniques such as the use of the glide scope, bronchoscope, Laryngeal Mask Airway, and the Gum Elastic Bougie should be made available in anticipation of these difficulties.

Renal[11,12]

Despite the loss of glomeruli (1/2 to 2/3 of those in younger patients), medullary interstitial fibrosis, glomerular sclerosis, dilatation of the collecting tubules, the reduction in renal blood flow caused by the subendothelial deposition of hyaline, and the reduction in glomerular filtration rate, the ageing kidney is still capable of maintaining homeostasis under normal circumstances. The older kidney is less capable of conserving sodium, perhaps due to lower aldosterone levels and diminished sodium reabsorption. This may be due to a co-existent renin deficiency as the response to Adrenocorticotropic Hormone (ACTH) stimulation is not impaired. The clinical significance is that the elderly do not respond immediately to sodium loading as younger patients do and they tend to develop hyperkalemia on a low sodium diet. The ability to conserve potassium is also restricted in the older patient as evidenced by a 20% reduction in total body potassium. These age related changes predispose the elderly to hyperkalemia particularly in association with acidosis as the aged kidney is slow to respond to the increase in serum hydrogen ion concentrations. Drugs with potential for the inhibition of renal potassium excretion, spironolactone, non-steroidal anti-inflammatory agents, β-blockers, and Angiotensin-Converting-Enzyme (ACE) inhibitors should be used with caution in older patients to avoid the risk of hyperkalemia. Serum levels of calcium are generally lower in the elderly and phosphate levels are higher. In the older patient the response to immobilization is exaggerated producing exceptionally high levels of calcium excretion in the urine. All these changes can be complicated by co-existing renal disease, hypertension, hyperthyroidism, malignancies, and diabetes. Drug dosing and administration must be adjusted in consideration of the changes in the senescent kidney. Many drugs have more direct toxic effects on the kidneys of older adults. These include Nonsteroidal Anti-inflammatory Drugs (NSAIDs), contrast agents used for imaging, aminoglycosides, methotrexate, and many others.

In the presence of renal insufficiency which is common in the elderly, drugs whose clearance is primarily through a renal mechanism should be administered with extreme caution while monitoring serum levels closely. Drugs that are not primarily cleared by renal excretion are preferable. Medications with known nephrotoxicity should be avoided if possible.

Standard estimates of renal function, i.e., serum creatinine and estimates of Glomerular Filtration Rate (GFR) commonly used today, may be misleading in the elderly. This compromises the ability to assess accurately baseline renal function and monitor the change in renal function in critically ill older patients.

The Cockcroft–Gault Equation (CGE) is less accurate, overestimating high GFR values and underestimating low values in older patients more so than the Modification of Diet in Renal Disease Formula (MDRDF). Some consider the Chronic Kidney Disease Epidemiology Collaboration formula (CKD-Epi) more accurate. The formulae are provided in Table 2. Considering the changes in creatinine metabolism associated with the loss of muscle mass in older patients, it has been suggested that determination of serum cystatin C alone or in combination with serum creatinine improves the ability to document renal function. Cystatin C is a cysteine proteinase inhibitor produced at a constant rate by all nucleated cells. It is freely filtered by the glomeruli and metabolized in the proximal tubule. Muscle mass and dietary protein intake have little to no effect on the serum levels of this substance. Many formulae have been proposed but unfortunately, the accuracy of using any of these in critically ill patients has not been validated. Further, their use in diabetic patients and the concurrent administration of some medications, e.g., corticosteroids, affect serum levels of this substance, while others interfere with the laboratory analysis.[13]

Table 2. Formula for estimating GFR in elderly patient.

Cockcroft–Gault Equation

$$\text{GFR} = \frac{140\text{–age} \times \text{Wt. (Kg)} \times (0.85 \text{ if } ♀)}{72 \times \text{Serum Cr}}$$

Modification of Diet in Renal Disease Formula

$$\text{GFR} = 175 \times (\text{SCr})^{-1.15} \times (\text{Age})^{-0.203} \times (0.742 \text{ if } ♀) \times (1.212 \text{ if African American})$$

Chronic Kidney Disease Epidemiology Collaborative Formula

$$\text{GFR} = 141 \times \min(\text{SCr}/\kappa,1)^{\alpha} \times \max(\text{SCr}/\kappa,1)^{-1.209} \times (0.993)^{\text{Age}} \times (1.018 \text{ if } ♀) \times (1.159 \text{ if Black})$$

$\kappa = 0.7$ for ♀; 0.9 for ♂

$\alpha = -0.329$ for ♀; -0.411 for ♂

$\min(\text{SCr}/\kappa,1)$ = minimum Serum Creatinine/κ, or 1

$\max(\text{SCr}/\kappa,1)$ = maximum Serum Creatinine/κ, or 1

Cystatin C Equation

$$\text{GFR} = 177.6 \times \text{Cr}^{-0.65} \times \text{CysC}^{-0.57} \times \text{Age}^{-0.57} \times (0.82 \text{ if } ♀) \times (1.11 \text{ if black})$$

Note: Results of all formula in mL/min/1.73 m^2. SCr = serum creatinine; CysC = serum cystatin C level.

Many elderly patients are chronically volume depleted from poor oral intake and chronic diuretic therapy. Isotonic hydration is preferred with careful attention to maintaining euvolemia while avoiding congestive HF from volume overload. Hypotension with a reduction in organ perfusion is especially deleterious to the aged kidney and must be avoided or promptly reversed. As indicated earlier, nephrotoxic drugs should be avoided or their serum level carefully monitored if they must be used. Multiple pharmacologic agents to prevent acute kidney injury have been studied with no conclusive results.

Hepatic[14]

Hepatic function appears to be reasonably well preserved in healthy older patients. However, liver disease accounts for a fourfold increase in mortality after the age of 40. The natural process of hepatic senescence is still poorly understood. Most data have been extrapolated from studies in animals, supporting the observation that there is a decrease in hepatic volume and a decrease in hepatic blood flow with increasing age. At the cellular level there is an increase in intracellular lipofuscin, precipitates of highly oxidized insoluble proteins, which can be identified by light microscopy and Hematoxylin and Eosin (H&E) stains. Lipofuscin is thought to interfere with many intracellular processes due to the trapping of metallic ions that facilitate oxidative damage. There also appears to be an age related decline in smooth endoplasmic reticulum, which is the site of many enzyme-mediated activities including glucose-6-phosphatase, xenobiotic, and lipid metabolism. Hepatic cells are thought to be intolerant of oxidative damage, perhaps through an increase in stress-induced transcription factors such as nuclear-factor kappa beta. The increase in nuclear DNA of hepatocytes, polyploidy, can be identified microscopically and may contribute to the increase in nuclear Deoxyribonucleic Acid (DNA) damage by oxidative or glycated damage. Telomere shortening, a marker for cellular senescence, appears to be enhanced in the presence of oxidative stress. Changes in the genetic expression of antioxidant and cytochrome p450 genes have been demonstrated in both rodent and human hepatic cells.

The clinical significance of these cellular and functional changes may be related to the inability of the older liver to regenerate under the stress of illness or injury. Clinical data supports the fact that viral disease (Hepatitis B Virus (HVB), Hepatitis C Virus (HVC), and Human Immunodeficiency Virus (HIV)) are poorly tolerated by the elderly as are the effects of alcoholic hepatitis and the survival following hepatic transplantation. For the elderly patient hospitalized in the ICU, the most clinically significant impact is on drug metabolism. The decline in p450 enzymes and the loss of smooth endoplasmic reticulum reduces Phase I metabolism. This may account for the increased susceptibility of adverse drug reactions in the elderly. The role of antioxidant pharmacotherapy is conflicting and to date no clinical recommendations can be made. However, in choosing drug therapy including parenteral nutrition, patients with hepatic insufficiency should be spared agents with known hepatotoxicity wherever possible and hepatic function should be monitored by appropriate liver function tests.

Gastrointestinal tract[15,16]

Sparse data exist regarding the effect of ageing *per se* on Gastrointestinal (GI) function. The changes described in humans may have little clinical significance in the absence of GI disease. Both the young and the elderly lose weight under the stress of starvation, illness, or injury but older patients do not recover lost weight as easily or as quickly. This may be due to the inability of the elderly to stimulate appetite.

There is a decrease in the amplitude of peristaltic pressure primarily in the upper third of the esophagus and an increase in non-propulsive contractions in the distal esophagus. Unless complicated by neurologic disease, compensation mechanisms, particularly the reduced pressure at the pharyngeal and lower esophageal sphincters, facilitates esophageal clearance. The duration of reflux episodes is extended in older adults but the number of reflux episodes does not appear to be increased. It is postulated that these motility changes may be due to a loss of enteric neurons in the aged esophagus. Clinically, these changes may make it more difficult for the elderly to overcome the dysphagia that is associated with naso- or oropharyngeal intubation, placing them at greater risk for aspiration when they are extubated. It is prudent to carefully assess swallowing function by bedside swallowing tests after removal of aerodigestive tubes and before initiating oral feedings.

Conflicting information regarding changes in gastric emptying are found in the current literature. Hypochlorhydria and atrophic gastritis are common, particularly in those patients who are *H. pylori-positive*. This may lead to bacterial overgrowth in the proximal small bowel and interfere with B_{12}, calcium, and iron absorption. It may be that the change in the microbiome in both the small bowel and colon may be more responsible for nutrient malabsorption than innate changes in GI morphology or physiology. No micro anatomic changes of clinical significance have been discovered.

Colonic dysmotility has been presumed due to the frequent complaints of constipation and excessive flatulence by older individuals. Whether this is due to the loss of myoenteric neurons, a reduction in neurotransmitters, e.g., nitric oxide or acetylcholine, or both remains speculative. There does appear an increase in opioid receptors in the older colons and specific opioid antagonists have some effect in accelerating colonic transit time. A decrease in *Firmicutes* species (producers of butyrate, a major source of short-chain fatty acids and primary source for colonic epithelial energy metabolism) and facultative anaerobes in the colon of older patients may stimulate the production of inflammatory cytokines, IL-1, IL-6, and IL-8. These are contributors to the chronic, low-grade inflammatory process, "inflammaging". Indiscriminate use of antimicrobials may not only predispose the elderly to overgrowth of *C. difficile* but perturb the microbiome to a greater degree particularly in the very old. Proton pump inhibitors and NSAIDs also change the microbiota of the colon contributing to harmful overgrowth of alternative bacterial species. The role of pro- and prebiotic use in the ICU is yet to be clearly defined, but good randomized data exist supporting its use in non-ICU hospitalized older adults.[17]

Issues Unique to the Geriatric Patient and their Impact on ICU Care

Central Nervous System[18,19]

Of all the aberrations in Central Nervous System (CNS) function operative in the elderly, none may have as detrimental an impact on outcomes as acute brain failure, more commonly labeled delirium. Most significant is the impact that delirium has on all outcome measures, morbidity, mortality (both short and long-term), length of ICU and hospital stay, costs of care, the increased likelihood of institutionalization and the frequency of relapse after discharge. Delirium is defined as change in cognition, consciousness, and attention span over the course of hours or days with a course that fluctuates. Both hyperactive and hypoactive forms exist, with the latter being of greater clinical significance and having more of a negative impact on outcome and less well recognized. The etiology, while poorly understood, is frequently multifactorial, commonly associated with systemic infections, pain, electrolyte abnormalities, medications (including polypharmacy), preexisting disabilities (cognitive, visual, hearing, physical, and functional), depression, mechanical ventilation, and severity of illness. Many elderly patients may experience delirium prior to ICU admission due to the nature and severity of their acute illness. The frequency of association with systemic infection lends credence to the theory that the inflammatory cytokine milieu released into the blood stream exacerbates the chronic inflammatory changes already in the CNS of the elderly. These inflammatory cytokines stimulate activation of neuronal and synaptic dysfunction resulting in neuro-behavioral changes. Despite its common occurrence in the ICU (up to 80% of elderly ICU patients), or following surgery, recognition by health care providers is frequently inadequate. Commonly it is the patient's family or an acquaintance who report that the patients "doesn't seem like themselves" or some other comment to suggest a change in mental status. Simple assessment methods include the Confusion Assessment Method (CAM) and an instrument designed to be more specific to the ICU environment, CAM–ICU (Figs. 1(a) and 1(b)).

Delirium is easier to prevent than to treat. Baseline cognitive screens can identify elderly patients at greatest risk. Having family members, friends, or recognizable personal items close at hand on a consistent basis is helpful. Avoidance of activities that interrupt normal sleep-waking cycles is advantageous. Removal of tethers, tubes, lines, restraints, etc., as permissible is advantageous. Avoidance of opioids, especially postoperatively, and benzodiazepines is prudent. Modifications of polypharmacy reduce adverse drug–drug interactions. Providing glasses and hearing aids normally utilized by the patient facilitates improved interactions with the environment. Attention to adequate pain control,[20] a frequently under-treated aspect of care of the elderly, is difficult especially in patients with cognitive impairment and those who cannot communicate with providers. Subtle signs, withdrawal, grimacing, agitation, aggressiveness, grabbing, mental status changes etc., may be the only clues to inadequate pain management.[21] Mobilization is one of the most effective pain management strategies that can be employed, but frequently difficult if not impossible for elderly patients in the ICU. Scheduled pain medications are superior to those provided on an "as needed" basis. Regional block, local anesthetics, and multimodal approaches can be helpful as well.

Pharmacologic prevention of delirium has not been universally successful, but some studies have shown that the duration of delirium has been reduced by oral haloperidol, utilized at low doses. Others have shown a reduction in the incidence of delirium with risperidone and olanzapine in select patient groups. However, current data do not allow extrapolation of these studies to ICU patients in general. Once delirium is identified management options are limited. Intravenous haloperidol in small incremental doses, i.e., 0.5 mg repeated as necessary, is usually effective treatment for

CONFUSION ASSESSMENT METHOD (CAM)
Shortened version worksheet

Evaluator: Date:

BOX 1

I. ACUTE ONSET AND FLUCTUATING COURSE

a) Is there evidence of an acute change in mental status from the patient's baseline? No __ Yes __

b) Did the (abnormal) behavior fluctuate during the day, that is tend to come and go or increase and decrease in severity? No __ Yes __

II. INATTENTION

Did the patient have difficulty focusing attention, for example, being easily distractible or having difficulty keeping track of what was being said? No __ Yes __

BOX 2

III. DISORGANIZED THINKING

Was the patient 's thinking disorganized or incoherent, such as rambling or irrelevant conversation, unclear or illogical flow of ideas, or unpredictable switching from subject to subject? No __ Yes __

IV. ALTERED LEVEL OF CONSCIOUSNESS

Overall, how would you rate the patient's level of consciousness?

Alert (normal) __

Vigilant (hyperalert) __
Lethargic (drowsy, easily aroused)
Stupor (difficult to arouse) __
Coma (unarousable) __

Do any checks appear in this box? No __ Yes __

If all items in Box 1 are checked and at least one item in Box 2 is checked a diagnosis of delirium is suggested.

Fig. 1(a). Confusion assessment method worksheet.

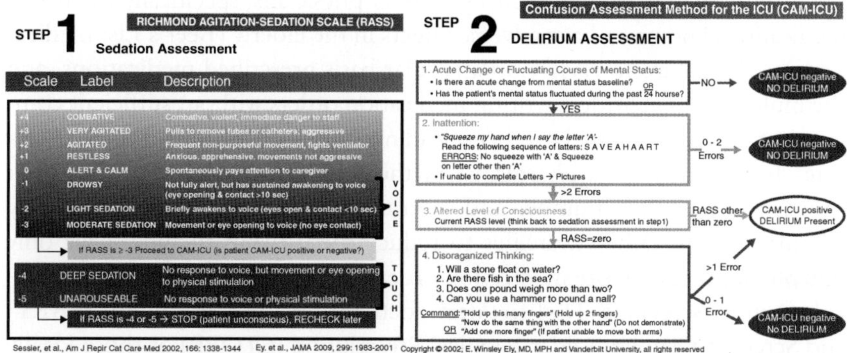

Fig. 1(b). Richmond agitation-sedation scale.

hyperactivity and may prevent the inadvertent removal of tubes and other devices necessary for patient care. Management in a unit dedicated to care of the geriatric patient has proven to be more effective than geriatric management teams, which provide collaborative rounds regularly on elderly patients with respect to outcomes. Few such units exist, however.

Polypharmacy[22–25]

Elderly patients take many medications, both by physician prescription and those self-prescribed over-the-counter supplements and herbal products. Many of these are inappropriate and even dangerous. Adverse Drug Events (ADEs) are responsible for one in six hospitalizations in individuals over 65-year old and one in three of those over 75. Drug–drug interactions account for more than 75% of all ADEs. Hypoglycemic agents and anticoagulants are the two classes of drugs that pose the greatest danger to the elderly. The elderly are at greatest risk due to a number of factors that include age alone, changes in pharmacokinetics due to changes in liver and renal function, the number of medications taken, inappropriate prescriptions, cognitive, and functional decline, levels of serum proteins, changes in body compositions (decrease in total body water and increase in body fat) with the associated changes in volume of distribution of drugs, the number of providers prescribing medications, associated comorbidities, and illness severity. Because of the number of medications utilized during a period of ICU care, ADEs are common in the ICU setting, occurring in up to 20% of all ICU admissions, 19.4 per 1,000 patient days. These events are probably underreported. ADEs lengthen hospital stay and increase costs. It is generally accepted that polypharmacy is a main contributor to these iatrogenic injuries. Inappropriate prescribing practices by ICU physicians, specifically the use of medications known to have adverse effects in the elderly (Beer's List medications),[26] the failure to review on a regular basis prescribed medications, and the multitude of providers writing medication orders without sufficient communication with others, have been leading causes of ADEs in the ICU setting. Involvement of a pharmacist in the multidisciplinary team has been shown to reduce the number and severity of ADEs but not to completely eliminate them. Other strategies to reduce these events include: have only one physician team write medication orders, adherence to prescribing protocols such as Screening Tool to Alert doctors to Right Treatment (START) and Screening Tool of Older Peoples' Prescription (STOPP) or those locally developed, institution of computerized monitoring of drug orders and administrations, discontinuation of all non-essential or duplicate medications, and repetitive medication reviews and reconciliation.

Frailty[27,28,31]

Frailty has been recently accepted as a geriatric syndrome but there is not yet consensus as to the definition or clinical findings necessary to make the diagnosis. Commonly accepted components include weakness, weight loss, anorexia, fatigue, falling or fear of falling, and sarcopenia. The presence of frailty in the elderly has been estimated to be as high as 45%. It is also accepted that frailty has a negative impact on short and long-term morbidity, mortality, speed of recovery, institutionalization at discharge, functional ability, and subsequent quality of life. Frailty is not synonymous with disability, but frailty can lead to disability if triggered by some external event, i.e., acute illness/injury, hospitalization or ICU admission, which may lead to deconditioning. In addition, frailty is not synonymous with multi-morbidity as it can exist in the absence of chronic disease(s). A number of frailty scales and scoring systems exist but they are cumbersome to use clinically. While hard to define, most health care providers, even with a modicum of clinical experience, can recognize it. Once recognized there are few specific interventions that are effective in reversing or managing it. Early and appropriate metabolic support, mobilization and physical/occupational therapy, avoidance of iatrogenic injury, e.g., ADEs, delirium risk modification strategies, multidisciplinary teams with specific expertise in geriatric care, etc. may be helpful but data quantitating the usefulness of such strategies does not exist.

Malnutrition[29,30]

Malnutrition, manifest by low Body Mass Index (BMI) (<20 Kg/m^2) or involuntary weight loss (>10 lbs. in six months, or 10%), has more of an impact on mortality in hospitalized elderly than multiple comorbidities or frailty by more than twice. While a simple history can identify malnutrition, current providers seem enamored with laboratory confirmation or anthropomorphic measurements. Serum prealbumin (<15 mg/dL), transferrin (<200 mg/dL), albumin (<3.5 g/dL), anemia and red cell distribution width (>15%), transthyretin (<258 or >316 mg/L), or serum micronutrient levels of iron, B_{12} or serum folate are commonly obtained. Multiple screening tools are also available, but provide little additional clinically useful information. Monitoring of improvement in nutritional status, practiced frequently by repeated laboratory testing, serves as reassurance for the physician, but has not been shown to have clinical significance. Monitoring of nutrient intake to assure estimated needs are being met is sufficient.

Other than the consideration of the early institution of metabolic support, preferentially via the gut, there are no strategies to overcome the effects of chronic malnutrition and reverse the impact on outcome for the elderly in the ICU. Specialized nutritional products, while appealing and sexy, have not been shown to improve outcome over less expensive, balanced formula that meet energy, protein, and micronutrient needs. Feed early and feed appropriately is the axiom. Probiotic and prebiotic are logical, but clinical evidence showing improvements in outcome are lacking, despite the popularity of their use in the ICU. This may be due to the heterogeneous nature of commercially available products, formulated more on ease of manufacturing than on sound scientific evidence.

Role of Decreased Immunity, Musculoskeletal Injuries, and Temperature Control in the Elderly ICU Patient

Decreased immunity

Many correlates of decreased immunity exist in the elderly: decreased cell mediated and humoral immune responses, decrease in thymic tissue, spleen and liver size and, possible alteration in granulocyte function. All these factors make the elderly less resistant to infection and alters the ability to recover from infections due to bacteria, viruses, and other pathogens. These patients particularly in the ICU environment must be protected from these pathogens by decreasing exposure through strict infection control strategies in the ICU. Infection in the elderly may present in unusual fashions such as a lack of fever or leukocytosis and diagnosis is frequently based on a high index of suspicion. Frequently, a change in level of consciousness, subtle drop in urine output, and even a decrease in temperature may herald an infection in the elderly. Aggressive search for a source of sepsis including chest X-ray, ultrasound and Computed Tomography (CT) of the abdomen as well as culture of urine, sputum, blood, wounds, vascular access are important. Antimicrobials should be directed at specific cultured organisms with measured sensitivity profiles, avoiding blind broad spectrum antimicrobials to prevent overgrowth of organisms and resistant infections. Failure to wean from the respirator is a frequent subtle sign of undrained sepsis which should prompt radiologic assessment and possible use of percutaneous sampling and drainage of collections to secure culture specimens and monitor response. When fever, leukocytosis, and tachycardia are present these should be monitored for evidence of infection and response to therapy.

Musculoskeletal injuries

Falls and fractures from mild or severe trauma are frequent causes of morbidity in the elderly. Decreased respiratory reserve increases the risk of pneumonia from simple rib fractures associated with pain and restriction of coughing and deep breathing, with inability to clear pulmonary secretions. Judicious use of analgesics including nerve blocks to decrease pain while not depressing cough and deep breathing and allowing vigorous chest physiotherapy is the mainstay of treatment and prevention of complications such as pneumonia and thromboembolic events.

Early operative fixation of fractures to encourage early ambulation and physiotherapy has been shown to decrease pulmonary complications, hospital as well as ICU stay in these elderly patients.

Temperature control

The decrease in subcutaneous fat and the thin skin as well as poor temperature homeostasis predispose the elderly to hypothermia, which carries a high mortality. Awareness of this possibility and prompt institution of preventive measures including a warm environment, warm blankets, warm fluids using fluid warmers for large volume infusions as frequently required in major surgical procedures, and blood transfusions, together with monitoring of core temperature are important measures in preventing hypothermia.

End-of-life Issues, Palliative Care and Withdrawal/Withholding Of Care[32,33]

Decisions concerning these issues vary widely around the world. Hospital/societal resources, religious beliefs, cultural norms, societal ethos, opinions about prognosis, bias, and emotions all influence these decisions. To admit, or not admit, the elderly to the ICU is the first difficult decision. Often when dealing with a critical or end-of-life issue, it is not possible for the patients to communicate their wishes to the health care team and communication is restricted to family members or surrogate decision makers. Participation by nurses in decision making is also variable. It has been suggested that leaving these decisions solely to critical care physicians is associated with early "burn out". Strategies that have been developed to assist with decision making and communication are listed in Table 3.

Table 3. Consensus principles regarding end-of-life, palliative, withholding, or withdrawing care.

- Autonomy, beneficence, and non-malfeasance are the principles establishing the foundation for decision making.
  - o Paternalism is out, shared decision making (patient, surrogate, family, and doctor) is in.
  - o Patient wishes are to be respected, despite the potential conflict with the value systems of others.
  - o Providing medical care against the patient's wishes is assault and battery, even if withholding treatment could lead to death.
  - o Respecting the patient's dignity despite conflicts with the value judgments of others is a priority consideration.
  - o The role of the physician is to honestly inform, not make value judgments.
  - o There is a significant difference between competence and capacity that must be considered.
  - o Surrogates are charged to make decisions based on what the patient would want, not what the surrogate feels is in the patient's best interest.
  - o Disagreements regarding the patient's wishes among family members, and sometimes providers, are not uncommon. The inclusion of all stake holders in a non-confrontational, unrushed, information sharing discussion is appropriate. Frequently a second opinion may be helpful. There may also be a role for consultation by hospitals' Ethics Committee.
- Limitations of Care are appropriate under certain circumstances.
  - o Advanced care planning is effective, when possible.
  - o ICU care can be beneficial and can also increase and prolong suffering.
  - o Elderly patient make judgments based on a different value system than younger individuals.
  - o Prolongation of life itself is not the primary objective in the minds of older people, particularly if it compromises quality-of-life, reduces functional status, impairs independence or prolongs pain and suffering.
  - o Limitations of care orders and DNR orders do not imply "no care".

(*Continued*)

Table 3. (*Continued*)

- o Decisions should be tempered by the projected benefits compared to the concept of prolonging suffering.
- o Often prolonging life is simply prolonging the dying process.

- Palliative Care
  - o There is no obligation to continue care that is judged to be futile.
  - o Alleviation of suffering by medications, even if it shortens life, is appropriate.
  - o Advanced care planning can help achieve a "good death" which is important to most elderly people.
  - o Prognostic tools are good for explaining outcomes in groups of patients, but are not appropriate in decision making for individual patients.
  - o Many hospitals have palliative care teams; use them.
  - o Health care providers should be attentive to the emotional needs of the patient's family and loved ones.

Sources: Consensus statements have been adapted from:
[32] *Best Pract Res Clin Anaesth* 2011; 25: 451–460.
[33] *NEJM* 2002; 346(14): 1061–1066.
[34] *Crit Care Med* 2008; 36: 953–963.

Older patients make decisions based on different value systems than younger ones. In general, concerns over functional status, quality of life, prevention of suffering, self-control, and independence take priority over concerns about death. For many older individuals there are far worse things than death itself. Physicians are legally and ethically responsible to protect our patients' autonomy and dignity, to act in their best interest (beneficence) and to avoid harm (non-malfeasance). Autonomy refers to the right of self-determination, to accept or refuse health interventions based on their own value system. Dignity refers to an individual's perception of self-worth, value system, and beliefs. Surrogates, relatives, and physicians are frequently guilty of inappropriately substituting their own value judgments under conditions that the patient would consider unacceptable.

Historically efforts have focused on documents, i.e., Medical Power of Attorney (MPOA), Advanced Directives, Living Wills, etc., more so than on candid and open discussion regarding the appropriateness of treatments and expectations with patients, including their family members when possible. Such discussions are time consuming and uncomfortable for many, especially for providers. The urgency of ICU care and the lack of capacity on the part of the patient to communicate their wishes complicate the matter. Surrogate decision makers frequently have the misconception that their role is to make decision that they think are in the best interest of the patient, and not based on the surrogates understanding of what the patient would have wanted. Studies have shown that the surrogate's judgment about what the patient would wish is frequently discordant with the patient's wishes.

Table 4 lists consensus principles regarding palliative or end-of-life care from Intensive Care Medicine Societies in the US, Canada, United Kingdom, Australia, and New Zealand. The principles are also applicable to withdrawal of care or the withholding of care deemed to be futile. Disagreements among family members are not uncommon and can interfere with providing care concordant with the patient's wishes. If such occurs, obtaining a second opinion, involvement of the hospital Ethics Committee and or the palliative care team may prove beneficial. Legal documents are less effective than honest, thoughtful discussion, and shared decision making. Often MPOAs, Advanced Directives and Living Wills are ignored by surrogate decision makers. Careful and comprehensive documentation in the medical record of medical opinions, decisions (and by whom they were made) and details of communication with the patient, surrogate, and family members is prudent. Physician judgment regarding prognosis is often paramount in influencing decision making. While prognostic indices may provide some data on which physicians may communicate their opinions to family members it must be remembered that the application of these indices to individual patients is not helpful.

Summary

Elderly ICU patients are not simply old adults. They have unique issues and physiologic changes that if ignored by the intensivist can lead to a deluge of adverse events that prolong ICU stay and negatively impact any outcome measure one choses to measure. Consequently, an understanding of the physiology of senescence is essential to avoid iatrogenic injury. Successful ICU care may require more aggressive and earlier interventions. Old patients benefit from ICU care and many are returned to their pre-hospital functional level. Evidence-based data regarding most aspects of ICU care for the elderly are lacking, but if needed future intensivists are to be expected to make rational decisions and provide appropriate care for this rapidly expanding cohort of the world's population. There will be difficult decisions to be made in the future regarding the financing of care for critically ill or injured elderly patients.

Table 4. Strategies for practice in the ICU regarding end-of-life care.

Policy

- Development of admission and discharge criteria.
- Development of policy for palliative, withdrawal, and withholding of care.
- Training for ICU physicians and other ICU health care providers in communication, ethics, and end-of-life issues.
- Open and liberal visitation policy.
- Develop guidelines for withdrawal or withholding of care.

Interdisciplinary team development and communication

- Establish a multidisciplinary team.
- Establish daily rounds with all members of the team.
- Daily review of progress, expectations, family concerns, and changes in prognosis.
- Frequent communication among all members of the team.

Family/surrogate involvement

- Open and liberal visitation policy.
- Daily communication and review of treatment plans.
- Frequent updates on progress or other changes in prognosis.
- Encourage family to join the team on rounds.
- Scheduled conferences with family members and the multidisciplinary team.

End-of-life education

- For all members of the multidisciplinary team.

References

1. Bagshaw SM, Webb SAR, Delaney A *et al.* Very old patients admitted to intensive care in Australia and New Zealand: A multi-center cohort analysis. *Crit Care* (London) 2009; 13(2): R45. Available online http://ccforum.com/content/13/2/R45.
2. Fuchs L, Chronaki CE, Park S *et al.* ICU admission characteristics and mortality rates among elderly and very elderly patients. *Intensive Care Med* 2012; 38: 1654–1661.
3. Halpern NA, Pastores SM. Critical care medicine in the United States 2000–2005: An analysis of bed numbers, occupancy rates, payer mix and costs. *Crit Care Med* 2010; 38: 65–71.
4. United Nations, Department of Economic and Social Affairs, Population Division (2013): World Population Prospects: The 2012 Revision. New York.

Available online http://www.un.org/en/development/desa/population/publications/pdf/ageing/WorldPopulationAgeing2013.pdf.

5. Pisani MA. Consideration is caring for the critically ill older patient. *J Inten Care Med* 2009; 24(2): 83–95.
6. Wunsch H, Angus DC, Harrison DA *et al.* Comparison of medical admissions to intensive care units in the United States and United Kingdom. *Am J Resp Care Med* 2011; 183: 1666–1673.
7. de Rooij SEJA, Bovers AC, Korevaar JC *et al.* Cognitive, functional and quality-of-life outcomes of patients aged 80 and older who survived at least 1 year after planned or unplanned surgery or medical intensive care treatment. *J Am Geriatr Soc* 2008; 56: 816–822.
8. Tabah A, Philippart F, Timsit JF *et al.* Quality of life in patients aged 80 or over after ICU discharge. *Crit Care* 2010; 14: R2. Available online http://ccforum.co/content/14/1/R2.
9. Leal MA, Field ME, Page RL. Ventricular arrhythmias in the elderly: Evaluation and medical management. *Clin Geriatr Med* 2012; 28: 665–677.
10. Siner JM, Pisani MA. Mechanical ventilation and acute respiratory distress syndrome in older patients. *Clin Chest Med* 2007; 28: 783–791.
11. Mulder WJ, Hillen HFP. Renal function and renal disease in the elderly: Part I. *Euro J Intern Med* 2001; 12: 86–97.
12. Haase M, Story DA, Hasse-Fielitz A. Renal injury in the elderly: Diagnosis biomarkers and prevention. *Best Pract Clin Anaesth* 2011; 25: 401–412.
13. Weinert LS, Damargo EG, Soares AA, Silveiro SP. Glomerular filtration rate estimation: Performance of serum cystatin C-based prediction equations. *Clim Chem Lab Med* 2011; 49(11): 1761–1771.
14. Schmucker DL. Age-related changes in liver structure and function: Implications for disease? *Exp Geront* 2005; 40: 650–659.
15. Salles N. Basic mechanisms of the aging gastrointestinal track. *Dig Dis* 2007; 25: 112–117.
16. Britton E, McLaughlin JT. Ageing and the gut. *Proc Nutrit Soc* 2013; 72: 173–177.
17. Duncan SH, Flint HJ. Probiotics and prebiotics and health in ageing populations. *Maturitas* 2013; 75: 44–50.
18. Balas MC, Happ MB, Yang W *et al.* Outcomes associated with delirium in older patients in surgical ICUs. *Chest* 2009; 135: 18–25.
19. Reade MC, Phil D, Finfer S. Sedation and delirium in the intensive care unit. *NEJM* 2014; 370: 444–454.
20. Graf C, Puntillo K. Pain in the older adult in the intensive care unit. *Crit Care Clin* 2003; 19: 749–770.
21. Brown D, Dip HP, PGCert LLL. Pain assessment with cognitively impaired older people in acute hospital setting. *Rev Pain* 2011; 3(3): 18–22. Available online http://www.sagepublications.com.

22. Kopp BJ, Erstad GL, Allen ME *et al.* Medication errors and adverse drug events in an intensive care unit: Direct observation approach for detection. *Crit Care Med* 2006; 34: 415–425.
23. Onder G, Tischa JM, van der Cammen TJM *et al.* Strategies to reduce the risk of iatrogenic illness in complex older adults. *Age Ageing* 2013; 42: 284–291.
24. Shi S, Klotz U. Age-related changes in pharmacokinetics. *Curr Drug Metab* 2011; 12: 601–610.
25. Pretorius RW, Gataric G, Sedlund SK, Miller JR. Reducing the risk of adverse drug events in older adults. *Am Fam Physician* 2013; 87(5): 331–336.
26. The American Geriatrics Society 2012 Beers Criteria Update Expert Panel. American Geriatrics Society updated Beers Criteria for potentially inappropriate medication use in older adults. *J Am Geriatr Soc* 2012; 60(4): 616–631.
27. Kane RL, Shamliyan T, Talley K, Pacala J. The association between geriatric syndromes and survival. *J Am Geriat Soc* 2012; 60: 896–904.
28. McDermid RC, Stelfox HT, Bagshaw SM. Frailty in the critically ill: A novel concept. *Crit Care* 2011; 15: 301–307.
29. Sheean PM, Peterson SJ, Chen Y *et al.* Utilizing multiple methods to classify malnutrition among elderly patients admitted to the medical and surgical intensive care units. *Clin Nutrit* 2013; 32: 752–757.
30. Young AM, Kidston S, Banks MD *et al.* Malnutrition screening tools: Comparison against two validated nutrition assessment methods in older medical patients. *Nutrit* 2013; 29: 101–106.
31. McDermid RC, Stelfox HT, Bagshaw SM. Frailty in the critically ill: A novel concept. *Crit Care* 2011; 15: 301–307.
32. Silvester W, Detering K. Advanced directives, perioperative care and end-of-life planning. *Best Pract Research Clin Anaesth* 2011; 25: 451–460.
33. Fried TR, Bradley EH, Towle VR *et al.* Understanding the treatment preferences of very ill patients. *NEJM* 2002; 346(14): 1061–1066.
34. Truog RD, Campbell ML, Curtis JR *et al.* Recommendations for end-of-life care in the intensive care unit: A consensus statement by the American Academy of Critical Care Medicine. *Crit Care Med* 2008; 36: 953–963.

Chapter 14

Ethical Issues in the Surgical ICU

Marshall Beckman, John Weigelt, Jameel Ali and Richard M. Bell

Chapter Overview

Technological advances in life sustaining devices with the attendant capability of prolonging life, complexity of diseases, comorbidities, differences in societal mores in the intensive care unit (ICU) patients all present major challenges to care givers in this increasingly complex environment. The surgical patient is also unique because treatment options are frequently invasive with potential for significant variations in outcome including iatrogenic harm. These factors demand a well-established infrastructure within the surgical ICU to address the inevitable ethical issues that arise. While variable in composition, the bioethics committee should have wide representation from medical staff, nurses, bioethicist, social worker, members of the clergy and lay people to help resolve issues. A totally transparent and free communication system is necessary among physicians, patients, family members, and ICU staff. Such communication allows voicing of concerns regarding choices of care, and potential outcome. One goal should be an attempt to bridge the gap between expectations and reality and the ability to modify plans in an ever changing care environment. Another ethical consideration in this communication is respecting cultural and religious sensibilities, acting with empathy in the best interest of the patient while providing understanding and a sense of deep caring for all individuals involved.

In this chapter, in order to assist the intensivist and staff caring for these patients we will briefly discuss general principles of biomedical ethics, their relation to rights, responsibilities, and the law. We will also discuss specific common ethical issues in the Surgical ICU and how these bioethics principles are applied to these issues.

Brief History, Hippocrates, Nuremburg, Belmont Commission[13,18]

As we have become more sophisticated in medicine, we have had further commentary on long held tenets of what is right and what is wrong as we deliver surgical critical care. Hippocrates (c. 460 B.C.), who is often referred to as the Father of Western Medicine, is well-known to for his Hippocratic Oath. It is a variation of this oath that medical students recite as they finish undergraduate medical education. This oath has morphed to make the first priority of a physician to not do harm.

This concept of no harm was surely tested during the reign of the Nazis in Europe during World War II. The Nuremberg Code resulted from the atrocities committed by physicians in Nazi Germany. This code is the first set of principles that guides research on human subjects that is recognized on an international basis (Flanagan).

After the controversial Tuskegee Syphilis Study, the National Commission for the Protection of Human Subjects in Biomedical and Behavioral Research, which is commonly referred to as the Belmont Report, was formed. This report, published in 1978, identified three principles for human subject research: "Respect for persons", "beneficence", and "justice". These principles dove tail into the four principles of Beauchamp and Childress in their book Principles of Biomedical Ethics, 2001. The principles are autonomy, beneficence, non-maleficence, and justice.

General Principles of Biomedical Ethics Applied to the Critical Care Environment[2,13,14,17,18]

(1) *Autonomy*: This refers to the right of the patient to decide for himself free from influence by others, how and what care is delivered. Many have regarded this principle to have the highest priority among the four principles. This notion of higher priority is not espoused by the original authors of these principles. The patient must have a clear understanding of the situation in order to make decisions. There is a fine line between education and informing the patient, which is a major function of the physician, and unduly influencing the patient through unjustified bias on the part of the physician. Part of that education is aimed at bridging the gap between the patient's

expectation and "reality" based on reliable scientific data. The right of the patient to decide also requires that the patient has the capacity to decide. In the ICU environment the patient may lack decisional capacity secondary to their level of cognition, level of consciousness, nature of injury etc. or metabolic derangements. Additionally, a patient's condition may hinder his/her ability to recognize the capacity to decide. Recognized mental competence testing may assist in resolving the situation. When a decision is made and the patient lacks the capacity to decide, there are several options.

An advance directive is one. This document is prepared and signed by the patient during a time when they had the capacity to decide which can be used to guide the decision making process. The patient's autonomy is thus preserved based on his previous level of mental competence. This appears to be a straight-forward solution to a difficult situation, but it is far from a perfect solution. Often the advance directive document is not specific enough to apply to a medical condition. Most directives designate a specific individual, (Power of Healthcare Attorney), to oversee the decision making process. The lack of a Power of Healthcare Attorney creates a void for decision making. Trying to decide who will be the substitute decision maker is difficult and controversial. Options for this substitute decision maker include a legal representative, a pastor, a member of the family, or even a friend. How this is decided is not easy when agreement among friends and family is not unanimous. Ethical issues can arise as family or friends believe that motives behind a decision are not shared by all. How these differences are mediated are unique to each patient or situation and may need legal involvement. The living will is another document which may contain elements of the Power of Healthcare Attorney as well as directives regarding disposal of assets etc. and would therefore also serve the purpose of the advance directive. More details on the living will are discussed below.

(2) *Beneficence*: This principle entails the obligation of the physician to do good things on behalf of his patient and to consider the welfare of his patient at all times without being viewed as being too paternalistic and/or manipulative. The risk of conflict between autonomy and beneficence commonly exists and safeguards against this conflict must be practiced by the physician with a clear aim of preserving the patient's welfare. The balance between risk and benefit is always present when a physician caring for a critically ill patient considers the beneficence principle. One example is that any intervention carries a potential benefit, but also risks. The moral duty of the physician is to ensure that the result is to the overall benefit of the patient.

In spite of the physician adhering to this principle of beneficence, the patient's perception may be different especially if the patient is reducing the risk and enhancing the benefit. In this situation, the physician must try to engender patient trust emphasizing that the doctor is trying to serve as the patient's advocate for his/her overall well-being. The earlier a physician can develop patient trust and understanding as well as demonstrate appropriate empathy, the more likely is the patient to accept physician recommendations.

A sense of beneficence and trust will encourage open communication so that the patient does not feel abandoned by the physician. A common scenario in the ICU is how to keep an entire family updated and involved in the patient's care. Ideally, at each meeting with care providers, all family members should be present. This is usually impossible. One solution is to have a policy for regularly scheduled family updates which are scheduled usually related to patient acuity. Another solution is short updates each day when convenient for a majority of family members and ICU staff and physicians. An additional step, especially with large families, is to have one or two individuals who the family designate as spokespersons to deliver information to the rest of the family. While these options are all applicable, no one solution will solve each family's needs for communication.

A final help in the field of beneficence is an institutional patient advocate. The institutional designated patient advocate serves the purpose of bringing patient's concerns to the attention of the treating team. They can be helpful in clarifying issues and reassuring patients. Depending on how they are organized within each institution they may be the ones setting up meetings, routinely communicating with families and even answering specific complaints. These individuals also learn that a frequent cause of complaints is miscommunication. They become very good at interpreting physician's communication with families and patients in terms they understand. Resolving patient and family complaints helps avoid painful interactions later including legal actions.

(3) *Non-maleficence*: The principle of non-maleficence emphasizes the physician obligation to avoid doing "bad things", i.e., things that could potentially harm the patient. So, on the one hand beneficence implies action to encourage good outcomes while the non-maleficence principle focuses on avoiding actions that could do harm. This emanates from the golden principle of "*primum non nocere*"-first do no harm. These two principles could potentially yield conflicts. In the extreme, if physicians do nothing in order to avoid harm, good interventions with acceptable risks could be omitted to

the detriment of the patient. For example a patient with major comorbidities and attendant high risk for postoperative complications may be denied an operative procedure such as appendectomy which could result in an improved outcome. Applying this principle is another risk benefit decision. As a critical care team elects to apply any intervention, a thoughtful review of the expected benefit versus any adverse event should occur. To give a simple example. A simple blood test has risks and benefits. If the test will not change anything, then why place the patient at risk for an invasive procedure as well as a lab error which could lead to further interventions. While simplistic it illustrates the non-maleficence principle.

(4) *Justice*: There are two components to this principle of Justice which may be in conflict with each other: Individual Justice and Distributive Justice.

Individual Justice involves doing the right or just thing for an individual with the assumption that the greater good will be served by the collective effect of these individual just acts whereas, Distributive Justice refers to the physician seeking out what is just or good for a group or population, e.g., an entire community. An assumption is made that more individuals will benefit if the general well-being of the community at large is served. These two principles are difficult since individual physicians generally serve individual patients and are advocates for these patients which may conflict with the general good of the community. A critical care issue that conforms to these principles is ICU bed use. Most hospitals have a limited number of ICU beds and the resources needed to proper staff them. How do we handle the situation where our patients exceed ICU bed capacity? The answer is always the least sick patient is transferred and a new patient is admitted who appears to be sicker. How often we are wrong in this assessment and patient harm occurs for the greater good. This is a difficult situation but all too real.[3]

Ethical Principles and the Law[4,17,19]

In most circumstances, application of ethical principles, clinical judgment, input from stake holders lead to consensus and resolution of ethical issues. These resolutions do not generally conflict with the law. However, occasionally our ethical deliberations result in a recommendation which could violate the law. For example, the "prudent decision" based on consensus may result in a recommendation for pursuing euthanasia as an option. The prevailing law in most countries considers euthanasia an illegal act. Where the recommended action conflicts with the law then the action is not pursued because the law of the land must prevail.

The legal system may also get involved when the parties in a conflict concerning the manner of care cannot agree on a course of action. This situation commonly arises when there is no power of healthcare attorney for a non-decisional patient and family and friends cannot agree among themselves as to what the patient would desire. The legal system often steps into this arena and appoints a power of healthcare attorney or more commonly a legal guardian depending on what is demanded by the state. Some measure of patient non-decisional status is established and once met, the legally appointed individual has the right to make choices for the patient. These choices are supposed to be in the best interest of the patient based on what the legal appointee believes to be true.

Independent action on the part of one party without legal opinion on the resolution of the conflict is considered a violation of the law while the matter still remains legally unresolved. This occurs frequently in situations where consideration is given to curtail treatment in patients with no realistic hope of recovering from a chronically vegetative state. Arguments then include what constitutes the vegetative state, the absolute likelihood of death and the value of life itself. Many consider preservation of life as a fundamental principle and thus life should be preserved at virtually all cost. Differing views on this issue give rise to major conflicts particularly in the intensive care unit. Patients, family members, and health care providers may view the continuation of aggressive medical interventions as prolonging suffering rather than prolonging life. Frequently, it becomes obvious to the health care team that the continuation of aggressive care is futile, that a patient's condition cannot be reversed and that continuing such efforts will not result in a meaningful survival. Unfortunately, this view may not be shared by family members or surrogate decision makers. Doctors are not required to continue providing care that they honestly believe will not be of value, but they are obligated to identify another provider who is willing to assume the patient's care. The most effective strategy to prevent this type of conflict and possible confrontations is through frequent and honest communication where expectations are openly discussed and information is shared by all those involved. Occasionally, a third party mediator may be required and this may involve another physician, the ethics committee or the legal system.

Physicians have a fiduciary responsibility to provide the highest standard of care. Fiduciary, from the Latin word ***fiducia*** for "trust" implies that the patient's wishes and values are placed above all others and that they will serve as the guiding principles. The physician must insure that the patient's best interest are primary, avoid conflicts of interest, maintain confidentiality, and practice in good faith. The historical premise that the physician "knows best", paternalism, has been replaced by the concept of shared decision-making. This is based on the concept of autonomy, previously discussed, and the right of self-determination which is rooted in common law. This includes the right to consent to treatment and the right to refuse it, even if such refusal may result in death or permanent harm. Patients today have accesses to a wealth of medical information; some of this information is accurate, but some of it is not. The role of the physician is to educate, honestly and without injecting the physician's personal bias or value system. The pitfall to overtly or subconsciously bias a patient's decision must be avoided.

Situations in the ICU frequently impair a patient's capacity to express their desires. Capacity is often confused with competency. The mental competency is a determination made by the legal system and a guardian is appointed by the court. The surrogate may also be a decision maker for the patient on the basis of "substituted judgment" and requests what he believes the patient would want. It is the duty of the health care team to remind the surrogate that his or her role is to facilitate the patient's preferences. Surrogates may be identified by a formal Medical Power of Attorney, advanced directives or a living will. A living will is a legal document in which the patient describes and defines what life-sustaining treatments he or she would want in the event of incapacity and terminal illness. Patients may also designate a power of attorney for healthcare; this person has the legal authority to make healthcare decisions on behalf of the patient. With or without this legal document, the surrogate, or proxy, is expected to use substituted judgment — to reconstruct what the patient would have wanted in a particular situation using formal and informal statements the patient may have made previously. The best interest standard requires the treating medical professional to act in accordance with current responsible and competent professional opinion when choosing treatment options for a patient who does not have decisional capacity and whose wishes are not known. When such designations have not been formally declared, state statutes list the order of family members who may act as surrogates. It is important to emphasize that the surrogates responsibility is to substitute a judgment based on what the patient would have decided under the circumstances, not what the surrogate thinks is best.[19]

Surrogate decision makers do not have absolute authority. Rather, they must demonstrate the ability to make the substitute judgment reflecting the patient's prior expressed values and wishes. It is also important to realize that the obligations of the physician are defined both by the wishes of the patient and the goals of medicine. If a physician believes that a surrogate's request is not in agreement with the goals of medical therapy, then he or she can refuse to comply with the surrogate's request. An ethics team may offer insight when the decision being made is questionable. The hospital's legal team may also become involved.

Withholding and Withdrawing Care[1,7,9,18]

As previously discussed, patients have the right to refuse care. Advanced directives can specifically state what the patient wishes to have done and not done, e.g., extended life support, feeding tubes, the extent of resuscitation efforts, etc. In many circumstances, families find it easier to withhold care rather than withdraw life-sustaining treatments once they have been initiated. Many medical ethicists view withdrawing care with the same guiding principles as withholding care, but this position is not shared by all. In Israel, orthodox Jewish law allows care to be withheld but forbids withdrawal of care once initiated. Others may view withdrawal of care as a form of physician assisted suicide, hastening death. Physician-assisted suicide is illegal in all states in the US except Oregon. Interestingly, only about half of the patients prescribed lethal doses of medication by their physician in that state actually use the medication to relieve their suffering by ending their life. There is a vast differences of opinion across cultures and differing religious beliefs regarding this issue. Catholics are more likely to accept withdrawal of care than Jews, Greek Orthodox or Muslims.[1,7] Most patients and families want, and expect, a good death, one free from pain and anxiety. Fortunately this can be accomplished in the majority of patients with opioids and anxiolytics. The assistance of a palliative care team can be immensely helpful in these circumstances.[6,8,15,16]

The concept of futility has been previously discussed. Physicians may find it useful to have discussions with patients and/or family members regarding expectations and to set limits on interventions with a scheduled time for reassessment of the patient's progress and prognosis rather than continuing an intervention indefinitely. Even this strategy is not consistently successful and often invasive strategies like mechanical ventilation are continued for extended periods of time. The critical care team must remember that the families of patient facing end-of-life care also need attention to their emotional and spiritual needs during these times of extreme stress.[12,16,20]

Clinical Research in the ICU[5]

Anyone who has attempted to do research involving human subjects has encountered the obstacles and hurdles imposed not only by the Federal Government, but by policies developed by the institutions in which the physician-researcher practices and their institutional review boards (IRBs). Conducting clinical research in the intensive care unit adds additional layers of requirements and ethical challenges. In addition to the fact there are no comprehensive guidelines that are universally accepted, or mandated, controversy and differences persist among medical ethicists, providers, and researchers. Flanagan and colleagues[5] have published and excellent review of the issues and the reader is referred to their work for more detail.

The ethical principles applicable to all human research apply to trials conducted in the ICU, but meeting federal and institutional requirements in this environment is fraught with difficulty. Four basic ethical considerations should be considered for all clinical trials in the ICU. First, the trial must have clinical value; second the trial must have scientific validity; thirdly, it should have efficiency and feasibility and lastly, protection of the participants. In addition, careful consideration must be given to benefits–risks ratio.

Common problems encountered in clinical research in the ICU include the fact that patients may lack the capacity to consent to participate due to a life-threatening illness, iatrogenic sedation and paralysis, loss of consciousness and a host of other issues. It has been argued that surrogate decision makers may not be aware of the patient's feeling about being involved in clinical trials even though they may have a clear understanding of the patient's preferences for medical care. A few studies have shown the discordant decisions between patients and their surrogates. Designing trials are much more difficult. The determination of a "control group" may be difficult if not impossible due to the heterogeneity of ICU populations, determining clinical equipoise (genuine uncertainty that one treatment has not been shown to be superior to another, or the lack of data regarding treatment options), frequent situations where the patient requires immediate life-saving intervention, and the concept that ICU patients might be considered a vulnerable population and therefore afforded extended protection by

Federal Mandate. There is inherent conflict between the physician's obligation to do what is best for the patient, i.e., therapeutic obligation, by applying the principle of standard of care and assigning patients to receive care that has not been proven. Another problem arises from therapeutic misconception where the patient or surrogate is under the presumption that the treatment under investigation is accepted therapy for the condition. Even the issue of data collection for Quality Improvement programs initiated by the institution is subject to the rules governing the use of human subjects as federal regulation states that "systematic data collection activity that is generalizable" is subject to IRB oversight and informed consent requirements.

Ethical dilemmas regarding research trials in the ICU remain and are not likely to be resolved without additional federal mandates. It is unlikely that even these will be universally accepted and no doubt controversy on many levels will persist for the foreseeable future.

Role of the Ethics Committee

One would expect that clearly delineated ethics principles and their application would resolve all ethical issues and ethics related conflicts in the ICU environment. However, it is clear that differences in understanding and application of these principles still exist. When pure application of these principles does not resolve the ethical issues, it is necessary to have a committee to assist with resolution of these issues. This Ethics committee should have members who are familiar with ethical principles and an interest in resolving ethical issues.

The members should have a prime interest in preserving the welfare of the patient and have no obvious socio-economic, racial or ethnic bias with a willingness to discuss and listen to frequently opposing views on the same topic and be prepared to assist in a totally transparent process. The members of the committee should have owned the respect of the medical and general community by virtue of their past history and recommendations. The committee should also have an integral role in drafting institutional guidelines for use of the Ethics Committee as well as assisting development of solutions for difficult clinical scenarios. How to handle organ donation after cardiac death is one example that is found within the ICU.

Although there is great variation in the composition of the Ethics committee, most centers have membership consisting of a bioethicist, a physician or surgeon, a social worker, a nurse, member of the clergy and a lay person. A patient advocate may also be a permanent member of the committee. At times a member of the family or the patient himself may be part of the deliberation process. A lawyer is not usually part of the committee but a legal expert should be advisory to the committee for legal matters and in cases before the court. Although most ethical issues in the ICU are resolved without input or convening of the Ethics Committee, it is essential to have a duly formed and functioning committee to assist with resolution of difficult and controversial issues. An *ad hoc* committee will not be sufficient. It should be noted that the Ethics Committee decision is not necessarily binding and if its recommendations are not to the satisfaction of the interested parties, other avenues of appeal including legal ruling may be required for resolution.

Summary

Many biomedical ethical issues present in the Surgical ICU. These require resolution in a supportive caring manner with transparency and involvement of all stakeholders. Adhering to general principles of biomedical ethics and applying them in a sound just manner is best achieved through a dedicated team effort of all staff with an established infrastructure. Patients, nurses, doctors, family members, and others involved in the care of the ICU patient all have their own and frequently different perspectives on the care of the patient. In such circumstances the potential for different approaches to care exists. Often these approaches involve ethical decisions. Traditionally, certain bioethical principles have been identified to guide resolution of these issues. The four commonly applied principles are: Autonomy, Beneficence, Non-maleficence, and justice.

References

1. Brierley J, Linthicum J, Petros A. Should religious beliefs be allowed to stonewall a secular approach to withdrawing and withholding treatment in children. *J Med Ethics* 2013; 39: 573–577.
2. Chen DT, Werhane PH, Mills AE. Role of organizational ethics in critical care medicine. *Crit Care Med* 2007; 35: S11–S17.
3. Curtis JR, Vincent JL. Ethics and end-of-life care for adults in the intensive care unit. *Lancet* 2010; 375:1347–1353.
4. Dorman T, Pauldine R. Economic stress and misaligned incentives in critical care medicine in the United States. *Crit Care Med* 2007; 35: S36–S43.
5. Flanagan BM, Philpott S, Strosberg MA. Protecting participants of clinical trials conducted in the intensive care unit. *J Int Care Med* 2011; 26(4): 237–249.

6. Garvin JR. Ethical considerations at the end-of-life in the intensive care unit. *Crit Care Med* 2007; 35: S85–S43.
7. Luce JM. Chronic disorders of consciousness following coma: Part two: Ethical, legal and social issues. *Chest* 2013; 144(4):1388–1393.
8. Luce JM. A history of resolving conflict over end-of-life care in the intensive care units in the United States. *Crit Car Med* 2010; 38(8): 1623–1629.
9. Luce JM. End-of-life decision-making in the intensive care unit. *Am J Resp Crit Care Med* 2010; 182: 6–11.
10. Mularski RA, Puntillo K, Erstad BL, *et al.* Pain management within the palliative and end-of-life experience in the ICU. *Chest* 2009; 135:1360–1369.
11. Nelson JE, Curtis JR, Mulkerin C, *et al.* Choosing and using screening criteria for palliative care consultation in the ICU: A report from the Improving Palliative Care in the ICU (IPAL–ICU) Advisory Board. *Crit Care Med* 2013; 41(10): 2318–2327.
12. Nelson JE, Hope AA. Integration of palliative care in chronic critical illness. *Resp Care* 2012; 57(6):1004–1012.
13. Rie MA, Kofke WA. Non-therapeutic quality improvement: The conflict of organizational ethics and societal rule of law. *Crit Care Med* 2007: 35: S66–S84.
14. Scheunemann LP, White DB. The ethics and reality of rationing in medicine. *Chest* 2011; 140(6):1625–1632.
15. Swetz KM, Rowley ME, Hook CC, Mueller PS. Report of 255 clinical ethics consultation and a review of the literature. *Mayo Clin Proc* 2007: 82(6): 686–691.
16. Swetz KM, Mansel JK. Ethical issues and palliative care in the cardiovascular intensive care unit. *Cardio Clin* 2013; 31: 657–668.
17. Szalados JE. Legal issues in the practice of critical care medicine. *Crit Care Med* 2007; 35: S44–S58.
18. Thompson DR. Principles of ethics: In managing a critical care unit. *Crit Care Med* 2007; 35: S2–S10.
19. Venkat A, Becher J. The effect of statutory limitations on the authority of substitute decision makers on the care of patients in the intensive care unit: Case examples and review of state laws affecting withdrawing and withholding life-sustaining treatment. *J Int Care Med* 2014; 29(2): 71–80.
20. Wigmore TJ, Farquhar-Smith P, Lawson A. Intensive care for the cancer patient-unique clinical and ethical challenges and outcome prediction in the critically ill cancer patient. *Best Pract Res Clin Anaesth* 2013; 27: 527–543.

SECTION 2
Specific Surgical Disorders

(a) TRAUMA

Chapter 15

Priorities in Multiple Trauma Management

Jameel Ali

Chapter Overview

Trauma patients admitted to the intensive care unit (ICU) are initially seen in the Emergency Department setting. A large percentage of these patients sustain injuries involving more than one body region. This is particularly so in motor vehicle crashes where the specific injuries may not be immediately obvious. Yet, management decisions need to be made and implemented before a specific diagnosis is made in order to ensure survival. This requires application of a priority system of intervention based on an understanding of the relative threat to life posed by the changes resulting from the injuries.

Although the trimodal distribution of deaths following trauma[1] has been modified as a result of institution of trauma systems, it is still useful to consider it broadly applicable in most situations. In the first peak of this trimodal distribution death occurs immediately after the injury and includes catastrophes such as decapitation, major brain tissue destruction, cardiac rupture etc. for which medical/surgical intervention is futile. During the second peak of this trimodal distribution death can result from abnormalities such as airway and ventilatory compromise, hemorrhage, cervical cord injury etc. Deaths in the third phase of the trimodal distribution results from complications of the trauma such as sepsis, renal failure, and multiple organ failure. Implementation of simple resuscitative measures during the second phase of this trimodal distribution can decrease deaths not only during the second phase but also indirectly during the third phase by prevention of complications, which may result from inadequate resuscitation. For example, late mortality from sepsis and organ failure secondary to prolonged hypo-perfusion states could be decreased by prompt treatment of contaminated wounds, open fractures, and early diagnosis and treatment of hollow viscous perforation within the abdomen as well as aggressive fluid resuscitation all of which should be instituted during the second phase of this trimodal distribution.

This chapter discusses the system of priority in multiple system trauma management, its rationale, methods of implementation, and its uniform application in all types of injuries.

The Order of Priorities

The order of priorities in the management of the multiple injured patient is based on the premise that early trauma deaths occur as a result of the effects of the injuries on the patient's biologic life sustaining systems and that the resulting effects consist of derangements in normal physiology. These physiologic changes may occur from varying types of injuries but with similar manifestations e.g., the airway may be compromised as a result of direct physical trauma to the airway or from a head injury interfering with the patient's ability to maintain patency of the airway. The end result and principles of management of the airway in both instances is essentially the same. Therefore, it is not necessary initially to know the specific cause of the airway compromise, but merely to know and identify airway compromise and to deal with it appropriately. Another important concept is that the degree of life threat posed by the physiologic derangements can be categorized in terms of time i.e., the greatest life threat is the one from which the patient will die most rapidly. An order of priority in assessing and managing the patient initially can then be based on this time-related sequence of life threat. The process of identifying this order of life threat in trauma is termed: The Primary Survey (2-Advanced Trauma Life support course).

This Primary survey may be considered a physiologic approach to management during which the immediately life threatening abnormalities are identified and resuscitation is instituted on a priority basis. This resuscitation phase is followed by the **Secondary Survey** which is an anatomic head to toe evaluation of the patient allowing identification and management of other injuries which may not be immediately life threatening but if left unattended could later pose a life threat or increase morbidity.

The third phase of assessment and management of the injured patient is the **Definitive Care and Transfer** phase when decisions are made regarding transfer to appropriate facilities and management of non-life-threatening injuries such as stable fractures.

Removal of the spine board

Most multi-trauma patients are brought to hospital stabilized on long spine boards. The patients should be removed from the spine board as early as possible to prevent decubitus ulcers and the spine board used thereafter only for transporting the patients. Spine stability is maintained on a flat firm mattress with frequent log rolling while maintaining in-line immobilization of the entire spine until a spine injury has been ruled out by clinical examination and definitive imaging.

The Primary Survey

The Primary Survey follows the ABCDE approach and the sequence is based on relative life threat as follows:

A — Airway and c-spine control — identification and correction of airway compromise with c-spine precaution.

B — Breathing with oxygenation and ventilation.

C — Circulation with hemorrhage control.

D — Disability (identification and correction of neurologic disability and prevention of secondary brain injury).

E — Exposure (total exposure for complete assessment while preventing hypothermia).

The order of these priorities is based on the degree of life threat in terms of time so that A is before B because there is less time to correct airway compromise before death or irreversible damage occurs compared to breathing or ventilation abnormalities. The same rationale applies to C, D, and E being in the order indicated. This order of priorities also allows abnormalities to be corrected as soon as they are identified because they are discovered in the order of life threat. Thus, assessment and resuscitation are conducted simultaneously.

In situations where more than one person is involved in managing the patient, different areas (e.g., airway and breathing) could be managed simultaneously. One person could, therefore, correct airway problems while another attends to breathing abnormalities. When more than one person is involved, it is important that one is designated a "team leader" who will coordinate the resuscitation and ensure that the order of priorities is maintained.

This order of priorities remains the same in all patients regardless, of gender, age or whether the patient is pregnant. However, in pregnancy there are two patients — the mother and the fetus — and the best treatment for the fetus is resuscitation of the mother by adhering to primary survey principles while monitoring the fetus. In the elderly, comorbidities, medications such as beta blockers, anticoagulants, pacemakers, and brittleness of the cardiorespiratory response to trauma and blood loss must be considered (see chapter on Geriatric Patient). The pediatric patient has a very strong compensatory response initially, but decompensation can be very rapid — these factors must be considered in resuscitating the pediatric patient (see chapter on Pediatric Trauma).

Adjuncts to the primary survey and re-evaluation

Although all the adjuncts mentioned here are not indicated in every patient, all multiple injured patients should have Oxygen (O_2) administered to maintain O_2 saturation of at least 95%, pulse oximetry, Electrocardiography (ECG), arterial line, large bore venous access (14–16 gauge), gastric intubation (orogastric route preferred when suspecting basal skull fracture), urinary catheterization to monitor urinary output (transurethral route is contraindicated when urethral injury is suspected e.g., blood at the urethral meatus, high riding prostate on rectal examination, perineal ecchymosis — urethrogram is then required to determine the integrity of the urethra), chest X-ray, and pelvic X-ray (if concerned about pelvic fractures as a source of hemorrhage).

Because the trauma patient's status could change at any time, constant monitoring is required to detect these changes as soon as they occur prompting re-assessment which begins with a repeat of the primary survey and institution of corrective measures.

Airway, oxygenation, ventilation, and cervical spine control

Loss of tone of the muscles supporting the tongue may occur from brain hypo-perfusion in shock or Central Nervous system (CNS) injury leading to one of the commonest causes of airway obstruction in the trauma patient because the tongue produces obstruction by receding into the pharynx. Movement of the tongue anteriorly by such simple maneuvers as the jaw thrust or chin lift will temporarily open the airway and allow suctioning of secretions and foreign material as well as delivery of administered oxygen. With prompt resuscitation maneuvers including volume infusion, if the patient is fully conscious, vocalizing clearly, and not in shock an artificial airway is not required. Caution should be exercised during the chin lift and jaw thrust maneuvers to protect the cervical spine. This is best accomplished by having one person maintain manual in-line stabilization of the cervical spine while the other secures and suctions the airway. The simplest technique should be used first for effective ventilation and oxygenation and in over 90% of cases endotracheal intubation is not necessary. In these circumstances suction of the airway is followed by insertion of an oropharyngeal airway device and 100% oxygen administered by a bag valve mask. Many patients who have an intact gag reflex would not tolerate an oropharyngeal airway and the oxygen is then administered without insertion of this device. This device should be inserted gently to avoid trauma and bleeding especially in elderly patients whose oral mucosa is quite friable. In the adult, the device is inserted first with the tip pointed upward and then rotated 180° when the tube reaches the base of the tongue, which is positioned anteriorly making space for the tube. Because of the risk of injury to the soft tissues this rotation technique is not practiced in the child. A nasopharyngeal tube may also be used, but all nasopharyngeal tubes should be avoided if there is concern about the presence of a basal skull fracture as evidenced by rhinorrhea, otorrhea, hemotympanum, battle's sign, or raccoon eyes. Other temporary airway devices may be used such as Laryngeal Mask Airway (LMA), Laryngo Tracheal Airway (LTA) and esophageal airway, but none of these devices are classified as a Definitive Airway which is defined as a secured cuffed tube placed in the trachea. When the patient is unable to spontaneously maintain a patent airway, a definitive airway is required and should be accomplished promptly and expeditiously, starting with pre-oxygenation using 100% oxygen delivered with a bag valve mask. Prolonged unsuccessful attempts at intubation should be avoided by intermittently providing manual bag valve mask ventilation with 100% oxygen to avoid hypoxia. All airway equipment should always be available and in proper working condition including laryngoscopes, LMA, Gum Elastic Bougies, glidescopes, and fiberoptic bronchoscopes together with appropriate drugs including topical anesthetic, sedatives, and short as well as medium acting neuromuscular paralyzing agents before proceeding to definitive airway. Whenever possible back up help must be available in anticipation of a difficult intubation. Marked obesity with a short fat neck, severe cervical spine arthritis, or limitation of cervical spine movements by other forms of disease, major facial trauma, and anatomical variations can all pose major challenges to successful intubation. One quick assessment to determine the likelihood of a difficult intubation also includes the LEMON[3] signs:

L — Look for outside signs e.g., beard, short fat neck, receded chin, etc.

E — Evaluate the 3-3-2 rule: Distance between the incisors should be at least three finger-widths; distance between the hyoid bone and the chin should be at least three finger-widths; distance between the thyroid notch and floor of mouth should be at least two finger-widths.

M — Mallampati score[4] visualization of the hypopharynx with the tongue protruded looking for the soft palate, uvula, fauces, and pillars.

In Class I, all four structures are clearly visible; Class II, only the first three structures;

Class III, only the soft palate and base of uvula visible; Class IV, only the hard palate is visible.

O — Obstruction due to trauma, inflammatory disorders edematous tissue, peritonsillar abscess etc. could make intubation technically very difficult.

N — Neck Mobility. If there are no signs of cervical spine trauma, neck mobility can be assessed by asking the patient to have the chin touch the chest and then attempt to look towards the ceiling. If the patient is able to accomplish this maneuver without difficulty, it suggest that mobility of the neck should not be an impediment to intubation.

The definitive airway is usually inserted orotracheally, but the nasotracheal route is sometimes used except when there is suspicion of a basal skull fracture as indicated earlier. The ideal technique is to visualize the vocal cords through the laryngoscope and directly see the tip of the tube pass between the cords. A useful technique for facilitating visualization of the cords during intubation is to have an assistant apply Backward, Upward and Rightwards Pressure (BURP) on the thyroid cartilage. An alternative "blind" intubation technique involves timing the advancement of the tube between the vocal cords when the patient inspires — this, of course, cannot be done when the patient is apneic. Another "blind" technique involves introducing a specially designed endotracheal tube through a lumen in an "intubating" laryngeal mask. Other techniques for placing a definitive airway include the use of a Gum Elastic Bougie which is easier to introduce into the trachea and this bougie can be used as a stylet over which the endotracheal tube is introduced into the trachea; a fiberoptic bronchoscope can also be visualized as it enters between the cords and the endotracheal tube introduced over the "scope; a glidescope, which is a modified llaryngoscope with a camera at its tip allows visualization of the cords on a monitor and this is also used to guide placement of the endotracheal tube .The intensivist should be familiar with several of these techniques and be prepared to have these as backups in anticipation of difficult intubations. Correct placement is suggested by visualization of the tube entering between the cords, observing chest wall movement with ventilation, auscultating for breath sounds at the apices and laterally, checking for the presence of CO_2 in end tidal gas through a capnograph or colorometric device, chest x-ray, and lack of borborygmy or gurgling sounds on auscultating over the epigastrium during bag ventilation.

Cricothyroidotomy

When the patient requires a definitive airway and this cannot be achieved by orotracheal or nasotracheal techniques access should be by cricothyroidotomy which may be either a needle or surgical cricothyroidotomy. The needle technique is preferred in children less than eight years of age because the cricoid cartilage is essential to the stability of the upper airway in infants and young children. This needle technique is a temporizing maneuver and allows 30–45 minutes of oxygenation until a formal surgical tracheostomy can be performed under ideal operating room conditions if required. This technique does not provide adequate ventilation and after 30–45 minutes, hypercapnea results. The surgical cricothyroidotomy[5] is more effective and preferred in adults. It involves placing a skin incision directly overt the cricothyroid membrane which is incised transversely, forceps are used to spread the opening and allow placement of an appropriately sized (6F or 7F) tracheotomy or endotracheal tube.

Caution-Iatrogenic Tension Pneumothorax

Once the definitive airway has been placed the patient is connected to a ventilator and positive pressure ventilation. If there is a pre-existing undiagnosed simple pneumothorax this will be immediately converted to a tension pneumothorax with immediate hemodynamic decompensation requiring urgent chest decompression.

Protection of the cervical spine

Until cervical spine injury is excluded, undue manipulation such as extension, flexion or rotation of the c-spine should be avoided to prevent spine injury or worsening of an already existing spine injury. In line immobilization of the neck in the neutral position should be maintained during intubation attempts. This may require use of airway adjuncts such as a Gum Elastic Bougie,[6] bronchoscope etc. as mentioned in the preceding paragraphs. All unconscious patients and multiple injured patients should be suspected of having spine injury and should have the c-spine immobilized in an appropriate c-collar until adequate spine clinical examination and imaging are conducted and shown to be normal as discussed in the Spinal Injury chapter. The patient should be off the spine board as early as possible to avoid decubitus skin changes and kept on a firm soft surface with frequent log rolling and the spine board should only be used thereafter for transporting the patient.

Breathing

Inspection, palpation, and auscultation of the chest together with a chest x-ray should allow assessment for pneumothorax, hemothorax, flail chest, cardiac tamponade, and lung contusion which are treated as outlined in the chapter on Thoracic Trauma. Suspicion of a tension pneumothorax should not require chest x-ray for confirmation before chest decompression. Open pneumothorax should be identified and an occlusive dressing applied followed by chest tube insertion. Paradoxical movement of the chest wall and underlying lung contusion should be detected by clinical and radiologic assessment. After maximum parenteral or epidural/intercostal analgesia, if oxygenation and/or ventilation are still compromised endotracheal intubation and mechanical ventilation may be necessary.

Circulation

Hemorrhage is the most common cause of circulatory compromise in the trauma patient. The approach to the patient with evidence of generalized hypoperfusion (shock) is, therefore, to first look for a source of hemorrhage, stop the hemorrhage and replace fluid. While the site of the bleeding is being sought, large bore IV access (14–16 gauge) is secured first in the peripheral sites such as the antecubital fossae and if not successful, central sites (internal jugular, subclavian, femoral veins) are sought for access. These central sites are ideally approached under ultrasound guidance[7] and more increasingly the intraosseous route is being used in both adults and children. Generally, it is best to avoid placing IV catheters in limbs with massive soft tissue trauma or bony injuries and to avoid lower limb vascular access when there is a major intra-abdominal source of hemorrhage. In children under six years, the intraosseous route is used before attempting central venous access. The internal jugular and subclavian access should be followed by chest x-ray to ensure proper placement as well as to rule out iatrogenic pneumothorax. At the time of vascular access blood is drawn for Complete Blood Count (CBC), cross type, toxicology, pregnancy test in the female patient and coagulation studies.

Clinical presentation of the hypoperfused state depends on factors such as age, comorbidities, duration, and magnitude of the blood loss. The physiologic response to hypovolemia includes catecholamine release leading to tachycardia, vasoconstriction which tend to maintain blood pressure even at higher than normal levels particularly in young patients in whom hypotension is a late sign of shock[2] (Advanced Trauma Life support course Chapter 3, Shock) compared to the older patient. Other signs of hypoperfusion should therefore be sought such as the level of consciousness, base deficit, location, and character of the pulse, skin color, capillary refill time, decrease in urine output. The patient who is alert, has a strong bounding radial pulse, warm skin, adequate urine output and a capillary refill time of less than 2 seconds would be considered not to have lost significant blood and the degree of deviation from these clinical parameters would correlate with the magnitude of blood loss.

Fluid resuscitation using warm Ringer's lactate is initiated as soon as vascular access is established. If the patient does not respond to 2 L of crystalloid wide open or if one suspects major blood loss, packed cells should be started as soon as it becomes available. Ideally, one should use cross typed blood, but if this is not available after the 2 L of IV fluid without a positive response, type specific blood, if available, should be administered and failing this, type O (O positive for males and O negative for females in the child bearing age) should be initiated. In patients who have suffered major blood loss, massive transfusion is anticipated and the "massive transfusion protocol"[8] should be followed which includes packed cells, platelets, fresh frozen plasma, and cryoprecipitate (see chapter on Massive Blood Transfusion) while monitoring clotting parameters, core temperature, and acid base status. The combination of hypothermia, acidosis, and hypocoagulability is lethal in these patients and should be prevented by treating patients in a warm environment, early use of fluid warmers and early activation of massive transfusion protocols. Major blood loss from the abdomen and thorax often require definitive surgical control of the bleeding source. In penetrating torso trauma, without head injury, hemodynamic endpoints of resuscitation may be modified to accept borderline hypotension in the neighborhood of 90 mmHg until definitive surgical control of internal hemorrhage is accomplished in order to decrease the preoperative magnitude of hemorrhage which may occur at higher systemic blood pressures.[9]

The hemorrhage will be either external or internal and total external physical examination including the back and extremities (by logrolling the patient while protecting the spine) should allow identification of external sources of blood loss which will usually respond to direct pressure without blind clamping or tourniquets. Occasionally, especially in the military, tourniquets may be required when the choice is between saving the patient's life and preserving the limb.[10]

The source of internal bleeding should be sought in the chest, abdomen, pelvis, or retroperitoneum. A combination of physical examination and chest x-ray (for a chest source), ultrasound of the abdomen (for an abdominal source) and x-ray of the pelvis (for a pelvic source) would identify the other sources of internal hemorrhage. The retroperitoneum as a source is best assessed by Computerized Tomography (CT) scan but should be done only if the hemodynamic status of the patient allows safe transfer to the CT scan suite. Detailed management of these sources and the indication for operative management of hemorrhage from these sites of hemorrhage are discussed in the chapters on Chest Trauma, Abdominal Trauma, and Pelvic Fractures.

Although volume deficit is the chief cause of hypoperfusion in the trauma patient, failure to respond to adequate volume infusion may represent cardiovascular decompensation. In such cases if causes such as cardiac tamponade and tension pneumothorax are excluded, it may be necessary to institute pharmacologic support of the circulation temporarily in the form of inotropes and vasoactive agents with close hemodynamic monitoring in the ICU.

Non-hemorrhagic causes of hypoperfusion in the trauma patient include cardiac tamponade, tension pneumothorax, myocardial injury, open pneumothorax. These entities as well as massive hemothorax are discussed in the Chest Trauma chapter.

One other source of hypoperfusion in the trauma patient is neurogenic shock resulting from sympathetic nervous system injury and presents with warm extremity, widened pulse pressure, hypotension and often bradycardia unless the cardiac sympathetics are spared. Although the cause is not blood loss these patients have a relative hypovolemia because of their expanded vascular space due to the vasodilatation. Initially, they require fluid infusion to fill this expanded vascular space and maintain perfusion which could be achieved at a lower than normal systemic blood pressure. If in spite of fluid infusion normal perfusion does not return then temporary vasopressor therapy may be required.

Differentiation of Non-hemorrhagic from Hemorrhagic Shock and Confounding Presentations

Apart from septic shock (which is a late complication of traumatic shock, often due to delayed identification and treatment of a septic focus) and neurogenic shock both of which present with warm extremities and a widened pulse pressure, all the other types of traumatic shock present with vasoconstriction, cold clammy extremities, narrowed pulse pressure, and hypotension as a late finding. The main difference between the hemorrhagic and these other non-hemorrhagic shock conditions is central venous distention manifested by distended neck veins in the non-hemorrhagic types of shock essentially represented by tension pneumothorax and cardiac tamponade. Differentiation of these two is based on physical examination of the chest with hyper-resonance, decreased breath sounds, and sometimes tracheal deviation in tension pneumothorax. The finding of muffled heart tones in cardiac tamponade is not very reliable particularly in the noisy emergency room or ICU setting. Hypotension, distended neck veins and hemopericardium on ultrasound suggest pericardial tamponade. Without ultrasound and if there is doubt about clinical differentiation between the presence of cardiac tamponade versus tension pneumothorax the approach should be to treat the condition as tension pneumothorax by chest decompression which will relieve the shock while at the same time confirming the diagnosis. If there is no improvement with chest decompression then the patient is treated for cardiac tamponade as discussed in the chapter on chest injuries.

As discussed in the earlier paragraphs of the chapter, young patients maintain their systolic blood pressure for a longer period of time but often there will be a decrease in pulse pressure because of a relative increase in diastolic pressure due to the intense peripheral vasoconstriction from catechol amine release[11] in response to the hypovolemia. Indeed, the volume of blood loss has been classified into 4 categories — Class I — up to 15%, Class II up to 30% and Class III up to 40% of total blood volume[2] and it is not until up to 40% or 2 L of blood loss in a 70 kg male does the blood pressure fall so that hypotension is a late finding in young patients with hemorrhagic shock and blood pressure should not be equated with cardiac output in hemorrhagic shock.[12] Base deficit is reported to be a better predictor of blood volume loss and requirement for blood transfusion[13] in hemorrhagic shock. Immediately after blood loss the Hemoglobin (Hb) level may be misleadingly normal until plasma refill or volume resuscitation has taken place so that although the Hb level should be checked initially as a baseline to follow changes with resuscitation it should not be used as an early indicator of blood loss. However, when hemoglobin level drops within minutes of injuries it signifies major blood loss requiring urgent intervention to stop hemorrhage.[14] During volume resuscitation, the clinical response in addition to correction of base deficit may be used as a measure of the degree of blood loss.[2] The Rapid Responder has lost minimal volume and will respond by return of normal capillary refill, decrease in tachycardia, improvement in urinary output, level of consciousness, and skin temperature with minimal fluid infusion. The Transient Responder will initially show signs of improvement in the same parameters but quickly reverse those findings suggesting recurrence or continuation of blood loss and increased fluid requirements. The Rapid Responder will usually respond to crystalloid alone but the Transient Responder will frequently require blood products as well. A test bolus of 2 L of warmed Ringer's lactate should allow differentiation of these two categories of responders and guide the requirement for starting blood infusion. The Non-responder is one that fails to respond to normal fluid boluses signifying either a non-hemorrhagic cause of the shock or massive blood loss requiring massive transfusion protocol[8] utilizing warm, packed red blood cells, fresh frozen plasma, platelets and cryoprecipitate as well as surgical intervention to stop the hemorrhage. Other confounding variables in monitoring the patient in shock is the failure to mount a tachycardia in spite of significant blood loss in patients on Beta blockers or the trained athlete whose baseline heart rate may be in the mid-40s and a 'normal' heart rate of 80 could represent a relative tachycardia in such patients.

The pregnant trauma patient may also present with misleading findings e.g., supine hypotension due to compression of the inferior vena cava from an enlarged gravid uterus (which should be manually displaced to the left). The catechol amine release in response to blood loss may have a more intensive vasoconrictive effect in the placental circulation than in the maternal circulation thus maintaining the mother's hemodynamics at the expense of fetal distress emphasizing not only resuscitation of the mother but also monitoring the fetus. The relative large maternal plasma volume to red cell mass is also reflected in a relative lowering of Hb level which could be mistakenly interpreted as blood loss.[15]

D-neurologic Deficit

After airway, respiratory, and circulatory issues have been addressed in the primary survey, attention is directed at the neurologic status. A change in the Level of Consciousness (LOC) is the prime indication for neurosurgical intervention. A baseline determination of LOC is therefore critical so that this can be compared with subsequent determinations of LOC. The mini-neurologic exam which consists of the Glasgow Coma Scale (GCS) score (see chapter on Head Injury), pupillary size, and reaction to light as well as any lateralizing sign serves as this initial quick determination of LOC against which any subsequent assessment is compared. Deterioration in LOC is an indication for neurosurgical consultation, CT scan and a more in-depth complete neurologic assessment which includes assessment of power, tone, coordination, sensation, and reflexes. The main goal of initial management of the head injured patient is to prevent secondary brain injury by maintaining, oxygenation, perfusion, controlling cerebral edema and intracranial pressure, and identifying and evacuating mass lesions. Further details on management of the Head injured patient are discussed in the Head Injury chapter.

E-exposure

Removal of the patient's clothing will allow total assessment of the patient after which the patient is covered with warm blankets and the room is kept warm to avoid hypothermia.[16] Complete physical examination of the patient includes assessment of the back. This requires log rolling of the patient to examine the back while protecting the spine.

The Secondary Survey

This begins after the patient has been resuscitated and the primary survey has been completed with airway, oxygenation ventilation, hemodynamics, and neurologic status maximized and stabilized. As aforementioned, the secondary survey is an in-depth head to toe assessment of the patient and also includes a history of allergies, medications, past illnesses, and details of the injury mechanism. Many details in the history may not be obtained directly from the patient but obtainable from pre-hospital personnel, family members etc.

Head and neck assessment

The entire head and face is examined including the eyes, ears, facial bones, cranial nerves, carotid vessels, trachea reassessing the jugular veins and the GCS score.

Chest

This is reassessed by inspection, palpation auscultation, and checking for volume of drainage from any chest tube as well as proper functioning of the chest tube.

Abdomen

Inspection, percussion, palpation, and auscultation of the entire abdomen should be conducted, checking for any new masses or tenderness and performing a CT scan if the hemodynamics have improved and there is still concern about occult intra-abdominal injury.

Perineum, rectum, vagina are assessed by inspection, digital and speculum examination seeking the help of a gynecologist in the female patient where appropriate and occasionally using lower gastro Intestinal (GI) endoscopy.

An in-depth musculoskeletal assessment looking for deformity and any neurovascular compromise reassessing splints to ensure they are not too tight as well as assessing the joints and ligaments and applying definite fracture treatment devices such as casts.

Adjuncts to the secondary survey include any investigation that is required including plain x-rays of extremities, CT scans, angiography, contrast urography as deemed necessary.

Transfer to Definitive Care

Decision to transfer a trauma patient to another facility is based on two main factors: the patient's needs and the treatment resources, including personnel, at the initial institution. When the patient's needs exceed the local capability, emphasis should be on resuscitation ensuring that cardiorespiratory status has stabilized and that it is safe to transfer the patient. Communication should be established with the referral institution and a decision made as to the safest, most rapid means of transport and the type of personnel required to accompany the patient. X-rays and other investigations which do not affect immediate care of the patient should not be conducted as these would result in unnecessary delay of the transport process. All investigations conducted and chart records including clinical assessments and interventions should accompany the patient.

Re-evaluation and Monitoring the Patient

A high index of suspicion is required in managing the multiple trauma patient because initially undiagnosed abnormalities could occur or the patient's clinical condition could deteriorate. This monitoring is frequently required in an ICU setting.

Patients may have initially contained hematomas which could suddenly rupture with deterioration in clinical findings. A fall in Hb level or drop in systemic blood pressure and new tachycardia may suggest new or continued bleeding. Any worsening of abdominal findings may suggest such conditions as undiagnosed perforation or intra-abdominal sepsis. One subtle sign of impending hemodynamic compromise is a fall in urine output or a change in base deficit. Deterioration in the respiratory status could suggest pulmonary embolism, a new pneumothorax or conversion of a simple pneumothorax to a tension pneumothorax with accompanying hemodynamic deterioration. A ruptured esophagus could present late with pain, hemodynamic/respiratory compromise with or without a pleural effusion. Traumatic abdominal compartment syndrome (discussed in the Abdominal Compartment Syndrome chapter) could also develop later with a deterioration in cardiorespiratory status and a fall in urine output. Late respiratory compromise could also occur in a patient with a ruptured diaphragm, the abdominal viscera being initially contained in the abdomen with later migration into the chest. These are only a few of the reasons why it is important to monitor and continually re-evaluate the multiple injured patient in the ICU.

Summary

The management of the multiple injured patient requires an organized approach which begins with identification of life threats with prompt application of resuscitative techniques. This is accomplished without necessarily having a definitive diagnosis initially. Once the patient's immediately life threatening abnormalities are corrected an anatomic detailed head to toe assessment to identify and treat other injuries and make specific diagnoses is conducted. Because of the possibility of change in the patient's status, reevaluation, and monitoring of these patients in the ICU setting is frequently necessary.

References

1. Demetriades D, Kimbrell B, Salim A *et al.* Trauma deaths in a mature urban trauma system: Is 'trimodal' distribution a valid concept? *J Am Coll* 2005; 201: 343–347.
2. American College of Surgeons Committee on Trauma: Advanced Trauma Life Support for Physicians. Chicago, IL , 2012.
3. Reed MJ, Dunn MJ, McKeown DW. Can an airway assessment score predict difficulty at intubation in the emergency department? *Emerg Med J* 2005; 22: 99–102.
4. Mallampati SR, Gatt SP, Gugino LD, Desai SP, Waraksa B, Freiberger D, Lui PL. A clinical sign to predict difficult tracheal intubation. *Canadian Anesthetists' Journal* 1985; 22: 429–434.
5. Narrod JA, Moore EE, Rosen P. Emergency Cricothyrostomy, technique, and anatomical considerations. *J Emerg Med* 1985; 2: 443–447.
6. Phelan MP. Use of the endotracheal bougie introducer for difficult intubations. *Am J Emerg Med* 2004; 22(6): 479–482.
7. Gilbert TB, Seneff MG, Becker RB. Facilitation of internal jugular venous cannulation using an audio-guided Doppler ultrasound vascular access device: Results from a prospective dual center, randomized, crossover clinical study. *Crit Care Med* 1995; 23: 60–64.
8. Riskin DJ, Tsai TC, Riskin L, Hernandez-Boussard T *et al.* Massive transfusion protocols: The role of aggressive resuscitation versus product ratio in mortality reduction. *J Am Coll Surg* 2009; 209: 198–205.
9. Bickell WH, Wall MJ Jr., Pepe PE *et al.* Immediate versus delayed fluid resuscitation for hypotensive patients with penetrating torso injuries. *N Engl J Med* 1994; 331: 1105–1111.
10. Walters TJ, Mabry RL. Use of tourniquets on the battlefield: A consensus panel report. *Mil Med* 2005; 170: 770–774.
11. Chernow B, Rainey TG, Lake CR. Endogenous and exogenous catecholamines. *Crit Care Med* 1982; 10: 409–413.
12. Eastbridge BJ, Salinas J, McManus JG, Blackburn L, Bugler EM *et al.* Hypotension begins at 110 mm Hg: Redefining "hypotension" with data. *J Trauma* 2007; 63: 291–298.

13. Davis JW, Parks SN, Kaups KL *et al.* Admission base deficit predicts transfusion requirements and risk of complications. *J Trauma* 1997; 42(3): 571–573.
14. Bruns B, Lindsey M, Rowe K, Brown S, Minei JP, Gentilello LM, Shafi S. Hemoglobin drops within minutes of injuries and predicts need for an intervention to stop hemorrhage. *J Trauma* 2007; 63(2): 312–315.
15. Tsuei BJ. Assessment of the pregnant trauma patient. *Injury* 2006; 37: 367–373.
16. Ferrara A, MacArthur JD, Wright HK *et al.* Hypothermia and acidosis worsen coagulopathy in pat massive transfusion. *Am J Surg* 1990; 160: 515–520.

Chapter 16

Thoracic Trauma

Col. (retd.) Mark W. Bowyer and Jameel Ali*

Introduction

Chest trauma is a frequent etiology for admission of patients to critical care units. In North America, blunt thoracic injury is responsible for about 8% of all trauma admissions and chest trauma (blunt and penetrating) account for one in four of all deaths from trauma, and is a contributing factor in another 25%.[1,2] Early deaths result from hemorrhage, or associated head, or abdominal trauma. Many of these patients die after reaching the hospital, and of those deaths, many might have been prevented with prompt diagnosis and treatment. The vast majority of thoracic injuries (90% blunt and 70–85% penetrating) can be managed without open surgical thoracotomy.[3] As such, the skills for dealing with thoracic trauma are well within the scope of intensivists who care for victims of trauma. All practitioners must be alert to the myriad of possible injuries that can occur in the chest, and facile in their treatment as recognition and treatment can be life-saving. The intensivist caring for patients with thoracic trauma should be skilled in establishing a patent airway, providing adequate ventilation and oxygenation, evacuation of fluid or air from the chest, diagnosing and temporizing cardiac tamponade

*The author is grateful to Ms. Elizabeth Weissbrod, MA, CMI for her expert illustrations contained in this chapter.

The views expressed herein are those of the authors and are not to be construed as official or reflecting the views of the Department of Defense, the Uniformed Services University, or the United States Government. The authors have nothing to disclose.

(pericardiocentesis), and providing vascular access for fluid administration. Recognition of when to seek surgical consultation/intervention in these patients is also an important principle for the critical care practitioner.

Classification of Thoracic Trauma

Generally, thoracic trauma may be classified into two broad groups: penetrating and blunt. It is important to remember that trauma to the chest is often not an isolated event and other structures can also sustain potentially life-threatening injuries as well.[4, 5] A penetrating missile entering inferior to the nipple line can produce diaphragmatic, intrathoracic, or abdominal injuries. Similarly, blunt injuries may disrupt intrathoracic contents as well as intra-abdominal contents either directly or indirectly through fractures of the lower ribs, which then puncture intra-abdominal organs such as the spleen, liver, and stomach. It is imperative when caring for these patients not to get "tunnel vision" and to rule in or out other potential life-threatening injuries outside of the chest.

A more practical (clinically relevant) method of classifying torso trauma involves two categories. The first category consists of injuries that are immediately life threatening and thus require immediate intervention because of cardiorespiratory or hemodynamic compromise. The other category includes injuries in a relatively hemodynamically normal patient that have the potential for adverse outcome if not promptly recognized and treated. As seen in Table 1, these two categories can be collectively referred to as the "**Deadly Dozen**" injuries of the chest which are further divided into the "**Fearsome Fatal Five**" and the "**Serious Seven**". The critical care practitioner caring for these patients must have a broad understanding of the diagnosis and treatment of all of these potential injuries. While one would hope that the recognition and initial treatment of the "Fearsome Fatal Five" would have occurred prior to a patient being admitted to the intensive care unit, the intensivist may be the one to make the diagnosis and in a position to render initial treatment, and will most certainly be involved in managing the aftermath of these conditions and their treatment. Additionally the intensivist may play a very important role in helping to identify and treat the "Serious Seven" injuries which may not be immediately apparent, and have the potential to be potentially life threatening if left unattended. It must also be kept in mind that some of these life-threatening thoracic injuries may result from complications of procedures done in the intensive care unit (ICU), e.g., simple or tension pneumothorax or hemothorax from central line insertion;

Table 1. The "Deadly Dozen" injuries of the chest.

The Fearsome fatal five (emergent, immediately life-threatening injuries that must be identified as part of the primary survey in addition to airway obstruction)	**The serious seven** (injuries that have a high potential to be life-threatening in a delayed fashion and should be found on secondary survey)
1. Complex Pneumothorax:	1. Pulmonary Contusion
a. Tension Pneumothorax	2. Blunt Cardiac Injury
b. Open Pneumothorax	3. Traumatic Aortic Disruption
c. Massive Pneumothorax	4. Esophageal Injury
2. Cardiac Tamponade	5. Traumatic Diaphragmatic Injury
3. Massive Hemothorax	6. Rib Fractures
4. Traumatic Air Embolism	7. Simple Hemo or Pneumothorax
5. Flail Chest	

rib fractures from chest compressions; cardiac tamponade from attempted pericardiocentesis; etc. The next sections will provide a detailed description of the multitude of injuries that can occur in the chest, the diagnostic adjuncts and the specific treatments and critical care considerations following treatment. In all cases it is imperative that the intensivist ensure a patent airway and adequate intravenous access.

Thoracic Injuries Requiring Immediate Intervention (The "Fearsome Fatal Five")

The initial treatment of all trauma patients is to ensure an adequate airway and intravenous access. In addition to upper airway obstruction, the following injuries require immediate recognition and intervention:

(1) Complex Pneumothorax:
  - (a) Tension Pneumothorax
  - (b) Open Pneumothorax
  - (c) Massive Pneumothorax/Broncho-pulmonary Disruption

(2) Cardiac Tamponade
(3) Massive Hemothorax
(4) Traumatic Air Embolism
(5) Flail Chest

Tension pneumothorax (one of the fearsome five)

Tension pneumothorax occurs when there is an injury to the lung with resultant air leakage into the chest cavity that cannot escape. This "one-way valve" phenomenon results in each breath increasing both the volume of air and the intrapleural pressure. As the pressure builds, structures in the chest are compressed and displaced with impairment of ventilation and venous return to the heart (see Fig. 1).

The resultant combination of hypoxemia and hypoperfusion can be rapidly fatal necessitating prompt recognition and immediate treatment. Tension pneumothorax is a common cause of preventable death in the pre-hospital environment. The diagnosis of a tension pneumothorax is a clinical one characterized by tachypnea, dyspnea, jugular venous distention, decreased air entry, hyperresonance on the affected side and tracheal deviation to the opposite side in a patient with hypotension. Tension pneumothorax should be considered in all patients with trauma to the

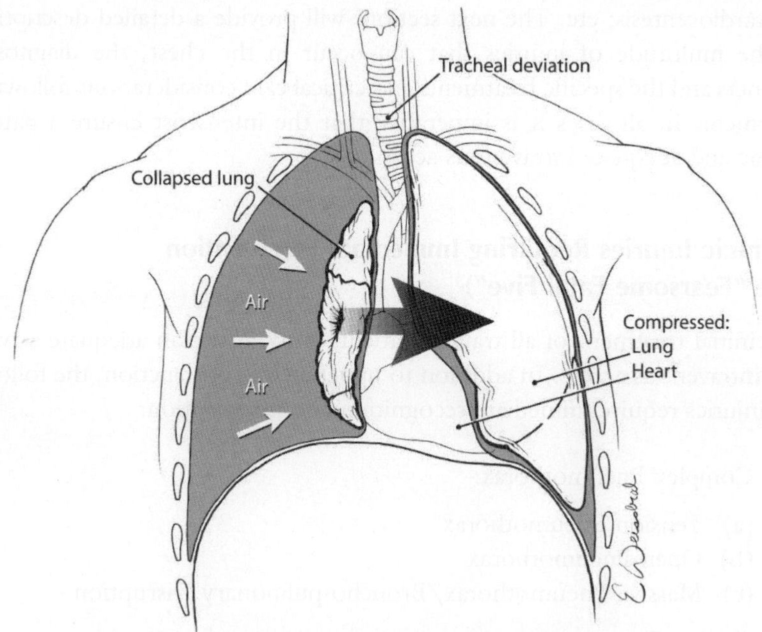

Fig. 1. Tension pneumothorax results when air leaking into the chest from an injured lung cannot escape with resultant compression and displacement of mediastinal structures and death if untreated.

thorax and ruled out in the initial assessment of the patient. It is important to note that patients placed on positive pressure ventilation after reaching the ICU can rapidly develop a tension pneumothorax, if they had an unrecognized or untreated occult or simple pneumothorax. Waiting to make or confirm the diagnosis with an X-ray is to be discouraged as the hemodynamic compromise associated with this process is rapidly fatal and delaying treatment for this reason would be a gross breach of standards of care. Additionally, distended neck veins may not be appreciated if the patient has concomitant hypovolemic shock. Likewise, tracheal deviation associated with tension pneumothorax may occur inferior to the jugular notch and may not be obvious, so its absence does not rule out this condition.

The treatment of tension pneumothorax is immediate decompression of the pleural space, which is accomplished initially by inserting a long large-bore needle into the pleural space at the second intercostal space in the line[6] or alternatively the fourth to fifth intercostal space just anterior to the midaxillary line[7] (see Fig. 2). The needle should be at least three inches in length in order to completely traverse the chest wall.[6] This procedure should be followed by formal insertion of a chest tube.

The ability to insert a chest tube is a mandatory skill for all clinicians working in the critical care arena, as surgical expertise is not always immediately available. The technique of chest tube insertion as diagramed in Fig. 3 require an incision of ~3 cm in the 4th to 5th intercostal space just anterior to the midaxillary line. If patient stability and time permits the area should be surgically prepped and draped, local anesthesia infiltrated, and the clinician appropriately gloved and gowned. The landmarks used for finding the site of the incision include the line of the nipple in males and the inframammary crease in females, though a potentially more reliable technique is to place the incision four fingerbreadths below the axillary crease (the width of a palm placed in the axilla). The incision is carried down onto the underlying rib and then a large blunt clamp (Kelley clamp) is popped into the chest above the rib though the intercostal muscle and pleura, enlarging the space by opening the clamp sequentially as it is removed. A gloved finger is then placed into the chest and rotated to first ensure that the chest cavity has been entered, and secondly to sweep away any potential adhesions of the lung up to the chest wall that might impede tube insertion. The chest tube is then inserted into the wound and pleural cavity aiming it towards the posterior apex of the chest cavity, such that the last hole on the chest tube is entirely within the chest (Fig. 3). The tube is then secured in place,

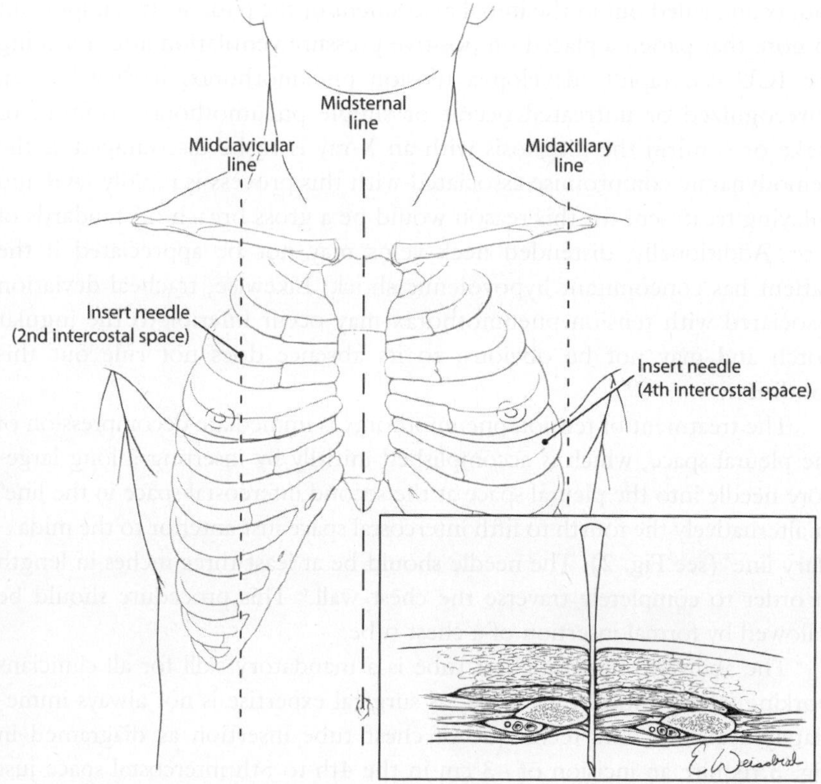

Fig. 2. Emergent treatment of a tension pneumothorax requires needle decompression of the chest using a large bore needle placed over the top of the rib in the 2nd intercostal space at the midclavicular line or alternatively in the 4th intercostal space just anterior to the midaxillary line.

dressed, and attached to an underwater seal device with application of suction (generally –20 cm water). The size of the chest tube should be geared to the problem being treated using larger bore chest tubes (36 French) if there is a need to drain blood from the chest, and smaller chest tubes if air is the primary focus. It should be kept in mind that blood drained from a chest tube can potentially be auto-transfused back to the patient and as such if one suspects a large hemothorax prior to placing a chest tube, an auto-transfusion bag should be placed on the chest tube in circuit with the underwater seal.

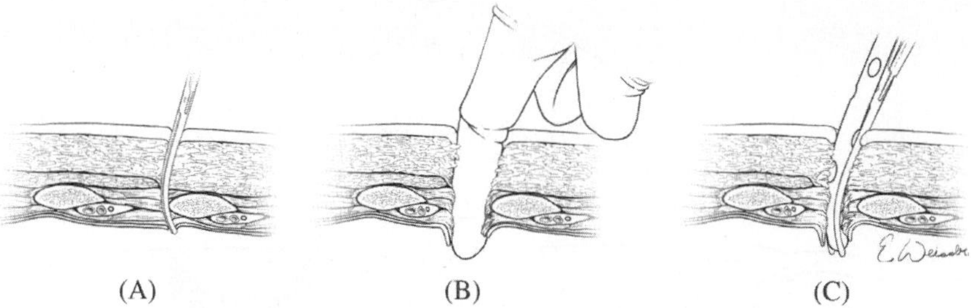

Fig. 3. Chest tube insertion is accomplished by puncturing the pleura of the lung with a clamp over the top of the rib (a) and spreading the clamp to enlarge the space sufficiently for a gloved finger to be passed into the chest (b) which is used to confirm entry into the chest and to sweep down any adhesions to the chest wall. A chest tube is then advanced into the chest (c) until the last hole of the chest tube is entirely within the chest cavity.

Open pneumothorax

The pathophysiology of open pneumothorax is similar to that of a tension pneumothorax with collapse of the lung and shift of the mediastinum resulting in hemodynamic and respiratory compromise. In the case of an open pneumothorax, which is also descriptively called a "sucking chest wound", there is free communication through a chest wall wound between the pleural space and the atmosphere. With each breath, air is "sucked" into the chest cavity through the wound in proportion to the size of the wound, preventing negative intrapleural pressure with resultant lung collapse. The communication of the pleural space to the atmosphere through the chest defect prevents generation of the negative pressure required for lung expansion during spontaneous inspiration. The net result is progressive collapse of the lung with each subsequent respiratory cycle. The larger the defect in the chest wall, the more pronounced this phenomenon will be. The diagnosis usually is obvious, with a visible open wound in the chest wall and a characteristic loud (sucking) noise created from atmospheric air entry into the pleural space.

The emergent treatment of a sucking chest wound is to occlude the open wound. Classically this is accomplished by tapping an occlusive dressing down onto the chest on three sides which allows for the egress of air from the plural space without further ingress (Fig. 4). Alternatively, a commercial device such as an Asherman or Bolin seal[8] can be placed over the open wound. After the wound has been occluded a chest tube should be placed

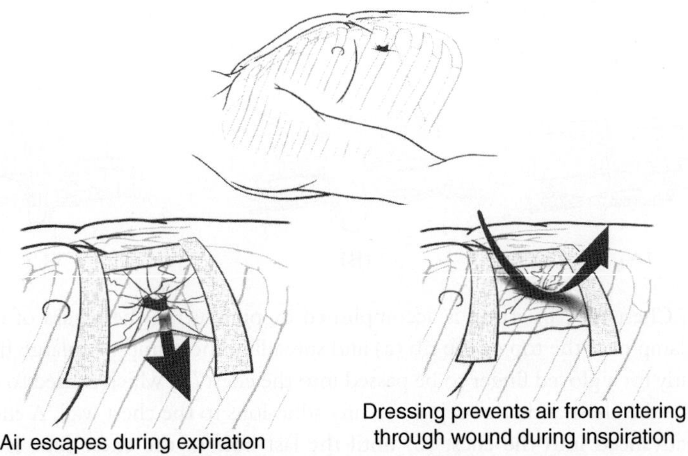
Air escapes during expiration
Dressing prevents air from entering through wound during inspiration

Fig. 4. The initial treatment of a "sucking" chest wound is to occlude the open wound by tapping an occlusive dressing down onto the chest on three sides which allows air to escape without further ingress.

through an incision separate from the wound as previously described. Wounds too large for simple occlusion will require endotracheal intubation and positive-pressure ventilation until formal surgical repair of the chest wall defect can be accomplished in the operating room (OR).

Massive pneumothorax/tracheobronchial disruption

Massive pneumothorax that occurs as a result of tracheobronchial disruption is a serious life-threatening problem that is reported to occur in about 1% of motor vehicle collision victims of whom 80% die before reaching the hospital. The injury to the bronchus is most commonly found on the right side within 2.5 cm of the carina. The typical presentation of patients surviving to hospital is mediastinal, deep cervical, and subcutaneous emphysema with persistent air leak and pneumothorax in spite of a functioning chest tube with associated hypoxemia and respiratory instability.

Patients with this suspected injury should be immediately placed on 100% oxygen, and for optimal outcome, patients with this injury should be taken emergently to the OR for repair by an experienced surgeon with a Computed Tomography (CT) scan and/or on table bronchoscopy to help delineate the site of the injury if time and patient stability permit. If there is massive destruction of the bronchus with failure to achieve an anastomosis or a high risk of subsequent stenosis, lung resection should be considered. Surgery remains the treatment of choice, however in very selected circumstances, based on strict clinical and endoscopic criteria conservative non-operative management has been advocated.[9]

Cardiac tamponade

Cardiac or pericardial tamponade results from accumulation of fluid (blood) into the pericardial sac around the heart that interferes with cardiac filling and restricts cardiac activity (Fig. 5). The diagnosis of cardiac tamponade should be considered in any patient who has penetrating or blunt trauma to the chest. Etiology in trauma patients is predominantly from a penetrating wound but can also occur in blunt trauma from cardiac rupture. Blunt cardiac rupture is immediately fatal in greater than 90%, and survivors usually have atrial injuries. The classic physical findings of cardiac tamponade described by Beck (Becks triad) of hypotension, distended neck veins, and muffled heart sounds are not always present and may be difficult to discern. The prevalence of portable ultrasound technology has made tamponade easier to diagnose as visualization of the heart via the epigastric pericardial view or parasternal view is sensitive for small amounts of fluid in the pericardial sac (see Fig. 6). Once the diagnosis of tamponade is made the patient should be taken promptly to the OR for surgical release of tamponade and correction of the underlying pathology which can be done either through an anterolateral thoracotomy or a sternotomy. If surgical expertise is not immediately available consideration should be given to performing a pericardiocentesis as relatively small amounts of blood (100 cc) will cause tamponade

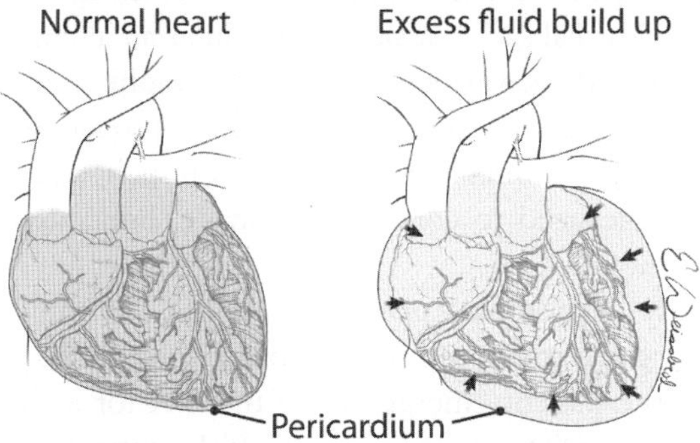

Fig. 5. Pericardial tamponade results from the accumulation of fluid (blood) in the intact pericardial sac with resultant compromise in cardiac function.

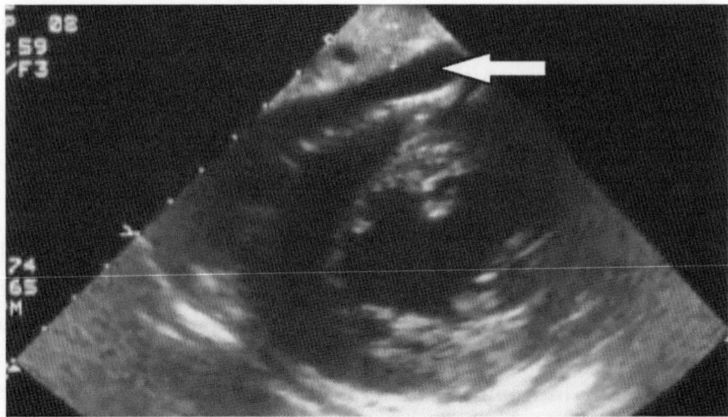

Fig. 6. Ultrasound of the heart demonstrates accumulation of blood (arrow) between the pericardium and the heart confirming the diagnosis of tamponade.

and removal of small amounts (15–20 cc) may be enormously beneficial. It must be kept in mind that pericardiocentesis is a temporizing measure only and that definitive treatment requires surgical opening of the pericardium with repair of the underlying injury.[10]

Pericardiocentesis is performed by inserting a long (> 6 inches) large bore (16 to 18 gauge) needle (preferably an angiocath) into the pericardial sac and aspirating the fluid therein with a large empty syringe with a three-way stopcock. The needle is inserted just below the xiphoid process a roughly a 45° angle and advanced cephalad toward the tip of the left scapula or the left nipple (Fig. 7). Gentle aspiration on the syringe is maintained as the needle is advanced with the return of non-clotting blood confirming entry into the pericardial sac. Classically, attaching an alligator clamp to the hub of the needle and then to an electrocardiographic lead is described to detect a "pattern of injury" if the needle is inserted too far and hits the heart. In actual practice the immediate availability of such equipment and the urgent nature of the need to correct tamponade, limits application of this "recommended" adjunct.

As previously mentioned, pericardiocentesis, is only a temporizing maneuver allowing for attempted restoration of the cardiac physiology long enough to take the patient emergently to the OR for a thoracotomy and definitive surgical repair of the cardiac injury. If the patient is in extremis, and will likely die before being transported, consideration should be given to opening the chest via a left anterolateral thoracotomy to relieve tamponade, at the bedside.[11]

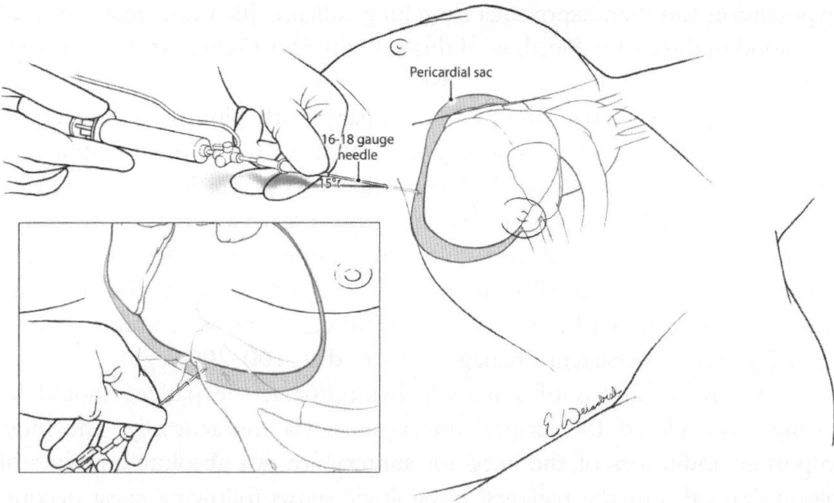

Fig. 7. Pericardiocentesis is accomplished by inserting a long (>6 inches) large bore needle below the xyphoid and aiming towards the left nipple to enter the pericardial sac and aspirate the fluid therein.

The anterolateral thoracotomy is conducted through an incision made from the edge of the sternum to the bed along the curve of the mid rib cage ideally positioned over the fifth intercostal space. The classically described landmark to identify the incision site is the nipple line (in males) or the inframammary crease (in females). The interspace is entered on top of the rib below, a rib spreader placed, and the pericardium is identified and opened longitudinally anterior to the path of the phrenic nerve which must not be injured. With the pericardium open, the tamponade can be released, and open heart massage, hemorrhage control, and surgical control accomplished as indicated. Though cardiac lacerations are ideally repaired with teflon pledgeted sutures, temporary control of hemorrhage can be obtained with finger occlusion, Foley catheter insertion into the wound with balloon inflation and gentle traction, or skin staples while awaiting experienced surgical assistance.

Massive hemothorax (one of the fearsome five)

Massive hemothorax is clinically defined as enough blood loss in the chest such that the patient becomes hemodynamically unstable. This generally occurs when 1200–1500 cc accumulate in the chest cavity with subsequent hypotension and then hxpoxemia from lung collapse due to the mass effect of the blood in the cavity. Bleeding of this magnitude is likely to be from disruption of a major central vasculature structure or laceration to an intercostals, or internal mammary artery and can accompany both blunt and penetrating injury.[2] In addition to hypotension and tachycardia the physical findings for massive hemothorax will also include dullness to percussion, decreased air entry over the affected hemithorax, and flattened neck veins. With enough blood, the mediastinum can also shift with tamponade physiology as a result. The diagnosis is confirmed by insertion of a large bore chest tube, through which a large volume of blood (>1200–1500 cc) is drained and further confirmed if there is persistent drainage of more than 100–200 cc/hr.

With the diagnosis of a massive hemothorax, the patient should be strongly considered for surgical intervention via thoracotomy. The most important indicators of the need for surgery are not absolute amounts of blood drained, but the patients' physiologic status following chest decompression. It is crucial that the intensivist caring for such patients carefully monitor the volume of blood from the drain and communicate this clearly to surgical colleagues both the amount and the physiologic consequences. If bleeding continues at a rapid rate, or the hemodynamic status cannot be rapidly corrected with blood and crystalloid infusion, the patient should be taken emergently to the OR for a thoracotomy. Once the chest is opened, blood is evacuated and a search for the bleeding is undertaken with surgical repair as indicated. Operative intervention may range from simple suture repair to wedge resection, staple tractotomy, lobectomy, and most extreme a pneumonectomy. It should also be kept in mind that the blood evacuated from the chest tube can be auto-transfused to the patient.

Traumatic Air Embolism

The diagnosis of traumatic air embolism should be suspected in any patient with sudden cardiovascular collapse who demonstrates a neurologic deficit after chest injury, especially if these signs occur with the initiation of positive-pressure ventilation.[12] In most cases, the diagnosis of traumatic air embolism is made at thoracotomy that is conducted on the basis of sudden collapse of a patient who has sustained major chest trauma. Occasionally, the patient may be initially stable, and when placed on positive pressure ventilation suddenly develop a focal neurologic deficit suddenly with cardiovascular collapse. The presence of bubbles within arterial blood drawn by arterial puncture also suggests the diagnosis. On occasion, air may be seen in the retinal arteries on funduscopic examination as well.

Traumatic air embolism occur secondary to a communication between the vasculature and the airway as a result of the traumatic event. The application of positive pressure ventilation forces the air into the exposed vasculature with entry into the cardiac circulation with the possibility of an "airlock" in the heart and embolization of air into the coronary arteries (generally fatal), or into the cerebral circulation with resultant stroke-like symptomology.

If suspected, an anterolateral thoracotomy should be performed on the side of the penetrating injury or on the left side if no penetration is apparent. Once in the chest the pulmonary hilum is cross clamped to prevent further embolization. This will require mobilizing the lung by talking down the inferior pulmonary ligament. An 18 gauge needle is then inserted into the most anterior surfaces of the left atrium, left ventricle, and ascending aorta to vent any air that may be present. This maneuver is followed by compressing the root of the aorta between the thumb and index finger, which are placed in the transverse sinus. The heart is then massaged in an attempt to drive air bubbles out of the coronary microvasculature.[13] Maintenance of a high systemic blood pressure, with α agonists if necessary, should help to force trapped air from the heart and brain through the microvasculature into the venous circulation. With reestablishment of cardiac activity, the left-sided chambers and the aorta should be vented once more. Attention is then directed to the pulmonary lesion, which will require repair by direct suture, stapled tractomoy, lobectomy, or pneumonectomy as necessitated by the nature of the injury. If available there may be a role for cardiopulmonary bypass in the management of this entity.[14]

Flail Chest

Flail chest arises whenever a portion of the chest wall becomes completely discontinuous from the rest of the rib cage. Classically this is defined as the fracture of three or more ribs in two or more places and typically results from blunt chest trauma (Fig. 8). The result is a free-floating segment of the chest wall that moves paradoxically in response to the ventilator cycle. During spontaneous breathing, the flail segment moves inward with the negative pleural pressure of inspiration and moves outward with expiration (Fig. 9). Paradoxical motion can be difficult to appreciate in patients with posterior fractures, prominent pectoral musculature, or who have limited respiratory

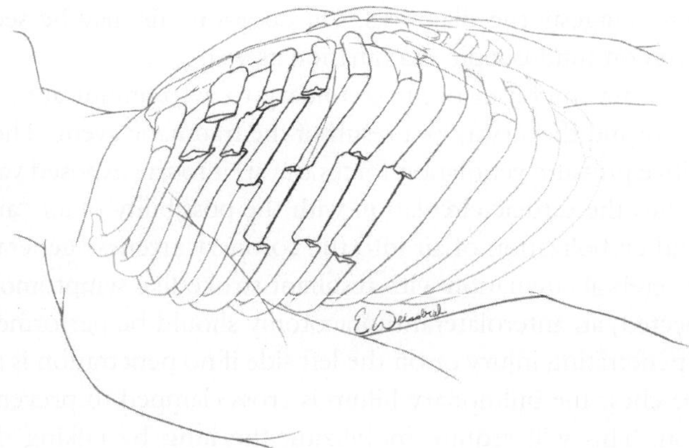

Fig. 8. A flail chest is classically defined as the fracture of three or more ribs in two or more places with a resultant free floating segment of the chest wall.

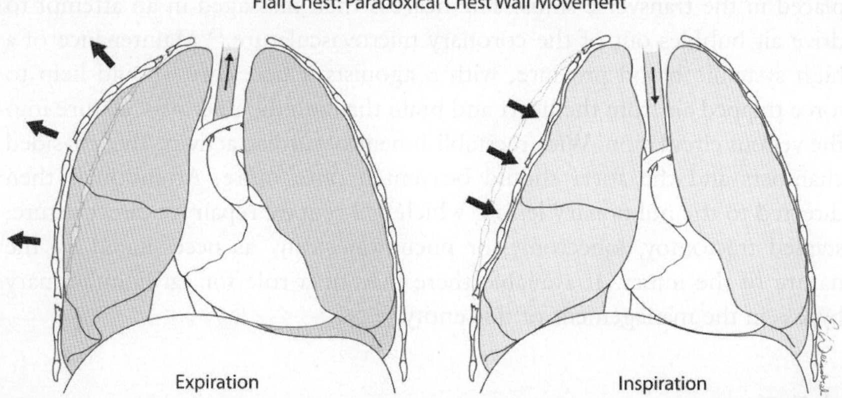

Fig. 9. Paradoxical movement of the chest can be seen with a flail chest where the flail segment moves inward with negative pleural pressure of inspiration and outward with expiration.

excursion due to pain, resulting in the diagnosis frequently being missed on initial exam. Additionally, if the patient has been intubated and placed on positive pressure ventilation, the paradoxical motion will not be seen. The presence of multiple adjacent rib fractures involving the same rib in different segments on chest X-ray or CT scan would suggest the presence of flail chest even if it is not apparent clinically. The clinical significance of the flail chest is that it can significantly impair gas exchange and hemodynamic stability and is proportional to the extent of the flail, the underlying lung contusion, and the restrictive effect of chest wall pain from the fractures. The presence of a flail chest is also a marker for potential underlying pulmonary contusion requiring a high index of suspicion that the patient has an increased likelihood of respiratory and hemodynamic compromise. In patients with the combination of flail chest and pulmonary contusion, up to 75% will require intubation and the associated mortality has been reported as high as 40%.[15]

In the severely hypoxemic patient with a large flail and/or hemodynamic instability, immediate endotracheal intubation and positive-pressure ventilation should be instituted. A chest tube should also be promptly inserted on the involved side to prevent a tension pneumothorax from developing on institution of positive-pressure ventilation. In most patients, adequate anesthesia via patient controlled analgesia, epidural, or intercostal blockade, will obviate the need for intubation and mechanical ventilation.[15, 16]

Though not yet standard of care, there is an increasing resurgence of interest in performing mechanical fixation of flail chest with rib platting techniques.[15, 17] The purported benefits of this are said to be decreased pain, and fewer ventilator and ICU days. In situations where thoracotomy is required for other reasons, it may be appropriate to reduce and plate the fractures involved, and input from a surgeon with appropriate expertise should be sought. Ventilated flail chest patients can be weaned from the respirator when the gas exchange abnormality associated with the underlying lung contusion is resolved, even if paradoxical movement remains.[18]

Thoracic Injuries that have the Potential to Become Life-Threatening in a Delayed Fashion (The "Serious Seven")

Although the following chest injuries do not immediately threaten life, early diagnosis and treatment are essential to prevent significant morbidity and later mortality:

(1) Pulmonary Contusion
(2) Blunt Cardiac Injury
(3) Traumatic Aortic Disruption
(4) Esophageal Injury
(5) Traumatic Diaphragmatic Injury
(6) Rib Fractures
(7) Simple Hemo or Pneumothorax

Because the pulmonary and hemodynamic consequences of the listed injuries can occur in a delayed fashion, the diagnosis may not be made or present with symptomology until the patient has been admitted to the ICU. As such, it is vital that all critical care practitioners be well-versed in the identification of and treatment or referral for treatment of these entities. A very brief discussion of the pathophysiology, diagnosis, and treatment of these entities follows.

Pulmonary contusion

Pulmonary contusion usually results from blunt injury (can also occur with penetrating injury) to the lung with bleeding into the parenchyma that can interfere with oxygenation (Fig. 10). This injury is arguably the most common life-threatening blunt chest injury with a reported mortality of 5–30%.[3,18] The danger of this injury is that it is often missed on initial presentation as the respiratory compromise that develops is not immediately evident and initial chest films may be completely normal even in the presence of significant injury. A high index of suspicion should be maintained in any patient with significant direct injury to the chest wall and especially in the presence

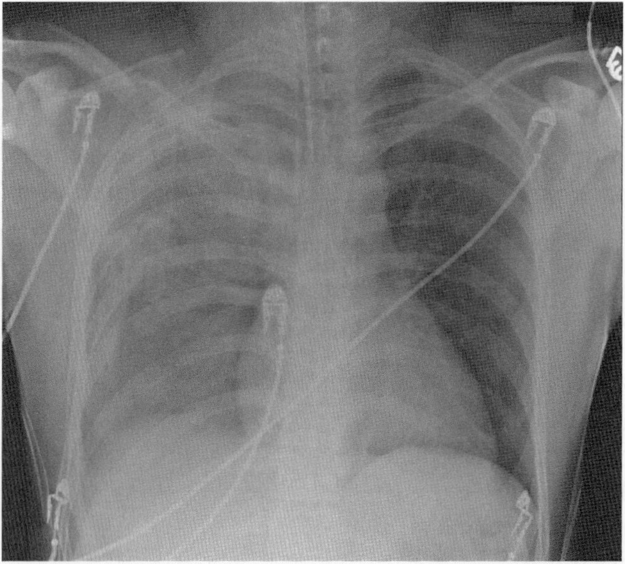

Fig. 10. This radiograph shows pulmonary contusion (increased opacity) of the right lung in addition to multiple rib fractures.

of a flail chest. Patients may initially have only chest pain and minimal dyspnea with slow deterioration of gas exchange and progressive development of radiographic abnormalities over a few hours (see Fig. 10).

The treatment of pulmonary contusion is generally supportive. A decision to intubate is based on the degree of underlying lung injury and the resultant respiratory impairment.[19] Though aggressive fluid resuscitation can exacerbate the respiratory compromise in these patients, fluid should not be restricted if the patient has altered hemodynamics. As such these patients require close attention to fluid balance with continuous monitoring of the hemodynamic and respiratory status. If there is no major hemodynamic or respiratory compromise, the patient will not require mechanical ventilation. Should there be any question, the patient should be promptly intubated and ventilated with a lung protective strategy.

Blunt cardiac injury (one of the serious seven)

The incidence of blunt cardiac injury has been reported in large series looking specifically for this to range from 10–20%.[20] The vast majority of these will be asymptomatic and clinically insignificant, with a very small minority developing symptoms (arrhythmias or pump failure) requiring treatment. The most common etiology is blunt trauma to the sternum, caused by steering wheel impact. In fact, whenever a fractured sternum is diagnosed in chest trauma, one must assume an underlying myocardial contusion. The patient's symptoms frequently are clouded by associated chest wall contusion and other causes for chest wall discomfort and cardiorespiratory dysfunction.

Evaluation, disposition, and treatment of patients with suspected cardiac contusion is based upon initial Electrocardiographic (ECG) evaluation. Current guidelines have discouraged the use of routine measurement of cardiac enzymes as the levels obtained following trauma are too inconclusive to allow a diagnosis of blunt cardiac injury and provide no information beyond that available by ECG.[21] ECG abnormalities may vary from few to multiple premature ventricular contractions, persistent tachycardia, dysrhythmias such as atrial fibrillation, bundle branch block, ST-segment changes, or even changes indistinguishable from those of acute myocardial infarction. None of these tests is specific for blunt cardiac injury.

Because of the propensity for certain life-threatening dysrhythmias, consideration should be given to monitoring patients with cardiac contusion in an ICU environment. The treatment of symptomatic patients will be similar to patients with myocardial ischemia in general. Oxygen and pain control are the mainstays with the use of inotropic agents, vasoactive drugs, and other forms of cardiac support as clinically indicated. Patients who develop bundle branch blocks may require temporary pacing, and intra-aortic balloon pump may be required in patients with low cardiac output. Most patients with minor degrees of contusion do not require ICU admission. Based on a review of the literature on this entity, the Eastern Association for the Surgery of Trauma (EAST) has recognized three levels of investigation. [22]

Level I

Admission Electrocardiogram (EKG) for all patients suspected of having blunt cardiac injury.

Level II

(a) An abnormal EKG requires monitoring for 24–48 hours.
(b) Hemodynamically unstable patients should have an echocardiogram (Transthoracic or Transesophageal)

Level III

Elderly patients with a cardiac history, unstable patients and those with abnormal admitting EKG may undergo surgery with appropriate monitoring including consideration for the placement of pulmonary artery catheter.

Traumatic aortic disruption (one of the serious seven)

Traumatic disruption of the thoracic aorta frequently is lethal with 70–80% of patients dying in the pre-hospital setting.[23] The remainder will make it to the hospital alive with a hematoma contained by an intact adventitial layer, and a significant risk of free rupture and exsanguination if not recognized and appropriately treated. The site of the aortic disruption is typically located at the point of fixation of the aorta just distal to the origin of the left subclavian artery at the ligamentum arteriosum, which represents the junction between a relatively fixed and mobile portion of the vessel (Fig. 11). This injury is most classically seen with acceleration–deceleration injuries, and should be suspected in all patients with significant blunt trauma to the chest. Because of the possibility of free rupture and exsanguination whenever this diagnosis is suspected, investigations and treatment should be prompt, only after dealing with other potentially life-threatening injuries.

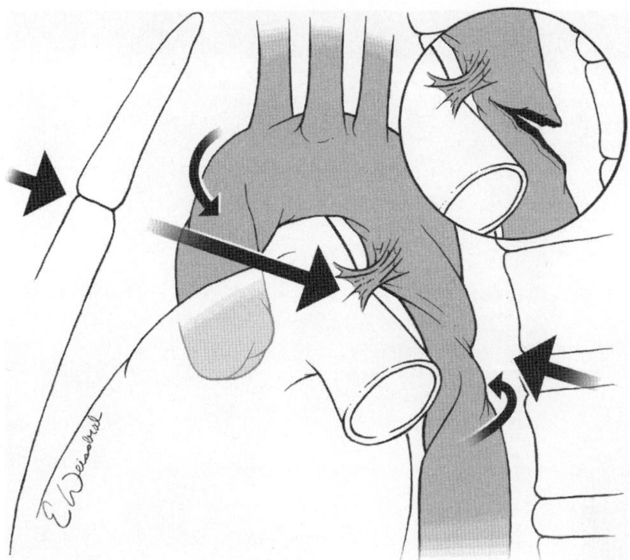

Fig. 11. The site of blunt aortic disruption is typically located at the point of fixation of the aorta at the level of the ligamentum arteriosum (long arrow).

Although several radiologic signs are described (such as widened mediastinum, fractures of the first and second ribs, obliteration of the aortic knob, deviation of the trachea to the right, presence of a pleural cap, elevation and rightward shift of the right main-stem bronchus, depression of the left main-stem bronchus, and obliteration of the space between the pulmonary artery and the aorta), frequently the only suggestive sign is a widening of the mediastinum on the plain chest film (Fig. 11). It is important to emphasize that a negative X-ray does not exclude aortic injury, and if the clinical suspicion based on mechanism is high additional studies must be undertaken to rule it out.

Helical CT Angiography (Fig. 13) has become diagnostic procedure of choice with 100% sensitivity, 99.7% specificity and 100% negative predictive value, and if totally normal, then further imaging is not warranted.[24,25] Angiography (the historic gold-standard) has 100% sensitivity and 98% specificity and may be useful in planning surgical approach, ruling out other vascular injury, and potentially therapeutic (endovascular stent placement). The use of transesophageal echocardiography[26] also has given excellent results in the diagnosis of aortic rupture, and in some centers it has virtually replaced angiography because of its accuracy and relative non-invasiveness, but there still remains a worrisome incidence of false positivity with this diagnostic tool.

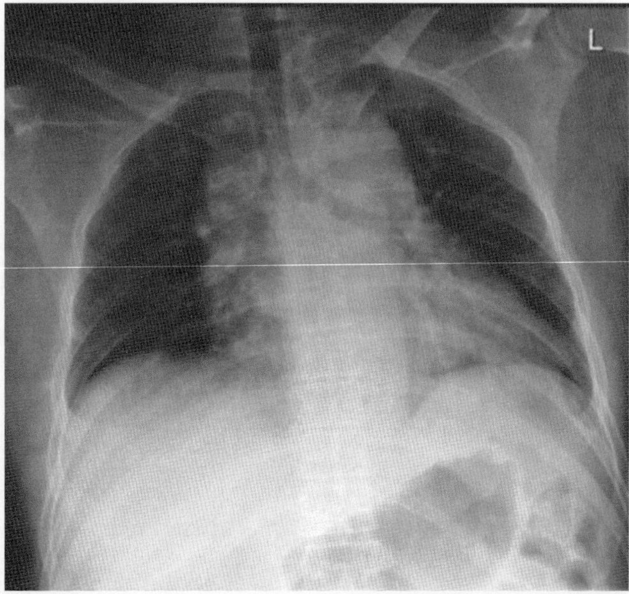

Fig. 12. Widening of the mediastinum as seen on this radiograph should raise the suspicion of traumatic aortic disruption and prompt further workup.

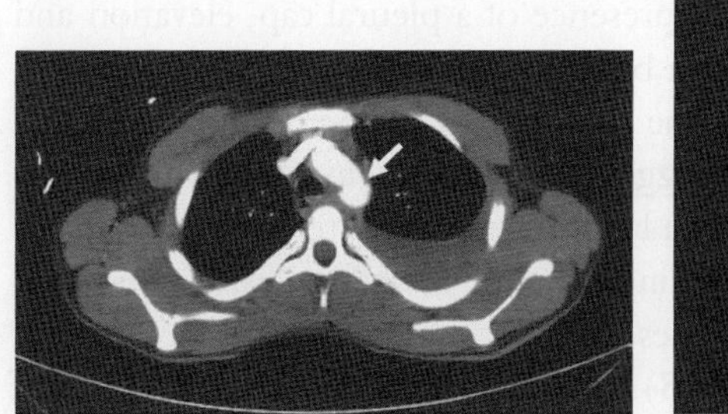

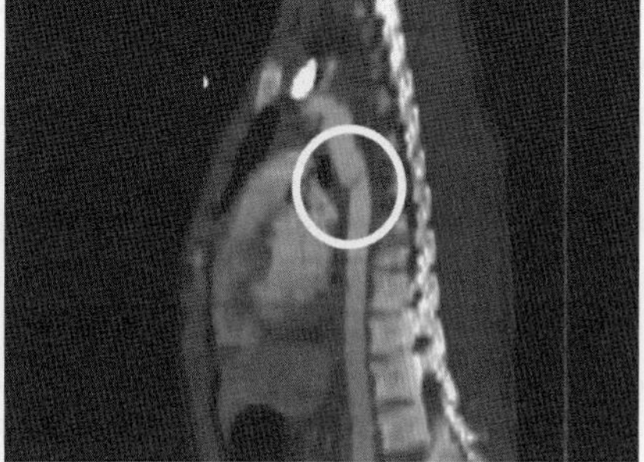

Fig. 13. CT Angiogram is the current diagnostic standard for traumatic aortic tears with the defect clearly seen on both the axial image on the left (arrow) and the reconstructed image on the right (circle).

The current management of choice for traumatic aortic injury is endovascular stenting.[27] In patients managed in centers without this expertize (or the ability to transfer the patient to such a center), or in whom endovascular repair may not be suitable, surgical resection with placement of a prosthetic graft would be necessary. If endovascular or surgical treatment is delayed because of associated major injuries or the need to transfer the patient, these patients should be managed with afterload reduction, β-Blockade, and maintenance of borderline hypotension.[28]

Esophageal Disruption

Iatrogenic injury as a result of endoscopy remains the most common cause of esophageal rupture, but can also result from both penetrating and blunt injury.[29] A severe blow to the upper abdomen in the presence of a closed glottis can result in a sudden increase in intraesophageal pressure with resultant rupture. Subsequent leakage of gastric contents into the mediastinum, causes severe mediastinitis with resultant systemic consequences. Patients with esophageal leakage present with complaints of severe retrosternal chest pain and very soon develop profound hypotension and tachycardia. Frequently, pneumothorax or hemothorax is evident without a rib fracture, and if a chest tube is inserted, particulate matter may appear in the drainage. The drainage of pleural fluid with a very low pH and high amylase content also should suggest the diagnosis. Other radiologic signs include the presence of mediastinal air. The diagnosis may be confirmed by gastrograffin swallow or esophagoscopy.

Early surgical repair via thoracotomy is the cornerstone of treatment, and perioperative management requires aggressive fluid resuscitation and broad spectrum antibiotic coverage. If the diagnosis is made late in the onset of the disease, direct repair of the laceration may not be possible, and esophageal diversion techniques may become necessary as part of the surgical therapy. This may require the formation of an esophagostomy in the neck, as well as a gastrostomy, pleural drainage through chest tubes, and parenteral nutrition, and antibiotic therapy.[30]

Diaphragmatic Rupture

Lacerations of the diaphragm may occur from blunt and penetrating injuries and are relatively infrequent (~3% of total injuries). Between 80–90% of these injuries result from motor vehicle crashes with blunt injuries, and can be large, irregular lacerations with herniation of intra-abdominal contents into the chest.[31] The injury is diagnosed most frequently on the left side but may occur with equal frequency on the right side. Penetrating injuries to the diaphragm tend to be small and sharply demarcated, making the diagnosis more challenging, but the repair easier. It is important to recognize that blunt diaphragm injuries are a marker of significant trauma and 80–100% of these patients will have other associated severe and potentially life-threatening injuries.

The diagnosis of diaphragmatic injury is often delayed with up to 50% not being recognized in the first 24 hours following the traumatic event. Chest X-ray findings suggestive or diagnostic of this injury include an elevated hemi-diaphragm, bowel pattern in the chest, or the presence of a nasogastric tube above the diaphragm. Unfortunately, the chest X-ray can be normal in up to 50% of cases.

Depending on the degree to which abdominal contents herniate into the thoracic cavity, the symptoms may be very minimal or very significant.[32] A patient with blunt chest or abdominal trauma who exhibits sudden deterioration in respiratory status when intra-abdominal pressure is increased should be considered as having a ruptured diaphragm. During peritoneal lavage, drainage of lavage fluid through a chest tube that is in place also indicates that diaphragmatic rupture is present.

The urgency of treatment depends on the degree to which the patient's hemodynamic and respiratory status is compromised. In most instances, an isolated diaphragmatic rupture can be repaired within several hours of admission, after the patient is resuscitated. Repair is done through a midline upper abdominal incision. This approach allows complete examination of the abdominal cavity. The hernia can be reduced quite easily and the repair conducted from within the abdomen.[32] Associated injuries, such as splenic rupture, also can be treated easily during the laparotomy. Although laparoscopy increases the risk of tension pneumothorax in the presence of a diaphragmatic rupture, recent reports have suggested that this technique may be employed cautiously in the diagnosis and treatment of diaphragmatic rupture when the laparoscope is used in assessment of the traumatized abdomen.[33] It is important to ensure that patients with stab wounds to the left lower chest/upper abdomen not have a missed diaphragmatic injury. Many centers have adopted a practice of routine diagnostic laparotomy or laparoscopy to evaluate for the presence of a diaphragmatic injury in such patients prior to hospital discharge.

Rib and Other Chest Wall Fractures

Rib fractures are the most common chest wall injury resulting from blunt trauma, and when present should heighten suspicion for other associated injuries. Trauma patients with a rib fracture have a risk of splenic injury of 1.7 fold, and a risk of liver injury 1.4 fold greater than a patient without.[1] Having more than three ribs fractures is associated with increased mortality, and fracture of the first rib is associated with heart and great vessel injuries in up to 15%, and head and neck injuries in up to 50% of cases. Rib fractures are frequently missed on X-ray examination unless special rib views are taken. However, the diagnosis is suspected when there is localized chest wall pain. The diagnosis is also suggested when one is able to elicit crepitus over the fracture site or auscultate a "click" with inspiration over the fracture site. Tenderness on compression of the chest wall is also suggestive of rib fractures.

The treatment of rib fractures primarily consists of analgesics, which may be administered orally, parenterally, or epidurally, depending on the degree of discomfort and the number of ribs involved. In the ICU setting, parenteral analgesics or regional blocks are preferable. Generally, the fractured ribs do not require any specific treatment. However, in the setting of a patient with preexisting pulmonary dysfunction, the restriction produced by fractured ribs can make the difference between normal gas exchange and severe respiratory failure. The mortality associated with rib fractures is much higher in the elderly (five times greater) due to their decreased pulmonary reserve and higher incidence of underlying pulmonary disease.[1] Close attention to maintenance of adequate respiratory function is the mainstay of treatment in these patients.

Other bones in the chest wall must be carefully evaluated in trauma patients as well specifically the sternum and scapulas. The presence of fractures to these structures is a marker of great force and should raise the index of suspicion of injury to other structures. In the presence of scapular fractures associated injuries to lung, great vessels, brachial plexus, and central nervous system are common and must be considered. With sternal fractures, associated injuries are common and high index of suspicion should be maintained for underlying visceral injuries (cardiac injury in 18–62%).[34] If unstable or displaced by more than 1 cm, they should be treated with open reduction and internal fixation.

Simple Hemopneumothorax

A simple pneumothorax is a non-expanding collection of air between the outside surface of the lung and the inside surface of the chest wall, and can occur in up to 24% of patients with blunt trauma. In contrast to a tension pneumothorax, the simple hemopneumothorax usually is diagnosed by a combination of physical examination and chest X-ray. The presence of rib fractures should prompt a careful search for pneumothorax. Chest X-ray is usually diagnostic but may miss small pneumothoraces. CT scanning is much more sensitive but the significance and treatment of a small or "occult pneumothorax" (seen on CT but not Chest X-ray) is controversial. It has been suggested that small pneumothoraces (those less than 20%) may be watched expectantly, unless patient is to undergo positive pressure ventilation or will be placed in a situation where close monitoring is not possible.[35] In general, if a hemothorax or pneumothorax is noted following trauma, a chest tube is inserted regardless of the size of the air or blood collection. This measure allows decompression of the pleural space, as well as monitoring of the drainage from the pleural space. It is particularly important that chest tube decompression of the pleural space be secured before mechanical ventilation is instituted or a general anesthetic administered.

A simple hemothorax is a collection of blood in the pleural space that does not cause hemodynamic or pulmonary compromise. Most hemothoraces are a result of rib fractures, lung parenchymal, and minor venous injuries, and therefore are usually self-limiting. Small hemothoraces are not detected by physical exam or Chest X-ray as it takes approximately 300 cc of blood to show up on an X-ray. FAST ultrasound has success in identifying smaller hemothoraces but is very user dependent. CT is very sensitive for finding small amounts of blood but this may not be clinically significant.

Chest tube placement (at least 36 French) is the first step in management and is definitive in up to 90% of cases. If there is retained blood in the chest there is an increased incidence of empyema and a thoracoscopic decortication and drainage is indicated in such circumstances.

Summary

Patients with thoracic trauma are frequently found in the ICU. It is imperative that the intensivist have a thorough understanding of the nature of these injuries, their expected course and the non-surgical and surgical management. Early recognition and intervention has the potential to greatly improve outcomes in these patients.

References

1. O'Connor JV, Adamski J. The diagnosis and treatment of non-cardiac thoracic trauma. *J R Army Med Corps* 2010; 156: 5–14.
2. Lim JY, Wolf AS, Flores RM. Thoracic vessel injury. *Minerva Chir* 2013; 68: 251–262.

3. LoCicero J, Mattox KL. Epidemiology of chest trauma. *Surg Clin North Am* 1989; 69: 15.
4. Moore JB, Moore EE, Thompson JS. Abdominal injuries associated with penetrating trauma in the lower chest. *Am J Surg* 1980; 140: 724.
5. Hirshberg A, Mattox KL, Wall MJ Jr. Double jeopardy: Thocoabdominal injuries requiring surgery in both chest and abdomen. *J Trauma* 1995; 39: 1.
6. Zengerlink I, Brink PR, Laupland KB, Raber EL, Zygunn D, Kortbeek JB. Needle thoracostomy in the treatment of a tension pneumothorax in trauma patients: What size needle? *J Trauma* 2008; 64: 111–114.
7. Rawlings R, Brown KM, Carr CS, Cameron CR. Life threatening haemorrhage after anterior needle aspiration of pneumothoraces. A role for lateral needle aspiration in emergency decompression of spontaneous pneumothorax. *Emerg Med J* 2003; 20: 383–384.
8. Arnaud F, Tomori T, Teranishi K, Yun J, McCarron R, Mahon R. Evaluation of chest seal performance in a swine model: Comparison of Asherman vs. Bolin seal. *Injury* 2008; 39: 1082–1088.
9. Carretta A, Melloni G, Bandiera A, Negri G, Voci C, Zannini P. Conservative and surgical treatment of acute posttraumatic tracheobronchial injuries. *World J Surg* 2011; 35: 2568–2574.
10. Lee TH, Ouellet JF, Cook M, Schreiber MA, Kortbeek JB. Pericardiocentesis in trauma a systemic review. *J Trauma Acute Care Surg* 2013; 75: 543–549.
11. Tan BK, Pothiawala S, Ong ME. Emergency thoracotomy: A review of its role in severe chest trama. *Minerva Chir* 2013; 86: 241–250.
12. King MW, Aitchison JM, Nel JP. Fatal air embolism following penetrating lung trauma: An autopsy study. *J Trauma* 1984; 24: 753.
13. Yee ES, Verrier ED, Thomas AN. Management of air embolism in blunt and penetrating thoracic trauma. *J Thorac Cardiovasc Surg* 1983; 85: 661.
14. Rawlins R, Momin A, Platts D, El-Gamel A. Traumatic cardiogenic shock due to massive pulmonary embolism. A possible role for cardiopulmaonary bypass. *Eur J Cardiothoracic Surg* 2002; 22: 845–846.
15. Dehghan N, de Mestral C, McKee MD, Schemitsch EH, Nathens A. Flail chest injuries: A review of outcomes and treatment practices from the National Trauma Data Bank. *J Trauma Acute Care Surg* 2014; 76: 462–468.
16. Vana PG, Neubauer DC, Luchette FA. Contemporary management of flail chest. *Am Surg* 2014; 80: 527–535.
17. De Jong MB, Kokke MC, Hietbrink F, Leenen LP. Surgical management of rib fractures: Strategies and literature review. *Scand J Surg* 2014; 103: 120–125.
18. Pettiford BL, Luketich JD, Landreneau RJ. The management of flail chest. *Thorac Surg Clin* 2007; 17: 25–33.
19. Richardson JD, Adams L, Flint LM. Selective management of flail chest and pulmonary contusion. *Ann Surg* 1982; 196: 481.

20. Tenzer ML: The spectrum of myocardial contusion: A review. *J Trauma* 1985; 25: 620.
21. Biffl WL, Moore FA, Moore EE *et al.* Cardiac enzymes are irrelevant in the patient with suspected myocardial contusion. *Am J Surg* 1994; 169: 523.
22. Pasquale M, Fabian TC, EAST Ad Hoc Committee on Practice Management Guideline Development. Practice management guidelines for trauma from the Eastern Association for the Surgery of Trauma. *J Trauma* 1998; 44: 94.
23. Hunt JP, Baker CC, Lentz CW *et al.* Thoracic aorta injuries: Management and outcome of 144 patients. *J Trauma* 1996; 40: 547.
24. Gavant ML, Menke PG, Fabian TC *et al.* Blunt traumatic aortic rupture: Detection with helical CT of the chest. *Radiology* 1995; 197: 125.
25. Cullen EL, Lantz EJ, Joohnson CM, Young PM. Traumatic aortic injury: CT findings, mimics, and therapeutic options. *Cardiovasc Diagn Ther* 2014; 4: 238–244.
26. Smith MD, Cassidy JM Souther S *et al.* Transesophegeal echocardiography in the diagnosis of traumatic rupture of the aorta. *New Engl J Med* 1995; 332: 356.
27. Branco BC, DuBose JJ, Zahn LX, Hughes JD, Goshima KR, Rhee P, Mills JL Sr. *J Vasc Surg*, 2014; Epub ahead of print.
28. Nagy K, Fabian T, Rodman G *et al.* Guidelines for the diagnosis and management of blunt aortic injury: an EAST Practice Management Guidelines Work Group. *J Trauma* 2000; 48: 1128.
29. Asensio JA, Chahwan S, Forno W *et al.* Penetrating esophageal injuries: Multicenter study of the American Association for the Surgery of Trauma. *J Trauma* 2001; 50: 289.
30. Nirula R. Esophageal perforation. *Surg Clin North Am*, 2013; 94: 35–41.
31. Brasel KJ, Borgstrom DC, Meyer P, Weigelt JA. Predictors of outcome in blunt diaphragm rupture. *J Trauma* 1996; 41: 484.
32. Ties JS, Peschman JR, Moreno A, Mathiason MA, Kallies KJ, Martin RF, Brasel KJ, Cogbill TH. Evolution in the management of traumatic diaphragmatic injuries: A multicenter review. *J Trauma Acute Care Surg* 2014; 76: 1024–1028.
33. Ali J, Qi W. 52. Ivatury RR, Simon RJ, Stahl WM. A critical evaluation of laparoscopy in penetrating abdominal trauma. *J Trauma* 1993; 34: 822.
34. Oyetunji TA, Jackson HT, Obireze AC, Moore D, Branche MJ, Grene WR, Cornwell EE 3rd, Siram SM. Associated injuries in traumatic sternal fractures: A review of the National Trauma Data Bank. *Am Surg* 2013; 79: 702–705.
35. Yadav K, Jalili M, Zehtabchi S. Management of traumatic occult pneumothorax. *Resuscitation* 2010; 81: 1063–1068.

Chapter 17

Abdominal Trauma

Jameel Ali

Chapter Overview

Missed or delayed diagnosis of intra-abdominal injuries accounts for a major cause of preventable deaths in trauma patients[1] because of the many diagnostic challenges in these patients. Management or monitoring in the intensive care unit (ICU) could potentially decrease this risk. In order to accomplish this, the surgical intensivist requires a clear understanding of the clinical features of initial presentation, the likelihood of change occurring later in the patient's course, general principles of abdominal trauma management as well as management of specific injuries affecting the intra-abdominal contents. These patients, particularly with blunt trauma may be difficult to assess because of altered sensorium (from drugs, alcohol, or head injury), altered sensation (from spinal injury), and injury to adjacent structures (pelvis, chest) that may present with abdominal findings.[2] ICU admission allows close observation during the preoperative as well as postoperative period during which important changes could occur that would prompt changes in management strategy including a return to the operating room (OR).

In this chapter, general principles of management of abdominal injuries are followed by description of the role of adjunctive studies and principles of management of specific injuries to guide the intensivist in caring for these patients.

General Principles

Abdominal injuries may be classified into two broad categories: blunt and penetrating which differ from each other in significant ways.

Penetrating injury may result from stabs or other sharp instruments, or from bullet or shotgun. Stab wounds tend to be the least serious because the organs involved are only those within the trajectory of the wounding instrument and surrounding organ injury is absent. Unless the stab wound penetrates a vascular structure directly, major hemorrhage is not as likely as in other forms of penetrating or blunt injury. Penetrating injuries from bullets or shotguns produce unpredictable injuries because of their variable trajectory since a straight line joining the points of entry and exit does not represent the path of the missile and multiple organ involvement is common. Low velocity missiles create less damage than high velocity missiles because of the lower kinetic energy transfer. In shotgun injuries much less damage occurs when the injury is sustained from far range than close range.

Blunt injury results from a crushing force producing irregular lacerations with multiple organ involvement. Diagnosis is more challenging and the treatment approach needs to be more aggressive because morbidity and mortality from major hemorrhage, devitalization of tissue and complications such as sepsis are much higher than in penetrating injuries.

The frequency of organ involvement is also different between penetrating and blunt injuries. In penetrating injuries the order of frequency of organ involvement is: liver, small bowel, stomach, colon, major vessels, and retroperitoneum. In blunt injuries the order is spleen, kidney, liver, and intestines.

Because of the variability in location of the diaphragm with the phases of respiration and the unpredictable trajectory of penetrating wounds to the abdominothoracic areas, it is prudent to consider the possibility of intra-abdominal injuries in all patients in whom there is impact to the chest or abdomen. In a hemodynamically compromised trauma patient, when the therapeutic decision is unclear, the combination of physical examination, chest X-ray, and chest tube insertion will frequently allow determination of whether the causative lesion is in the chest. With a negative chest X-ray and no chest tube drainage in the absence of cardiac tamponade or traumatic air embolism laparotomy should be considered to identify and treat a possible intra-abdominal cause of the hemodynamic compromise.

The entire abdomen, chest, and upper thigh should be prepped and draped in preparation for the laparotomy to allow access to both the abdomen and chest as well as to deal with possible lesions in either cavity, access to the supradiaphragmatic aorta for temporary control of massive intraperitoneal hemorrhage as well as access to the groin for possible venous graft harvesting. In most instances where abdominal aortic control is deemed necessary, this is accomplished through the intra-abdominal approach. Preoperative antibiotics to cover aerobic and anaerobic organisms should be administered preferably prior to the incision[3] to prevent septic complications. In the absence of fecal contamination, the antibiotics should not be continued after the operation. However, when there is contamination, antibiotics should be continued until the temperature returns to normal without a leukocytosis. An increase in temperature and leukocytosis during antibiotic treatment or after cessation of antibiotics suggests residual sepsis often in the form of an undrained abscess warranting intervention — operative or minimally invasive — or a change in antibiotics (see chapter on Intra-abdominal Sepsis).

Although with the availability of the multitude of reliable diagnostic modalities a specific diagnosis is usually made prior to laparotomy, in most instances a specific preoperative diagnosis is not required. In general, signs suggestive of peritonitis, hemorrhage, perforation, or penetration warrant consideration for exploration of the abdomen. These signs may be elicited during assessment in the ICU.

Peritonitis is suggested by pain, localized, generalized, or rebound tenderness, guarding with or without rigidity.

Hemorrhage is detected by many modalities and depends also on the magnitude of blood loss. Intraperitoneal hemorrhage occasionally but not always results in clinical signs of peritoneal irritation. Other signs include subtle drop in Hemoglobin (Hb), tachycardia, and a decrease in urine output and in major hemorrhage, signs of shock. In blunt trauma without evidence of hollow viscus injury and with bleeding that is likely to stop spontaneously, selective nonoperative management is an acceptable option.[4] Such patients must be monitored in an ICU setting with readily available surgeons to take the patient to the OR promptly when indicated by worsening of hemorrhage as manifested by a continued fall in Hb, worsening vital signs, and urine output. The threshold for laparotomy in penetrating injury with hemorrhage is much lower.

Penetration of the abdomen in stab wounds is diagnosed by wound exploration under local anesthesia. The wound is visually explored with good lighting and appropriate retractors. If it is determined that the peritoneum has been violated, in most instances laparotomy is conducted. Others have combined wound exploration with peritoneal lavage when the wound exploration suggests peritoneal penetration and if the peritoneal lavage is also positive, proceeding to laparotomy.[5–7] All bullet wounds to the abdomen are generally treated by laparotomy.[8] However, a selective approach which involves scanning of the abdomen and using abdominal wall radio-opaque markers has been used to identify tangential wounds which do not penetrate the peritoneum, thus, sparing laparotomy.[9–10] All these patients should still be observed very carefully in the ICU for delayed signs of hollow viscus perforation which can be missed and also can occur from blast injury without evidence of peritoneal violation on imaging. The safest approach, however, is to subject all gunshot wounds to laparotomy.

In general, physical examination and history would determine the need for the trauma laparotomy. However, when the history and physical signs are equivocal, unreliable, or impossible to elicit because of neurologic deficits from drugs, spinal cord, or brain injury — ultrasound, peritoneal lavage, Computed Tomography (CT) scan, and laparoscopy are very useful adjuncts in deciding on the need for laparotomy.[9–12]

Role of Peritoneal Lavage, CT, Ultrasound, and Laporoscopy in Assessing Abdominal Trauma

Non-therapeutic laparotomy for penetrating abdominal trauma has been reported to be as high as nearly 60%.[11] If the decision is made from wound examination the incidence of non-therapeutic laparotomy is 57%, from CT is 24%, from diagnostic peritoneal lavage is 31%, focused abdominal sonogram for trauma (FAST) is 40%, and systematic clinical assessment with blood cell count is 33%. So, clinical assessment with blood cell count which could be easily accomplished by the intensivist without need for extra imaging would result in a significant decrease in non-therapeutic laparotomy when compared to wound examination (from 57% to 33%). The most specific modality among ultrasound, CT and peritoneal lavage is CT scan. The disadvantage of CT is that it requires movement of the patient to the CT scan suite and is therefore not appropriate for hemodynamically compromised patients. The advantages of ultrasound are its portability, ease of application, repeatability, rapidity, and sensitivity but it is operator dependent and requires a well-trained experienced operator of the equipment, who does not need to be a radiologist.[13] Although peritoneal lavage is very sensitive it is not very specific-this plus its relative invasiveness limits its application and in most institutions where ultrasound is immediately available, peritoneal lavage is seldom used.

Selecting the Diagnostic Modality in Blunt Abdominal Trauma

Intra-abdominal hemorrhage is the prime indication for laparotomy in blunt abdominal trauma. A diagnostic test such as ultrasound is most attractive because of its relative accuracy, rapidity, non-invasiveness, and minimal cost. However, there is still a role for other modalities such as CT and peritoneal lavage. With a negative ultrasound the patient may be observed by clinical examination. Change in the patient's hemodynamic status warrants a repeat ultrasound or CT. In a stable patient with equivocal ultrasound findings CT should be done. An unstable patient with equivocal ultrasound should be considered for a peritoneal lavage or taken directly to the OR. When the ultrasound in a hemodynamically normal patient is positive for hemoperitoneum, CT scan should be conducted to assist in the decision for non-operative management of solid organ injury. The unstable patent with hemoperitoneum on ultrasound requires laparotomy.

There are variable results with using laparoscopy[14] in abdominal trauma and there are no uniform recommendations for its use. Its most practical application is in the patient with equivocal findings who may be taken to the OR and the laparoscopy conducted prior to any planned open laparotomy with a view to abandoning the laparotomy if the laparoscopic findings do not indicate the need for a therapeutic laparotomy. When the decision for nonoperative management is made based on the above guidelines, these patients should ideally be monitored in an ICU setting unless there is another unit where the patient could be closely observed.

General Conduct of the Trauma Laparotomy

After cardiorespiratory resuscitation, usually in the emergency room, including insertion of two large bore IV's, availability of blood and blood products, administration of fluids through a fluid warming device, insertion of a urinary and gastric catheter, insertion of an arterial line where appropriate, the patient is taken to the OR where a general anesthetic is administered, IV antibiotics administered as described, and the abdomen, chest, and groin are prepped and draped as indicated earlier. The anesthetist is notified of the intent to begin and to ensure that the fluids, including blood and blood products as well as warming and monitoring devices are ready. A generous midline incision from xiphisternum to pubis is then made.

Based on the principles enunciated in the Advanced Trauma Operative Management (ATOM) Course,[15] the goals of the trauma laparotomy are to:

(1) Control hemorrhage
(2) Control contamination
(3) Definitive repair of injuries/damage control as required.

(1) Control of hemorrhage: The major cause of mortality in the multiple injured patient is hemorrhage with the major source being from abdominal trauma. The main initial focus on opening the abdomen is therefore to identify and stop bleeding while administering IV fluids. The site of the intra-abdominal bleeding is frequently not immediately obvious and a systematic approach is essential. Two large suctions and sponges are used to remove blood while packing with large radio-opaque sponges, starting with packing above and below the solid organs in the upper abdomen (spleen and liver), then displacing the intestines from the lateral gutters towards the midline and packing laterally, followed by moving the bowel upward from the pelvis and tightly packing the pelvis. These maneuvers allow temporary control of the bleeding and provides the opportunity to "catch up" with fluid/blood administration. The packing is then removed in sequence and bleeding controlled by direct means as required. If on removal of packing from the liver and spleen bleeding recurs and cannot be controlled definitively it may be necessary to replace the packing and decide later whether a "damage control" approach (see in the following paragraphs) is required. Other techniques of hemorrhage control includes application of topical hemostatic agents, electro coagulation, vascular clips and agents such as the Argon beam, proximal and distal control of vessels with ligation or repair.

(2) Control of contamination: Gross spilled intestinal contents, devitalized necrotic tissue are suctioned out and perforations are identified and marked with temporary clamps, large sutures or staples initially and a decision made later as to whether formal repair, resection, anastomosis are appropriate depending on the patients overall clinical status.

(3) Definitive repair/damage control: Once hemorrhage and contamination are controlled, a reassessment of the patient's clinical status is made, including core temperature, coagulation, hemodynamic, and acid–base status. If these parameters are acceptable then definitive surgical repair of injuries is conducted.

The presence of hypothermia, acidosis, hypocoagulability and/or continued hemodynamic/respiratory compromise are indications for a switch in the management theme from definitive repair to "Damage Control" mode. This requires transferring the patient to the ICU with packing in place, temporary skin closure or "open abdomen" using such techniques as temporary mesh to cover the edematous bowel while leaving the skin wound open to prevent "Abdominal Compartment Syndrome" (see in the succeeding paragraphs). In the ICU, resuscitation and monitoring are continued to return metabolic abnormalities, temperature, hemodynamics, coagulation to normal before returning to the OR in 48–72 hours for continued attempts at definitive treatment. If the patients hemodynamic status does not improve and there is concern about continued bleeding, prompt return to the OR is required to reassess for the source and control of the bleeding sites. In patients who are able to maintain reasonable hemodynamics, another option is angiography to identify bleeding sources and allow selective embolization to stop hemorrhage where appropriate.

Abdominal compartment syndrome

Abdominal compartment syndrome is characterized by organ dysfunction occurring secondary to intra-abdominal hypertension. In trauma this increased intra-abdominal pressure results from a multitude of factors including intra-abdominal bleeding from injuries themselves, bowel edema from the trauma or manipulation of the intestines as occurs during laparotomy and handling of the bowel, massive fluid administration as occurs during fluid resuscitation in shock or third spacing of fluid during prolonged surgery.

Pathophysiology — the basic process begins with increasing intra-abdominal pressure from the above causes. The increased pressure leads to: increased airway pressure, pulmonary barotrauma leading to hypoxemia and hypocapnea; collapse of hollow viscus such as small bowel, the portocaval system leading to ischemia and further edema with worsening of the intra-abdominal hypetension; vascular thrombosois; decreased renal and splanchnic perfusion; bowel infarction; metabolic acidosis from anaerobic metabolism; release of vasoactive agents such as serotonin and histamine leading to increased capillary permeability and further edema as well as translocation of bacterial products and multiple organ dysfunction with death if the intra-abdominal tension is not relieved promptly.

The diagnosis should be anticipated in the presence of any of the aforestated predisposing situations in the trauma patient. If during attempts at abdominal closure there is increased airway pressure, difficulty ventilating the patient, hypotension or decreased urine output, primary closure of the abdominal wall should be abandoned and temporary closure effected by such techniques as application of a mesh, a plastic bag, or other devices. The abdominal closure is then attempted after the inciting agent or abnormality has been reversed. Many techniques are then utilized for secondary closure of the abdomen. Intra-abdominal pressure may increase insidiously in the ICU and many centers routinely monitor intra-abdominal pressure continuously through the insertion of a Foley catheter into the bladder connected to a pressure transducing device. At the first sign of significant increase in intra-abdominal pressure above 25 mmHg the abdomen should be decompressed through an abdominal incision and temporary packing or mesh applied while monitoring for return of normal intra-abdominal pressure when closure is then attempted by the many techniques available.

Nonoperative Management of Abdominal Trauma

Following the demonstrated successful nonoperative management of pediatric trauma patients with solid intra-abdominal injury,[16] more and more adult trauma centers have resorted to this technique of management in adult abdominal trauma patients whose hemodynamic status normalizes after temporary instability and with minimal fluid and blood administration. The key to success of this technique is proper patient selection based on expectation that bleeding will stop and hemodynamics will return to normal without surgical intervention. Factors such as the severity of the injury, degree of hemodynamic compromise, "vascular blush" on CT angiography, blood transfusion requirements have been recommended as guidelines for institution of nonoperative management but the most important determinant is the hemodynamic status of the patient. Return to and maintenance of normal hemodynamics with minimal blood replacement normal temperature, normal acid–base status, urine output, and coagulation status are indices that should be monitored very closely in the ICU setting to guide the decision to continue nonoperative management which may include the use of angiographic control of bleeding. Failure of nonoperative management is heralded by evidence of continued bleeding which requires return to surgical management techniques.

Highlights in Management of Specific Intra-Abdominal Injuries

Stomach injuries: These injuries occur with blunt impact or penetrating wounds to the epigastric area or in the context of multiple injuries from other mechanisms. Epigastric and shoulder tip pain with free intraperitoneal air (if there is perforation), tenderness, and bloody aspirate from the gastric tube may be present. Frequently the diagnosis is made at laparotomy in a multiple trauma patient. There is usually minimal spillage or hemorrhage. Surgical treatment consists of debridement of devitalized tissue and primary suture. The entire stomach should be assessed including the posterior wall to avoid missing lacerations.

Duodenal injuries: These are frequently associated with other injuries. Because of its partial retroperitoneal location, signs of perforation may be minimal and late. A high index of suspicion is required to avoid missing these injuries which may present with retroperitoneal air on a plain abdominal film. At laparotomy, complete mobilization of the entire duodenum with a Kocher maneuver, inspecting for bile staining. Intramural hematomas may present as gastric outlet obstruction and are seen on contrast studies of the stomach and duodenum. These hematomas resolve spontaneously with gastric suction. If the lesion is found at laparotomy evacuation of the hematoma is easily accomplished through a duodenal wall incision. With other injuries, after debridement of devitalized tissue the defect can be closed primarily if there is no tension. Defects may also be closed by serosal patch from adjacent small bowel, Roux-en-Y anastomosis between the duodenal ends and small bowel, pyloric exclusion with a gastrojejunostomy or duodenal diverticulization.[17–20]

Pancreatic injuries: These usually occur after blunt trauma with impact of the pancreas against the vertebral column. Because of its retroperitoneal location diagnosis is frequently late because of lack of peritoneal signs and the injury is frequently found at laparotomy. An early increase in serum amylase may suggest the diagnosis and this is confirmed by contrast CT of the abdomen. Simple contusions are treated by drainage after complete assessment of the entire pancreas. It is important to determine if there is ductal injury which is usually diagnosed by careful detailed assessment during laparotomy beginning with unroofing of pancreatic hematomas with full mobilization of the pancreas and duodenum. Distal ductal jury is best treated by distal pancreatectomy usually using a staple device which allows closure of the ductal end. In most instances this is combined with a splenectomy. When the head of the pancreas is involved, Roux-en-Y anastomosis of the pancreatic segment to small bowel is required. In severe combined pancreaticoduodenal injury, a Whipple procedure may be required but this carries a very high mortality[21–23] and less aggressive surgical procedures such as a diverticulization of the duodenum, gastro-jejunostomy and wide drainage may be safer. Placement of a jejunal feeding tube at laparotomy facilitates enteric feeding postoperatively.

Postoperative complications of pancreatic injury such as pancreatic abscess and pseudocyst may occur, the former presenting as a septic process with pain and a mass on CT and requires percutaneous drainage and antibiotic coverage. Pseudocyst may present with pain from the mass or gastric outlet obstruction; such symptoms warrant decompression of the pseudocyst. In asymptomatic patients the mass may resolve over several weeks, but if after six weeks there is continued enlargement of the mass, decompression by internal or external, open or percutaneous routes should be considered.[24]

Intestinal injuries: Blunt impact injury with acceleration/deceleration produces injuries at points of fixation e.g., ligament of Treitz, ileo-cecal junction, and the recto-sigmoid areas. Blowout perforations of small bowel from sudden increase in intraluminal pressure can occur at any point and is frequently seen with seatbelt injuries presenting with a seatbelt imprint and contusion on the abdominal wall. The presence of peritoneal signs necessitates laparotomy. In multiple trauma situations aggressive imaging with contrast CT is required to minimize missed small bowel injury.[25–27]

Blowout injuries of the ***small bowel*** are treated by controlling hemorrhage, debridement of devitalized tissue, and primary closure. With wide areas of devitalized tissue, resection and primary anastomosis is accomplished with excellent results.

Surgical treatment of ***colonic injuries*** depends on time from injury, degree of contamination, stability of the patient, associated injuries, and comorbidities. With minimal contamination, short duration — less than six hours, no associated injuries or shock, primary closure after debridement or resection of devitalized bowel with primary anastomosis is recommended. Otherwise, defunctioning ostomy, exteriorization with resection, and mucus fistula are options.[28,29]

Extraperitoneal ***rectal injuries*** require procto-sigmoidoscopic assessment followed by debridement with or without defunctioning colostomy and primary repair.[30,31] Intraperitoneal rectal injuries are treated essentially the same as other colonic injuries.

Any patient who has had bowel injuries treated surgically should be monitored very closely for signs of sepsis and aggressive contrast imaging used to identify undrained septic collections which can usually be treated percutaneously.

Liver injuries: Intra-abdominal hemorrhage following trauma is frequently due to blunt or penetrating liver injuries and the diagnosis may be made by CT or Ultrasound but frequently is a finding at laparotomy for other injuries. The objectives of surgical treatment is to control hemorrhage (by such techniques as packing, topical hemostatic agents, coagulation, staples, etc.), removal of devitalized tissue, and wide drainage. Frequently damage control techniques as described earlier are required to treat liver injuries. Prevention of complications requires administration of warm fluids, massive transfusion protocol where required and careful monitoring for postoperative signs of sepsis followed by percutaneous drainage of identified drainable collections.[32–38]

Spleen injuries: Many patients with splenic injuries present with other injuries and the splenic injury is masqued by signs of the other injuries. Isolated splenic injury may present with lower left rib fractures, left shoulder tip pain, and left upper quadrant abdominal pain. Occasionally, the patient may present in hemorrhagic shock from massive intraperitoneal hemorrhage when splenectomy is usually required. Patients who are able to maintain adequate hemodynamics with minimal requirements for blood transfusion are treated nonoperatively as described previously. Such patients should be monitored very closely in the ICU for signs of continued blood loss as mentioned. If the decision is made to proceed to laparotomy, frequently splenectomy is conducted because these patients have failed conservative management and the bleeding is not likely to be controlled by splenic salvage procedures.[39–41] Postoperative splenectomy patients should receive hemophilus, meningococcal, and pneumococcal vaccines prior to discharge to protect against post splnectomy sepsis syndrome.[42]

Extra-hepatic biliary tract injuries: These injuries are infrequent and are often combined injuries involving the porta hepatis, liver, and duodenum with associated high mortality. Vascular injuries take priority and a Pringle maneuver would allow better identification. If portal vein injury is identified attempts should be made to repair it by lateral venorrhaphy, resection, and anastomosis or interposition graft. Portal systemic shunting should be avoided because of the high risk for severe encephalopathy. Common hepatic artery injury should be repaired wherever possible, with ligation as an absolute last resort. Common bile duct injury which involves less than 50% of the circumference should be treated by debridement, primary closure, and stent. If more than 50% of the circumference is involved a biliary enteric anastomosis will decrease the stricture rate from 50% with primary repair to 5%.[43,44]

Gallbladder injuries are frequently associated with other injuries and the gallbladder injury is usually treated at laparotomy by cholecystectomy.

Retroperitoneal hemorrhage: Trauma patients are frequently taken to the OR before complete imaging could be completed because of the urgent need for exploration of the abdomen based on clinical findings alone. When evidence of retro peritoneal hemorrhage is identified during laparotomy certain guidelines must be followed to allow appropriate care. The approach is based on the location and nature of the hemorrhage. This requires an understanding of the anatomic division of the retroperitoneum into three zones and the rationale for this division. These zones are: Central upper (Zone1), Lateral (Zone 2), and Pelvic (Zone 3).

In Zone 1, injury may involve the pancreas and major retroperitoneal vascular structures. Hematomas in this area need to be explored to identify injuries involving these structures and to treat them appropriately.

Zone 2 hematomas that are not pulsatile or expanding should not be explored because of the risk of increasing bleeding by decompressing the hematoma leading to unnecessary procedures such as nephrectomy to control the hemorrhage which if left undisturbed will not pose a threat to the patient. Further investigation to identify the nature of the injury can then be conducted during the postoperative period. Zone 2 hematomas that are pulsatile or expanding require exploration in the OR to identify the cause of the expanding or pulsatile lesion and treat accordingly.

Zone 3 hematomas are frequently associated with a pelvic fracture and exploration is not recommended because this will remove the tamponading effect of the intact retroperitoneum on the pelvic hemorrhage which will stop spontaneously because its source is usually venous. Restriction of pelvic volume by external fixators or binders combined with fluid resuscitation will result in correction of the hemodynamic abnormality unless the bleeding is from an arterial source when angiography with embolization is conducted to control the bleeding.

Genito-urinary injuries: Urinary tract injury may result from both blunt and penetrating mechanisms and the commonest present in finding is hematuria, although the absence of hematuria does not rule out injury to the genitourinary tract. IV pyelography is no longer standard for investigating post-traumatic hematuria because of its low yield for significant injury, allergic reactions to contrast, and the lack of impact on management decisions. Based on these considerations and the fact that microhematuria without shock has not been shown to be associated with lesions requiring surgery whereas gross hematuria or microhematuria with shock requires surgery in up to 10% of cases, guidelines for imaging have been formulated. High resolution spiral CT is the diagnostic modality of choice. Imaging is recommended when: (1) there is gross hematuria or microhematuria with shock (2) there is hematuria in the presence of major abdominal injury, and (3) there is a penetrating injury in the vicinity of the urinary tract even without hematuria. The main indication for surgery is major hemorrhage in which the patient's hemodynamics cannot be maintained with blood and crystalloid. Otherwise most renal trauma patients are treated nonoperatively initially with close monitoring of hemodynamic status in an ICU setting — when there is hemodynamic deterioration in spite of blood and crystalloid infusion surgical intervention is pursued. Failure to visualize both kidneys on contrast CT is followed by angiography to identify a possible renal artery thrombosis or intimal flap that is amenable to surgical correction. The main goals of surgical exploration are to control hemorrhage and preserve kidney function which is best achieved by exploring the kidneys only in the presence of an expanding or pulsatile hematoma. The best bleeding control is by isolating the renal pedicle and occluding it with a clamp before the repair and if after repair attempts and release of the occluding clamps there is still continued hemorrhage, nephrectomy is conducted when there is an opposite functioning kidney.[45, 46] Suspicion of bladder injury is investigated by cystography using three views one of which is conducted after emptying the bladder. This is superior to CT cystography. Extraperitoneal laceration of the bladder may be treated by catheter drainage alone whereas intraperitoneal rupture requires open surgical repair. Postoperative care requires maintenance of renal perfusion by adequate volume resuscitation and monitoring of hemodynamics, clearing of hematuria and maintaining urine output in the ICU. Occult urinary tract injury may present with septic complications from an infected urinoma which is identified by CT or Ultrasound followed by drainage of the urinoma.[47,48]

Summary

Abdominal injury is a frequent cause of preventable trauma related death. An understanding of the mechanism of injury prompting suspicion for specific injuries will decrease the risk of missing injuries. Recognizing the early signs of penetration, hemorrhage, and perforation and choosing the imaging modality for confirming the presence of significant injury will lead to earlier diagnosis, prevention of complications, and improved outcome. Knowledge of the clinical features of abdominal injury in general and specific abdominal organ injuries will enhance the intensivist's ability to make sound therapeutic decisions when managing these patients in the ICU.

Patient monitoring in the ICU is very useful in nonoperative management of abdominal trauma, early detection of complications and the need for return to the OR. Patients undergoing damage control laparotomy benefit significantly from ICU monitoring to determine return of normalcy to vital signs, coagulopathy, acidosis, hypothermia, and the timing of return to the OR for definitive surgery.

References

1. Sung CK, Kim KH. Missed injuries in abdominal trauma. *J Trauma* 1996; 41: 28–33.
2. Brooks A, Holroyd B, Riley B. Missed injury in major trauma patients. *Injury* 2004; 35: 407–412.
3. Goldberg SR, Anand RJ, Como JJ. Prophylactic antibiotic use in penetrating abdominal trauma: An Eastern Association for the Surgery of Trauma practice management guideline. *J Trauma Acute Care Surg* 2012; 73: S321–S324.
4. Al-Mulhim AS, Mohammad HA. Non-operative management of blunt hepatic injury in multiply injured adult patients. *Surgeon* 2003; 1: 81–86.
5. Fabian TC, Croce MA. Abdominal trauma, including indications for laparotomy, n Mattox LK, Feliciano DV and Moore EE (eds). Trauma. East Norwalk, Appleton & Lange, 2000, 583–602.
6. Huizinga WK, Baker LW, Mtshali ZW. Selective management of abdominal and thoracic stab wounds with established peritoneal penetration: The eviscerated omentum. *Am J Surg* 1987; 153: 564–568.
7. Robin AP, Andrews JR, Lange DA. Selective management of anterior abdominal stab wounds. *J Trauma* 1989; 29: 1684–1689.
8. Moore EE, Moore JB, van Duzer-Moore S. Mandatory laparotomy for gunshot wounds penetrating the abdomen. *Am J Surg* 1980; 140: 847–852.
9. Demetriades D, Velhmahos GC, Comwell EE III. Selective non-operative management of gunshot wounds of the anterior abdomen. *Arch Surg* 1997; 132: 178–184.
10. Velmahos CG, Demetriades D, Toutouzas KG *et al.* Selective non-operative management in 1,856 patients with abdominal gunshot wounds. Should routine laparotomy still be standard of care? *Ann Surg* 2001; 234: 395–401.
11. Liu M, Lee C, Veng F. Prospective comparison of diagnostic peritoneal lavage, computed tomographic scanning and ultrasonography for the diagnosis of blunt abdominal trauma. *J Trauma* 1993; 35: 267–277.
12. McAlvarak MJ, Shaftan GW. Selective conservatism in penetrating abdominal wounds: A continuing re-appraisal. *J Trauma* 1978; 18: 206–211.

13. Rozycki GS, Ochsner MG, Schmidt JA *et al.* A prospective study of surgeon performed ultrasound as the primary adjuvant modality for injured patient assessment. *J Trauma* 1995; 39: 492–499.
14. Neugebauer E, Suaerland S. Guidelines for emergency laparoscopy. *World J Emerg Surg* 2006; 1: 31–36.
15. Lenworth M Jacobs, Stephen S Luk, in Advanced Trauma Operative Management, 2nd ed. Woodbury, Ciné-Med Publishing, Inc., 2010.
16. Paddock HN, Tepas JJ, Ramenofsky ML. Management of blunt pediatric hepatic and splenic injury: Similar process, different outcome. *Am Surg* 2004; 70: 1068–1072.
17. Fullen WD, Selle JG, Whitely DH *et al.* Intramural duodenal hematoma. *Ann Surg* 197; 179: 549–552.
18. Cogbill TH, Moore EE, Feliciano DV *et al.* Conservative management of duodenal trauma: A multicenter perspective. *J Trauma* 1990; 30: 1469–1473.
19. Shorr RM, Greaney GC, Donovan AJ. Injuries of the duodenum. *Am J Surg* 1987; 154: 193–199.
20. Degiannis E, Krawcrykowski D, Velmahos GC *et al.* Pyloric exclusion in severe penetrating injuries of the duodenum. *World J Surg* 1993; 17: 751–755.
21. Cogbill TH, Moore EE, Kashuk JL. Changing trends in the management of pancreatic trauma. *Ann Surg* 1978; 187: 555–560.
22. Feliciano DV, Martin JD, Cruse PA *et al.* Management of combined pancreaticoduodenal injuries. *Ann Surg* 1987; 205: 670–673.
23. Mckone TK, Bursch LR, Schoelten DJ. Pancreaticoduodenectomy for trauma: A lifesaving procedure. *Am Surg* 1998; 54: 361–369.
24. Bradley EL III, Clements JL Jr, Gonzales AC. The natural history of pancreatic pseudocysts: A unified concept of management. *Am J Surg* 1979; 137: 135–141.
25. Wisner DH, Chun V, Blaisdell FW. Blunt intestinal injury: Key to diagnosis and management. *Arch Surg* 1990; 125: 1319–1326.
26. Scherk J, Shatney C,Sensaki K *et al.* The accuracy of computer tomography in the diagnosis of blunt small bowel perforation. *Am J Surg* 1994; 168: 670–675.
27. Hackam D, Ali J, Jastaniah S. Effects of other intra-abdominal injuries on the diagnosis, management and outcome of small bowel trauma. *J Trauma* 2000; 49: 606–610.
28. Stone HH, Fabian TC. Management of perforating colon trauma: Randomization between primary closure and exteriorization. *Ann Surg* 1979; 190: 430–441.
29. Nelson R, Singer M. Primary repair for penetrating colon injuries. *Cochrane Database of Systematic Reviews* 2003, Issue 3, Art No CD002247. DOI: ID. 1002/14651858.
30. Ivatury RR, Licata J, Gunduz Y *et al.* Management options in penetrating rectal injuries. *Ann Surg* 1991; 57: 57–64.
32. Ali J. Abdominal trauma with specific reference to hepatic trauma. *Can J Surg* 1978; 21: 512–517.

33. Feliciano DV, Mattox KL, Jordan GL Jr. Intra-abdominal packing for control of hepatic hemorrhage: A reappraisal. *J Trauma* 1981; 21: 285–291.
34. Pachter HL, Knudson MM, Esrig B *et al.* Status of non-operative management of blunt hepatic injuries in 1995: A multicenter experience with 404 patients. *J Trauma* 1996; 40: 31–40.
35. Malhotra AK, Fabian TC, Croce MA *et al.* Blunt hepatic injury: A paradigm shift from operative to non-operative management in the 1990's. *Ann Surg* 2000; 231: 804–810.
36. Shapiro MB, Jenkins DH, Schwab CW *et al.* Damage control: Collective review. *J Trauma* 2000; 49: 969–982.
37. Moore EE, Thomas G. Orr Memorial lecture: Staged laparotomy for the hypothermia acidosis and coagulopathy syndrome. *Am J Surg* 1996; 172: 405–412.
38. Bryan A, Cotton MD, Brigham K *et al.* Predefined massive transfusion protocols are associated with a reduction in organ failure and postinjury complications. *J Trauma* 2009; 66: 41–49.
39. Smith JS, Cooney RN, Mucha P. Non-operative management of the ruptured spleen: A revalidation of criteria. *Surgery* 1996; 120: 745–751.
40. Sclafani SJA, Shaftan GW, Scalea TM *et al.* Non-operative salvage of computed tomography-diagnosed splenic injuries: Utilization of angiography for triage and embolization for hemostasis. *J Trauma* 1995; 39: 818–826.
41. Powell M, Courcoulas A, Gardner M *et al.* Management of blunt splenic trauma: Significant difference between adults and children. *Surgery* 1997; 122: 654–659.
42. Francke EL, Neu HC. Post splenectomy infection. *Surg Clin North Am* 1981; 61: 135–141.
43. Sheldon GF, Lim RC, Yee ES *et al.* Management of injury to the porta hepatis. *Ann Surg* 1985; 202: 539–546.
44. Ivatury RR, Rohman M, Nallathambi M. The morbidity of injuries of the extrahepatic biliary system. *J Trauma* 1985; 225: 967–974.
45. Thomason RB, Julian JS, Mortellar HC *et al.* Microscopic hematuria after blunt trauma — Is pyelography necessary? *Am Surg* 1989; 55: 145–149.
46. Mee SL, McAninch JW, Robinson AL *et al.* Radiographic assessment of renal trauma: A 10 year prospective study of patient selection. *J Urol* 1989; 141: 1095–1101.
47. Haas CA, Brown SL, Spirnak JP. Limitation of routine spiral computerized tomography in the evaluation of bladder trauma. *J Urol* 1999; 162: 51–58.
48. Carroll PR, Mc Aninch JW. Major bladder trauma: Mechanism of injury and a unified method of diagnosis and repair. *J Urol* 1984; 132: 254–262.

Chapter 18

Head Injury

Jameel Ali, Lyne Noël de Tilly and R. Loch Macdonald

Chapter Overview

Head injuries account for a large percentage of worldwide trauma related mortality and morbidity. In North America over 90% of pre-hospital trauma deaths have an associated head injury and of those head injuries which are admitted to hospital, roughly 75% sustain mild injuries, 15% moderate, and 10% severe head trauma.[1,2] The outcome in patients with mild injuries is generally good but mortality and morbidity increase progressively in the moderate and severe categories.[1] Head injury is among the leading causes of death worldwide and is the leading cause of death among adults under 45-years in the United States. Thus, an important impact on survival could be achieved by aggressive management of moderate and severe head injuries. Ideally, such care is frequently provided in the intensive care environment. Proper management of these injuries requires a clear understanding of the unique anatomical and physiologic features of the brain as they are affected by trauma. Generally, medical/surgical intervention is not effective in reversing the primary tissue damage resulting from the direct brain trauma itself. The main focus of management is therefore prevention of secondary brain injury.

In this chapter, we will discuss the unique features of intracranial anatomy and physiology, how they affect the presentation of head injuries and how they may be manipulated to preserve brain function in the head injured patient. Classifications and investigation of head injuries, their clinical presentation as well as principles of medical and surgical management will also be discussed.

Anatomic Considerations

The brain is confined within a fixed space by a rigid non-yielding bony skull. Addition of mass to the intracranial contents as would occur from hemorrhage in trauma will eventually lead to increased intracranial pressure (ICP), which will reduce cerebral blood flow and affect brain function. The unyielding rigid surface of the skull also predisposes to direct (coup) as well as contra coup tissue injury on movement of intracranial contents resulting from force applied to the skull and shearing of brain tissue.

To understand intracranial changes following trauma, the intracranial contents may be considered to consist of brain, cerebrospinal fluid (CSF) and blood. The meninges which cover the brain consist of three layers; the duramater, arachnoid mater and pia mater

The dura mater is a two-layered tough fibrous layer of tissue closely applied to the inner surface of the skull. The potential space between the skull and dura (epidural or extradural space) houses the meningeal arteries and veins. Skull fractures can lacerate these vessels leading to rapidly fatal epidural hematomas. This commonly occurs, secondary to a temporal bone skull fracture overlying the middle meningeal artery. At specific sites the dura splits into two leaves to accommodate the venous sinuses. Massive hemorrhage can occur from injury involving these sinuses.

The arachnoid mater is a thin layer of translucent tissue deep to the dura. It is only loosely adherent to the dura by dural border cells which results in a potential space (the subdural space) between the dura and arachnoid within which hemorrhage from bridging veins can occur (acute or chronic subdural hematoma). Cerebral atrophy in elderly patients causes the brain to recede from the skull which increases the potential for a subdural space to develop and be filled with blood from veins bridging from the brain to the dura after minor trauma. Bridging veins are believed to tear at the point where they traverse the potential subdural space because their walls are thinnest in this segment. The arachnoid membrane encases the brain but does not by and large enter the sulci. The arachnoid is a water tight barrier between it and the third meningeal layer, the pia mater.

The pia mater is tightly attached to the entire brain and spinal cord surface. The space between these two (subarachnoid space) contains CSF which is formed in party by the choroid plexus in the cerebral ventricles at the rate of approximately 20 ml per hour. The CSF circulates over the entire brain and spinal cord surface before entering the systemic circulation through the arachnoid granulations. Bleeding into the subarachnoid space (subarachnoid hemorrhage) is frequently seen with brain contusions or major vessel injuries. When such bleeding obstructs the arachnoid granulations CSF flow can be impeded, giving rise to CSF accumulation in the ventricular system or traumatic hydrocephalus. This adds mass to the cranial cavity and can lead to increased ICP.

The tentorium cerebelli separates the brain into two main compartments — one above the tentorium or supratentorial compartment and the other below or the infratentorial compartment. The midbrain passes through an aperture in the tentorium, the incisura or hiatus which allows continuation of the supraratentorial with the infratentorial compartment. The oculomotor nerve with parasympathetic fibers on its surface courses along the edge of the tentorium.

If a supratentorial hematoma or hydrocephalus displaces the brain medially and inferiorly through the tentorialincisura, transtentorial herniation develops. There is a classic sequence of events starting with decreased level of consciousness due to bi-hemispheric cortical dysfunction from the brain shift. It is important to realize that ICP may not be increased early on. The parasympathetic fibers of the oculomotor nerve, which are responsible for pupillary constriction, are compressed leading to ipsilateral pupillary dilation. The motor fibers of the cortico spinal tract in the adjacent cerebral peduncle of the midbrain are also compressed giving rise to contralateral motor paralysis. Paralysis is contralateral because these fibers decussate lower in the medulla. Next there is occlusion of the cerebral aqueduct which obstructs CSF outflow and further aggravates the now increased intracranial pressure and compression of the posterior cerebral artery resulting in infarction of this vascular territory. Progressive rostral-caudal deterioration ensues with dilation of the other pupil, midbrain Duret hemorrhages, loss of corneal reflexes, lower brainstem reflexes and eventually brain death. The critical early signs from an intracranial mass lesion such as traumatic hemorrhage are therefore ipsilateral pupillary dilation and contralateral motor paralysis. In about 10% of cases, the hemiparesis may be on the same side due to the Kernohan notch syndrome.[3]

Another herniation syndrome from lateral displacement of the brain by a unilateral hematoma is subfalcine herniation where the cingulate gyrus and associated anterior cerebral arteries are pushed across under the falx cerebri.

Physiologic Considerations

The interplay of cerebral blood flow and metabolism, ICP, systemic hemodynamics, and arterial blood–gas changes is crucial in determining the patient's response to head trauma and understanding the basic concepts involved provides a solid guide to therapeutic interventions. The brain consumes 25% of oxygen used by the body and is highly dependent on a continuous supply of oxygen and glucose-rich blood. Cerebral perfusion pressure (CPP) (mean blood pressure minus ICP) ensures this. As in any fixed rigid container such as the skull, the internal pressure is determined by the volume of its contents. The relevant contents under consideration are the brain, blood, and CSF; the pressure is the Intracranial Pressure (ICP). Normal ICP is approximately 10 mmHg and usually lower. While there is some controversy as to whether increased ICP after head injury is a cause of poor outcome or a consequence of severe irreversible injury, sustained ICP above 20 mmHg is associated with poor outcome and would be expected to reduce CPP and cause brain injury.

The pathophysiology of increased ICP and reduced CPP after Traumatic Brain Injury (TBI) includes brain swelling and cerebral edema due to the injury that reduces cerebral blood flow, causes ischemia and then further brain swelling, and edema. There are two approaches for treatment based on this. The most common is ICP- or CPP-based. The ICP based approach is to prevent and reduce increased intracranial pressure by elevating the head of the bed (with spine precaution), sedation, pharmacologic paralysis, treatment of hypertension, CSF drainage, osmotic diuretics, and occasionally barbiturates.[4] A variation of this focuses on maintaining adequate CPP and uses flat position in bed, no sedation, hyperventilation or barbiturates, and elevating the blood pressure to maintain CPP if necessary. At the opposite end of the spectrum is the Lund concept, where the goal is to reduce cerebral edema by flat head position, sedation, aggressive blood pressure reduction, no pharmacologic paralysis and no hyperventilation, osmotic diuretics, or barbiturates.[4]

Autoregulation of cerebral blood flow: The cerebral vasculature dilates or constricts in response to variations in mean systemic arterial blood pressure, maintaining stable cerebral blood flow over a range of mean systemic arterial blood pressures from about 50–150 mmHg. Cerebral blood flow cannot easily be measured in the clinical setting except intermittently by techniques such as computed tomographic or magnetic resonance perfusion, xenon Computed Tomography (CT) or positron emission tomography or focally, and continuously by implanted thermodilution probes. Furthermore, the adequacy of cerebral blood flow depends on metabolic demand of the brain. Thus, in practice, CPP tends to be used as a surrogate for cerebral blood flow recognizing that the two are not linearly related. Autoregulation may be disrupted in severe brain injury.[5] Other indirect methods of monitoring brain perfusion are discussed in the following paragraphs.

Another determinant of cerebral blood flow is the arterial blood gases; particularly the arterial Partial Pressure of Carbon dioxide (PCO_2). Hypocarbia stimulates vasoconstriction and can decrease cerebral blood flow. The constriction reduces the volume of blood in the cranium and thus can decrease ICP. However, this hypocarbia has the potential to induce ischemia that if prolonged, could result in cerebral infarction and potentially worsen outcome. Thus, when used to decrease ICP, hyperventilation should be applied for very brief periods such as when a patient has transtentorial herniation and has not been taken to surgery yet to evacuate a mass lesion.

The Monro–Kellie doctrine depicts the relationship between ICP and volume (Fig. 1). Under normal conditions the ICP is low with normal intracranial volumes of blood, CSF, and brain tissue.[6] The total intracranial volume is constant. If there is an increase in the volume of one component there initially is a compensatory decrease in the other volumes resulting in a homeostatic mechanism directed at maintaining normal ICP. With addition of a mass such as an intracranial hematoma, the compensatory mechanisms include decreased blood and CSF volume. Eventually, compensatory mechanisms are exhausted and ICP rises. It follows that to decrease ICP in patients with an intracranial hematoma:

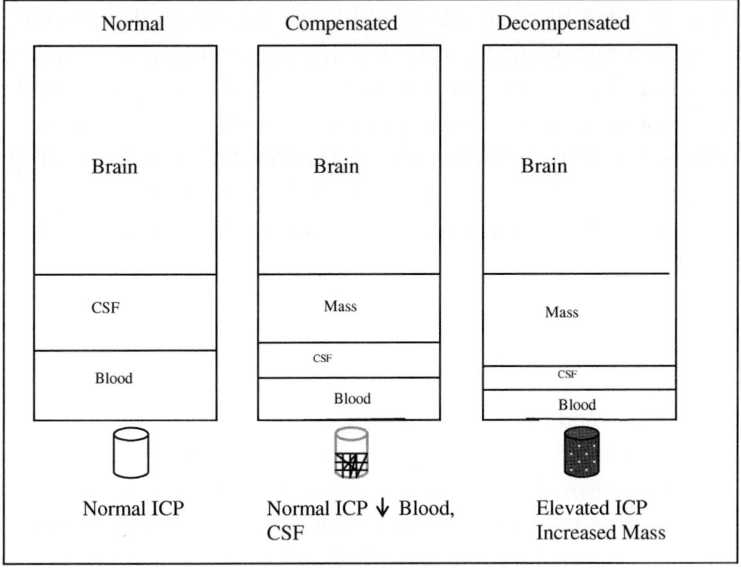

Fig. 1. Monro–Kellie Doctrine.

1. Blood volume could be decreased by raising the head of the bed, sedation/pharmacologic paralysis to reduce intracranial venous pressure and volume, as well as hypocarbia induced vasoconstriction.
2. CSF volume could be decreased by drainage from a ventricular catheter.
3. Brain mass could be diminished by agents such as mannitol or hypertonic saline.
4. The intracranial mass could be evacuated.

Each of these would decrease the overall intracranial volume to accommodate the added intracranial mass and maintain normal ICP and cerebral perfusion and function. However, when the added intracranial mass enlarges further or the effects of the interventions and compensatory mechanisms are exhausted there is a precipitous rise in ICP that leads to transtentorial herniation with increased ICP and death of the patient. The key to management is to intervene before this terminal event.

Another response to head injury is the Cushing reflex whereby an increase in ICP is associated with bradycardia. There is usually an increase in mean systemic arterial pressure which is less consistent than the bradycardia and which may be a compensatory mechanism to preserve cerebral perfusion pressure. In general, it should be recognized that this reflex is a compensatory response and attempts to lower the blood pressure should be avoided because this would lower the cerebral perfusion pressure. The best treatment for this systemic hypertension is to reduce the increased ICP. The combination of increased ICP from a head injury and systemic hypotension from inadequate resuscitation plus inadequate oxygenation is a well recognized situation associated with poor prognosis and can prove lethal for these patients. This is the basis for focusing on prevention of secondary brain injury by maintaining adequate perfusion and oxygenation.

Classification of Head Injuries

There are many methods of classifying head injuries. The first distinction is between primary and secondary injury. The primary injury can be classified based on mechanism. Primary injuries are shearing injuries (a spectrum from concussion on the mild end to diffuse axonal injury on the severe end) and each of the types of bleeding described below. Head injury also can be categorized by morphology and severity.

Classification based on mechanism

Primary injuries

As in other anatomic areas brain injuries may be classified into direct impact, acceleration–deceleration, blast and penetrating.

DIRECT IMPACT INJURY includes scalp laceration and contusion, skull fracture, epidural hematoma, and brain contusion. Scalp lesions and skull fractures are pathognomonic of something hitting the head or the head hitting something. Acceleration–deceleration injuries could arise from direct impact but the head does not have to hit anything to undergo this, for example, in a restrained occupant of a motor vehicle crash. The fundamental damaging process is rotational or angular acceleration–deceleration about the center of rotation of the head that causes shearing of axons and blood vessels. The role of contact of the intracranial contents against the irregular inner surface of the skull is likely less important. Shearing of blood vessels leads to contusions. Contusions are:

1. Coup contusions under the site of impact.
2. Contra coup, usually in the basal frontal lobes and anterior temporal lobes, since they are farthest from the brain center of rotation and experience the greatest shearing.
3. Gliding contusions in the superior parts of the hemispheres.
4. Contusions in the corpus callosum and superior cerebellar peduncle.

SHEARING MECHANISMS occur on a continuum from mild, causing transient loss of consciousness, to severe which is called diffuse axonal injury and is characterized by white matter lesions in the corpus callosum and brainstem, petechial contusions, axon retraction balls, coma, usually no increased ICP, and often poor outcome.

PENETRATING INJURIES arise from gunshots, knife or other penetrating missiles. Low velocity penetrating injuries such as from knives and such, will not cause shearing injury but will only cause injury by direct disruption of brain tissue or by hemorrhage from damaged blood vessels. Gunshots and shrapnel, however, carry kinetic energy that is dissipated in the brain. Kinetic energy is equal to ½ of the mass of the projectile multiplied by the velocity squared. Thus, velocity is more important than mass. Although cranial gunshot wounds are highly mortal overall, the dependency on velocity explains why high velocity military guns are even more lethal than civilian hand guns.

Penetrating bullet injuries cause brain damage along the tract of the bullet plus by producing cavitation and shock waves that propagate away from the bullet trajectory and through the brain and further by hemorrhage from damaged blood vessels.

BLAST INJURIES are due to pressure waves from explosions.[7] The pressure waves propagate through the head and body tissues, each of which has a different acoustic impedance. Mechanical disruption of tissues occurs at the interfaces between tissues with different impedances. In addition, the pressure waves cause sudden changes in ICP that cause cavitations in the brain damaging axons and blood vessels.

Classification Based on Morphology

1. ***The tissue plane of injury***: Scalp lacerations, contusions and avulsions — these are obvious on examination and indicate the head hit something or something hit the head.
2. ***Skull fractures***: They occur in 10% of severe head injuries and are classified as closed or open: linear, depressed, diastatic, or basal.

Closed, open and linear fractures are self-explanatory.

Depressed fractures mean the inner table of the skull is deeper inside the head than normal. Infants can have 'ping–pong' depressed fractures because their skulls are thin and soft, resulting in indentation as would occur when a ping–pong ball is pressed.

Diastatic fractures are traumatic separation of the skull along a suture line, usually in children and young adults because the sutures have not fused yet.

Basal skull fractures are most commonly through the temporal bone or the basal frontal bones. They may be difficult or almost impossible to image even on CT scan and diagnosis may rely on clinical features. Basal temporal bone fractures are characterized by retroauricular ecchymosis (Battle sign), hemotympanum, otorrhea, and facial or vestibulocochlear cranial nerve palsies. Anterior frontal fossa basal fractures may cause raccoon eyes and rhinorrhea. Basal skull fractures may traverse the carotid canal giving rise to carotid artery injuries which would require CT angiography or standard contrast angiography for diagnosis. Fractures also increase the likelihood of intracranial hematomas.

INTRACRANIAL LESIONS — ***may be diffuse, localized or both.***

Diffuse lesions — these vary from concussion in which there is a transient loss of brain function as detected by altered mental status or transient loss of consciousness, normal CT scan and no major sequelae to diffuse axon injury characterized by coma, diffuse shearing injury to the brain, and poor prognosis.

Localized lesions are named according to the location of the hematoma — epidural hematoma, subdural hematoma, subarachnoid hemorrhage, contusions, and intracerebral hemorrhage.

1. *Epidural hematoma* — On axial CT imaging these are biconvex hyper dense hematomas adjacent to the inner table of the skull, and if sizable, associated with compression and shift of the underlying brain (Fig. 2). Since the dura is more firmly adherent to the skull at the cranial sutures, they usually do not (although they can) extend across sutures. Epidural hematomas are almost always acute complications of head injury, only rarely do they increase in size days after the injury. They are uncommon and complicate less than 5% of head injuries.

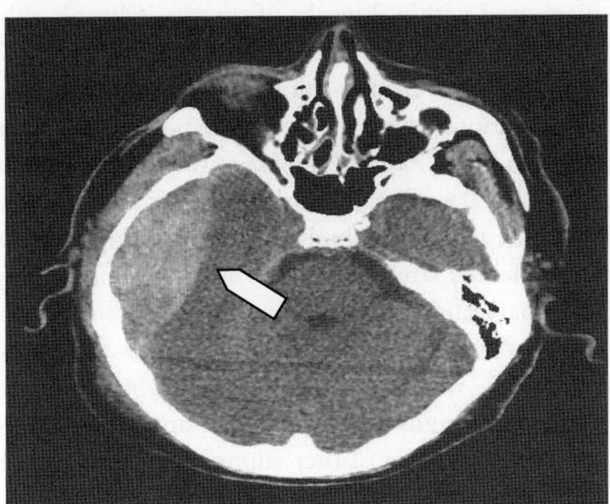

Fig. 2. Right temporal epidural hematoma (arrow head) demonstrates a medial convexity.

Epidural hematomas classically arise from a blow to the temporal skull with resultant fracture and laceration of the underlying middle meningeal artery leading to rapid arterial bleeding into the epidural space. There is usually loss of consciousness due to the acceleration/deceleration inertial injury to the head imparted by the initial blow. The patient may regain consciousness because the initial injury is mild but they then develop the syndrome of transtentorial herniation as described earlier. This transient awakening is called the lucid interval. In such cases, death can occur rapidly unless emergent evacuation of the hematoma is accomplished. The epidural hematoma may sometimes occur through laceration of the venous sinuses from an associated fracture. The key to outcome in the epidural hematoma is rapid surgical evacuation of the hematoma but when there is laceration of a major venous sinus, catastrophic uncontrollable bleeding can accompany attempts to evacuate the hematoma and surgery should be attempted in such cases only if absolutely necessary and with preparations for this risk in mind. The prognosis of patients with epidural hematomas is often good because there is usually no severe underlying inertial, shearing type of brain injury.

2. *Subdural hematomas* are more common than epidural hematomas and result from laceration by stretching and shearing forces of the bridging veins over the cerebral cortex. Acute subdural hematomas are hyperdense on CT scan and are diagnosed within 3 weeks of trauma. Chronic subdural hematomas are of variable density on CT scan and present more than 3 weeks after trauma or in patients who cannot recollect any traumatic event. Subdural hematomas are not confined by suture lines and on axial imaging have a concave inner margin (Figs. 3a and 3b). Acute subdural hematomas are common and occur in 10–20% of head injuries. They frequently occur in elderly patients with some degree of cerebral atrophy resulting in retraction of the brain from the skull thus stretching the bridging veins making them very vulnerable to minimal trauma. The resulting bleeding is not as rapid as in the epidural hematoma of arterial origin but in cases of acute subdural hematoma the prognosis is worse because of underlying brain injury. These patients also present with signs of increased ICP and require rapid evacuation of the hematoma in addition to other supportive measures which are discussed in the following paragraphs.

3. *Subarachnoid hemorrhage* — This is characterized by high density acute blood in the normally hypodense CSF-filled subarachnoid space. It may be focal on the surface of the brain over contusions, or more diffuse (Fig. 4).

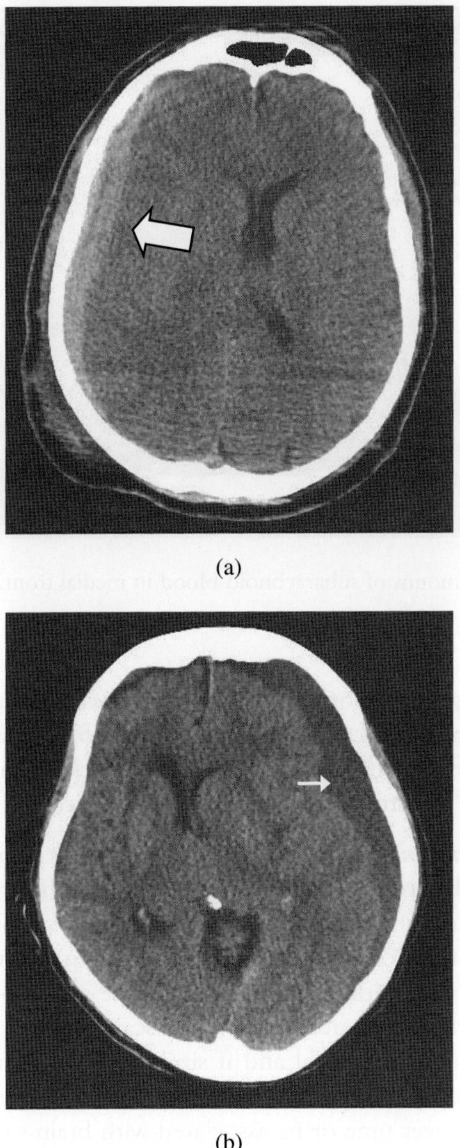

(a)

(b)

Fig. 3. (a) Right Frontal parietal subdural hematoma (arrow) shows a crescentic configuration. (b) Large chronic left hemispheric subdural hematoma (arrow) causing compression of the left lateral ventricle and shift of the midline structures toward the right.

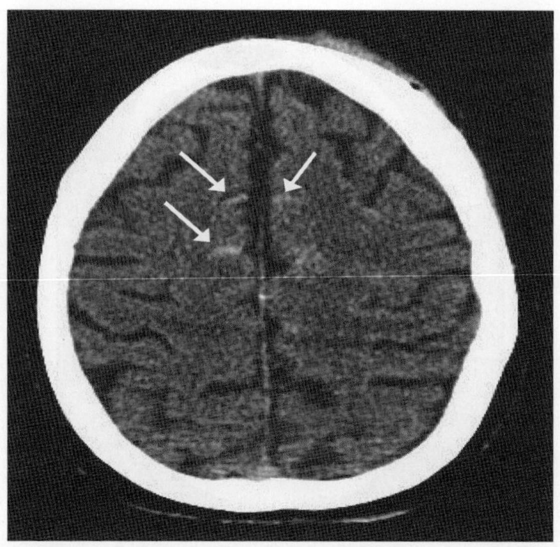

Fig. 4. Small amount of subarachnoid blood in medial frontal sulci (arrows).

It occurs on CT scan in about 10% of head injuries although small amounts of subarachnoid bleeding can be detected in the CSF by lumbar puncture in a much higher percent of patients with head injuries. Traumatic subarachnoid hemorrhage is virtually always an acute complication of head injury.

4. *Cerebral contusions and intracerebral hematomas*: Contusions are small confluent or patchy areas of acute hyperdense hemorrhage on CT under the site of injury (coup), in the frontal and temporal lobes (contra-coup) or the convexity areas of the cerebral hemispheres (gliding). Contusions can coalesce into hematomas within the brain substance and appear as radiodense opacities within the brain substance on CT scan (Figs. 5, 6). They may be single or more often multifocal and if sizable, require surgical evacuation. Like subdural and unlike epidural or subarachnoid bleeding, they can progressively enlarge over time or be associated with brain swelling and edema that develops days after the injury. They are common after severe TBI. The intracerebral hematomas often begin as contusions from blunt force to the head usually over the frontal or temporal lobes although they may occur in any part of the brain. If there are no lateralizing signs and midline shift or signs of increased ICP these patients are monitored in the intensive care unit (ICU) with frequent checking of the neurologic status, maintenance of

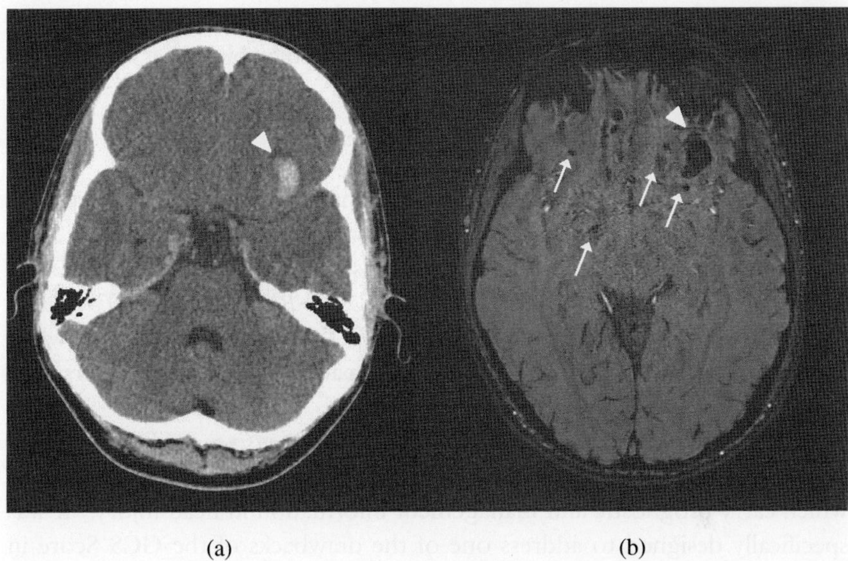

(a) (b)

Fig. 5. (a) CT shows a small inferior left frontal lobe contusion (arrow head). (b) Magnetic Resonance Imaging (MRI) shows the same hematoma (arrow head) and additional multiple small hemorrhagic foci (small arrows) in bilateral inferior frontal lobes and medial right temporal lobe.

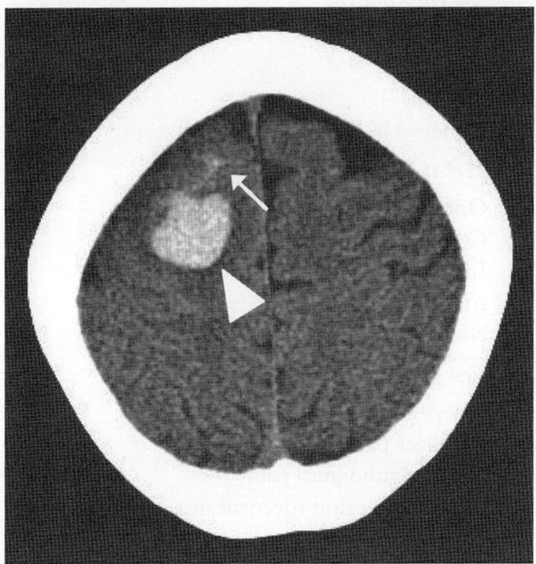

Fig. 6. Small high posterior left frontal hematoma (arrow head) and adjacent subtle subarachnoid blood (arrow).

oxygenation and perfusion and repeat CT scans if neurologic deterioration ensues. The prognosis is quite variable and unpredictable.

Classification based on severity of injuries

This is a classification based on the level of consciousness on clinical examination. A common method to assess consciousness is the Glasgow Coma Scale (GCS) score (Table 1). According to this classification, *MILD BRAIN INJURY* — GCS Score of 13–15, *MODERATE BRAIN INJURY* — GCS Score of 9–12 and *SEVERE BRAIN INJURY* — GCS Score of 3–8 when the GCS is assessed after stabilization of the patient classically six hours after the injury.

Another scoring system (*Full Outline of Unresponsiveness* (*FOUR*) *Score*) was developed to incorporate brainstem reflexes and respiratory pattern which carry prognostic and management information in head injury.[8] It was specifically designed to address one of the drawbacks of the GCS Score in

Table 1. Glascow Coma Scale (GCS).

Assessment area	Score
Eye Opening (E)	
Spontaneous	4
To speech	3
To pain	2
None	1
Verbal Response (V)	
Oriented	5
Confused conversation	4
Inappropriate words	3
Incomprehensible sounds	2
None	1
Best motor response (M)	
Obeys commands	6
Localizes pain	5
Flexion withdrawal pain	4
Abnormal flexion (decorticate)	3
Extension	2
None (flaccid)	1

intubated patients when the GCS verbal score is simply assigned a '1T' level. The Full Outline of UnResponsiveness (FOUR) score is a 17-point scale assessing more detailed eye responses, verbal responses, brain stem reflexes, and breathing pattern. Although it has been validated with reference to the GCS score in neurocritical care units, by intensive care nurses, medical intensive care units and the Emergency department, it has not yet replaced the GCS score as the international standard for classifying head injuries based on clinical severity.

Interpretation of the CT Scan in Brain Injury

There are many systems for assessing the CT scan. It is important to have one system so that it will always be applied in the same manner in order to avoid missing injuries. One system is to assess the images from the outside in:

1. Ensuring that the images are of the correct patient and of good quality without intravenous contrast.
2. Examine each of the following on each slice of the CT scan.
3. Skin and subcutaneous tissue should be assessed for hematomas, air, and edema.
4. The next layer is the bone. Although skull fractures could be identified by plain X-rays, a cranial CT scan together with the clinical presentation usually allow diagnosis of fractures. The bone window settings should be reviewed separately to diagnose skull fractures.
5. The next layer is the dura which is usually not visible on the scan but if one thinks "dura" then this prompts looking for epidural and then subdural collections. Two distinct entities: radiolucencies and radiodensities are sought. Acute blood is radiodense or high density on CT scan, although with acute ongoing bleeding there may be radiolucent areas inside the hyperdensity.
6. The arachnoid and subarachnoid spaces are then assessed for high density areas that indicate subarachnoid bleeding. The subarachnoid space is normally filled with hypodense CSF.
7. The sulci and gyri are next, looking for clarity, delineation and any suggestion of distortion. Look for hyper and hypodensities on each slice. It is helpful to compare adjacent areas on the right and left sides in order to detect subtle density changes.
8. Look for preservation of the gray–white matter interface next, which is obscured by cerebral edema or other pathology, although if it is diffuse

this may be difficult. Assessment of the gray–white matter differentiation is often difficult in the acute stage because the patient lies on the trauma board which creates artifacts.

9. The other sign to look for is mass effect or brain swelling as obliteration of the cisterns around the midbrain.
10. Look next for intracerebral hyperdensities such as contusions, hematomas or foreign bodies in penetrating injuries or hypodensities such as air.
11. The midline structures should then be assessed to look for midline shift that indicates a unilateral lesion of some type. Midline shift is usually measured at the level of the foramen of Monro by determining how many millimeters the septum pellucidum is shifted.
12. The next areas are frequently neglected but should be assessed viz: the orbits, facial bones, sinuses, and foramen magnum.

Brain MRI is sometimes performed in assessing head injury. It allows a much better evaluation of the extension of the brain hemorrhages (see Fig. 5b) including contusions and especially DAI, and is more sensitive than CT in the detection of infarcts, especially along the infratentorial brain (brain stem and cerebellum). CT is however much easier to perform and remains the imaging modality of choice in the setting of acute head trauma.

Management of the Head Injured Patient

General principles

Many head injuries occur in the setting of multiple trauma in which case the principles of resuscitation based on the Airway, breathing, Circulation, Disability, Exposure (ABCDE) approach of the Primary survey of the Advanced Trauma Life Support Program apply. Thus, securing the airway while not manipulating the cervical spine, providing adequate ventilation, controlling bleeding, and management of shock take priority over the head injury. If a head CT is required this is conducted after airway, ventilation, and hemodynamic issues are addressed. If urgent surgical intervention is anticipated for the head trauma in a patient who also requires surgical intervention for torso trauma then the head CT should be done prior to taking the patient to the operating room (OR) if the cardio respiratory status of the patient allows safe transfer to the CT scanner; otherwise control of life threatening hemorrhage takes priority. Such decisions require rapid ongoing consultation between the neurosurgical and other surgical services involved. Where possible, consideration can be given to simultaneous surgical approaches to the torso and head such as combined intracranial hematoma and intra-abdominal hemorrhage, the goals being to save the patient's life by controlling hemorrhage while maintaining perfusion and oxygenation to prevent secondary brain injury and at the same time dealing with the intracranial pathology. In penetrating torso trauma, borderline hypotension has been advocated prior to definitive surgical control of bleeding in order to minimize preoperative blood loss.[9] This principle does not apply in the head injured patient with penetrating torso trauma because it violates the goal of preventing secondary brain injury by maintaining cerebral perfusion and oxygenation. The risk of increasing bleeding from the penetrating torso trauma by maintaining normal systemic blood pressure is accepted in order to prevent secondary brain injury from decreased brain perfusion and oxygenation.

A plain head CT provides crucial information for accurate diagnosis of head trauma and guiding therapy. It is conducted in all patients with moderate or severe brain injuries after airway, ventilation, and hemorrhage control. Essentially all these patients are admitted to hospital.

There are a number of decision tools to guide physicians in determining whether or not a CT scan is indicated in patients presenting with mild head injury (GCS 13–15). The Canadian CT head rule applies to patients with mild head injury, 16 years old or older, no coagulopathy or anticoagulants, and no obvious open skull fracture.[10] These patients are classified in two categories:

1. High risk for neurosurgical intervention (GCS less than 15 at two hours, suspected open or depressed skull fracture, signs of basal skull fracture, more than two episodes of vomiting, age over 65).
2. Moderate risk (more than five minutes loss of consciousness, 30 minutes pre-impact amnesia, dangerous mechanism of injury [pedestrian motor vehicle collision, occupant ejection, fall from height >three feet or five stairs]).

CT scan is considered mandatory in high risk patients. In general, patients with the above features are admitted to hospital with neurosurgical consultation if there are abnormal CT findings, if the patient remains symptomatic or continues to have neurologic abnormalities. A CT scan is usually repeated 24 hours later, although the utility of this has been questioned and it may be acceptable to rely on a change in the neurological examination to indicate need for repeat CT imaging.[11] Asymptomatic, fully awake and alert patients with no neurologic deficits after several hours of observation may be discharged home with written instructions and a companion to observe them over at least 24 hours and to return promptly in the extremely unlikely event that worsening such as headache, focal neurologic deficit or depression in mental status occurs.

In Moderate brain injury (GCS 9–12) after cardiorespiratory stability is achieved, a head CT scan is conducted followed by prompt neurosurgical consultation and admission to the ICU for further monitoring and management. If the first CT scan is abnormal further CT follow-up is required within 24 hours or as soon as there is any deterioration in neurologic status.

In Severe brain injury (GCS 3–8), after cardiorespiratory resuscitation, CT scan and admission to the ICU, frequent neurologic assessment, repeated CT scan usually around 24 hours after the injury and after any deterioration in neurologic status as well as other therapeutic interventions (such as placement of a ventricular catheter or craniotomy) is required. The focus is prevention of secondary brain injury by maintaining oxygenation and brain perfusion, controlling ICP (may require ICP monitoring), instituting measures to control cerebral edema, and identify any mass lesion which requires evacuation. These patients require intubation and mechanical ventilation because of their inability to protect the airway.

The mini-neurologic examination

The initial level of consciousness as determined by the GCS, along with pupillary responses and any lateralizing or focal neurologic signs are the fundamental parameters needed in patients with TBI. Abnormalities detected on the mini-neurologic assessment prompt further more detailed neurologic assessment such as power, tone, coordination, sensation, and reflexes in order to accurately localize the site of neurological injury. Although changes detected in the clinical assessment lead to changes in medical or surgical management, it can be difficult to detect neurologic changes in comatose, severely head injured patients and even some with moderate TBI so in these cases, sophisticated frequently invasive, monitoring techniques are often used.

Monitoring Techniques

The main goals of monitoring the severely brain injured patient are early identification of signs of worsening of brain function from secondary brain injury and to guide therapeutic interventions. The Brain Trauma Foundation has provided several iterations of guidelines for implementation of these monitoring techniques in the severely brain injured patient.[12]

General monitoring parameters

As in most other ICU patients and as discussed in other chapters, the head injured patient requires such monitoring as electrocardiography, pulse oximetry, arterial blood pressure, core temperature, urine output, arterial blood gases, electrolytes and frequently, at least in the early phases of hemodynamic assessment, invasive or non-invasive cardiac output, and central venous pressure monitoring.

Specific monitoring

As discussed earlier, there are at least two management strategies for patients with TBI, mainly applicable to severe TBI. Most physicians rely on an ICP or CPP based approach, fewer use the Lund concept approach.

Monitoring is typically aimed at measuring indices of cerebral perfusion, oxygenation, metabolism, and electrophysiologic function, the importance of which has been identified in our preamble. These indices include ICP, jugular venous oxygen saturation, brain tissue oxygen, brain tissue biochemistry, cerebral blood flow, cerebral blood flow velocity, electrophysiology, cerebral oxygenation, and brain temperature.[12]

ICP monitoring

Guidelines from the Brain Trauma Foundation indicate that ICP should be monitored in all salvageable severely brain injured patients with an abnormal brain CT scan (level 2 evidence) and in severe TBI patients with a normal CT and two or more of: age >40, motor posturing or systolic blood pressure <90 mmHg (level 3 evidence).Theoretically, such monitoring should benefit the patient by earlier detection of mass lesions, drainage of CSF to reduce ICP, avoidance of ineffective potentially harmful therapy and improvement of cerebral perfusion pressure. In general, an intraventricular catheter is the best method to measure ICP since it is most accurate, inexpensive and allows drainage of CSF to control ICP. Non-invasive techniques such as transcranial Doppler, tympanic membrane displacement, optic nerve sheath diameter, CT scan/MRI and fundoscopy have been used to assess ICP but none provide real-time continuous assessment of ICP.[13] Their advantage is they would avoid complications such as hemorrhage and infection from the invasive techniques like ventricular catheters or parenchymal ICP monitors. Treatment aimed at decreasing ICP should generally begin at pressures between 15–20 mmHg or a CPP below 50 mmHg depending on the cause of the increased ICP. CPP is generally recommended to be kept below 70 mmHg. ICP monitoring has become standard in treating severe brain injuries in many trauma centers based on the known relationship between high ICP and poor outcome. However, there are no randomized clinical trials comparing patients with severe TBI managed with or without ICP monitors. One randomized trial did show no difference in outcome between such patients managed with ICP monitors compared to those monitored closely with clinical and radiologic examinations.[14]

Jugular bulb venous oxygen saturation

Placement of an internal jugular vein catheter allows measurement of the jugular venous oxygen saturation which is used as an indicator of the relation between cerebral blood flow and cerebral metabolic rate of oxygen utilization. The measurement may be continuous by fiber-optic technique or intermittent based on repeated blood sampling. The normal range is 55%–71% and sustained saturation less than 50% is associated with poor outcome. Monitoring of jugular oxygen venous saturation allows early detection of brain ischemia which occurs after sustained hyperventilation to low PCO_2 in order to decrease ICP. This could be used as a trigger for modifying the degree of hyperventilation and its vasoconstrictive effect on the cerebral vasculature. Brain trauma guidelines concluded there was insufficient data to recommend or not to recommend the use of this method, but level 3 evidence suggested if measured, it be kept >50%.[15]

Brain tissue oxygen tension

This differs from jugular venous oxygen saturation in that it measures focal cerebral oxygenation while the jugular sample measures global cerebral oxygenation. It requires an invasive probe placed into the brain and is used for measuring specific brain tissue oxygenation in targeted vulnerable areas which may not be reflected in the measurement of global oxygenation. The normal range is 35–50 mmHg and a value of less than 15 mmHg is considered a threshold for intervention. Uncontrolled studies have suggested better outcome when brain tissue oxygenation is monitored in combination with ICP/CPP- based therapy than with the latter alone.[16]

Near infrared spectroscopy

This technique is based on the differential absorption properties of hemoglobin and cytochrome oxidase. It provides[17] a continuous non-invasive monitor of cerebral oxygenation and cerebral blood volume. However, it is less accurate than the jugular bulb venous saturation in measuring cerebral oxygenation. Its use in the clinical setting is still evolving and it has not found general acceptance as a monitoring tool for brain injury in the critical care unit.

Transcranial Doppler (TCD) Ultrasonography

This allows non-invasive measurement of cerebral blood flow velocity and is useful in identifying complications which may occur in severe traumatic brain injury such as angiographic vaso spasm, decreases in cerebral perfusion pressure, elevations of ICP, carotid dissection, and cerebral circulatory arrest. This technique has been suggested as a non-invasive alternative to the invasive ICP and CPP measurements which carry higher risk for complications but evidence for its use in traumatic brain injury is limited.[18]

Electrophysiologic monitoring

The depth of coma can be monitored by the electroencephalogram (EEG). This also allows the detection of subclinical seizures including in paralyzed patients and the diagnosis of brain death which is important in the ICU setting in the context of organ donation. In many centers continuous EEG monitoring is used in paralyzed patients to detect post-traumatic seizures which are thought to be injurious to brain tissue and may not be clinically apparent in such patients because of the neuromuscular blockade. Strip electrodes placed on the brain surface after TBI have shown cortical spreading depolarizations associated with brain ischemia — this remains an experimental tool.[19]

Sensory evoked potentials may be useful in predicting outcome from severe brain injury. The combination of somatosensory, auditory and visual evoked potentials yields the highest prognostic accuracy. While its use is very limited in early management of severe head injury, it is useful in the late phases for predicting outcome and decisions regarding discontinuation of aggressive treatment regimes.

Brain Temperature

Elevated brain temperature results in secondary brain injury. Invasive and non-invasive methods for continuous measure of brain temperature are commercially available but their ICU use is not widespread.

Brain tissue biochemistry

An invasive microdialysis device inserted into the brain parenchyma allows bedside monitoring of biochemical changes in susceptible brain tissue. Glucose, lactate, pyruvate, glycerol, glutamate, and lactate/pyruvate ratios are measurable with microdialysis probes. The lactate/pyruvate ratio is used as an index of local brain tissue ischemia. However, it is not widely applied in most ICU's.

The Emergency Neurological Life Support (ENLS) Algorithm for Initial Management of Intracranial Hypertension

As indicated earlier, sustained intracranial hypertension, if left untreated, leads to catastrophic outcome in head injury. Maintenance of perfusion and oxygenation and measures aimed at deceasing intracranial hypertension are the chief methods of preventing secondary brain injury and improving outcome. The ENLS has proposed a stepwise management algorithm (Fig. 7) utilizing the interventions presented earlier to guide treatment and prevention of intracranial hypertension.[20] The inflection point of the intracranial pressure–volume relationship (Fig. 8) signifies an exponential rise in ICP after the compensatory mechanisms have been exhausted. At Tier 0, usual medical measures such as head elevation, oxygenation, ventilation, fluid, and electrolyte normalization are instituted and head CT is assessed. Tier 1 involves PCO_2 manipulations, mannitol, CSF drainage, and consideration of additional monitoring. Failure to respond prompts repeat CT and Tier 2 interventions such as sedation with propofol, thiopental, and a revision of ICP and MAP goals. Finally at Tier 3, pentobarbital, hypothermia, and decompression are therapeutic considerations. These measures are discussed further following consideration of surgical management.

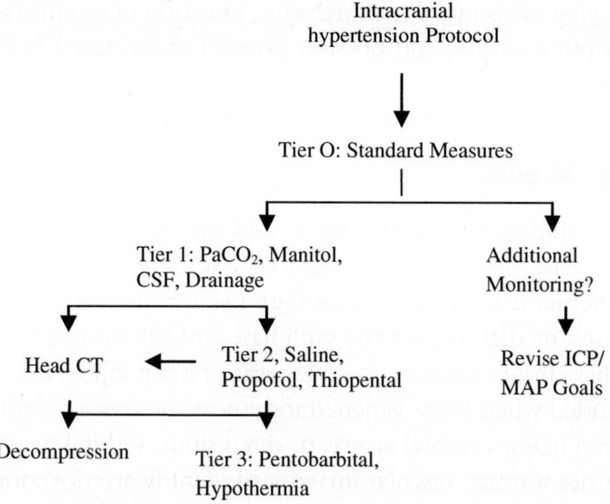

Fig. 7. ENLS Protocol.

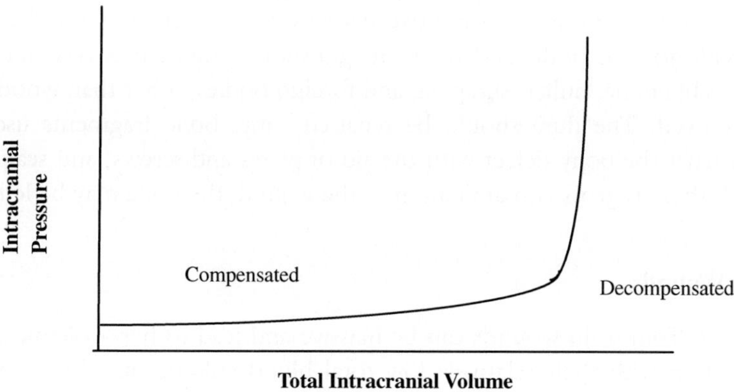

Fig. 8. Relation between intracranial volume and intracranial pressure

Surgical Management

General principles

The initial principles of management after airway, ventilation, and hemodynamic resuscitation is to control any hemorrhage, remove devitalized tissue, control contamination with antibiotics and timely wound repair, removal of space-occupying intracranial hemorrhages, insertion of monitors as indicated in the description earlier, and possibly control of increased ICP by decompressive craniectomy.

Penetrating Wounds

All patients with penetrating wounds should have broad spectrum antibiotics for about five days. They should undergo CT scanning to assess the trajectory of injury, whether it traverses areas at high risk for vascular injury such as the venous sinuses, medial parts of the skull base and Sylvian fissures, presence of foreign bodies, and to identify possible areas of brain injury. CT angiography is recommended when there is penetration near the base of skull, Sylvian fissure, or near a major cerebral artery, or dural sinus. Orbital or pterional penetrating injuries warrant vascular imaging to identify arteriovenous fistulas or traumatic aneurysms requiring endovascular or surgical repair. Penetrating objects should be left in place until vascular injury is ruled out and should be removed only in the sterile well equipped OR by a qualified surgeon. The principles then are to remove the penetrating object as well as debride the entry and exit wounds and remove necrotic tissue, hematoma and readily accessible foreign body, and bone. In gunshot wounds, it is accepted that inaccessible bone, bullet, shrapnel, and foreign bodies, other than wood, not be removed. The dura should be repaired, large bone fragments used to reconstruct the bony defect with the aid of plates and screws, and scalp closure. If there is gross contamination of the wound, the bone may be left out.

Scalp Wounds

Bleeding from scalp wounds can be massive and lead to hypovolemic shock in children with their relatively low total blood volume but this is rare in adults. Temporary hemostasis with pressure, skin clips, cautery, and sutures should be applied followed by more definitive surgical methods of hemorrhage control after thorough cleansing and debridement. The wound should be carefully inspected for underlying fracture, CSF leak, or foreign material.

Depressed skull fractures

A CT Scan should be used to determine the degree of depression of the skull fracture. If the degree of depression is greater than the thickness of the adjacent skull, traditionally operative elevation is suggested. Open depressed fractures may be treated by simple scalp repair if they are not depressed more than 1 cm, there is no involvement of the frontal sinus, dural laceration, underlying hematoma requiring evacuation, gross deformity, or wound contamination. Nonoperative management is also an option for closed depressed fractures when cosmesis is not a major issue.

Intracranial mass lesions

All patients with intracranial mass legions require neurosurgical consultation.

An epidural hematoma of >30 ml should be removed regardless of the GCS. Observation and serial CT scanning is reasonable for smaller epidural hematomas with less than 15 mm thickness, less than 5 mm midline shift, and GCS >8.

A subdural hematoma with thickness >10 mm or midline shift of 5 mm or greater should be removed regardless of the GCS. Removal of subdural hematomas that are thinner or associated with less midline shift in patients with GCS <9 may also be indicated especially if there is abnormal pupillary reactivity, deterioration in level of consciousness, or increase ICP. Whether or not the bone flap should be left out after craniotomy for subdural hematoma is controversial.

Subarachnoid hemorrhage generally does not require early surgical intervention for evacuation of hemorrhage. In late phases, development of traumatic hydrocephalus may warrant surgical procedures to control the hydrocephalus by such techniques as ventriculo-peritoneal shunting.

Intracerebral hemorrhages should generally be evacuated if there is progressive neurological deterioration, increased ICP that is medically refractory or mass effect on CT scan. Usually such hematomas will be greater than 20 ml or so in the temporal lobe or 50 ml in other areas, and associated with more than 5 mm midline shift.

Decompressive Craniectomy

Intracranial hypertension is highly associated with morbidity and mortality in severe brain injury and much of the management assumes this relationship is causal, mainly based on the logical association between increased ICP, usually low CPP, and the potential for brain ischemia. Prompt and early surgical treatment involving evacuation of a mass lesion which is responsible for the intracranial hypertension is effective in reducing ICP and improving outcome.

Decompressive craniectomy[21] may be considered in two main situations. The first is when an intracranial hematoma, usually a subdural hematoma or occasionally intracerebral hemorrhage is removed. Usually a large, unilateral craniectomy is performed. Level 3 evidence suggests it may be beneficial but randomized trials are needed to determine this. At this point, it is not a widely used treatment option.

The second situation is when the elevated ICP is due to diffuse brain swelling and/or cerebral edema in the absence of a mass lesion which could be evacuated. In these cases, efforts are aimed at controlling the ICP by aggressive medical intervention to be discussed in the following paragraphs. Despite these efforts, however, many severe brain injured patients continue to have progressive rise of the ICP and eventual death. In such circumstances, a theoretically attractive treatment strategy is to allow the edema to run its course but protect the brain from increased intracranial pressure effects by temporarily removing the restricting calvarium. This could be a unilateral craniectomy or if there is no midline shift in the presence of bilateral brain swelling, a bifrontotemporal craniectomy may be performed. This surgical technique of decompressive craniectomy has been tried and studied with inconsistent results. In a controlled prospective randomized trial involving 155 patients with severe traumatic brain injury and refractory intracranial hypertension, decompressive craniectomy compared to standard care yielded lower ICP and length of stay but with similar unfavorable outcomes after adjusting for prognostic factors and similar death rates at six months — 19% in the craniectomy group and 18% standard care group.[21] The effectiveness of this therapy is therefore debatable, controversial and should be considered on a case-by-case basis. At present, there is another clinical trial in progress which may identify appropriate candidates for this procedure.

Medical Management

Apart from standard resuscitation techniques to maintain adequate oxygenation and perfusion to prevent secondary brain injury, many non-surgical measures are implemented in the preoperative, operative, postoperative, and other phases of brain injury management with monitoring as outlined earlier.

General intensive care measures

The blood pressure should be monitored and the systolic blood pressure kept >90 mmHg. Hypoxia should be avoided. Frequent turning to prevent decubitus ulcers, physiotherapy for chest and maintenance of musculoskeletal function, eye, ear and mouth care hygiene, bowel regime to prevent constipation, frequent airway suctioning, stomach decompression by orogastric tube initially, and later using the tube for enteral nutrition. Enteral feeding should begin at least within seven days of the injury. A Foley catheter for monitoring hourly urine output and later conversion to condom catheter, arterial catheter for initial continuous hemodynamic and arterial blood gas monitoring as required. Regular monitoring of hemoglobin, white blood cell count, serum electrolytes, magnesium, phosphate, and calcium to detect and correct abnormalities is required. Specific to the head injured patient, venous thrombo-embolism prophylaxis using graduated compression stockings or intermittent pneumatic compression devices is indicated in bedridden moderate TBI and all severe TBI patients unless there are lower extremity injuries that preclude their use or some other contraindication. Pharmacologic prophylaxis is controversial but is often used after intracranial bleeding has been shown to be stable over 24 or more hours. If there are no thoracolumbar spine injuries that preclude it, elevation of the head of the bed to about 30° to reduce ICP and maintain CPP is recommended, keeping the head and neck in the neutral position, and avoiding neck vein compression from tight collars or tapes. Glucocorticoid steroids are not indicated in patients with TBI.

Other measures

Analgesics and sedatives assist with controlling pain and limit increase in ICP associated with maneuvers such as suctioning. Morphine and fentanyl are frequently used for these purposes and pain control is important for both mobilization of the patient and control of increased ICP. Sedatives are only indicated as necessary to control agitation, permit ventilation and in the management of increased ICP. Selection of the sedative is based on the hemodynamic profile of the agent. Propofol is a good agent because it is easily titratable and rapidly reversible but it should be avoided in hypotensive or hypovolemic patients and testing for propofol infusion syndrome (rhabdomyolysis, metabolic acidosis, renal failure, and bradycardia) should be considered. Benzodiazepines such as midazolam and lorazapam are alternate agents. Brain Trauma Foundation guidelines also suggest barbiturates to control increased ICP when it is not controlled by other measures.

Fluid and electrolytes

The goal is to maintain euvolemia with isotonic solutions mainly normal saline while monitoring serum electrolytes. Hypotonic solutions should be avoided in resuscitation. Glucose solutions should be avoided in the first 24–48 hours unless there is hypoglycemia from other causes because hyperglycemia has direct deleterious effects on the injured brain and anaerobic cerebral metabolism of glucose leads to acidosis and free water production which could worsen cerebral edema. Hypo and hypernatremia should be identified and treated promptly. Hypophosphatemia and hypomagnesemia occur commonly in head injured patients and lower the seizure threshold. Close monitoring and correction by appropriate replacement is important.

Hyperglycemia has been associated with worse outcome after TBI. However, tight glycemic control with intensive insulin therapy has not been associated with uniformly better outcome and remains controversial.[22] A reasonable recommended approach is to monitor blood glucose while maintaining the level between 80 and 180 mg/dl.

Blood transfusion

While there is evidence that outcome from severe brain injury is worse with anemia, there is no consensus on a specific transfusion threshold for these patients and no evidence that this threshold should be different from that in other critically ill patients. At present transfusion should be individualized based on hemodynamics and other clinical parameters. In general critical care, a transfusion threshold of 7–8 g/dL is standard but in patients with brain injury, it may be warranted to transfuse if the hemoglobin is less than 10–11 g/dL. The brain injured patient is also susceptible to coagulopathy as in other trauma patients. This topic is discussed in greater detail in the textbook.

Ventilation

Hyperventilation decreases ICP by decreasing cerebral blood volume by causing cerebral vasoconstriction. However, vasoconstriction could lead to ischemia, brain swelling, and cerebral edema, leading to increased ICP. The recommendation is therefore to use hyperventilation to reduce ICP only for brief periods (15–30 minutes of PCO_2 at 30–35 mmHg) and to monitor cerebral oxygenation by some method if hyperventilation is used. Hyperventilation is a temporizing measure before moving to barbiturate coma or neurosurgical procedures as indicated earlier. Otherwise, the ventilator settings should achieve an (oxygen) O_2 saturation of at least 95% and a PCO_2 of 35–40 mmHg. Positive end expiratory pressure (PEEP) increases partial pressure of oxygen (PO_2) for the same inspired oxygen concentration and it has been suggested that the increased intrathoracic pressure impedes cerebral venous drainage thus increasing ICP. This effect of PEEP, however, is only significant at levels greater than 15 cm H_2O. Nevertheless the level of PEEP used should be the lowest that achieves adequate oxygenation except in cases of refractory hypoxemia. Usual levels of PEEP at 5–8 cm H_2O to achieve acceptable oxygenation is ideal.[23]

Hyperosmolar therapy

The standard for hyperosmolar therapy to decrease brain edema and ICP has been mannitol but recent studies have suggested that hypertonic saline may have a similar or safer profile and be more or at least as effective.[24] Both of these agents are effective in decreasing ICP and are associated with hemodynamic blood volume and electrolyte imbalances and should not be used prophylactically but generally as a temporizing measure when transtentorial herniation is suspected or occurring before surgery and when ICP is increased or CPP is decreased and other measures have been exhausted. Administration of mannitol or hypertonic saline requires monitoring of systemic volume status and serum electrolytes.

Barbiturate coma

Barbiturates reduce cerebral metabolism and as a result, cerebral blood flow. Thus, they lower ICP and have been shown to be effective in treating increased ICP that is refractory to other interventions.[25] Pentobarbital or thiopental may be used but they are contraindicated in the hypovolemic hypotensive patient because of their hypotensive side effect. Another significant side effect is immune suppression that may increase the risk of infection. Nevertheless, barbiturates may be used when other measures to control increased ICP have failed.

Hypothermia

Decreasing brain metabolism, cerebral blood flow and allowing time for cell recovery under hypothermic conditions form the basis for treating refractory intracranial hypertension by cooling patients to temperatures of 32–34°C.[26] Cooling for 48 hours and other time periods have been studied and there is no consensus on its utility in the brain injured patient. This therapeutic modality is now used sporadically and its effectiveness requires further clinical trials.

Anti-seizure therapy

Patients with GCS score < 9, cortical contusions, depressed skull fractures, subdural hematomas, intracerebral hematomas, penetrating brain injury, and seizures within 24 hours of injury are at high risk for seizures. It is recommended that patients with severe TBI receive seizure prophylaxis. If a patient has a risk factor as noted earlier and mild or moderate TBI, whether or not to administer seizure prophylaxis is uncertain. In all cases, it is not recommended to continue antiepileptic drugs for more than seven days after the ictus unless the patient has more than one seizure in the first week. The most commonly used agent is phenytoin starting with a loading dose of 15–20 mg/kg intravenously over 30 minutes followed by 100 mg every eight hours for seven days. Levetiracetam is also frequently used; no randomized studies have assessed them.

Conclusion

The main focus of therapy for post-traumatic brain injury is the prevention of secondary insult to the brain. This requires an understanding of the mechanism of not only the brain injury but also the potential benefits of intervention in preserving brain function. Thus by far, our efforts are based on controlling brain oxygenation and perfusion, decreasing intracranial hypertension, cerebral edema, and evacuating mass lesions. Optimum care requires collaboration among neurosurgeons, anesthetists, and critical care practitioners.

References

1. Bruns J Jr, Hauser WA. The epidemiology of traumatic brain injury: A review. *Epilepsia* 2003; 44 Suppl 10: 2–10.
2. Rickels E, von WK, Wenzlaff P. Head injury in Germany: A population-based prospective study on epidemiology, causes, treatment and outcome of all degrees of head-injury severity in two distinct areas. *Brain Inj* 2010; 24: 1491–1504.

3. Codd PJ, Agarwalla PK, Berry-Candelario J *et al.* Kernohan-woltman notch phenomenon in acute subdural hematoma. *JAMA Neurol* 2013; 70: 1194–1195.
4. Muzevic D, Splavski B. The Lund concept for severe traumatic brain injury. *Cochrane Database Syst Rev* 2013; 12: CD010193.
5. Dagal A, Lam AM. Cerebral blood flow and the injured brain: How should we monitor and manipulate it? *Curr Opin Anaesthesiol* 2011; 24: 131–137.
6. Mokri B. The Monro–Kellie hypothesis: Applications in CSF volume depletion. *Neurology* 2001; 56: 1746–1748.
7. Rosenfeld JV, McFarlane AC, Bragge P *et al.* Blast-related traumatic brain injury. *Lancet Neurol* 2013; 12: 882–893.
8. Stead LG, Wijdicks EF, Bhagra A *et al.* Validation of a new coma scale, the FOUR score, in the emergency department. *Neurocrit Care* 2009; 10: 50–54.
9. Bickell WH, Wall MJ, Pepe PE *et al.* Immediate vs delayed fluid resuscitation for hypotensive patients with penetrating torso injuries. *N Engl J Med* 1994; 331(17): 1105–1109.
10. Stiell IG, Wells GA, Vandemheen K *et al.* The Canadian CT Head Rule for patients with minor head injury. *Lancet* 2001; 357: 1391–1396.
11. Almenawer SA, Bogza I, Yarascavitch B *et al.* The value of scheduled repeat cranial computed tomography after mild head injury: Single-center series and meta-analysis. *Neurosurgery* 2013; 72: 56–62.
12. Guidelines for the management of severe traumatic brain injury. *J Neurotrauma* 2007; 24 Suppl 1: S1–106.
13. Forsyth R, Wolny S, Rodrigues B. Routine intracranial pressure monitoring in acute coma. *Cochrane Database Syst Rev.* 2010; pCD002043.
14. Chesnut RM, Temkin N, Carney N *et al.* A trial of intracranial-pressure monitoring in traumatic brain injury. *N Engl J Med* 2012; 367: 2471–2481.
15. Cruz J. The first decade of continuous monitoring of jugular bulb oxyhemoglobin saturation: management strategies and clinical outcome. *Crit Care Med* 1998; 26: 344–351.
16. Adamides AA, Cooper DJ, Rosenfeldt FL *et al.* Focal cerebral oxygenation and neurological outcome with or without brain tissue oxygen-guided therapy in patients with traumatic brain injury. *Acta Neurochir* (*Wien*) 2009; 151: 1399–1409.
17. Lewis SB, Myburgh JA, Thornton EL *et al.* Cerebral oxygen monitoring by near-infrared spectroscopy is not clinically useful in patients with severe closed-head injury. A comparison with jugular venous bulb oximetry. *Crit Care Med* 1996; 24: 1334–1338.
18. Bellner J, Romner B, Reinstrup P *et al.* Transcranial Doppler sonography pulsatility index (PI) reflects intracranial pressure (ICP) *Surg Neurol* 2004; 62: 45–51.
19. Dreier JP. The role of spreading depression, spreading depolarization and spreading ischemia in neurological disease. *Nat Med* 2011; 17: 439–447.

20. Stevens RD, Huff JS, Duckworth J *et al.* Emergency Neurological Life Support: Intracranial Hypertension and Herniation. *Neurocrit Care* 2012. DOI 10.100.107/812-9754-5.
21. Cooper DJ, Rosenfeld JV, Murray L *et al.* Decompressive craniectomy in diffuse traumatic brain injury. *N Engl J Med* 2011; 364: 1493–1502.
22. Zafar SN, Iqbal A, Farez MF *et al.* Intensive insulin therapy in brain injury: a meta-analysis. *J Neurotrauma* 2011; 28(7): 1307–1317.
23. Hesdorffer D, Ghajar J, Iacono L. Predictors of compliance with the evidence-based guidelines for traumatic brain injury care: A survey of United States Trauma Centres. *J Trauma* 2002; 52: 1202–1209.
24. Marko NF. Hypertonic saline, not mannitol, should be considered gold standard medical therapy for intracranial hypertension. *Crit Care* 2012; 16(1): 113–116.
25. Kassel NF, Hitchon PW, Gerk MK *et al.* Alterations in cerebral blood flow, oxygen metabolism, and electrical activity produced by high dose sodium thiopental. *Neurosurgery* 1980; 7: 598–603.
26. Clifton GL, Valadka A, Zygun D *et al.* Very early hypothermia induction in patients with severe brain injury (the National Acute Brain Injury Study: Hypothermia II): A randomized trial. *Lancet Neurol* 2011; 10: 131–139.

Chapter 19

Spine and Spinal Cord Injury

Safraz Mohammed, Shelly Wang and Jameel Ali

Chapter Overview

The exact incidence of traumatic spinal cord injury (SCI) is not known but is estimated to be between 35–40 cases per million people in North America. The actual incidence is greater because reported statistics usually do not include pre-hospital deaths which may account for up to 30% of cases. In the United States, the annual incidence is about 10,000 per year. The annual cost of taking care of SCI patients is estimated at over $8 billion.

The life-long morbidity and disability is devastating since the most commonly affected individuals are young adults. The most consistent predictor of long-term outcome is the severity of neurologic injury, which can be characterized by both the level and completeness of motor and sensory loss. The contributors of mortality include respiratory disorders, cardiovascular disorders, pulmonary embolism (PE), and infections, in addition to suicide, which highlights the devastating emotional impact on the patients.

SCI patients may require ICU treatment in the context of multiple trauma or for the isolated spinal injury itself because of cardio-respiratory and other effects of the injury which requires treatment and monitoring in the ICU setting. To assist the intensivists in managing these patients, this chapter discusses the anatomic, physiologic and clinical features of SCI.

Anatomical Considerations

The following is a review of the anatomy and physiology of the spine and spinal cord.

The spinal column consists of 33 vertebrae — seven cervical, 12 thoracic, five lumbar, five fused sacral vertebrae (which forms the sacrum), and four fused coccygeal vertebrae (which forms the coccyx or tailbone). These bones are held together by an elaborate series of ligaments, intervertebral discs and facet joints. With regards to mobility, the cervical spine and the thoracolumbar spine are the most mobile, and thus subject to the highest incidence of fractures. Of all spinal fractures, the cervical spine accounts for 55%, while the thoracic spine, thoracolumbar junction and the lumbar spine each accounts for 15%.

The spinal cord extends from the medulla at the skull base to the intervertebral disc between L1 and L2 in adults and between L2 and L3 in pediatric age group generally. Axial sections of the spinal cord reveal the typical H-shape gray matter intimately surrounded by white matter, made up of somatotopically arranged ascending and descending tracts. Generally the cervical fibers are found medially with the lumbosacral fibers placed laterally within the motor tracts. Of the many white matter tracts only three are of clinical significance, because they can be tested. These include: (1) the anterolateral spinothalamic tract, that transmits information of pain, temperature, light touch, and pressure sensation of the contralateral side, (2) the posterolateral corticospinal tract that transmit motor control to the ipsilateral side, (3) the posterior columns that transmit touch, vibration and propioceptive sensation.

The spinal cord receives its blood supply by a single anterior and two posterior spinal arteries. The anterior spinal artery originates from two branches of the vertebral arteries just prior to their union to form the basilar artery. The spinal arteries are subsequently augmented by radicular branches of the thyrocervical, costocervical, intercostal, and lumbar vessels. The artery of Adamkiewicz, is a major contributor to the anterior spinal artery and usually comes of the left posterior intercostal artery between T8 and L1 vertebral segments in about 78% of cases. It helps to supply the lower two thirds of the spinal cord via the anterior spinal artery. The anterior spinal artery supplies the anterior two thirds of the spinal cord, while the posterior one third of the spinal cord is supplied by the two posterior spinal arteries. The venous drainage goes to the internal and external vertebral plexuses that ultimately run into the caval systems. The spinal cord blood flow is very similar to the cerebral blood flow, with an average rate of 40–60 mL per 100g of tissue per minute. Auto regulation occurs between mean arterial pressures of 60 and 150 mmHg, and this is lost when the spinal cord is injured.

Levels

In describing spinal disorders, an understanding of the designation of levels is important. These levels are:

Neurologic level: The most caudal segment with normal sensory and motor function on both sides.

Sensory level: The most caudal segment with normal sensory function on both sides.

Motor level: The most caudal segment with normal motor function on both sides.

Skeletal level: Radiographic level of greatest vertebral damage.

The C1 spinal root exits the spine at the atlanto–occipital junction. The C2 nerve root exits above C2. The C8 nerve root exits below C7 vertebra. The T1 nerve root exits below T1 vertebra, and so forth, the L1 nerve root exits below the L1 vertebra.

An important distinction must be made with regard to spinal levels. As noted before, the spinal cord ends at the L1–L2 interspace. This means that the spinal cord is much shorter than the spine itself. So an injury at a particular vertebral level may have neurological examination different to what is expected. The First two cervical cord segments roughly match the first two cervical vertebral levels. C3–C8 segments of the spinal cords are situated between C3 through C7 bony vertebral levels. Similarly in the thoracic spinal cord, the first two thoracic cord segments match the first two thoracic vertebral levels. However, T3 through T12 cord segments are situated between T3 to T8 vertebral levels. The lumbar cord segments are roughly situated from T9 through T11 levels while the sacral segments are situated from T12 to L1. The tip of the spinal cord or conus medullaris is situated at L1–L2 interspace and below this there are only spinal roots, called the cauda equina.

Dermatomes and Myotomes

The following table is a quick guide that can be used in the clinical exam of a patient with SCI.

Spinal level	Key sensory area	Action	Myotome
C5	Radial antecubital fossa	Elbow flexors	Biceps, brachialis, brachioradialis
C6	Thumb	Wrist extensors	Extensor carpi radialis longus and brevis
C7	Middle finger	Elbow extensors	Triceps
C8	Little finger	Finger flexors	Flexor digitorum profundus
T1	Ulnar antecubital fossa	Hand intrinsics	Interossei
L2	Mid-anterior thigh	Hip flexors	Iliopsoas
L3	Medial femoral condyle	Knee extensors	Quadriceps
L4	Medial malleolus	Ankle dorsiflexors	Tibialis anterior
L5	Dorsal first/second toe web space	Big toe extensors	Extensor hallucis longus
S1	Lateral heel	Ankle plantar flexors	Gastrocnemius, soleus

Etiology

Motor vehicle crashes are the most common cause of SCI, accounting for 41% of all injuries, of which 70% are subsequent to vehicle rollovers where ejections occurred in 35–39% of cases. Fall (27%) account for the second most common cause, followed by violence (15%), sports/recreation (8%) and others (collectively 9%).

Pathophysiology

Acute SCI involves two pathological processes: Primary and secondary. The primary cord injury is caused by the direct initial trauma. The secondary SCI can be either iatrogenic or natural. Iatrogenic injury results from cord manipulation and compression with movement, for example improper log roll. The natural secondary cord injury may result from: (1) spinal cord ischemia from hypoxia, hypotension, vascular compromise, impaired vasomotor function, hemorrhage, vasospasm, and thrombosis, (2) inflammatory response with release of chemokines, eicosanoids, cytokines, and leucocyte infiltration, (3) cellular dysfunction with ATP depletion, free radical generation, lipid peroxidation, and mitochondrial insufficiency. Secondary SCI is best seen on MRI which demonstrates spinal cord edema, which peaks 3–6 days after the trauma and takes several weeks to resolve. SCI may progress even further due to apoptotic cell death, glial scar formation, and cystic cavity formation. The effects of the secondary SCI can be mitigated by the correction or prevention of hypoxia, hypotension, shock, hyperthermia, hypercoagulability, and catecholamine release.

Clinical Features and Presentations

One categorization of SCI depends on whether the injury is above or below T1. Injury to the first eight segments results in neurological deficit in all four limbs: Quadriplegia. Injuries below T1 result in paraplegia. This has significant impact on not only the acute management but also the rehabilitative process.

Injury Severity may be categorized as:

— Incomplete quadriplegia (incomplete cervical injury)
— Complete quadriplegia (complete cervical injury)
— Incomplete paraplegia (incomplete thoracic injury)
— Complete paraplegia (complete thoracic injury)

Complete injury means that there is no motor or sensory function below the level of the injury. In an incomplete injury there is some preservation of long tract signs. These include any sensation or motor controlling the lower extremities and sacral sparing. The sacral segments must be thoroughly examined for sensation and motor power. Sacral sparing is demonstrated by perianal sensation, rectal motor activity, and great toe flexor activity. Sacral reflexes such as the bulbocavernosus reflex or anal wink are not components of sacral sparing.

Preservation of sacral function may be the only indication of an incomplete cord lesion which predicts some sort of recovery. If the patient is paralyzed and has no signs of sacral sparing, then the patient is considered to have a complete cord lesion. However, a decision as to whether a lesion is complete should not be made in the presence of spinal shock which is a loss of all motor and sensory functions which may include loss of sacral sparing and occurs soon after the injury to the spinal cord.

The duration of this spinal shock state is quite variable. The bulbocavernosus reflex is spinal mediated through S2–S4 and is positive when there is anal sphincter contraction in response to squeezing the glans penis or clitoris or tugging on an indwelling bladder foley catheter. This reflex may also be lost during spinal shock and is one of the first reflexes to return after spinal shock is over. The persistent loss of all motor and sensory function below the cord lesion on return of the bulbocavernosus reflex (heralding the end of spinal shock) suggests complete cord injury. Spinal shock which is a neurologic phenomenon must be differentiated from neurogenic shock which is a hemodynamic abnormality resulting from loss of sympathetic tone.

Spinal Cord Syndromes

Due to the well-defined vascular territories within the spinal cord and the somatotopically arranged white matter tracts, there are commonly encountered and easily recognized injury patterns with associated prognostication for recovery.

***Anterior cord syndrome*:** This is characterized by paraplegia, sensory loss, loss of pain and temperature sensation while position, deep pressure and vibratory sensation are intact. This syndrome is brought about by the infarction of the anterior two thirds of the spinal cord which is the territory supplied by the anterior spinal artery. This syndrome has the poorest prognosis for recovery, among all the incomplete syndromes.

***Central cord syndrome*:** is characterized by a patchy sensory loss, with weakness in all four limbs, the upper limbs being weaker than the lower limbs. Central cord syndrome is thought to be caused by ischemia of the central aspect of the cord; a vascular territory of the anterior spinal artery. Since the cervical motor fibers are more centrally located in the cord, ischemia in this territory results in preferential weakness of the upper limbs. This syndrome is commonly seen in hyperextension injury with pre-existing cervical canal stenosis from degenerative spine disease. Prognosis is somewhat better than other incomplete injuries. Patients generally gain the ability to walk but have limited improvement in upper limb function, especially the hands.

***Posterior cord syndrome*:** This is the least common of the incomplete injuries, and is due to dorsal column injury resulting in loss of proprioception and vibratory sense, with preservation of motor function. Many patients are unable to walk because of the impairment in proprioception.

***Brown-Séquard syndrome*:** Occurs as a result of hemisection of the spinal cord with subsequent unilateral disruption of the corticospinal tract, spinothalamic tract and dorsal columns. This results in ipsilateral loss of motor control, proprioception and light touch sensation with contralateral loss of pain and temperature sensation below the level of the lesion. Prognosis is generally good.

Investigations: X-ray, CT, MRI

Radiographs

Standard cervical spine radiographs include the antero-posterior, lateral, and odontoid views. Lateral films identify up to 85% of unstable fractures. Radiographs should ideally be interpreted in a systematic manner to avoid missing injuries. The lateral cervical spine X-ray should be assessed for adequacy (defined by clear visualization of the base of the skull, all seven cervical vertebrae, and the C7–T1 junction), abnormalities in vertebral alignment, vertebral fractures, intervertebral disc space, and prevertebral soft tissue swelling.

Computed tomography

CT is the most commonly used for detecting spinal injuries especially in poly-trauma patients and if the spine is not adequately visualized on plain radiographs, or if there is a high clinical suspicion of injury despite normal looking X-rays.[1]

Magnetic resonance imaging

MRI is the modality of choice for assessing acute cord injury and soft tissue/ ligamentous injury. It is less sensitive than CT or plain films in distinguishing bony abnormalities, in particular, those of the upper portion or posterior portions of the spine. MRI (T2-weighted and STIR — Short Tau Inversion Recovery-sequences) is very useful in detecting spinal cord edema and hemorrhage, ligamentous injury, and other non-osseous changes that can be missed with CT.[2]

Specific Traumatic Spine Injuries

Following is a brief summary of the different spinal column injuries, described in anatomical sequence

1. *Occipital condyle fracture*

The occipital condyles are oval-shaped paired prominences which form the lateral aspect of the foramen magnum, and articulate with Cl lateral masses. Condylar fractures are seen in about 1–3% of patients with blunt craniocervical trauma. Diagnosis is best made with CT, as opposed to plain radiographs. These types of fractures are associated with head injuries and cervical spine injuries in up to 30% of cases. Intrinsic ligaments within the spinal canal are essential to the integrity of the atlanto-occipital joint. Thus condylar fractures with associated significant ligamentous injury are unstable. Anderson and Montesano have classified occipital condyle fractures as follows: type I — Impaction-type fracture with combination of the occipital condyle; type II — Basilar skull fracture that extends into one- or both occipital condyles; type III — Avulsion fracture of condyle in region of the alar ligament attachment. Types I and II are generally regarded as stable, and can be managed in a rigid collar for 6–12 weeks. Type III is unstable in over 50% of cases, due to the craniocervcal disruption, and depending upon the degree of stability can be treated with rigid collar, halo or occipit-C2 instrumented fusion.[3]

2. *Cervical*

The cervical spine accounts for 55% of all spinal traumas. And can occur as a result of one or more of the following injury mechanisms — axial loading, flexion, extension, rotation, lateral bending and distraction. The following is a brief summary of the different spinal column injuries that can occur, outlined in anatomical sequence.

a. Atlanto-occipital dislocation

These are very uncommon injuries and often fatal due to brainstem compression and, seen in up to 19% of fatal cervical spine injuries. These injuries include subluxations, dislocation, often with fractures of the occipital condyles, and the mechanism of injury is one of severe flexion and distraction at the occipito–cervical junction. Diagnosis can be suspected on imaging. The rule of 12's indicate the basion-dental interval (BDI) and the basion-posterior axial line interval (BAI), in a normal individual is less than 12 mm. the Power's ratio can also be used, but this is useful primarily in determining anterior occipito-cervical dislocations and subluxations. Powers ratio = distance from basion to posterior arch/distance from anterior arch to opisthion. Normal is approximately 1. If the ratio is > 1.0 then there is concern for anterior dislocation. If the ratio < 1.0 then this raises concern for posterior atlanto-occipital dislocation, odontoid fractures or fractures of the ring of atlas. There are three classes of atlanto-occipital dislocation — Type I (anterior dislocation), Type II (longitudinal dislocation) and Type III (posterior dislocation). Traction is to be avoided; instead temporary halo immobilization can be done while hemodynamic status is addressed, until definitive operative stabilization is performed.

b. Atlas fracture

The C1 ring is thin with broad articular surfaces. It makes up ~7% of all cervical spine fractures. The risk of neurologic injury is low, since the fragment is spread apart rather than compress the neural elements. These fractures can be commonly missed due to inadequate imaging of occipito-cervical junction, and the lack of neurological deficit. Mechanisms of injury include hyperextension, lateral compression, but are most commonly the result of heavy axial compression. It is important to note that atlas fractures are associated with other spine fractures; 50% have an associated spine injury, and 40% associated with C2 fracture. The three most common types of atlas fractures are classified as follows: Type 1 — isolated anterior or posterior arch fractures where the articulating lateral masses do not spread apart; Type 2 — burst fracture or Jefferson fracture, where the lateral masses spread apart and there is bilateral anterior and posterior arch fractures, the rule of Spence dictates that if the combined overhang of the lateral masses is more than 7 mm then the transverse alar ligament must be disrupted and the facture is highly unstable; Type 3 — Unilateral lateral mass fractures where the stability is determined by integrity of transverse ligament.

c. Atlanto-axial instability

There are two common types — sagittal or rotational instability.

C1–C2 sagittal instability — atlanto axial subluxations occurs when the transverse alar ligament is injured, and there is abnormal translation of the odontoid with respect to the atlas. This subluxation is best demonstrated on lateral radiographs. A distance greater than 4 mm between the posterior aspect of the anterior arch of C1 and the anterior aspect of the odontoid process is indicative of injury.

C1–C2 rotatory instability — while this type of injury is most commonly seen in children, it can occur in adults with even after minor trauma. Patients present with torticollis. The injury is best diagnosed with an open mouth odontoid view, which shows an asymmetry in the gap between the lateral aspect of the odontoid process and the lateral masses of C1 on each side. There may be accompanying decrease in the joint space between C1 and C2 lateral masses.

d. Axis fractures

The C2 vertebra is the largest of the cervical vertebrae and certainly the most peculiar in shape. Axis fractures account for 18% of all cervical spine fractures. Of the axis fractures 60% are odontoid fractures, 20% percent are Hangman's fracture and the remaining 20% are fractures of the body, pedicles, lateral masses, laminae, and spinous processes.

Odontoid fractures — the odontoid process is the bony protuberance of C2 that projects upwards and is held in contact with C1 by the transverse alar ligament. Fractures can be easily identified in lateral and open-mouth view radiographs but are best characterized by CT scan. These fractures are classified into three types by Anderson and D'Alonzo.[4] Type I fracture is an avulsion of the tip of the odontoid process by the apical ligament, and is generally stable. Type II fractures occur at the waist region of the odontoid process where the vascular supply is a watershed region. As a result of the propensity for poor healing and non-union, intervention is usually required. Type III fractures extend into the body of C2 and do require intervention. Bone healing is generally good in this type. Risk factors for non-union include systemic factors, such as osteoporosis, diabetes mellitus, smoking, and rheumatoid arthritis; and local factors, such as >11 degrees angulation, >5 mm displacement, and posterior displacement. Treatment varies from rigid collar, to halo to surgery.

e. Hangman's fracture

Also referred to as traumatic spondylolisthesis of the axis, this type of fracture is usually caused by a hyperextension type mechanism sometimes associated with an axial load. The fracture involves the posterior elements, more specifically the pars inter-articularis bilaterally. Patients usually present with neck pain and more often are neurologically intact. Hangman's fractures are classified into types I, II, IIA, and III, by Levine and Edwards, depending upon the amount of displacement, the degree of angulation, and integrity of the C2–3 intervertebral disc. Treatment varies from rigid collar, to halo to surgery.

f. Sub-axial spine fractures (C3–7)

Injuries that can occur in the sub-axial cervical spine include fractures, subluxations, dislocations, compressions and a combination of those. The most common sub-axial vertebra that is fractured is C5, while the C5–6 level is the most common site of sub-axial subluxations. The reason for this is that in the cervical spine the greatest flexion and extension occurs at the C5–6 levels.

Sub-axial Injury Classification (SLIC) Scale[5]

This is a now widely used scoring system to help direct management of sub-axial spinal injury. It constitutes three aspects of the injury — fracture morphology, disco-ligamentous complex, and neurological status. Fracture morphology can be compression, burst, distraction and rotation or translation. The disco-ligamentous complex refers to the soft tissues that hold the spine together and include the intervertebral discs, facet joint capsule, ligamentun flavum, interspinous and supraspinous ligaments. The disco-ligamentous complex can be rated as intact, disrupted or indeterminate. The neurological status is scored on intact, root injury, complete cord injury, incomplete cord injury and continuous cord compression with neurological deficit. The sum of scores in each category is obtained. Total score <4 suggests nonoperative management, >4 operative management and score of 4 is equivocal.

3. *Thoracic spine fractures (T1–T10)*[6]

Thoracic spine injury mechanisms are similar to those of the cervical spine. There are certain common injury morphologies associated with the thoracic spine. These include compression fractures, burst fractures, Chance fractures and fracture-dislocations. The thoracic spine is however innately stable due in part to facet joint alignment, in addition to the presence of the rib cage and sternum that function as a strut. This inherent stability means that high energy forces are required to produce injury with neurological deficit. The very narrow spinal canal, less than usual arterial blood supply to the thoracic cord and high energy force required for unstable fractures to be produced, all contribute to significant neurological deficit when thoracic spinal fractures occur. Due to the high energy forces many unstable thoracic spine fractures are accompanied by other organ injury such as cardiac contusion, pulmonary contusions, rib fractures, cardiac tamponade, pneumothoraces, sternal fractures and large vessel injury many of which require ICU admission for monitoring and management.[7]

a. **Anterior Wedge Compression Fractures** — are the result of axial loading and are the most frequent type of thoracic fractures especially in older osteoporotic patients. These fractures are rarely associated with neurological injury and are usually managed conservatively, with or without a brace. About 50% loss in body height and greater than 30° angulation suggest instability.
b. **Burst Fractures** are usually produced from an axial loading mechanism, where the anterior and middle columns are injured. There may be accompanying middle column retropulsion and resulting spinal cord compression. The loss of height of the vertebral body causes a shearing force on the lamina and occasional vertical lamina fractures that may result in dural tears and entrap nerves. Unstable fractures are defined by those with neurological deficit or those that have greater than 50% height loss, greater than 30° angulation or greater than 40% retropulsion.[8] Unstable fractures are treated with brace or if there is movement in the brace, by surgical intervention.
c. **Flexion–Distraction injury** — also known as Chance fractures, and involve the middle and posterior columns. These types of fractures have been divided into ligamentous or bony Chance fractures. Injury through the posterior ligaments and into the intervertebral discs almost always warrants surgical intervention. Injury through the bone however with less than 30° angulation, may be treated with a brace. Log roll precautions must be strict here as rotational forces can worsen the fracture with ensuing SCI. CT and MRI scans are very useful to assess the degree of ligamentous versus bony injury.
d. **Fracture-Dislocation** — involves all three columns and is highly unstable. Neurological deficits are common, and surgical intervention must always be considered. Mechanisms include a combination of flexion, rotation and subluxation.

4. *Thoracolumbar junction fractures (T11–L1)*[6]

Although a relatively short segment of the spine, this junction has a high injury rate because it is where the relatively immobile thoracic spine meets a highly mobile lumbar spine. Mechanism of injury usually includes hyperflexion with some degree of rotation. These kinds of fractures are very susceptible to rotational forces and thus log roll precautions must be meticulously applied. Because the spinal cord terminates (conus medullaris) at this level, compression of the cord will produce not only motor weakness and sensory loss in lower limbs, but also bowel and bladder dysfunction accompanied by perineal numbness.

5. *Lumbar fractures*

Morphology and mechanisms of injury are very much similar to that of the thoracic and thoracolumbar spine.[6,8] The difference however is that instead of the spinal cord, the cauda equina is involved, thus the chance of complete neurological deficit is very low.

Thoracolumbar Injury Classification and Severity Score (TLICS)[9]

This is similar to the previously described SLIC system. The aim of the scoring system is also to aid in guiding treatment. This scale also focuses on three characteristics of the injury–fracture morphology, posterior ligamentous complex and neurological status. Morphology can be compression, burst, rotation or translation and distraction. Posterior ligamentous complex can be intact, injured or indeterminate. Neurologic status is classified into intact, root injury, complete, incomplete and cauda equina. Total score <4 suggests nonoperative management, >4 operative management and score of 4 is equivocal.

Penetrating Injuries

Penetrating injuries to the spine, while a relatively uncommon cause of SCI, is on the rise. The usual causes are gunshot wounds (GSW) and knife injuries. In general these injuries tend to be stable, unless a large portion of the vertebra is destroyed. Studies have shown that of the unstable spinal cases due to GSWs, 75% were found to be cervical.

The pathway of the bullet or knife is very useful in helping to determine which structures may be involved, and thus what investigations should be ordered. For example a penetrating injury to the neck may warrant further investigations such as angiography, esophagoscopy, gastrograffin swallow and bronchoscopy to rule out trauma to vessels or hollow viscous. The extent of injury of a bullet is determined somewhat by the amount of kinetic energy it possesses. The kinetic energy of an object is related to the mass (m) and velocity (v) which is the most important determinant as given by the formula: $\frac{1}{2}mv^2$. Low-energy bullets, example from a handgun, travel at speeds between 1000–2000 ft/s. High-energy bullet e.g., from an assault rifle, travel at speeds over 2000 ft/s. Bullets that remain within the body tend to do significantly more harm than those that exit the body because all of the kinetic energy is transferred from the bullet to the body when the bullet remains lodged within the patient.

Bullets cause injury by laceration, crush, cavitation and blast mechanisms. Neurological injury can also occur when bullets either traverse the neural structures or pass near them. Neurological recovery from GSW is very limited. Surgical decompression is sometimes warranted, but there is usually a high incidence of CSF leaks, and infections. Perhaps the most reasonable indication for bullet removal is a patient with an intra-canal bullet who presents with an incomplete injury. There is no role for steroids in penetrating SCI.

Vascular Injuries

Injury to the carotids and vertebral arteries are seen in up to 25% of patients with head and neck trauma. Vascular injuries are more likely in the following situations: C1–3 fractures, cervical subluxation and fractures involving the foramen tranversarium. The vertebral artery enters the foramen transversarium at the C6 level in 94% of individuals, and in C7 in less than 2%.

Carotid injury — While blunt trauma can cause carotid injury by direct blow, hyper-rotation, hyperextension and bone fragments, more than 90% of carotid injuries is caused by penetrating trauma. Mortality ranges from 10–30%, and permanent neurological deficit from 15–55%. Penetrating trauma can cause partial or complete transection of the carotid, pseudoaneurysm and arteriovenous fistula. Expanding pseudoaneuryms can lead to airway obstruction, and compression of neural elements such as the brachial plexus. Blunt trauma can cause intimal flaps, carotid wall hematomas, and carotid dissection leading to complete occlusion of the vessel. Clinical signs that will suggest a vascular injury include: Expanding neck hematoma, absent carotid pulse, vascular neck bruit, Horner's syndrome, cranial nerve dysfunction (IX–XII), unilateral upper limb neurological deficits. Up to half of the patients with vascular injury may not be recognized because of the often concomitant head injury, recreational drug use, alcohol intoxication or shock.

Vertebral artery injury — the incidence is very low, 2–8%. It occurs mainly with penetrating trauma, especially GSW. Blunt trauma, such as motor vehicle accidents, near hangings, and extreme chiropractic manipulation can cause vertebral artery injury be means of sudden rotation, hyperextension, fractures and subluxations.

Diagnosis and treatment — CT angiography is the best tool to diagnose vascular trauma in cervical spine injuries. Active pulsatile bleeding with expanding hematoma may warrant immediate surgical intervention if directed external pressure does not stop the bleeding. Penetrating carotid injury and completely occluded blunt carotid injury are best treated with primary repair. If distal circulation is normal and there is no active bleeding then conservative management should be considered. Blunt carotid and vertebral artery injury with intimal tears that are extra cranial, can be treated with systemic anticoagulation, first with IV heparin, and then followed by oral anticoagulation for at least 3 months. This is provided when there are no contraindications to anticoagulation at the time of injury. The aim of treatment in the acute phase is to prevent thrombus formation, propagation and embolization, and to maintain cerebral perfusion. In vertebral artery injury, angiographic embolization is the preferred treatment, and surgery is only indicated rarely if bleeding persists or embolization has failed.

SCIWORA

SCI without Radiographic Abnormality is the term given to the occurrence of acute SCI without evidence of trauma radiographically. This phenomenon is typically described in the pediatric age group where the very mobile joints, flat facets, disproportionally large head, growth plates not fused, and elastic ligaments all facilitate abnormal movements without bony injury. While associated with good prognosis, long-term sequelae do occur in some patients.

Non-Traumatic SCI

There are many non-traumatic causes of acute SCI. These include spinal infections, tumors and other compressive lesions, vascular causes, demyelinating conditions, toxins, autoimmune diseases and nutritional deficiencies. Infections produce acute myelopathy by means of spinal epidural abscess, with a relatively low incidence of 0.2–1.2 per 10,000 admissions. Risk factors for developing spinal epidural abscesses include diabetes mellitus, IV drug use, spinal instrumentation, urinary tract infections, immunosuppression, dental caries, degenerative joint disease and inflammatory bowel disease. The most common site of infection is the thoracic spine. About 50% are from hematogenous spread from distant source of infection. The most infections are ***Staphylococcus aureus***, followed by ***Streptococcus*** and Gram-negative Bacilli.

Spinal cord tumors produce SCI either by direct compression or by invasion into the cord. Tumors are classified by location, (extradural, intradural extra-medullary and intramedullary). Each location has a differential diagnosis. Extradural tumors are usually metastases from the paired organs (lung, breast, prostate). Myeloma is the only primary tumor that will invade into the spine. Intradural extra medullary tumors include schwannoma, meningioma and neurofibrom as common examples. Intramedullary tumors include ependymoma and astrocytoma. The symptomatology from tumor compression tends to occur over a period of time and include motor and sensory loss, with proprioception, bladder and bowel dysfunction.

Vascular events such as acute spinal cord ischemia can occur with aortic dissection, aortic surgery with prolonged clamp times, spinal dural arteriovenous fistula or arteriovenous malformations. Symptoms can present acutely when there is hemorrhage, but typically presents over a prolonged course due to progressive venous congestion.

Scales and Grading

American Spinal Injury Association (ASIA) Impairment Scale — All spinal cord lesions can be classified using the ASIA Scale. This scale distinguishes incomplete from complete SCI. Incomplete injuries have relatively good prognosis for recovery and influence timing of surgical intervention. Patients with complete injuries have a 3% chance of some return of motor function in the first 24 hours and no chance of return of function after 24–48 hours.

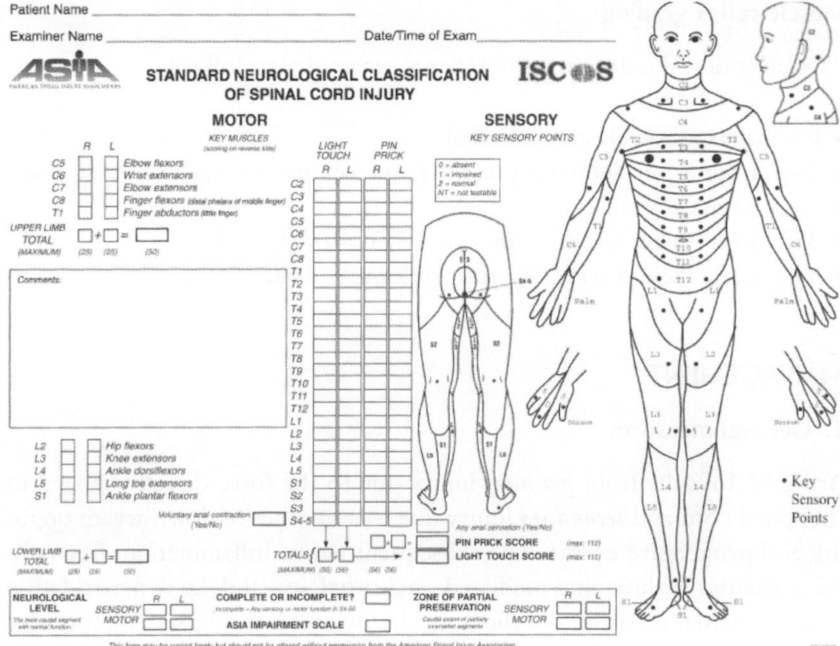

Patient Name

Examiner Name Date/Time of Exam

ASIA — STANDARD NEUROLOGICAL CLASSIFICATION OF SPINAL CORD INJURY — ISCoS

MOTOR

KEY MUSCLES

	R	L	
C5			Elbow flexors
C6			Wrist extensors
C7			Elbow extensors
C8			Finger flexors (distal phalanx of middle finger)
T1			Finger abductors (little finger)

UPPER LIMB TOTAL (MAXIMUM) (25) + (25) = (50)

Comments:

	R	L	
L2			Hip flexors
L3			Knee extensors
L4			Ankle dorsiflexors
L5			Long toe extensors
S1			Ankle plantar flexors

Voluntary anal contraction (Yes/No)

LOWER LIMB TOTAL (MAXIMUM) (25) + (25) = (50)

SENSORY

KEY SENSORY POINTS

LIGHT TOUCH R L — PIN PRICK R L

C2, C3, C4, C5, C6, C7, C8, T1, T2, T3, T4, T5, T6, T7, T8, T9, T10, T11, T12, L1, L2, L3, L4, L5, S1, S2, S3, S4-5

0 = absent
1 = impaired
2 = normal
NT = not testable

Any anal sensation (Yes/No)

TOTALS (MAXIMUM) (56) (56) (56) (56)

PIN PRICK SCORE (max: 112)

LIGHT TOUCH SCORE (max: 112)

NEUROLOGICAL LEVEL — The most caudal segment with normal function — SENSORY R L, MOTOR R L

COMPLETE OR INCOMPLETE? — Incomplete = Any sensory or motor function in S4-S5

ASIA IMPAIRMENT SCALE

ZONE OF PARTIAL PRESERVATION — Caudal extent of partially innervated segments — SENSORY R L, MOTOR R L

This form may be copied freely but should not be altered without permission from the American Spinal Injury Association.

This form may be copied freely but should not be altered without permission from the ASIA.

Muscle Strength Grading

Muscle strength is graded by the Medical Research Council (MRC) scale

Grade	Description
0	No contraction
1	Flicker or trace of contraction
2	Active movement with gravity eliminated
3	Active movement against gravity
4*	Active movement against gravity and resistance
5	Normal power

* Grades 4–, 4, and 4+ are sometimes used to indicate movement against slight, moderate and strong resistance respectively.

Muscle reflex grading

By convention the deep tendon reflexes are graded as follows:

- 0 = no response; always abnormal
- 1+ = a slight but definitely present response; may or may not be normal
- 2+ = a brisk response; normal
- 3+ = a very brisk response; may or may not be normal
- 4+ = a tap elicits a repeating reflex (clonus); always abnormal

MANAGEMENT

1. General measures

Acute SCI results from *primary* injury due to the force directly applied to the spinal cord and *secondary* injury due to a number of downstream ongoing and progressive events. The subsequent neuro-inflammation, free radical formation, glutamine-mediated excitotoxicity, and lipid peroxidation lead to gradual expansion of the initial lesion and astrogliosis. Additionally, spinal cord edema and reduced spinal cord blood flow worsen ischemic injury.

The management of SCI is directed at limiting secondary injury, creating environments favorable for cellular survival and regeneration, and optimizing neurologic outcomes. Furthermore, appropriate management of the challenges unique to SCI patients, including airway management in an unstable cervical spine, cardiorespiratory complications of sympathetic interruption, and sequelae of long-term immobility, are essential to improving survival. Principles of management for SCI include medical and intensive care therapy, pharmacotherapy, surgical decompression, and stabilization.

2. Surgery

Goals of surgical management in patients with traumatic spine and SCI are (1) to decompress neural tissue and (2) to prevent cord injury by ensuring mechanical stability of the spine. Options include initial bed rest in traction, external immobilization, and open reduction with internal fixation. Many clinicians have abandoned traction because of the complications associated with prolonged bed rest.

Unique Challenges in SCI Management

1. Airway

Airway management challenges in cervical spinal injury patients include maintenance of stability, prevention of repeated injury, and concurrent management of associated facial, neck, and pharyngeal injuries while establishing and maintaining patency of the airway. Rapid-sequence intubation with in-line spinal immobilization is the preferred method of intubation when a definitive airway is urgently required (see chapter on priorities in multiple trauma for further details on airway management). Manual in-line stabilization is imperative during spinal manipulation, and has been shown to limit cervical spine movement and is thought to be safer than axial traction. In elective scenarios, awake fiberoptic intubation with local anesthesia is preferred as it offers direct visualization without any movement of the cervical spine. Induction of anesthesia during airway management must be performed with special attention to maintain hemodynamic stability and avoid hypoxia, both of which can produce further injury to the spinal cord.

2. Respiratory management

Acute SCI patients, especially those with complete cervical injury, encounter a unique set of ventilation challenges. Depending on the level of injury, patients may experience interruption of phrenic (C3–5), intercostal (T1–11), and abdominal (T12–L1) innervation. In the most severe scenario, complete SCI above C3 leads to diaphragmatic paralysis and apnea, which is rapidly fatal. The loss of intercostal muscle innervation with preservation of the diaphragm allows for adequate tidal volume and resting breaths, but an inability to take breaths to the full inspiratory capacity. Flaccid paralysis of the intercostals lead to mechanically inefficient and work-intensive breathing because a significant proportion of the respiratory effort is lost to intercostal and chest wall in drawing. Finally, loss of the abdominal muscle function prevents forced exhalation and cough. Concomitant pulmonary injuries, including pneumothorax, hemothorax, and pulmonary contusions further diminish respiratory function. Chest wall injuries, rib fractures, and flail chest may further impair ventilation through mechanical compression and pain leading to poor cough or splinting of the chest wall. The combination of these factors results in varying degrees of respiratory failure warranting measures as discussed in other sections of the text including mechanical ventilation.

3. Cardiovascular system

Cardiac arrhythmias, abnormal cardiac contractility, sinus bradycardia, and neurogenic shock are commonly associated with SCI. The most pronounced cardiovascular changes are observed initially and often gradually improve over the next 2–6 weeks post injury. The careful management of hemodynamic instability can minimize secondary injury and improve clinical outcomes.

Various arrhythmias, including repolarization changes, atrioventricular blocks, supraventricular tachycardia, ventricular tachycardia, and primary cardiac arrest have been described, although sinus bradycardia is the most common cardiac abnormality in SCI patients. Bradycardia results from unopposed vagal stimulation and sympathetic interruption from SCI above T6. Atropine, a parasympatholytic anticholinergic agent, can be used to improve sinoatrial node pacing and atrioventricular conduction. A transcutaneous pacemaker or a temporary endocardial pacemaker electrode can be considered for symptomatic bradycardia refractory to conservative management.

Potential causes of hypotension in SCI patients with concomitant injuries include hemorrhagic shock, tension pneumothorax, myocardial injury, pericardial tamponade, and early sepsis. Neurogenic shock is specific to SCI above T6, and results from sympathetic disruption, decreased systemic vascular resistance (SVR) and pooling of blood in the arterioles and venous system; this results in a clinical picture of hypotension refractory to fluid resuscitation, relative bradycardia, and warm skin. Approximately 25% of cervical SCI patients experience a component of neurogenic shock, and patients with complete SCI are more likely to develop refractory hypotension. Treatment of neurogenic shock and maintenance of spinal cord and systemic perfusion has been shown to lead to favorable outcomes. The AANS (American Association of Neurological Surgeons) guidelines support the prevention of hypotension (systolic blood pressure <90mm Hg) and maintenance of a mean arterial pressure (MAP) of >85mm Hg for the first seven days after SCI.

Intravenous fluid resuscitation is the initial management, especially in the case of concomitant hemorrhagic shock. Crystalloids are preferred over colloids, especially in patients with concomitant TBI.[10] For neurogenic shock unresponsive to initial crystalloid resuscitation, vasopressors should be considered early to avoid iatrogenic fluid overload. To address both peripheral vasodilatation and bradycardia, a vasopressor with both α and β adrenergic activity should be selected. Dopamine, norepinephrine, and epinephrine will provide vasoconstriction and increase in heart rate, and are common first-line agents for treatment of neurogenic shock. Phenylephrine should be avoided due to its exclusive α-receptor activity and propensity to exacerbate reflex bradycardia through peripheral vasoconstriction and baroreceptor stimulation.

4. Venous thromboembolism

Deep venous thrombosis (DVT) and PE are common complications of SCI. The development of Venous Thromboembolism (VTE) is likely due to a multifactorial combination of stasis, hypercoagulability, vessel intimal injury, impaired circadian variations of hemostatic and fibrinolytic paramaters, and changes in platelet dysfunction and fibrinolytic activity.[11] In untreated acute SCI patients, the prevalence of VTE approaches 100% in some studies, with the greatest incidence between 3 and 14 days post injury.[12]

Low molecular weight heparin (LMWH) is preferred over oral anti-coagulation and unfractionated heparin (UFH), due to its efficacy, decreased bleeding risk, and short half-life. LMWH should be initiated within 72 hours of SCI, and continued for a 3 month period or until restoration of mobility. Despite LMWH administration, the risk of VTE continues to be 6–9%; mechanical prophylaxis, include rotating beds, intermittent pneumatic compression (IPC) stockings and electrical stimulation can be used concomitantly for decreased VTE risk.[13]

Despite pharmacologic and mechanical prophylaxis, VTEs continue to account for 10% of all deaths within the first year following SCI.[14] Due to the high risk of VTE development especially in tetraplegic patients, clinicians should have a low threshold for VTE screening and treatment.

5. Gastrointestinal system

SCI patients are at high risk for stress ulceration due to increased parasympathetic vagal tone. Gastrointestinal hemorrhage occurs in 3% of SCI patients during initial hospitalization, and are more common in older (>age 50) and tetraplegic patients. Prophylaxis with H2 antagonists is recommended upon admission for 4 weeks.[15]

Patients unable to take oral feedings should be started as soon as tolerable on enteral feeds to maintain nutritional status. (NOTE- don't need to have bowel sounds or 'motility' to start feedings. For patients intolerant of enteral feeds, parental nutrition may be started in seven days with vigilance for catheter related and metabolic complications.

6. Integumentary system

In immobilized SCI patients, decubitus ulcers are prevalent in both acute and rehabilitation settings, and are most common in the sacrum and heels. Backboards should be used only to transport patients with potentially unstable spinal injury and removed as soon as possible, after which a thorough skin check should be performed for identification of ulcers. After spinal stabilization, the patient should be repositioned frequently. Specialized rotating beds can be used to dissipate impact and avoid ulcerations. Furthermore, identification and management of any underlying medical conditions and treatment of malnutrition and diabetes may contribute to optimal healing.[16]

7. Autonomic dysreflexia

Autonomic dysreflexia is a potentially life-threatening clinical symptom characterized by an unopposed reflex sympathetic discharge and acute hypertension. It is often provoked by a strong noxious sensory input below the level of SCI, usually in the form of urinary retention or fecal impaction. Among patients with SCI above T6, the incidence of autonomic dysreflexia was 48–90%, most commonly in the subacute period.

Patients with autonomic dysreflexia present with acute hypertension, headache, profuse sweating, facial erythema and blurred vision. Without prompt recognition, the hypertensive crisis can lead to end organ injury including retinal and cerebral hemorrhage, myocardial infarction and pulmonary edema. During episodes of autonomic dysreflexia, upright positioning to evoke orthostatic hypotension, prompt survey for precipitating causes, frequent monitoring of blood pressure, and administration of fast-acting antihypertensive medications are key. Hypertension resolves after correction of the underlying cause.

8. Orthostatic hypotension

Orthostatic hypotension, defined as either a symptomatic or a significant drop (>20 mm Hg systolic BP or >10mm Hg diastolic BP) in blood pressure within 2–5 minutes of upright positioning, results from excessive venous pooling in the lower extremities and viscera. It is commonly seen in the subacute period after SCI, and results from reduced efferent sympathetic output and the loss of reflex vasoconstriction below the level of injury. This results in reduction of end-diastolic volume and ventricular stroke volume, which manifests as a decrease in blood pressure and symptoms of light-headedness, dizziness, fatigue, dyspnea, and syncope. In SCI patients, prolonged immobility and recumbency lead to muscular and cardiovascular deconditioning which can exacerbate orthostatic hypotension. Other contributory factors include rapid positional change, decreased circulatory volume, heavy meals, and medications (diuretics, antidepressants, α-blockers, and narcotics).

Orthostatic hypotension can be managed with maintenance of euvolemia, compression stockings and abdominal binders to prevent peripheral pooling of blood, gradual tilt-table implementation, maintenance of head-up tilt during sleep, and use of reclining wheelchair. Medications shown to be of benefit include midodrine, an oral α-agonist, and fludrocortisone, a mineralocorticoid that protects intravascular fluid volume through sodium retention. Caution should be taken in treatment of patients with pre-existing congestive heart failure, and patients with persistent bradycardia as these conditions can be aggravated.

9. Corticosteroids therapy

Methylprednisolone sodium succinate (MPSS) is a synthetic glucocorticoid with proposed neuroprotective mechanisms including stabilization of neuronal membranes, decreasing TNF-α release, improving spinal cord perfusion, and reducing neuronal calcium influx. It has been investigated in several human RCTs including the landmark National Acute SCI Study (NASCIS) I–III. Analysis of these trials demonstrates that corticosteroids administered within 8 hours of SCI may provide benefit. However, adverse complications including increased rates of wound infections, sepsis, pulmonary complications, gastrointestinal complications, urinary tract infections, and steroid myopathy were more consistently seen.

In the context of inconsistent benefits and clear complications, the AANS guidelines do not support the use of corticosteroids for the treatment of acute SCI. However, corticosteroid use in SCI continues to be a topic of contention, and some clinicians may administer it for a 24 or 48 hour period in a selective population, specifically young, non-diabetic, non-immunocompromised patients presenting within 8 hours of non-penetrating, incomplete cervical SCI, where benefits are most appreciable.

10. Spasticity

Spasticity is very common in SCI, but is not an inevitable long-term sequelae. Onset is variable and occurs weeks after the injury. There are many different definitions for spasticity, the most popular being — "Spasticity is a motor disorder characterized by a velocity-dependent increase in tonic stretch reflexes (muscle tone) with exaggerated tendon jerks, resulting from hyper-excitability of the stretch reflex, as one component of the upper motor neuron syndrome". About 65–80% of patients with SCI develop spasticity. There are no reliable predictors of spasticity; however it is found that the spinal level and ASIA grade are correlated with the development of spasticity. For patients with ASIA A grade, 93% develop spasticity in the cervical level patients while 78% reported spasticity in the thoracic level patients. Additionally, of the cervical level patients, those with ASIA B–D, 73% develop spasticity, compared to the 93% previously mentioned for ASIA A patients.

Management

(1) Physical Therapy and Rehabilitation are essential parts of spasticity treatment, and should ideally be started as early as possible, and continued in the long term. Some of the techniques used include positioning, range of motion exercises, stretching, weight bearing and muscle strengthening.
(2) Systemic pharmacological treatments is another option. Most medications that help alleviate spasticity can be grouped into three major classes — (a) Drugs that act at interneurons that use the neurotransmitter gamma-aminobutyric acid (GABA) in the central nervous system (CNS), such as baclofen and diazepam; (b) alpha-2-adrenergic medications that act at alpha-2 receptors in the CNS such as tizanidine and clonidine and (c) peripheral acting drugs that act at the neuromuscular level such as dantrolene.

In individuals that do not respond to oral medications or if the side effect profile is too severe for continued administration then intrathecal baclofen is an option. A pump, with a built-in reservoir is surgically implanted in the subcutaneous tissue of the anterior abdominal wall. This pump is connected to a tube that allows direct delivery of baclofen into the cerebrospinal fluid. The dosage can be adjusted with an external computer. By circumventing the blood–brain barrier baclofen concentration of up to four times the amount delivered by oral means can be achieved with only 1% of the oral dose. Intrathecal baclofen pumps are widely considered to be the most popular and most successful modality of treating spasticity. Other less commonly used therapies include phenol and ethanol injections into the spinal cord, botulinum toxin injections into the muscles (used mainly for focal spasticity), surgical management (selective rhizotomy and tendon lengthening procedures).

11. Pain management

There are many different sources of pain in a spinal cord injured patient. Pain may be primary and arise from the initial trauma to pain sensitive soft tissues and bones acutely. This can be treated with narcotics, acetaminophen and non-steroidals. Judicious use of non-steroidal anti-inflammatory medications should be considered with caution because they can negatively impact on bone healing, particularly if instrumented fusion is performed on the patient. Addressing the patients' pain may be difficult initially because many times the patient may not be able to express their pain due to sedation, associated head injury or the patient may be intubated. A spinal cord injured patient, who is unable to communicate, may present with tachycardia, increase in blood pressure but not necessarily with an increase in heart rate, agitation and confusion. Many of these signs and symptoms can be explained by other treatable medical conditions such as pneumonia, urinary tract infections, DVT's and PE, and thus these need to be investigated and ruled out.

In contrast to acute pain, chronic pain is much more difficult to treat. Studies have shown that up to 82% of spinal cord injured patients have pain at 25 years post injury. The pain is divided into two broad categories: Musculoskeletal and neuropathic pain. In complete SCI the musculoskeletal pain is only experienced above the level of the lesion, however in incomplete SCI, musculoskeletal pain can be experienced below the level of the lesion. Treatment of musculoskeletal pain is aimed at treatment of the underlying condition — such as poor posture, overuse and spasticity.

Neuropathic pain is much more difficult to treat than musculoskeletal pain. It can occur at or below the level of the lesion, and varies in presentation, e.g., allodynia (pain evoked by normally non-noxious stimuli) and hyperalgesia (an increased response to noxious stimuli). Neuropathic pain is a diagnosis of exclusion, and other causes of pain should be ruled out, such as disc herniation from injury, Charcot arthropathy and post-traumatic syrinx formation. There are 4 categories of neuropathic pain — pain that occurs below the level of injury, transition zone pain that occurs at the level of injury (usually bilateral), radicular pain (usually unilateral), and visceral pain. Pharmacological agents in the management of neuropathic pain fall into three classes — analgesics (opiods), antidepressants (amitriptyline, trazodone) and anticonvulsants (gabapentin, pregabalin, lamotrigine, valproaic acid, and tegretol).

12. Emerging neuroprotective therapies

A variety pharmacologic neuroprotective agents, cell replacement therapies, and interventional techniques have emerged over the past few decades and are actively undergoing human clinical research for establishment of safety and efficacy.

Minocycline, a synthetic tetracycline antibiotic with anti-inflammatory and anti-apoptotic properties, and riluzole, a benzothiazole sodium-channel blocker which inhibits presynaptic glutamate release, can be administered orally to mitigate neurotoxicity and neuroinflammation. A number of other experimental therapies, including cethrin, Mg–PEG (polyethylene glycol), and fibroblast growth factors (FGF) can be directly applied to the dura during laminectomy. Cethrin is a combination of fibrin sealant Tisseel and Rho-inhibtor BA-210, which works to prevent collapse of regenerating axonal growth cones. Mg–PEG is a combination of magnesium, a physiologic antagonist of NMDA receptors, and PEG, a hydrophilic polymer used for drug delivery, with independent neuroprotective properties. Lastly, FGF are a family of growth factors that have been shown to attenuate astrocyte activation, neuroinflammation, and scar formation. These pharmacologic therapies have all demonstrated efficacy and safety in animal studies and phase I trials, and are undergoing active investigation in larger human trials.

Stem cell transplantation is also an active area of research for SCI, as it offers a method of neuroprotection (in the form of anti-apoptotic and pro-angiogenic trophic factor secretion) and cell replacement. In addition to supporting and preserving surviving cells, they replace damaged neurons and glial cells, remyelinate surviving axons, and bridge lesion cavities across gliotic and scarred tissue. Bone marrow stromal cells, olfactory ensheathing cells, Schwann cells, activated autologous macrophages, human embryonic stem cells, and tissue derived adult neural stem cells have all been investigated in preclinical studies.[17]

Non-invasive or minimally invasive interventions have also captured interest for a possible role in SCI. Therapeutic hypothermia has been intensively studied in animal models and human conditions of cardiac arrest and TBI, and has been shown in laboratory studies to reduce cellular energy requirements, slow enzymatic activity, and decrease cerebral metabolic rate and glucose requirements. Additionally, CSF drainage to decrease intrathecal pressure, is investigated for its role in increasing spinal cord perfusion pressure, attenuate ischemia and provide neuroprotection. Both the techniques of therapeutic hypothermia and CSF drainage are undergoing human clinical trials for establishment of efficacy.

References

1. Harris TJ, Blackmore CC, Mirza SK *et al.* Clearing the cervical spine in obtunded patients. *Spine* 2008; 33(14): 1547–1553.
2. Muchow RD, Resnick DK, Abdel MP *et al.* Magnetic resonance imaging (MRI) in the clearance of the cervical spine in blunt trauma: A meta-analysis. *J Trauma* 2008; 64(1): 179–189.
3. Anderson PA, Montesano PX. Morphology and treatment of occipital condyle fractures. *Spine* 1988; 13(7): 731–736.
4. Anderson LD, D'Alonzo RT. Fractures of the odontoid process of the axis. *J Bone Joint Surg Am* 1974; 56(8): 1663–1674.
5. Vaccaro AR, Hulbert RJ, Patel AA *et al.* The subaxial cervical spine injury classification system: A novel approach to recognize the importance of morphology, neurology, and integrity of the disco-ligamentous complex. *Spine* 2007; 32(21): 2365–2374.
6. Magerl F, Aebi M, Gertzbein SD *et al.* A comprehensive classification of thoracic and lumbar injuries. *Eur Spine J* 1994; 3(4): 184–201.
7. Bailey CS, Dvorak MF, Thomas KC *et al.* Comparison of thoracolumbosacral orthosis and no orthosis for the treatment of thoracolumbar burst fractures: Interim analysis of a multicenter randomized clinical equivalence trial. *J Neurosurg Spine* 2009; 11(3): 295–303.
8. Denis F. The three column spine and its significance in the classification of acute thoracolumbar spinal injuries. *Spine* 1983; 8(8): 817–831.
9. Vaccaro AR, Lehman RA, Hurlbert RJ *et al.* A new classification of thoracolumbar injuries: The importance of injury morphology, the integrity of the posterior ligamentous complex, and neurologic status. *Spine* 2005; 30(20): 2325–2333.
10. Finfer S, Bellomo R, Boyce N *et al.* A comparison of albumin and saline for fluid resuscitation in the intensive care unit. *N Engl J Med* 2004; 350(22): 2247–2256.
11. Furlan JC, Fehlings MG. Cardiovascular complications after acute spinal cord injury: Pathophysiology, diagnosis, and management. *Neurosurg Focus* 2008; 25(5): E15.

12. Merli GJ, Crabbe S, Paluzzi RG *et al.* Etiology, incidence, and prevention of deep vein thrombosis in acute spinal cord injury. *Arch Phys Med Rehabil* 1993; 74(11): 1199–11205.
13. Ploumis A, Ponnappan RK, Maltenfort MG *et al.* Thromboprophylaxis in patients with acute spinal injuries: An evidence-based analysis. *J Bone Joint Surg Am* 2009; 91(11): 2568–2576.
14. DeVivo MJ, Krause JS, Lammertse DP. Recent trends in mortality and causes of death among persons with spinal cord injury. *Arch Phys Med Rehabil* 1999; 80(11): 1411–1419.
15. Wuermser LA, Parquier JN, Preiser JC *et al.* Spinal cord injury medicine. 2. Acute care management of traumatic and nontraumatic injury. *Arch Phys Med Rehabil* 2007; 88(3): S55–S61.
16. Olsen, M.A, Nepple JJ, Riew KD *et al.* Risk factors for surgical site infection following orthopaedic spinal operations. *J Bone Joint Surg Am* 2008; 90(1): 62–69.
17. Sahni V, Kessler KA. Stem cell therapies for spinal cord injury. *Nat Rev Neurol* 2010; 6(7): 363–372.

Chapter 20

Pelvic Fractures

Jameel Ali and Jeremie Larouche

Patients with pelvic fractures may have major hemorrhage from the fracture itself or from other major injuries and will often require care in the ICU at some point. Management of the hemodynamic, cardiopulmonary, coagulation, metabolic, acid–base and hypothermic derangements that frequently occur in such patients are discussed elsewhere in this textbook. Understanding issues specific to the pelvic fracture is crucial to optimize management of these patients. In this chapter, we discuss the clinical presentation, diagnosis, classification and principles of management that will guide the intensivist in caring for these patients.

Initial assessment of mechanical stability, as well as the application of a pelvic binder in hemodynamically compromised patients is a crucial first step in managing individuals with a pelvic fracture. For those injuries associated with ongoing hemodynamic compromise, clinicians must differentiate arterial from venous hemorrhage and urgently determine in consultation with the appropriate specialist whether the patient would benefit most from arterial embolization or retroperitoneal packing. Definitive management often involves both internal and external fixation options, the timing and priority of which requires consultation with the orthopedic surgeon.

Introduction

The care of pelvic fractures has evolved significantly over the last 50 years. As highlighted by Flint and Cryer,[1] the recognition of retroperitoneal bleeding associated with pelvic fractures as well as the difficulties in controlling it have lead to vastly different approaches. Initial enthusiasm for exploration of the hematoma and attempts at direct control of the source of bleeding quickly lost popularity as surgeons realized that there was often no discreet bleeding vessel and decompression of the hematoma too often resulted in exsanguination of the patient.[2] Instead, four major therapeutic modalities have evolved in the management of acute pelvic fractures. Various commercial and improvised pelvic binders, minimally invasive surgery via external fixators or percutaneous screw fixation, the use of Transcatheter Arterial Embolization (TAE), and retroperitoneal pelvic packing.

Despite these advances, there is no universally accepted algorithm in the management of the hemodynamically compromised patient with a pelvic fracture. A review of the literature reveals very contrasting practices by different institutions, with certain regional preferences. Regardless of the algorithm used, the challenge lies in adequately resuscitating the patient while identifying and controlling the hemorrhage. Three possible sources of bleeding exist[3]: (1) venous, from tearing or puncturing of pre-sacral venous plexuses, (2) from the cancellous surface of bone, and (3) arterial, from disruption of the anterior or posterior trunk of the internal iliac arteries or their branches. Patients may often have multiple sources of hemorrhage occurring simultaneously. Tamponade can normally be achieved in low pressure venous bleeding but it is not as effective in significant arterial bleeding. Conversely, non-specific embolization of supplying arteries does not decrease venous blood loss, and carries significant complications.[4] It is therefore imperative that physicians who are managing these severely injured patients collaborate as part of a multidisciplinary team, and consider each patient individually.

Classification

The pelvic ring is formed by three components: the left ilium, the right ilium, and the sacrum (Fig. 1). These are joined posteriorly by the left and right sacroiliac ligaments and anteriorly at the pubis symphysis. The sacrospinous and sacrotuberous ligaments, as well as the pelvic floor musculature provide further stability. Disruption at any one particular aspect of the ring usually leads to failure at a second point, and clinicians should be weary of diagnosing isolated pelvic ring injuries.

Injuries to the pelvic ring are normally classified according to one of two systems: the Young–Burgess classification (Table 1), or the Tile classification

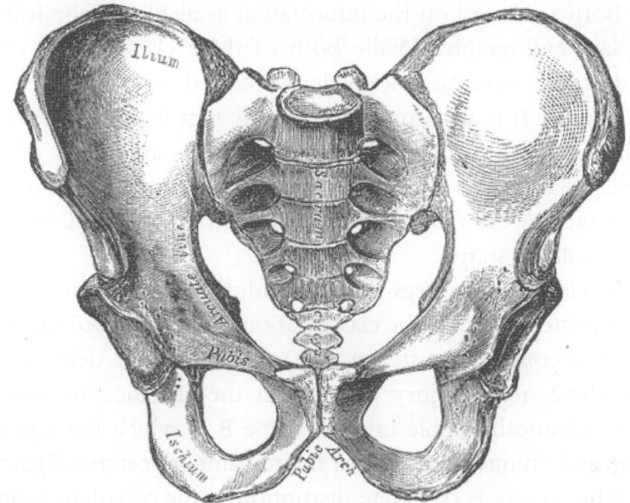

Fig. 1. Drawings of pelvic osseous anatomy.

Table 1. Tile classification of pelvic ring fractures.

Type A: Pelvic ring is stable	
A1	Fractures not involving the ring (avulsions, iliac crest or wing fractures)
A2	Stable, minimally displaced fractures of the pelvic ring
Type B: Pelvic ring is rotationally unstable, but vertically stable	
B1	Open book
B2	Lateral compression injury
B2-1	Anterior ring displacement through ipsilateral rami
B2–2	Anterior ring displacement through contralateral rami
B3	Anterior ring injury to bilateral rami
Type C: Pelvic ring is both rotationally and vertically unstable	
C1	Unilateral
C1-1	Posterior ring injury is iliac fracture
C1-2	Posterior ring injury is through sacroiliac fracture/dislocation
C1-3	Posterior ring injury is through sacral fracture
C2	Bilateral pelvic injury with one type B and one type C
C2	Bilateral pelvic injury with both sides type C

(Table 2). Both are based on the information available by physical examination and plain radiographs. While both of these classification systems are widely used, studies have historically demonstrated very little inter- or intraobserver reliability.[5] It is also important to note that fracture classification has little predictive ability to determine which patients are at risk of significant hemorrhage.[1,6] Physicians should therefore take into account not only the X-ray appearance of the fracture, but also the mechanism of injury and the patient's physiologic status.

The Tile classification uses the acetabulum to divide the pelvis into an anterior and posterior arch. The classification system is based on the stability of the sacroiliac complex (posterior arch) and is useful in determining treatment. The three major injury patterns in the classification are: Type A, which are mechanically stable injuries; Type B in which the anterior pelvis can open up and "hinge" on some of the remaining posterior ligaments; and Type C in which there is complete disruption of the osteoligamentous complex both anteriorly and posteriorly, resulting in both rotational and vertical instability.

The Young–Burgess classification focuses on the vector of force at the time of injury, and the resultant bony displacement. This force is divided into three categories: anterior to posterior compression that can result in "open book" injuries, lateral compression injuries with fractures through the ilium or the sacrum, and lastly vertical shear injuries in which one hemi-pelvis becomes detached from the remaining skeleton (Table 2).

Table 2. Young–Burgess classification of pelvic fractures.

(A) (B) (C) (D)

(E) (F) (G)

Epidemiology

There is an estimated incidence of 23 pelvic fractures per 100,000 persons per year in the USA.[5] Of these, approximately half are low energy, with a propensity to occur in geriatric patients with low bone mineral density. Reported mortality for these patients is <1%.[1] The other half occurs in younger patients in the setting of a high-energy trauma, and is associated with a higher injury severity score, a higher propensity for massive hemorrhage, and a mortality rate ranging from 19–50%.[2,5]

In their series of 174 patients with unstable pelvic ring injuries, O'Sullivan *et al.*[6] have demonstrated an association between mortality and an Injury Severity Score >25, a Triage-Revised Trauma Score less than 8, age over 65, systolic blood pressure <100 mmHg, a GCS <8, and a requirement for more than 10 units of blood in the first 24 hours. Morphology of the fracture was not predictive of mortality.

Physical Exam

All trauma patients should initially undergo a complete and thorough assessment according to the latest Advanced Trauma Life Support (ATLS) guidelines. Between 60–80% of patients with a pelvic ring injury will possess another musculoskeletal injury, and 8% will possess a lumbosacral plexus injury.[5] Assessment of pelvic injuries is a critical part of determining the source of hemorrhage in any hemodynamically compromised patient. It has been estimated that the retroperitoneum can accommodate up to 4L of blood prior to physiological tamponade of venous bleeding.[2] If there is significant disruption of the retroperitoneal muscle compartment, or if arterial bleeding exists, the patient may completely exsanguinate in the absence of acute intervention.

Assessment of pelvic stability

Determination of pelvic stability is required as part of the initial assessment of a polytraumatized patient. This should be done only once and performed gently to minimize pain and the disturbance of any clot that may have formed. It should be carried out by the most experienced physician available. It is performed by first having the examiner's thumbs placed over the anterior superior iliac spines of the patient, which are to be used as a reference point. The palms of the examiner then come to rest on the anterior inferior iliac spines, and from there, both a distraction and compression force may be applied (Fig. 2). Any movement of one hemi-pelvis compared to the contralateral side constitutes a positive examination. Fluoroscopy, if available in the trauma bay, may be a useful adjunct in this examination.

Application of Pelvic Binder

Any pelvis that is deemed to be mechanically unstable should have a pelvic binder applied immediately. While many physicians are concerned about the

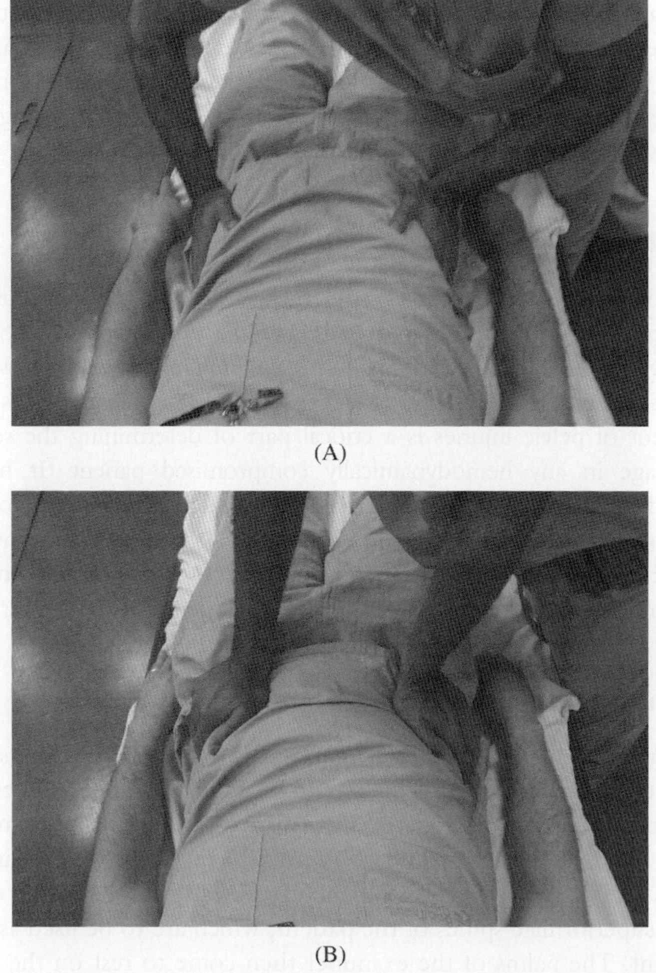

(A)

(B)

Fig. 2. Picture of how to assess for pelvic stability.

theoretical risk of inappropriately applying a binder to a lateral compression-type fracture and "over-reducing" the fragments, this must be weight against the possibility of not reducing a fracture that may directly affect the patients chance of survival. We therefore recommend the immediate application of a pelvic binder to any pelvis fracture that is mechanically unstable, which should be followed up with an anterior–posterior radiograph of the pelvis when possible to judge the quality of the reduction.

Applied properly, pelvic binders achieve two important goals. First, they reduce pelvic volume allowing for tamponade of a retroperitoneal hematoma. Secondly, they provide mechanical stability to the fracture, minimizing further soft tissue damage and alleviating pain. Three modalities are available to accomplish this goal: A folded bed sheet secured with towel clips, commercial binders such as the T-Pod or Sam Splint, or lastly via the use of a C-clamp or external fixator (Fig. 3). Circumferential bed sheets and commercial splints reduce the volume of the pelvis via an indirect reduction by applying pressure over the greater trochanters, and are easily applied in both a pre-hospital setting or in the trauma bay. The C-clamp, on the other hand, applies direct pressure on the outer table of the ilium, and must be applied by a surgeon in a controlled environment. Further stability in all three techniques may be obtained by taping the knees and ankles together to avoid significant external rotation forces upon the lower extremities (Fig. 4). It is also important to note that Tile C or Vertical Shear pelvic injuries may also require longitudinal traction to reduce the vertical component of the displacement, which should be performed prior to the application of a pelvic binder.

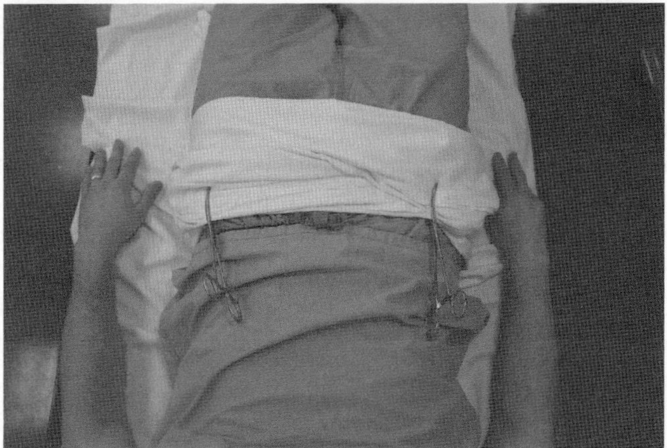

Fig. 3. Pictures of folded bed sheet, commercial binder, C-clamp.

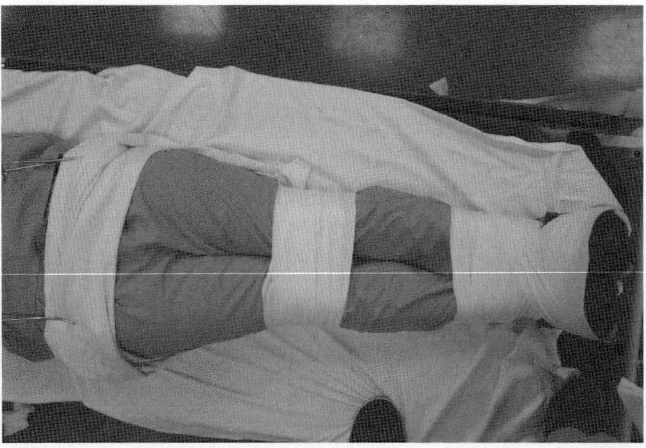

Fig. 4. Taping of knees and ankles to prevent external rotation.

Proper application of a circumferential pelvic binder ideally requires three personnel, but may be done with two, as the mechanical force generated by tightening the pelvic sheet is often inadequate to reduce the pelvis on its own.[7] Therefore, a manual reduction must be performed first, with the binder used secondarily to maintain the reduction. It is also imperative that the binder be placed over the trochanters and not directly over the abdomen. Binders which are placed too high are not only ineffective in reducing pelvic volume, but also are more likely to be removed during the resuscitation process as other physicians attempt to gain access to the abdomen.[7] If access to the groin is required, a hole may be cut in the binder without removing it. (Fig. 5) reveals the proper application of a pelvic sheet binder, as well as an example of how access to the femoral vein and artery may be obtained with a binder ***in situ***.

When comparing all three methods of pelvic stabilization, Pizanis *et al.* reported the experience from the German trauma registry in 207 hemodynamically compromised patients with pelvic ring injuries. They noted a significantly higher rate of lethal pelvic bleeding when sheet wrapping was used compared to binders or C-clamps (23% versus 4% versus 8%).[7] No significant difference in gender, fracture type, blood transfusion, blood hemoglobin concentration, arterial blood pressure, and injury severity score were observed among the three groups. In their conclusion, the authors suggest that the sheet wrapping may be a less appropriate mechanical tool as compared to available commercial binders and C-clamps, that they are more

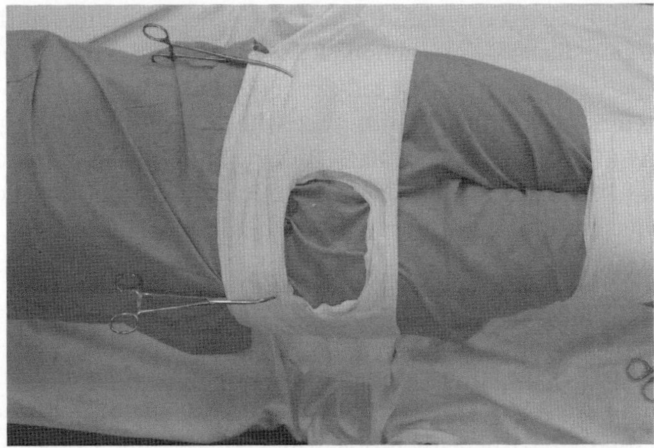

Fig. 5. Proper application of pelvic blinder with access to vessels.

commonly inappropriately applied, and that they are often removed prematurely to gain access to the abdomen to perform further diagnostic and therapeutic interventions. Despite these findings, it is extremely important to obtain an early and effective reduction of the pelvis regardless of the method used. Therefore, all physicians involved in the care of polytraumatized patients should familiarize themselves with any commercial splints that are available at their institution, and also review the proper technique of applying a circumferential binder.

Assessment of the lower urinary tract

Injuries of the lower urinary tract are commonly associated with pelvic ring trauma, with the literature often reporting 4% rate of bladder injury and a 2% rate of urethral injuries.[1] Physicians should perform a careful urological examination looking for blood at the urethral meatus, perineal ecchymosis, or lacerations surrounding the perineum. In men, a high riding or 'boggy' prostate should be ruled out while performing the digital rectal examination. As part of the trauma resuscitation protocol, an attempt should be made to pass a Foley catheter transurethrally if there is no clinical contraindication. If any resistance is encountered, a retrograde urethrogram should first be performed to avoid further damage to the urethra.

Historically, urethral disruptions have been treated with the placement of a suprapubic catheter and a delayed repair. This technique, however, is associated with certain complications, such as stricture formation that often require surgical dilatation and a high rate of sexual dysfunction. More recent evidence has demonstrated that early endoscopic repair of urethral disruption versus delayed treatment is associated with an earlier return to spontaneous voiding (35 days versus 229 days), decreased rate of stricture formation (14% versus 100%) and improved long term sexual function.[1] Early consultation with the urologist in managing these injuries is recommended.

Open Pelvic Injuries

An open pelvic fracture is not only one that penetrates the skin but also one that communicates with adjacent structures such as the bladder and bowel. These fractures are particularly problematic, both because of their increased risk of infection and their tendency to be associated with increased bleeding as the hematoma is decompressed.[1] When an open pelvic fracture with active bleeding is encountered, the initial response should be to pack the injury with sterile, radio-opaque sponges to allow tamponade of the bleeding. If multiple sponges are required, they may be tied together so as to facilitate their retrieval, and the number of sponges used recorded in the chart. The more difficult diagnosis to establish is that of the occult open pelvic fracture, which can often occur through the perineum, the vaginal vault, or through the rectal mucosa. It is therefore essential to prove that all high-energy pelvic fractures are not open, and a detailed physical examination must be performed. This examination should not, however, compromise pelvic stability or displace pelvic binders that are already in place. Occasionally, this detailed examination may have to be deferred until provisional stability of the pelvis is obtained.

As part of the examination, inspection of the perineum should be carried out to assess for open fractures. Even small puncture wounds or lacerations should be assumed to represent an open fracture, particularly if they are associated with ongoing venous bleeding. In all patients, a digital rectal examination should also be performed to assess for the possibility of an open fracture. If ambiguity exists, sigmoidoscopy should be performed for more complete assessment.[1] In women with suspected pubic bone fractures, a vaginal speculum exam should be undertaken.

If an open fracture is suspected, antibiotic prophylaxis should commence immediately, and the orthopedic surgeon notified so that he or she may plan for a thorough irrigation and debridement. A tetanus booster should also be administered if appropriate. Lastly, the role of fecal flow diversion in an open pelvic fracture is controversial. Discussion between the orthopedic and general surgeon should occur to review each case individually.

Neurological examination

Approximately 20% of patients sustaining a pelvic fracture will present with a neurological abnormality. These often account for the most common long term disabilities after a pelvic fracture, and include neurogenic pain, parasthesias, muscle wasting, and erectile dysfunction.[1] The mechanisms of these injuries are either from traction to the lumbar plexus during displacement of one hemi-pelvis, or due to direct neural injury sustained secondarily to a sacral fracture affecting the nerve roots as they exit the neural foramina.

The basic principles guiding the management of these injuries are to: minimize ongoing insult to the neural elements and prevent secondary injuries. As such, all displaced pelvic fractures should be rapidly reduced, and temporarily stabilized with the use of a pelvic binder. A detailed neurological exam should be performed both pre- and post-reduction. Careful attention should be paid to cross-sectional imaging to determine if there is ongoing compression of the neural elements that may be amenable to surgical decompression.

Radiographic Assessment

A plain AP radiograph of the pelvis as part of the trauma assessment of the patient provides sufficient information for clinicians to diagnose an unstable pelvic fracture in the vast majority of cases. One exception to this rule is where X-rays have been obtained with a pelvic binder already in place, as it is possible to reduce a rotationally unstable pelvis so that it appears anatomic on radiographs. It there is any doubt as to whether a subtle injury exists, a second X-ray should be obtained after the pelvic binder has been removed.

As part of the trauma work-up, computed tomography (CT) scans are performed in most institutions, and purportedly reduce the time from diagnosis to treatment.[8] Although definitive evidence is lacking, whole body CT scans will increasingly become a part of the assessment of polytraumatized patients because of claims that whole body CT scans may reduce trauma related mortality. This must be considered in the context of the theoretical increased risks associated with the radiation itself. CT scans of the pelvis reveal fractures as well as significant hematoma formation. With intravenous contrast agents, active extravasation (identified by a 'blush') of the contrast medium may signify an arterial injury. This technique has been further refined by multiphasic techniques, which often include a delayed phase revealing contrast pooling, as well as the adjunct use of a formal CT angiography.

It is important for physicians to note that the presence of a blush on CT scan does not necessarily mandate an intervention. Given the sensitivity of multi-detector computed tomography (MDCT) scanners, it is often possible to detect contrast extravasation that does not carry any clinical significance. Verbeek *et al.* reviewed 162 polytrauma patients with pelvic fractures and 134 patients with isolated pelvic fractures looking for a pelvic blush. They determined that 42% and 40% of these patients, respectively, had a positive pelvic blush on MDCT. Only half of these patients (47% and 51%) required either a surgical or radiological procedures for pelvic hemorrhage control.[8] They therefore concluded that many patients with a positive blush and stable vitals could be managed conservatively, and that the need for an intervention in the setting of a pelvic blush should be reserved to those with clinical signs of ongoing bleeding.[8]

Initial Management of the Hemodynamically Compromised Patient with a Pelvic Fracture

The primary goal in managing a hemodynamically compromised patient with a pelvic ring injury is the prevention of death secondary to hemorrhage. As such, while acute resuscitative efforts are underway, identification and control of internal hemorrhage is of paramount importance. Physicians should be aware that high-energy pelvic fractures rarely occur as an isolated injury. Patients should be carefully screened for abdominal, thoracic, and head injuries. Approximately 70% of patients with a pelvic ring disruption will also sustain other musculoskeletal injuries, which may also contribute to ongoing blood loss.

When managing a hemodynamically compromised patient, physicians should recognize that hemorrhage from disruption of the pelvic ring can occur through three different sources, and more than one modality may be required to achieve hemostasis. Bleeding from displaced cancellous bony surfaces responds best to reduction and immobilization of the fracture. Bleeding from venous origin also typically responds to fluid resuscitation and the reduction of the fracture through the application of a pelvic binder. In cases where there is only a transient response or no response, pelvic packing against a stabilized pelvis may be required. Lastly, bleeding of arterial origin responds best to direct embolization of the vessel in question. It is often impossible to distinguish the relative contribution of each of these sources based on physical examination and imaging assessment. As such, constant monitoring of the patients response to resuscitative efforts is required, and more than one type of intervention may be necessary.

Arterial Inflow Arrest

Arterial inflow arrest has been utilized as a means to temporarily occlude blood flow to the distal torso, pelvis and legs, allowing the trauma team to "catch-up" with resuscitative efforts. It allows blood flow to be redistributed to the coronary vessels, lungs, and brain. It is typically performed through one of two methods; direct cross clamping of the descending thoracic aorta through an emergency thoracotomy, or via percutaneous balloon technique. Arterial inflow arrest should be reserved only for patients who are imminently on the verge of exsanguination, and discontinued as soon as hemostasis and adequate resuscitation are achieved.

Pelvic Packing

Patients with ongoing bleeding from either cancellous bone surfaces or from venous plexuses can effectively be managed with pre-peritoneal pelvic packing (PPP). Cothren *et al.*[9] describe a standard technique whereby the pelvis is initially stabilized with either an anterior external fixator or a C-clamp. A midline incision is then made starting from the pubis symphysis is then extended 6–8 cm cephalad. From there, the fascia is divided in the midline. The pelvic hematoma is encountered once the transversalis fascia is opened. Surgeons must be careful to avoid entry into the pelvic peritoneum. Three standard laparotomy sponges are then inserted in the true pelvis on either side of the bladder. The fascia is closed with a 0-PDS suture, and the skin is closed with staples (Fig. 6).

The advantage of this technique is that it allows rapid tamponade of venous bleeding, which historically accounts for approximately 80–95% of all pelvic fracture patients who are hemodynamically compromised.[2,9,10] It may also be performed in conjunction with a trauma laparotomy, using the same positioning and surgical preparation. In their study, Cothren *et al.* reported a significant decrease in the number of red blood cell units required before PPP as compared to the next 24-hour period (12 ± 2.0 versus 6 ± 1.1; $p = 0.006$),

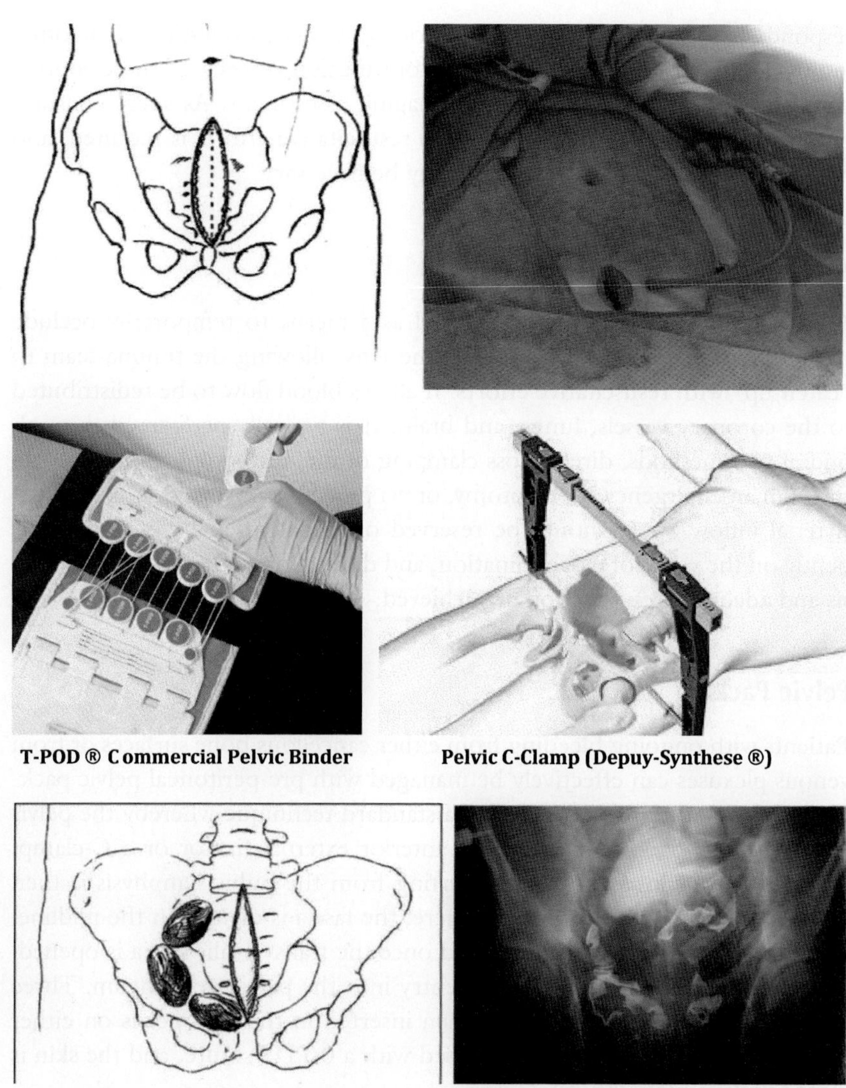

T-POD ® C ommercial Pelvic Binder
Pelvic C-Clamp (Depuy-Synthese ®)

Fig. 6. Pelvic packing.

and they concluded that PPP appears to reduce mortality in this select, high-risk group of patients. It is important to note that PPP may not, however, be sufficient to occlude bleeding of arterial origin. Ongoing hemodynamic compromise after pelvic packing warrants further investigation and treatment.

Embolization

The use of TAE for hemorrhage control from pelvic fractures has been in use since the 1970s and is the mainstay of treating these patients in numerous institutions.[1,10] It involves gaining access to the arterial system and using platinum embolization coils or gelatin sponge particles to occlude vessels that display ongoing contrast extravasation during angiography. The main advantage of this procedure is that it is minimally invasive and that it addresses arterial bleeding that would not otherwise be amenable to tamponade in contrast to the low-pressure venous system. After conducting a meta-analysis of the available evidence for the use of TAE in controlling retroperitoneal arterial hemorrhage in patients with unstable pelvic fractures, Papakostidis *et al.* found that its efficacy ranged from 81–100%.[10] The rate of associated complications in this study had a pooled estimate of only 1.1%. These complications include gluteal muscle necrosis, surgical wound breakdown, deep infection, bladder necrosis, and impotence.[4] Of note, these complications are significantly more common when bilateral embolization is performed, or if non-selective embolization is conducted.[4]

There are, however, a few notable drawbacks while proceeding with TAE in the hemodynamically compromised patient. First, there is often a significant delay in mobilizing the interventional radiology team. In a retrospective comparison of two matched cohorts, Osborn *et al.* found that the average time to proceed to the operating room was only 45 minutes as compared to 130 minutes for interventional radiology.[11] Physicians should therefore consider the time required for mobilization of their own interventional radiology team during trauma team activations in their decision-making. The same study also noted that there was a statistically significant reduction in the number of PRBC required in the first 24 hours for patients who underwent PPP, but not for those who had TAE (6.9 versus 10.1). Despite this difference, both groups had similar mortality. Lastly, taking a hemodynamically compromised and actively bleeding patient to the interventional radiology suite is not without risk. An ICU outreach team with appropriate equipment, readily available drugs for resuscitation, fluid, and blood with warming devices should accompany the patient. Given the possibility of a patient exsanguinating from continued uncontrolled bleeding from an arterial source in the emergency department and the chance of controlling that hemorrhage in the interventional radiology suite, the decision to transfer to the radiology suite is acceptable provided appropriate precautions are taken. Too often this decision is delayed to the detriment of the patient because of the reliance on continued transfusion, which leads to hypocoagulability, acidosis and hypothermia from which the patient frequently succumbs.

Definitive Management of Pelvic Fractures

Nonoperative management of an unstable pelvic injury is associated with poor long-term functional results.[5] In order to maximize pain-free walking and the ability to return to work, early definitive fixation, particularly of the posterior elements, is critical.[1] As such, the standard treatment for these injuries includes anatomic reduction of the pelvic ring and internal fixation, external fixation or a combination thereof. Typically, Tile A pelvic fractures which by definition are both rotationally and vertically stable do not require surgery and patients may be weight-bearing as tolerated. Tile B fractures, which are rotationally unstable, require fixation of the anterior disruption of the pelvic ring only. Tile C fractures require both anterior and posterior ring fixation.

The timing of pelvic ring fixation is controversial. Compared to femur fractures, which should be treated urgently to minimize complications, patients with pelvic fractures that have been provisionally reduced using a binder or C-clamp and that are hemodynamically normal may benefit from a "cooling off" period to ensure adequate resuscitation.[1] Excessive delays beyond two weeks, however, may hamper the surgeon's ability to obtain an anatomic reduction as callous formation beings to interfere with fracture mobilization. Patients who have been stabilized with a sheet or binder should also undergo regular examination to ensure that the pressure of the binder is not compromising their soft tissues. Lastly, prior to proceeding to the operating room, it is imperative to ensure adequate IV access and resuscitation as well as correction of any coagulopathies, as removal of the pelvic binder may disturb the clot that has formed, causing new bleeding.

Postoperative Considerations

Patients who have undergone surgical fixation of a pelvic injury face the standard postoperative orthopedic risks, including infection, thromboembolic disease, damage to neurovascular structures, and non-union/mal-union of the fracture. Consultation with the treating orthopedic surgeon as well as the remainder of the trauma team is required to determine when anticoagulation should be initiated, if postoperative antibiotic prophylaxis is required, and what the patients weight-bearing status should be. Certain transfer aids, such as ceiling lifts, may be contraindicated following pelvic fixation. Weight-bearing restrictions may be advised for three months or longer depending on the severity of the injury and the fixation method. Once the patient is able to cooperate, a repeat neurological examination should be carried out post-operatively, paying particular attention to the lower lumbar and sacral nerve root distributions.

Summary and recommendations for acute management of pelvic fractures

1. All trauma patients undergo an assessment of pelvic stability as part of their initial survey.
2. All patients with a clinically unstable pelvic fracture immediately undergo stabilization with the use of a pelvic binder, pelvic sheet, or C-clamp.
3. Patients who are on the verge of an imminent cardiac arrest secondary to pelvic hemorrhage may be considered for temporary arterial inflow arrest via cross clamping of the aorta or by percutaneous balloon techniques.
4. Patients who are hemodynamically compromised and have an unstable pelvic fracture should be considered for an urgent external fixator as well as pre-peritoneal pelvic packing or an urgent TAE procedure based on institutional standards and availability.
5. Patients with ongoing hemodynamic compromise following pre-peritoneal pelvic packing or patients who have radiographic evidence of a significant arterial injury in the setting of an unstable pelvic fracture should be considered for emergent TAE.
6. Presence of a positive 'blush' on contrast CT is not necessarily an indication for TAE unless there is evidence of continued bleeding and unresponsiveness to standard resuscitation.

References

1. Flint L, Cryer HG. Pelvic fracture: The last 50 years. *J Trauma* 2010; 69(3): 483–488.
2. Giannoudis PV, Pape HC. Damage control orthopedics in unstable pelvic ring injuries. *Injury* 2004; 35: 671–677.

3. Dyer GSM, Vrahas MS. Review of the pathophysiology and acute management of haemorrhage in pelvic fracture. *Injury* 2006; 37(7): 602–613.
4. Matityahu A, Marmor M, Elson JK *et al.* Acute complications of patients with pelvic fractures after pelvic angiographic embolization. *Clin Orthop Relat Res* 2013; 471(9): 2906–2911.
5. Wong JM-L, Bucknill A. Fractures of the pelvic ring. *Injury* 2013.
6. O'Sullivan R, O'Sullivan REM, White TO, Keating JF. Major pelvic fractures identification of patients at high risk. *J Bone Joint Surg Br.* 2005; 87–B(4): 530–533.
7. Pizanis A, Pohlemann T, Burkhardt M, Aghayev E, Holstein JH. Emergency stabilization of the pelvic ring: Clinical comparison between three different techniques. *Injury* 2013; 44(12): 1760–1764.
8. Verbeek DOF, Zijlstra IAJ, Van der Leij C, Ponsen KJ, Van Delden OM, Goslings JC. Management of pelvic ring fracture patients with a pelvic "blush" on early computed tomography. *J Trauma Acute Care Surg* 2014; 76(2): 374–379.
9. Cothren CC, Osborn PM, Moore EE, Morgan SJ, Johnson JL, Smith WR. Preperitonal pelvic packing for hemodynamically unstable pelvic fractures: A paradigm shift. *J Trauma* 2007; 62(4): 834–839.
10. Papakostidis C, Kanakaris N, Dimitriou R, Giannoudis PV. The role of arterial embolization in controlling pelvic fracture haemorrhage: A systematic review of the literature. *Eur J Radiol* 2012; 81(5): 897–904.
11. Osborn PM, Smith WR, Moore EE *et al.* Direct retroperitoneal pelvic packing versus pelvic angiography: A comparison of two management protocols for haemodynamically unstable pelvic fractures. *Injury* 2009; 40(1): 54–60.

Chapter 21

Extremity Fractures

Jeremy Hall and Jeremie Larouche

Chapter Overview

During the initial assessment of a polytraumatized patient, the priorities of resuscitation focus on life threatening abnormalities. The time-sensitive and complex nature of this initial treatment often leads physicians to overlook subtle non-life-threatening peripheral injuries. A decreased level of consciousness, distracting injuries, and the requirement to sedate and intubate patients often create an even greater diagnostic challenge. If neglected, these missed injuries can increase hospital stay, become a source of long-term pain and disability, and are also the leading cause of medicolegal action following trauma. Major extremity trauma, on the other hand, has the potential to become a significant source of both morbidity and mortality, and its management priority must be carefully considered within the context of the patient's overall status.

Many polytraumatized patients are treated in the ICU where the main reason for this admission is usually not the musculoskeletal injury itself but rather associated injuries or their systemic consequences. Long bone fractures are often associated with a significant blood loss, which may significantly tax the cardiovascular system. The care of these patients necessitates a close working relationship between the intensivist and the orthopedic surgeon in order to ensure that each understands the patient's physiological reserves and the predicted demands of the surgery. To assist the intensivist in managing orthopedic injuries in the ICU, this chapter will first briefly review the initial assessment and treatment of extremity trauma. Secondly, general considerations in the timing of surgery, the role of "early total care" versus "damage control surgery" as well as decisions surrounding the care of the mangled extremity will be summarized. Lastly, systemic complications associated with extremity trauma will be discussed.

Introduction

The widely used Advanced Trauma Life Support (ATLS) guidelines have standardized the approach to trauma patients, and divided the examination into three different phases. The primary survey focuses on life threatening injuries, and is carried out expeditiously upon the arrival of the patient to the trauma bay. The injured limb requires urgent attention in the primary survey during the "C" or circulatory phase of the ABCDE approach when identification and control of hemorrhage is necessary. This control is secured usually by the application of direct pressure and avoiding blind clamping. In situations where the bleeding is from an amputated or near amputated limb, judicious and appropriate temporary application of tourniquets may be required as a life saving measure in addition to fluid resuscitation, while accepting the potential risk of limb loss.

A secondary survey is then performed after completing the ABCDE assessment, which is aimed at detecting other injuries that may not present an immediate threat to life but could lead to late deaths and/or complications. Lastly, a tertiary survey is performed after 24 hours of the patient's arrival to hospital in an effort to examine them once their level of consciousness has improved, and to ensure no injuries have been missed. Despite these redundant exams, injuries to the extremities are quite commonly missed. In a cohort of 1,124 patients, Giannakopoulos *et al.* have reported 122 missed injuries, with the majority of these injuries occurring in the extremities.[1] Furthermore, 59% of these injuries remained undetected during the tertiary survey. Factors associated with these missed injuries included traumatic brain injuries, as well as an Injury Severity Score (ISS) greater than 16. It is therefore imperative that clinicians pay particular attention to a detailed extremity exam, particularly in the setting of an ICU patient with a decreased level of consciousness.

Clinical Assessment

All extremities should undergo a detailed clinical exam as part of a tertiary survey, once the patient regains consciousness and is able to participate in the examination. The orthopaedic dictum of "Look, Feel, Move" should be applied, with a careful examination for deformity, ecchymosis, edema, and skin compromise circumferentially to all four extremities. Sequential palpation of every bone and joint should then be carried out to ensure that no crepitus is felt and no abnormal pain response is detected. Lastly, all major joints should undergo a full passive range of motion to ensure stability and symmetrical movement as compared to their contralateral side. All suspected fractures or dislocations should be imaged with two orthogonal views using X-ray. All but the simplest intra-articular fracture are usually further characterized by a computed tomography scan.

Any disruption in the skin integrity in the same area as a fracture should be considered an open fracture. These are graded according to the Gustilo classification (Table 1). It is important to remember that with reduction of the fracture, the bone end responsible for the puncture of soft tissues may be located a distance away from the skin laceration. It is therefore sometimes difficult to determine if a small laceration in the skin represents an outside-in injury versus a grade I open fracture. Typically, soft tissue defects associated with an open fracture will continue to hemorrhage even after light pressure is applied, as they communicate directly with the intramedullary canal of long bones which are richly vascularized. The management of open fractures is discussed later in this chapter.

Careful assessment of peripheral pulses, capillary refill and extremity temperature should be documented. Any suspected vascular abnormality should be investigated using an Ankle Brachial Index (ABI) at the very least, and possibly via the use of Duplex ultrasound, CT angiogram, or formal angiogram based on institutional standards. For further details on vascular injuries, please refer to the chapter on vascular injuries in this book.

If the patient is able to cooperate, a screening exam should assess sensation, motor, and reflexes in all four extremities. To begin, the terminal motor

Table 1. Gustilo classification.

Type I	Clean wound, less than 1 cm in length
Type II	Wound >1 cm in length but without extensive soft tissue damage
Type IIIA	Extensive soft tissue damage includes massively contaminated, severely comminuted or segmental fractures. Soft tissue is adequate for primary closure.
Type IIIB	Same as IIIA, but requires flap coverage for closure.
Type IIIC	Same as IIIA, but associated with an arterial injury requiring repair for limb salvage.

and sensory function of each major peripheral nerve should be evaluated. Any abnormality must further be investigated to determine if it relates to an injury to the peripheral nerve itself, or to a more proximal source such as a plexus, a nerve root, the spinal cord, or an injury to the central nervous system itself. In the upper extremity, the ulnar, median, axillary, radial nerve proper and posterior interosseous branch of the radial nerve should be assessed for both motor and sensory function. In the lower extremity, the femoral, obturator, tibial, saphenous, sural, and both the deep and superficial branches of the peroneal nerves should be assessed. Should a deficiency be identified which does not correlate to a peripheral nerve, physicians should instead assess each myotome and dermatome to see if the deficit corresponds to a nerve root or spinal cord injury instead.

Initial Treatment

All fractures and dislocations should be reduced as soon as clinically possible to alleviate pain, minimize bleeding, and prevent further damage to soft tissues. Non-anatomical alignment of a limb can lead to interruption of distal vascular flow, neural injury, and increased pressure on soft tissues leading to eventual necrosis (Fig. 1). Furthermore, imaging studies which are obtained prior to a reduction being performed are often difficult to interpret, and must be repeated once a reduction is performed. This is particularly true of cross-sectional imaging, such as computed tomography scans and magnetic resonance imaging.

Once reduced, most fractures require immobilization through the use of a splint, cast, or traction. It is customary to initially use a plaster splint (non-circumferential) so as to facilitate repeat examination of the limb and to prevent compartment syndrome. In their experiment, Capo *et al.* have demonstrated how a forearm immobilized in circumferential plaster can reach compartment pressures of 50 mm Hg with the addition of only 19 mL of volume.[2] This is in comparison to the 77 mL that was required to achieve the same compartment pressure of the non-wrapped arm. Given the possibility of missing a compartment syndrome in an obtunded trauma patient, physicians should be weary of applying circumferential plaster or fiberglass to an extremity injury in a trauma setting.

Due to the large muscle mass located in the thigh, diaphyseal fractures of the femur tend to be initially immobilized in traction while awaiting definitive treatment. Typically, this involves using skin traction tape attached to a weight or to a Thomas splint (Fig. 2). The advantage of the Thomas splint is that patients may easily be transferred across different stretchers and

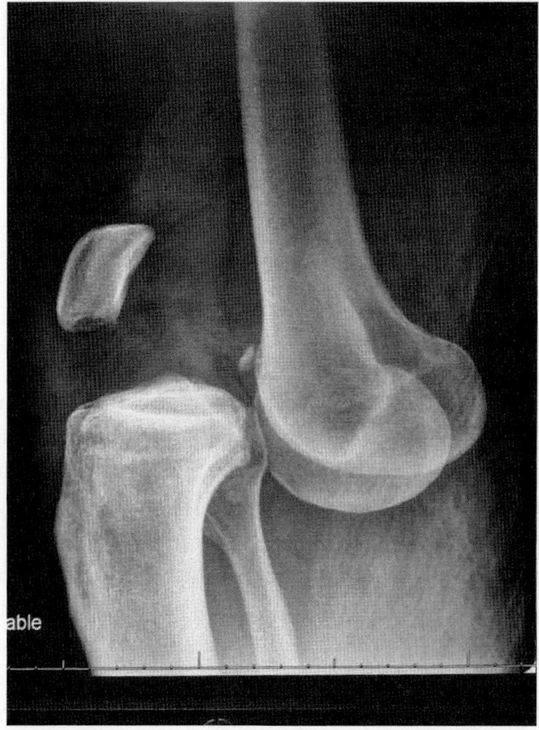

Fig. 1. Knee dislocation association with ongoing compression of the popliteal artery. Note that the common peroneal nerve in this injury was completely disrupted.

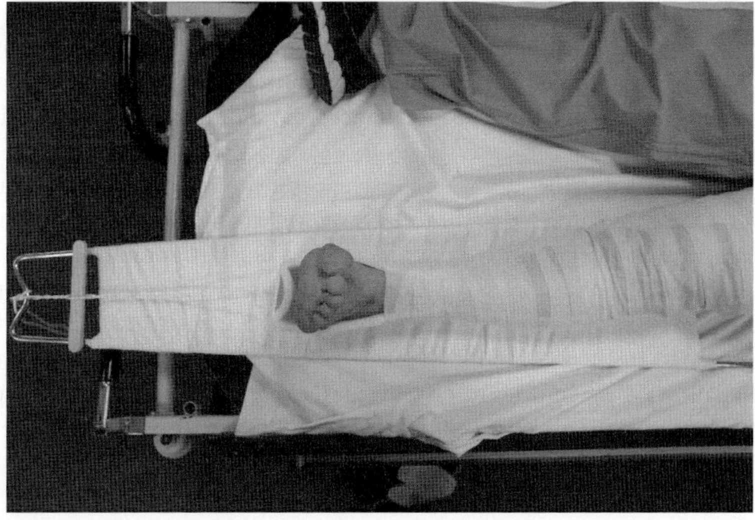

Fig. 2. Application of Thomas splint.

or beds without requiring the traction to be removed. This alleviates pain, prevents fracture shortening, and facilitates reduction at the time of surgery. Note that recent meta-analysis found no benefit to such traction for hip fractures (described as fractures of the proximal femur).[3] Skin traction should be checked regularly to ensure the integrity of the integumentary system, especially in geriatric patients with frail skin. Skeletal traction, which is applied through a metal pin transfixing the bone, may be applied indefinitely as long as the pin sites do not demonstrate any signs on infection.

Open Fractures

The treatment of open fractures focuses on the timely administration of antibiotics, tetanus prophylaxis, surgical debridement and irrigation, and finally the provision of stability across the fracture to facilitate soft tissue healing. Numerous studies have confirmed the importance of early and appropriate antibiotic administration. In their Cochrane Review Database article, Gosselin *et al.* concluded that early antibiotic administration reduced by more than half the rate of infection following an open fracture (absolute risk reduction of 0.07).[4] The American Academy of Orthopaedic Surgeons currently recommends the administration of a first generation cephalosporin to cover gram-positive infections, as well as the addition of an aminoglycoside to cover gram-negative bacteria. If anaerobic organisms are suspected, such as when a fracture occurs in conjunction with a vascular injury and ischemia is present, or when a farm injury occurs, penicillin or ampicillin should also be administered.

The timing of the debridement and irrigation remains more controversial. The "six hour rule" has long been the standard across numerous institutions, and states that all open fractures should undergo definitive management within the first six hours. More recent evidence, however, brings this dictum into question. In their cohort of 791 open fractures, Weber *et al.* concluded that time to surgery was not associated with an increase rate of infection.[5] Instead, increasing Gustilo grade of injury, and open tibia/fibular fractures proved to be a risk for the development of infection. The authors were careful to point out that that this evidence does not support elective delay of surgical treatment for open fractures, but instead allows these injuries to be treated in more convenient daytime operating theatres by an experienced team of surgeons and nurses to achieve the best possible results.

Noteworthy exceptions to the management of open fractures are those caused by gunshot wounds. While the path of the bullet through the skin and into bone technically constitutes an open fracture, it is thought that the heat for the propellant effectively sterilizes the bullet as it leaves the barrel. Low velocity gunshot wounds, such as those from most handguns, can therefore be treated conservatively if the fracture characteristics allow it. The exception to this rule includes high velocity rounds (such as those from a military or hunting rifle), the presence of wadding material in the wound, intra-articular bullet fragments, or a bullet trajectory through contaminated tissue (such as large bowel).

General Management Principles

While the scope of this handbook is insufficient to address the ideal management of each type of fractures, some basic considerations for different categories of fractures are listed below. It is important to remember that each fracture has its own peculiar characteristics, and based on other mitigating factors such as the health and associated injuries of the patient, the ideal management for any given injury may vary from case to case.

Intra-articular Fractures: Most displaced intra-articular fractures benefit from achieving anatomical reduction and absolute stability that is only possible through open reduction with internal fixation. Non-displaced intra-articular fractures may occasionally be treated conservatively, but careful follow up must be obtained to ensure that late displacement does not occur.

Diaphyseal Long Bone Fractures: Diaphyseal fractures of the femur and tibia are generally treated with intramedullary nailing. This provides patients with the ability to mobilize quickly, and minimizes the surgical insult that is associated with the exposure required for plate fixation. Many of these patients may begin weight bearing immediately postoperatively. Fractures of the radial and ulna diaphysis also tend to be treated surgically in adults to restore the exact anatomy, which is required to preserve range of motion. This is especially important if accompanied by a dislocation of radio-humeral or distal radio-ulnar joints. Humeral diaphyseal fractures, on the other hand, can tolerate a significant amount of malalignment, and tend to heal quite readily with conservative management. Individually, they may be treated conservatively, but numerous surgeons will elect to fix them in the setting of polytrauma to facilitate mobilization.

Metaphyseal Fractures: The treatment required for fractures that predominantly involve the metaphysis usually depends on their effect on the length, alignment, and rotation of the limb. Each joint can tolerate a certain amount of malalignment, and therefore each fracture must be considered individually. Should these fractures be treated surgically, they normally require a plate and screw construct, and as a result, will often require modified weight bearing for several weeks following fixation.

Timing of Surgery

There have been several paradigm shifts within the field of orthopaedics with respect to the timing of surgical fixation in the polytraumatized patient. In the early 1980's, as surgeons discovered that patients who had their femur fractures promptly addressed had lower mortality rates and shorter hospital stays,[6] the concept of "Early Total Care" evolved. As Giannoudis points out, "the previously held belief that the patient was too sick to operate on was now replaced with the opposite view that the patient was too sick ***not*** to operate on".[6]

In a rush to adopt this new standard, numerous surgeons started to notice an increased rate of pulmonary complications, particularly after reamed femoral nailing in patients with pre-existing chest trauma.[7] The prevailing theory to account for this finding was that the initial trauma established a baseline systemic inflammatory response, and that surgery became the "second hit" which overwhelmed the patient, and frequently lead to Acute Respiratory Distress Syndrome (ARDS) and Multiple Organ Failure (MOF). A new concept of "Damage Control Orthopaedics" was then established, whereby surgeons would perform the minimal amount of surgery to stabilize the patient (usually in the form of external-fixators), allow the patient to recover in the ICU for a period of time, and then plan definitive fixation at a later stage.

In an effort to answer the question as to when a patient should ideally undergo definitive surgery, Nahm *et al.* reviewed 750 skeletally mature patients who suffered femur fractures, 492 of which had an ISS >18.[8] After accounting for age and ISS, they noted that early definitive fixation in patients with multiple injuries was associated with fewer complications than delayed stabilizations (18.9% versus 42.9%). They concluded that they were unable to find any group for which early treatment had more complications then delayed treatment, and strongly advocated for "Early Appropriate Care" once the patient was stable enough to proceed to the operating room.

The Mangled Extremity

The decision whether to proceed with a primary amputation versus attempts at limb reconstruction is often a difficult one, even for experienced surgeons. While the scope of this chapter is insufficient to fully address this issue, it is important to review basic considerations that the trauma team should consider when faced with a mangled extremity. Much of the information currently used to guide decisions surrounding this issue has been derived from the Lower Extremity Assessment Project (LEAP). In their seminal study, MacKenzie and Bosse assessed 601 patients at two and seven years after they sustained major lower extremity injuries. They found no difference in functional outcomes at two years between patients who underwent primary amputation versus limb salvaging operations, both being rated as poor.[9] They found that patients who underwent reconstruction were more likely to have a secondary hospitalization for a major complication as compared to those who underwent primary amputation (47.5% versus 33.9%). About half of patients who underwent either amputation or reconstruction were able to return to work (53% versus 49% respectively). The most important determinant of the patients' ability to return to work and cope with their injury was their "Self-Efficacy" score, which is described as the confidence to be able to perform specific tasks or activities. Not surprisingly, a high rate of post-traumatic stress disorder, chronic pain, and depression is common in this patient population.[9]

In an effort to provide surgeons with a valid clinical decision making tool, numerous extremity injury-severity scores have been developed over the years. These include the Mangled Extremity Severity Score, the Limb Salvage Index, the Predictive Salvage Index, the Hanover Fracture Scale (1997 version) and the Nerve injury, Ischemia, Soft Tissue Injury, Skeletal Injury, Shock and Age of Patient (NISSA) score. In a prospective study, Bosse *et al.* attempted to determine the clinical utility of all five of these scores in predicting the need for an amputation within six months of the injury.[10] All five of these scores looked at common variables in assorted combinations, which are included in Table 2. Scores were assessed by both including and excluding limbs that required immediate amputations. The authors concluded that their analysis did not validate any of the five extremity injury-severity scores assessed, which unfortunately leaves clinicians with very few tools to guide these challenging decisions.

Given the lack of standard guidelines, it is therefore always advisable to obtain and document the opinions of various colleagues as to what they

Table 2. Components of extremity ISS.

Age
Shock
Warm Ischemia Time
Bone Injury
Muscle Injury
Skin Injury
Nerve Injury
Deep-vein Injury
Skeletal/soft-tissue Injury
Contamination
Time to Treatment

believe to be the best course of action given the patient's particular circumstances and hemodynamic status. The assessment of the intensivist and anesthesiologist as to whether or not the patient is able to tolerate multiple lengthy operations necessary to proceed with reconstructive efforts must also be carefully considered. Lastly, and perhaps most importantly, the patient's personal wishes must be respected whenever possible.

Systemic Complications

Thromboembolic disease

The risk of thromboembolic disease following extremity fractures continues to be an ongoing concern for clinicians. It has been estimated that deep vein thrombosis (DVT) can occur in as many as 60% of polytraumatized patients.[11] Godzik *et al.* reviewed 199,952 patients from the National Trauma Data Bank with pelvic and lower extremity fractures, and found a rate of pulmonary embolism of 0.46% (12% of which were associated with patient death during hospitalization). They found the risks of pulmonary embolisms to be associated in patients with multiple fractures (odds ratio 1.89, $P < 0.001$),[11] and not the location of the fractures. Furthermore, obese patients, prior history of Warfarin use, surgery, and ICU stay were also associated with increased rates of pulmonary embolism.

The American College of Chest Physicians Evidence-Based Clinical Practice Guidelines ninth edition is currently the standard by which most institutions determine their management protocol. The recommendations for anticoagulation pertinent for major orthopedic procedures[12] are summarized in Table 3. Clinicians should ensure they stay current with the most recent guidelines, as with the introduction of new pharmaceutical agents, this field of medicine is constantly evolving.

Fat emboli syndrome (FES)

FES, first described over 100 years ago, consists of the triad of cerebral dysfunction, petechial rash, and acute respiratory insufficiency.[13] As Bugler *et al.* point out, it is important to distinguish between fat embolism, and

Table 3. Selected recommendations from CHEST guidelines 9th edition.[12]

In patients undergoing hip fracture surgery (HFS), we recommend use of one of the following rather than no antithrombotic prophylaxis for a minimum of 10 to 14 days: LMWH, fondaparinux, LDUH, adjusted-dose VKA, aspirin (all Grade 1B), or an IPCD (Grade 1C).
For patients undergoing major orthopedic surgery (THA, TKA, HFS) and receiving LMWH as thromboprophylaxis, we recommend starting either 12 hours or more preoperatively or 12 hours or more postoperatively rather than within 4 hours or less preoperatively or 4 hours or less postoperatively (Grade 1B).
2.3.2. In patients undergoing HFS, irrespective of the concomitant use of an IPCD or length of treatment, we suggest the use of LMWH in preference to the other agents we have recommended as alternatives: fondaparinux, LDUH (Grade 2B), adjusted-dose VKA, or aspirin (all Grade 2C).
2.4. For patients undergoing major orthopedic surgery, we suggest extending thromboprophylaxis in the outpatient period for up to 35 days from the day of surgery rather than for only 10 to 14 days (Grade 2B).
2.5. In patients undergoing major orthopedic surgery, we suggest using dual prophylaxis with an antithrombotic agent and an IPCD during the hospital stay (Grade 2C).
2.8. In patients undergoing major orthopedic surgery, we suggest against using inferior vena cava (IVC) filter placement for primary prevention over no thromboprophylaxis in patients with an increased bleeding risk or contraindications to both pharmacologic and mechanical thromboprophylaxis (Grade 2C).
3.0. We suggest no prophylaxis rather than pharmacologic thromboprophylaxis in patients with isolated lower-leg injuries requiring leg immobilization (Grade 2C).

FES. Fat embolism refers to fat globules found in the general circulation as well as the lung parenchyma after a long bone or pelvic fracture. Using various techniques, these can be detected in more than 90% of trauma patients with a major fracture as well as those undergoing intramedullary nailing. Fat Embolism Syndrome, on the other hand, is much less common, with approximately 1% of major trauma patients demonstrating the triad of symptoms.[14] Other less common causes of FES include severe burns, massive soft tissue injury, median sternotomy, bone marrow transplant, bone marrow biopsy, cardiopulmonary resuscitation, and liposuction (Shaikh 2009).

The diagnosis of FES is normally made on the basis of Gurd's major and minor criteria (Table 4). To confirm the diagnosis, it is suggested that the patient have at least one major and four minor criteria. These criteria were later reviewed in a cohort of 27 patients with established diagnosis of FES. Fabian *et al.* noted that 96% of these patients were hypoxic, 59% suffered from a decreased level of consciousness, and 33% demonstrated petechiae. Only 15% of patients demonstrated all three major signs.[14]

The treatment of FES remains primarily supportive. Mortality as a result of FES is thought to be 5.5%, and it has been implicated as a contributing factor to a further 10% of deaths in trauma patients.[13] Early intubation to prevent further respiratory compromise or aspiration may be clinically warranted. Attempts at treatment such as heparin, low molecular-weight dextran, albumin, steroids, and hyptertonic glucose with insulin have failed to provide any benefit in limited studies[14] and are not recommended.

Table 4. Gurd's diagnostic criteria for fat embolism syndrome.

Major	Minor
Hypoxia	Tachycardia > 120 bpm
Central nervous system depression	Fever > 39°C
Petechiae	Unexplained anemia or thrombocytopenia ($<150 \times 10^9$/L)
	High erythrocyte sedimentation rate
	Retinal changes
	Jaundice
	Fat present in urine or oliguria
	Fat Macroglobulinemia

Summary and Recommendations for the Acute Management of Extremity Trauma

1. The first priority in managing the traumatized extremity is identification and control of bleeding followed by prevention of sepsis.
2. A detailed examination of the extremities is critical in all polytraumatized patients, particularly in those with a decreased level of consciousness, given the prevalence of missed injuries.
3. All dislocations and displaced fractures should undergo an urgent closed reduction and immobilization to minimize further damage to the soft tissues, minimize further blood loss, alleviate pain, and allow for better imaging.
4. Femur fractures should be placed in skin or skeletal traction until definitive fixation can be obtained.
5. All open fractures should receive appropriate antibiotic prophylaxis and if required, tetanus prophylaxis early.
6. Polytraumatized patients with long bone fractures should receive "Early Appropriate Care" and undergo definitive fixation as soon as is considered possible.
7. The treatment of mangled extremities must be considered on an individual basis. Opinions of multiple physicians should be sought whenever possible.
8. Patients with long-bone fractures and multiple fractures are at risk for thromboembolic disease, and the initiation of DVT prophylaxis should be discussed with both the orthopaedic surgeon as well as the intensivist.

References

1. Giannakopoulos GF, Saltzherr TP, Beenen LFM *et al.* Missed injuries during the initial assessment in a cohort of 1124 level-1 trauma patients. *Injury* 2012; 43(9): 1517–1521.
2. Capo JT, Renard RL, Moulton MJR *et al.* How is Forearm Compliance Affected by Various Circumferential Dressings? *Clin Orthop Relat Res* 2014; 472(10): 1–7.
3. Handoll HHG, Queally JM, Parker MJ. Pre-operative traction for hip fractures in adults. *Cochrane Database Syst Rev* 2011; 12, Issue 12. Art. No.: CD000168. DOI: 10.1002/14651858.CD000168.pub3.
4. Gosselin RA, Roberts I, Gillespie WJ. Antibiotics for preventing infection in open limb fractures. *Cochrane Database Syst Rev* 2004; 1, Issue 1. Art. No.: CD003764. DOI: 10.1002/14651858.CD003764.pub2.

5. Weber D, Dulai SK, Bergman J, Buckley R, Beaupre LA. Time to Initial Operative Treatment following Open Fracture does not impact Development of Deep Infection: A Prospective Cohort Study of 736 Subjects. *J Orthop Trauma* 2014; 28(11): 613–619.
6. Giannoudis PV. Surgical priorities in damage control in polytrauma. *J Bone Joint Surg Br* 2003; 85(4); 478–483.
7. Pape HC, Auf'm'Kolk M, Paffrath T, Regel G, Sturm JA, Tscherne H. Primary intramedullary femur fixation in multiple trauma patients with associated lung contusion — a cause of posttraumatic ARDS? *J Trauma* 1993; 34(4); 540–547.
8. Nahm NJ, Como JJ, Wilber JH, Vallier HA. Early appropriate care: Definitive stabilization of femoral fractures within 24 hours of injury is safe in most patients with multiple injuries. *J Trauma* 2011; 71(1); 175–185.
9. Mackenzie EJ, Bosse MJ. Factors influencing outcome following limb-threatening lower limb trauma: Lessons learned from the Lower Extremity Assessment Project (LEAP). *J Am Acad Orthop Surg* 2006; 14(10 Spec No.); S205–210.
10. Bosse MJ, Mackenzie EJ, Kellam JF *et al.* A Prospective Evaluation of the Clinical Utility of the Lower-Extremity Injury-Severity Scores. *J Bone Joint Surg Am* 2001; 83(1); 3–3.
11. Godzik J, McAndrew CM, Morshed S, Kandemir U, Kelly MP. Multiple lower-extremity and pelvic fractures increase pulmonary embolus risk. *Orthop* 2014; 37(6); e517–524.
12. Falck-Ytter Y, Francis CW, Johanson NA *et al.* Prevention of VTE in orthopedic surgery patients: Antithrombotic Therapy and Prevention of Thrombosis, 9th ed: American College of Chest Physicians Evidence-Based Clinical Practice Guidelines. *Chest* 2012; 141(2 Suppl); e278S–325S.
13. Meyer N, Pennington WT, Dewitt D, Schmeling GJ. Isolated cerebral fat emboli syndrome in multiply injured patients: A review of three cases and the literature. *J Trauma* 2007; 63(6); 1395–1402.
14. Fabian TC, Hoots AV, Stanford DS, Patterson CR, Mangiante EC. Fat embolism syndrome: Prospective evaluation in 92 fracture patients. *Crit Care Med* 1990; 18(1); 42–46.
15. Shaikh, N. (2009). Emergency management of fat embolism syndrome. *Journal of Emergencies, Trauma and Shock*, 2(1), 29–33. http://doi.org/10.4103/0974-2700.44680.

Chapter 22

Extremity Compartment Syndromes

Col. (retd.) Mark W. Bowyer

Chapter Overview

All clinicians caring for critically ill patients must be able to recognize and treat (or refer for treatment) Compartment Syndrome (CS) of the extremities. CS results from a variety of etiologies (traumatic and non-traumatic) with the final common pathway being increased compartmental pressure that exceeds the arterial inflow with resultant ischemia and necrosis. Failure to identify and treat CS in a timely fashion is associated with preventable morbidity and mortality, and is a common source of litigation. The diagnosis of CS is largely clinical, but measurement of compartment pressures may be useful in patients with equivocal findings or altered level of consciousness. The below-knee lower extremity is most commonly affected, followed much less frequently, by the forearm, thigh, foot, and hand. This chapter will review the pathophysiology, epidemiology, diagnosis, relevant anatomy, and treatment of CS, emphasizing the proper performance of a fasciotomy, and the complications associated with this vital limb and potentially life-saving procedure.

Introduction

CS is a condition in which increased pressure within a limited space compromises the circulation and function of affected tissues.[1,2] This limb and potentially life-threatening condition may result from several possible etiologies

Table 1. Factors implicated with the development of acute limb CS.[1,3,4,7]

Restriction of compartment size	Increased compartment volume
	<u>From Hemorrhage</u>
	Fractures
Casts	Vascular Injury
Splints	Drugs: (anticoagulants)
Burn Eschar	Hemophilia; Sickle Cell
Tourniquets	<u>From Muscle Edema/Swelling</u>
Tight Dressings	Crush — trauma, drugs or alcohol
Fracture Reduction	Rhabdomyolysis/Blast injury
Closure of Fascial Defects	Sepsis
Incomplete Skin Release	Exercise induced
Military Antishock Trousers	Envenomation or Bee Sting
Prolonged Extrication Trapped Limb	Massive resuscitation
Localized External Pressure	Intra-compartmental fluid infusion
Long Leg Brace	Phlegmasia caerulea dolens
Automated BP monitoring	Electrical burns
Malpositioning on OR table	Reperfusion Injury
	Post Partum Eclampsia

(Table 1),[1,3,4,7] with which every clinician should be familiar. Failure to identify and treat CS properly, leads to tissue necrosis, permanent functional impairment, possible amputation, and potential renal failure and death.[1,3,4] In a nine-year review of extremity trauma, Feliciano *et al.*[5] found that 75% of amputations in the lower extremity were related to a delay in performing fasciotomy or an incomplete fasciotomy.

Not only is disability resulting from CS of great consequence to the patient, but failure to diagnose or properly treat CS is one of the most common causes of medical litigation.[6] Bhattacharyya and Vrahas[6] reported an average indemnity payment of $426,000 in nine cases settled between 1980 and 2003 in Massachusetts, and awards as high as $14.9 million have been made in cases of missed CS.

Optimal outcomes result from early recognition of CS and aggressive, properly performed fasciotomy. Proper fasciotomy requires extensive knowledge of the anatomical landmarks and anatomy of the muscle compartments of the extremities.

Pathophysiology

Groups of muscles and their associated nerves and vessels are surrounded by thick fascial layers that define the various compartments of the extremities which are of relatively fixed volume. CS occurs either when compartment size is restricted or when compartment volume is increased. It is imperative that all clinicians working in critical care settings be aware of the numerous non-traumatic causes (Table 1) of extremity CS, especially sepsis, massive resuscitation, and reperfusion as the diagnosis of CS in these settings is often delayed, as it is frequently not considered by many otherwise well-trained physicians.

As pressure increases, venous flow decreases and narrows the arterio-venous perfusion gradient, resulting in diminished blood flow. This condition is self-perpetuating, leading to a continuous loop that must be broken with the timely initiation of definitive care. Cellular hypoxia is the final common pathway of all compartment syndromes. As ischemia continues, irreparable damage to tissue ensues and myoneural necrosis occurs. Development of CS depends on many factors, including the duration of the pressure elevation, the metabolic rate of the tissues, vascular tone, associated soft tissue damage, and local blood pressure.[11] Nerves demonstrate functional abnormalities (paresthesias and hypoesthesia) within 30 minutes of ischemic onset. Irreversible functional loss will occur after 12 to 24 hours of total ischemia.[1] Muscle shows functional changes after 2 to 4 hours of ischemia with irreversible loss of function beginning at 4 to 12 hours.[1] Clinically, there is no precise pressure threshold and duration above which significant damage is irreversible and below which recovery is assured.

Tissue previously subjected to intervals of ischemia is especially sensitive to increased pressure. Bernot and colleagues[8] showed that tissue compromised by ischemia prior to an elevated compartment pressure has a lower threshold for metabolic deterioration and irreversible damage. Polytrauma or otherwise critically ill patients with low blood pressures can sustain irreversible injury at lower compartment pressures than patients with normal blood pressures, and a very high index of suspicion should be maintained in this group.

Epidemiology/risk factors

Given the consequences of missing a CS, it is important to identify the population at risk. Trauma is the major cause of extremity CS requiring fasciotomy. In a 10-year retrospective review of over 10,000 trauma patients sustaining extremity injury, Branco *et al.*, described a fasciotomy rate of 2.8%.[3] During this period 315 fasciotomies were performed on 237 patients with 68.4% done below the knee, 14.4% on the forearm, and 8.9% on the thigh. In a review of 294 combat injured soldiers undergoing 494 fasciotomies, Ritenour *et al.* reported the calf as the most common site (51%) followed by the forearm (22.3%), thigh (8.3%), upper arm (7.3%), hand (5.7%), and the foot (4.8%).[9]

Branco *et al.*[3] found that incidence of fasciotomy varied widely by mechanism of injury (0.9% after motor vehicle collision to 8.6% after a gunshot wound). Additionally, the need for fasciotomy was related to the type of injury ranging from 2.2% incidence for patients with closed fractures up to 41.8% in patients with combined venous and arterial injuries. Young males, with penetrating or multi-system trauma, requiring blood transfusion, with open fractures, elbow or knee dislocations, or vascular injury (arterial, venous, or combined) are at the highest risk of requiring a fasciotomy after extremity trauma.[3]

Diagnosis

Diagnosis depends on a high clinical suspicion and an understanding of risk factors, pathophysiology, and subtle physical findings. The diagnosis of CS is often based on subtle changes in symptoms and vague clinical findings. Time to diagnosis and treatment are the most important prognostic factors. Incomplete knowledge of the natural history and signs and symptoms primarily account for delays in diagnosis.[10] The aim is to recognize and treat raised intra-compartmental pressure before irreversible cell damage occurs.

Numerous authors have stated that the diagnosis of CS is a clinical diagnosis.[1,7,10,11] The classically described five "Ps" — pain, pallor, paresthesias, paralysis, and pulselessness are said to be pathognomonic of CS. However, **these are usually late signs and extensive and irreversible damage may have taken place by the time they are manifested.** In the earliest stages of CS, patients may report some tingling and an uncomfortable feeling in their extremity followed closely by pain with passive stretching of the muscles of the affected compartment. The most important symptom of CS is ***pain greater than expected due to the injury alone.***

Nerve tissue is affected first by the subsequent hypoxia causing pain on passive motion seen early in the development of CS, sparing distal pulses until late in the course.[7] The loss of pulse is a late finding, and the presence of pulses and normal capillary refill do not rule-out CS! **The presence of open wounds does *not* exclude CS**. In fact, the worst open fractures are actually more likely to have a CS.

All clinical signs have inherent drawbacks in making the diagnosis. Pain is an unreliable and variable predictor, and the pain of the obvious injury can mask that of an impending CS and cannot alone be relied upon for diagnosis. Wide consensus in the literature suggests that the clinical features of CS are more useful by their absence in excluding the diagnosis, than when they are present in confirming the diagnosis.

Since clinical findings may be absent in patients with altered sensorium (common in the intensive care setting), under the influence of drugs or alcohol, distracting injuries, or paralysis, many authors advise using tissue pressure measurements as an adjunct to clinical findings.[12] There are also some who advocate the use of compartment pressure measurement as a principle criterion for the diagnosis of CS.

In actual practice, tissue pressure (compartment pressure) measurements have a limited role in making the diagnosis of CS. However, in polytrauma patients with associated head injury, drug and alcohol intoxication, intubation, spinal injuries, use of paralyzing drugs, extremes of age, unconsciousness, or low diastolic pressures, measuring compartment pressures may be of use in determining the need for fasciotomy.

The pressure threshold for making the diagnosis of CS is controversial. A number of authors recommend 30 mmHg, and others cite pressure as high as 45 mmHg. Many surgeons use the "Delta-P" system. The compartment pressure is subtracted from the patient's diastolic blood pressure to obtain the Delta-P. Whitesides in 1975 proposed that muscle was at risk when the compartment pressure was within 10–30 mmHg of the diastolic pressure.[12] If the Delta-P is less than 30, the surgeon should be concerned that a CS may be present. For instance, if the diastolic blood pressure was 60 and the measured compartment pressure was 42 (60 – 42 = 18), the "Delta-P" would be 18 and the patient is likely to have CS.

A variety of techniques have been used to measure compartment pressures but many suffer from the cumbersome nature of setting them up and user variability. A commercially available portable hand-held, self contained,

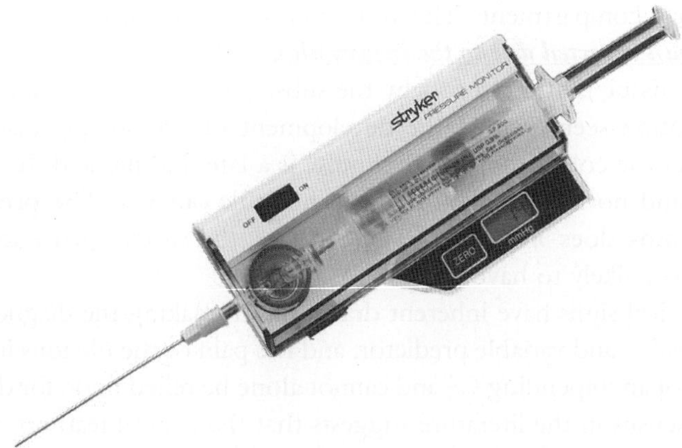

Fig. 1. Intra-Compartmental Pressure Monitor System manufactured by Stryker® Surgical, Kalamazoo, Michigan.

Source: Figure courtesy of Stryker® Instruments. Kalamazoo, Michigan.

electronic pressure monitor with a digital display is available (Stryker® Intra-Compartmental Pressure Monitor System, Stryker® Surgical, Kalamazoo, Michigan) has replaced most less reproducible devices as the current standard (Fig. 1). An alternative approach is to use an 18-gauge needle attached to a side-port arterial line set-up inserted into the compartment.

The use of pressure measurements to decide if fasciotomy is necessary can be very useful if the pressure is significantly elevated, but there are several potential pitfalls. The pressure in one compartment could be normal whilst that in the compartment immediately adjacent could be elevated.

Many other non-invasive techniques have been proposed for making the diagnosis of CS such as near-infrared spectroscopy, laser dopler flowmetry, pulsed phase-locked loop ultrasound, magnetic resonance imaging, skin quantitative hardness measurement, vibratory sensation, and scintigraphy using 99Tcm-methoxyisobutyl isonitril (MIBI). Though some of these techniques have shown early promise, none have reached clinical use outside of protocols.[13]

CS remains primarily a clinical diagnosis fueled by a high index of suspicion, and supported by objective examination. The reliance on clinical examination with a low threshold for fascial release may result in unwarranted fasciotomies, but it avoids the grave consequences of a missed diagnosis.

Treatment

The definitive treatment of CS is **early and aggressive fasciotomy.** In patients with vascular injury in whom a fasciotomy in conjunction with a vascular repair is planned, it is advisable to perform the fasciotomy **before** doing the repair. The rationale for this is that the ischemic compartment is likely to be already tight and thus will create inflow resistance to the vascular repair, making it susceptible to early thrombosis.

Surgeons caring for injured patients must fully understand the anatomy of the extremity compartments and the technique of fasciotomy for each. As previously mentioned in the series reported by Feliciano *et al.*, 75% of amputations of the lower extremity were related to a delay in performing, or performing an incomplete fasciotomy.[5] In a recent large review of combat patients, Ritenour *et al.*, reported that patients who had incomplete or delayed fasciotomy had twice the rate of major amputation and three times the rate of mortality.[9] In spite of these alarming numbers, many otherwise well trained surgeons continue to make these mistakes. The following section will focus on the recommended technique for performing fasciotomy of the lower extremity emphasizing the landmarks, relevant anatomy, and pitfalls.

Fasciotomy of the Lower Leg

The lower leg (calf) is the most common site for CS requiring fasciotomy. The preferred technique for fasciotomy of the below the knee CS is the two incision, four compartment fasciotomy. An alternative single incision approach in which the fibula is resected has been championed by some, but has been condemned by others as being unnecessarily mutilating, more likely to result in injury to the peroneal nerve, and likely to result in incomplete release of the compartments.

The two incision, four compartment fasciotomy is not performed frequently by the majority of general or even vascular surgeons, and the rate of delayed, incomplete or improperly performed fasciotomy is alarmingly high with preventable morbidity and mortality.[9] The most commonly missed compartments are the anterior followed closely by the deep posterior,[9] and this likely occurs as a result of incomplete knowledge of the anatomy of the lower extremity. Successful fasciotomy of the lower extremity requires a thorough understanding of the anatomy and the relevant landmarks. The lower leg has four major tissue compartments bounded by investing muscle fascia (Fig. 2).

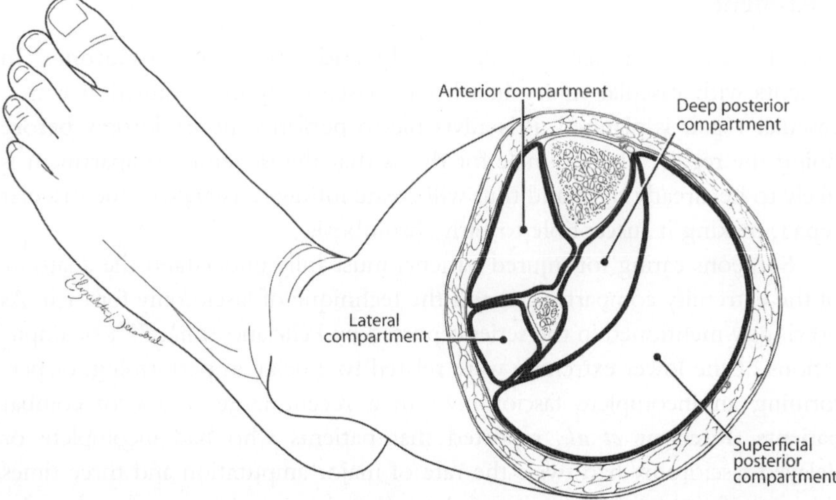

Fig. 2. Cross sectional anatomy of the mid-portion of the left lower leg depicting the four compartments that must be released when performing a lower leg fasciotomy.

It is not necessary to remember the names of all the muscles (Fig. 3) in each compartment, but it is useful to remember — that the anterior compartment contains the anterior tibial artery and vein and the deep peroneal nerve; the lateral compartment the superficial peroneal nerve; the superficial posterior compartment the soleus and gastrocnemius muscles; and the deep posterior compartment the posterior tibial and peroneal vessels and the tibial nerve (Fig. 4).

There are several key features that will enable performance of a successful two incision four compartment fasciotomy. Proper placement of the incisions is essential. As extremities needing fasciotomy are often grossly swollen or deformed marking the key landmarks will aid in placement of the incisions. The tibial spine serves as a reliable midpoint between the incisions. The lateral malleous and fibular head are used to identify the course of the fibula on the lateral portion of the leg (Fig. 5). The lateral incision is usually made just anterior (~1 fingerbreadth) to the line of the fibula, or ***A FINGER IN FRONT OF THE FIBULA***. It is important to stay anterior to the fibula as this minimizes the chance of damaging the superficial peroneal nerve. The medial incision is made one thumb-breadth below the palpable medial edge of the tibia, or ***A THUMB BELOW THE TIBIA*** (Fig. 6). The extent of the

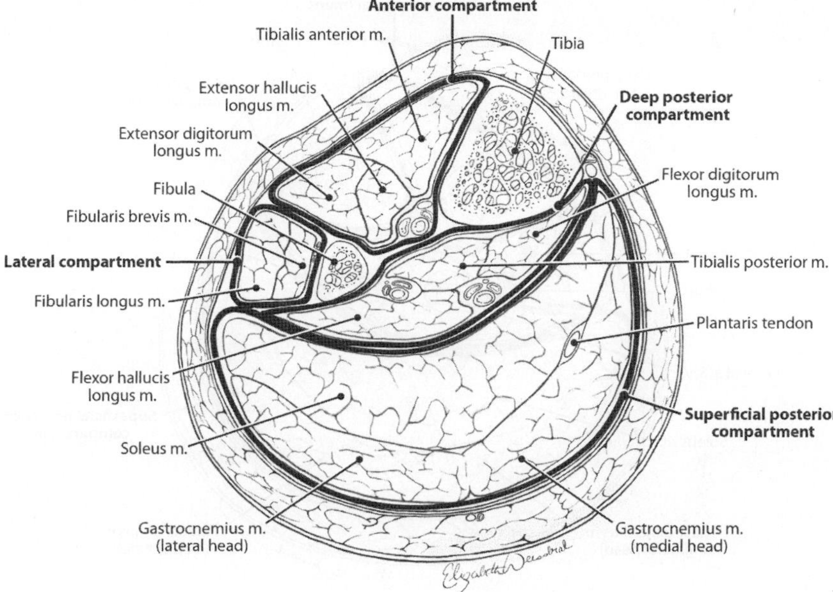

Fig. 3. Cross-sectional anatomy of the mid-portion of the left lower leg depicting the contents of the four compartments and their relationship to the tibia and fibula.

skin incision should be approximately three fingerbreadths below the tibial tuberosity and above the malleolus on either side.

It is very important to mark the incisions on both sides prior to opening them, as the landmarks of the swollen extremity will become distorted once the incision is made.

The lateral incision of the lower leg

The lateral incision (Fig. 5) is made **one finger in front of the fibula** and should in general extend from three fingerbreadths below the head of the fibula down to three fingerbreadths above the lateral malleolus. The exact length of the skin incision will depend on the clinical setting and care must be taken that it is long enough so that the skin does not serve as a constricting band. The skin and subcutaneous tissue are incised to expose the fascia encasing the lateral and anterior compartments. Care should be taken to avoid the lesser saphenous vein and peroneal nerve when making these skin incisions.

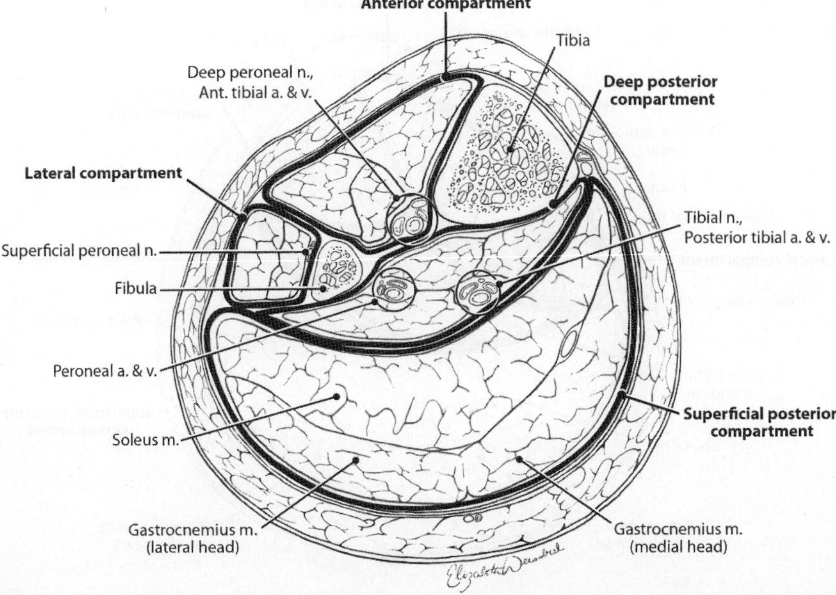

Fig. 4. Cross-sectional anatomy of the mid-portion of the left lower leg depicting the key structures and relationships that must be kept in mind when performing a two incision four compartment fasciotomy.

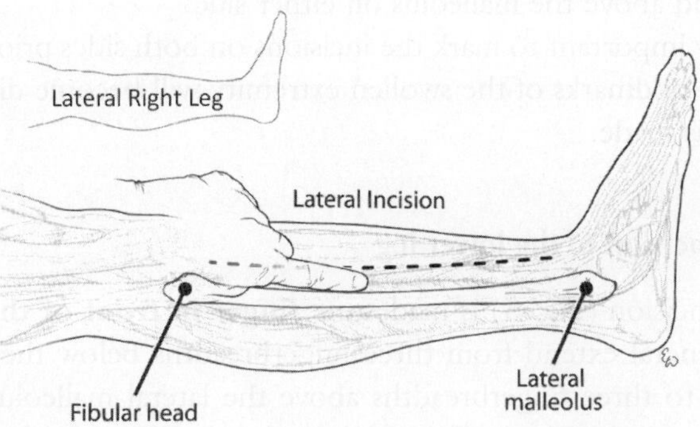

Fig. 5. The fibular head and lateral malleolus are reference points to mark the edge of the fibula and the lateral incision (dotted line) is made one finger in front of this. FINGER IN FRONT OF THE FIBULA

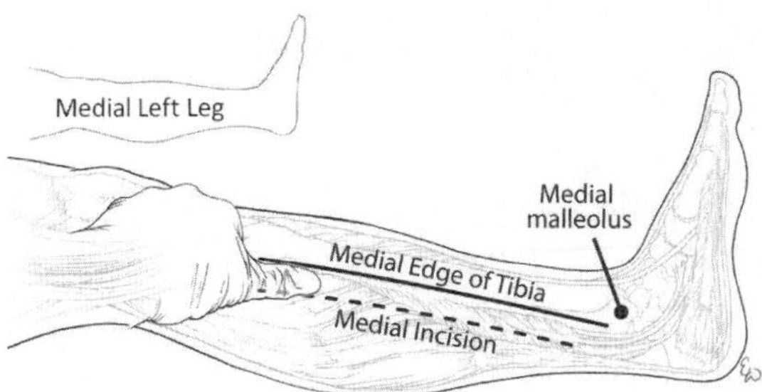

Fig. 6. The medial incision (dotted line) is made one thumb breadth below the palpable medial edge of the tibia (solid line).
THUMB BELOW THE TIBIA

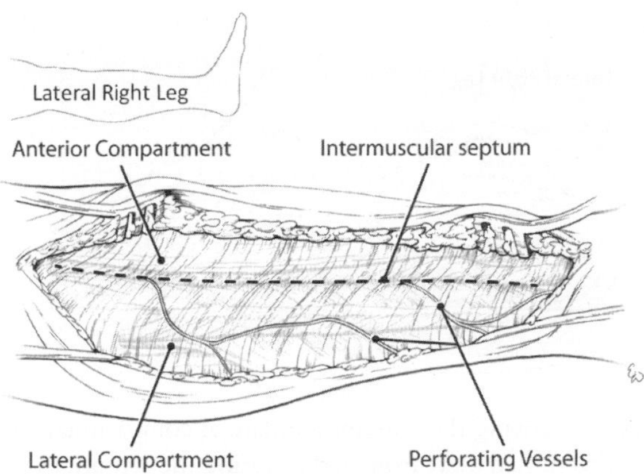

Fig. 7. The intermuscular septum separates the anterior and lateral compartments and is where the perforating vessels traverse. This is a representation of the lateral incision of the right lower leg.

Once the skin flap is raised the intermuscular septum, which divides the anterior and lateral compartments, is identified. In the swollen or injured extremity it may be difficult to find the intermuscular septum. In these circumstances, the septum can often be found by following the perforating vessels down to it (Fig. 7). Classically the fascia of the lower leg is opened using an "H" shaped incision (Fig. 8). This will be accomplished by making the cross piece of the "H" using a scalpel which will expose both

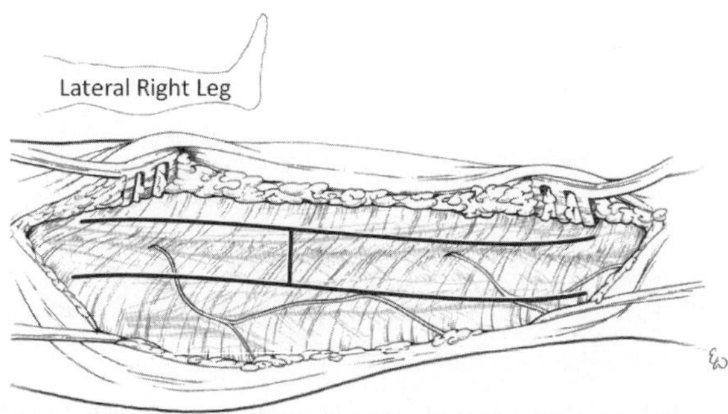

Fig. 8. The fascia overlying the anterior and lateral compartments is opened in an "H" shaped fashion.

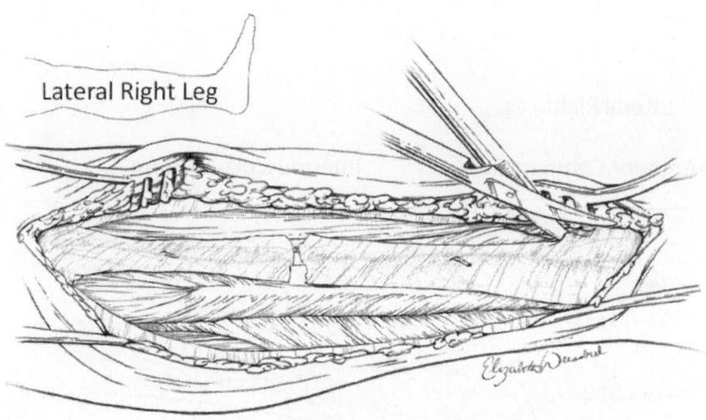

Fig. 9. The fascia overlying the anterior and lateral compartments is opened using scissors with the tips turned away from and elevating the septum to avoid damage to underlying nerves.

compartments and the septum. The legs of the "H" are made with curved scissors using just the tips which are turned away from the septum to avoid injury to the underlying nerves (Figs. 8 and 9). It is important to identify the intermuscular septum and open the fascia at least one centimeter from it on either side, because the terminal branch of the deep peroneal nerve perforates the septum in the distal one third of the lower leg and this could be cut if care is not taken.

The fascia of the anterior and lateral compartments should be opened by pushing the partially opened scissor tips in both directions on either side of the septum opening the fascia from the level of the head of the fibula down

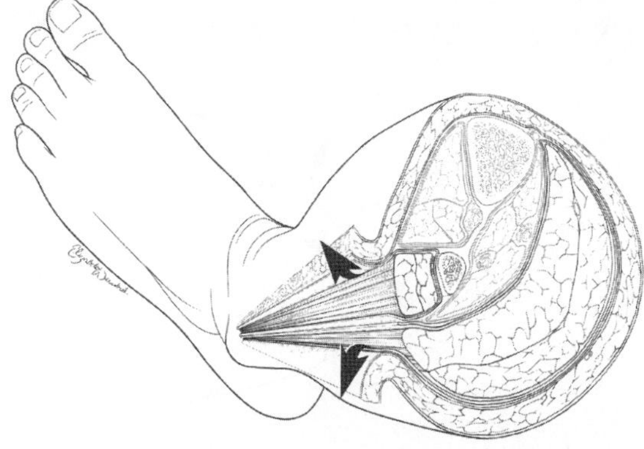

Fig. 10. When the lateral incision is made too far posterior, the septum between the lateral and superficial posterior compartments may be mistaken for that between the anterior and lateral leading to the anterior compartment not being opened.

to the level of the lateral malleolus in a line that is 1–2 cm from the septum. Inspection of the septum and identification of the deep peroneal nerve and/or the anterior tibial vessels confirms entry into the anterior compartment. The skin incision should be closely inspected and extended as needed to ensure that the ends do not serve as a point of constriction.

The anterior compartment can be missed by making the incision too far posteriorly, either directly over or behind the fibula. When the incision is made in this manner the septum between the lateral and the superficial compartment may be directly below the incision and is erroneously identified as the septum between the anterior and lateral compartments (Fig. 10). When the lateral incision is made ONE FINGER IN FRONT OF THE FIBULA, the intramuscular septum between the anterior and lateral compartments is found directly below the incision resulting in successful decompression (Fig. 11).

The medial incision of the lower leg

The medial incision is made one fingerbreadth below the palpable medial edge of the tibia (Fig. 6). When making this incision it is important to both, identify and preserve the greater saphenous vein, as well ligate any perforators to it, as these can bleed profusely. After dividing the skin and subcutaneous tissues the fascia overlying the superficial posterior compartment which

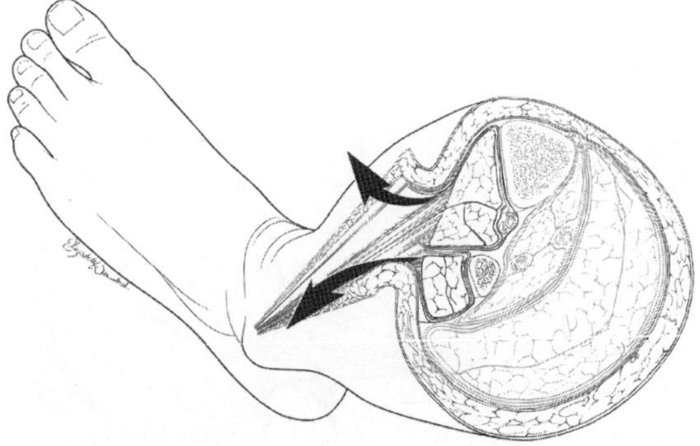

Fig. 11. When the lateral incision is made one finger in front of the fibula, the septum between the anterior and lateral compartments is more readily identified allowing for adequate decompression of both the anterior and lateral compartments.

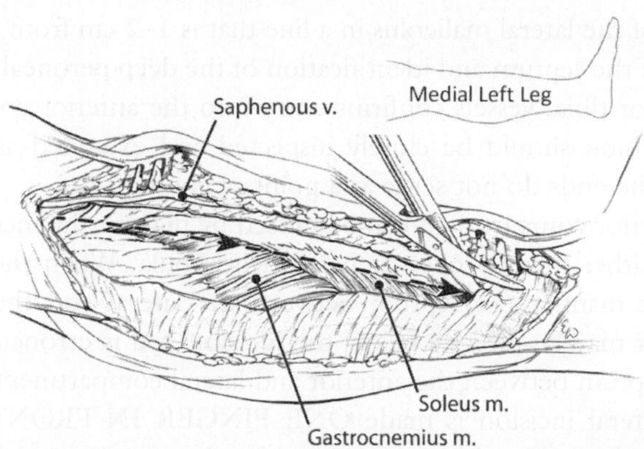

Fig. 12. The fascia overlying the superficial posterior compartment is opened with partially closed scissors from the tibial tuberosity to the medial malleolus.

contains the soleus and gastrocnemius muscle is exposed. The fascia should be opened with partially opened scissors from the level of the tibial tuberosity to the level of the medial malleolus to effectively decompress this compartment (Fig. 12). The key to entering the deep posterior compartment is the soleus muscle. The soleus muscle attaches to the medial edge of the tibia, and dissecting these fibers (the "soleus bridge") off the underside of the tibia

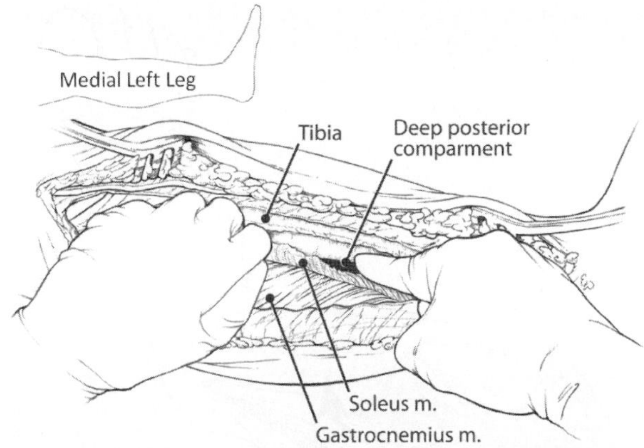

Fig. 13. The deep posterior compartment is entered by taking the soleus fibers down off the underside of the tibia.

enables entry into the deep posterior compartment (Fig. 13). Identification of the posterior tibial neurovascular bundle confirms that the compartment has been entered.

The deep posterior compartment can also be missed, and thorough understanding of the anatomy is the key to ensuring that this does not happen. One potential way to miss the deep posterior compartment is to get into the plane between the gastrocnemius and soleus muscles thinking that the compartment has been released (Fig. 14). Proper decompression of the deep posterior compartment requires that the soleus fibers be separated from the underside of the tibia (Figs. 13 and 15).

Wound Care

The muscle in each compartment should be assessed for viability. Viable muscle is pink, contracts when stimulated, and bleeds when cut. Dead muscle should be debrided back to healthy viable tissue when necessary. Generally, fasciotomy wounds are not closed at the time of the initial procedure. These wounds are often large and tissue swelling, skin retraction, or tissue loss make these wounds impossible to close at the initial setting, and closure would also defeat pressure decreases obtained by fasciotomy.

Wound management focuses on swelling control, allowing recovery of injured tissues and minimizing skin retraction. Patients are generally returned

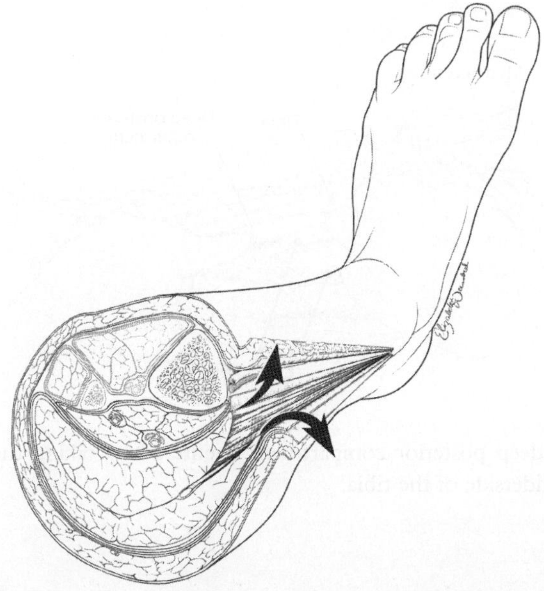

Fig. 14. A potential pitfall when doing the medial incision is to develop a plane between the gastrocnemius and soleus muscles and believing that this represents the plane between the superficial and deep posterior compartment.

to the operating room every 24–72 hours for dressing changes, reevaluation of muscle viability, and gradual closure of the wound. If the wounds cannot be primarily closed within 7–10 days, Split-Thickness Skin Grafts (STSG) may be required when both the patient and the wound are stable. Several techniques have been described to minimize skin retraction and obviate the need for STSG.

The vessel-loop or shoelace technique is commonly performed.[14] It involves using vessel loops interlaced over the wound through staples placed at the skin edges. Although it uses equipment readily available, it suffers from several drawbacks. The thin vessel loops frequently do not have adequate tensile forces to allow minimal skin retraction in severe injuries because of the significant soft-tissue swelling.

Subatmospheric (negative pressure) wound dressings (e.g., Wound V.A.C.™, Kinetic Concepts, Inc. (KCI) , San Antonio, TX) have been used successfully to provide fasciotomy and open-wound control.

Singh and colleagues[15] described their experience caring for war casualties in Iraq using a dynamic wound-closure device (Dynamic Wound Closure

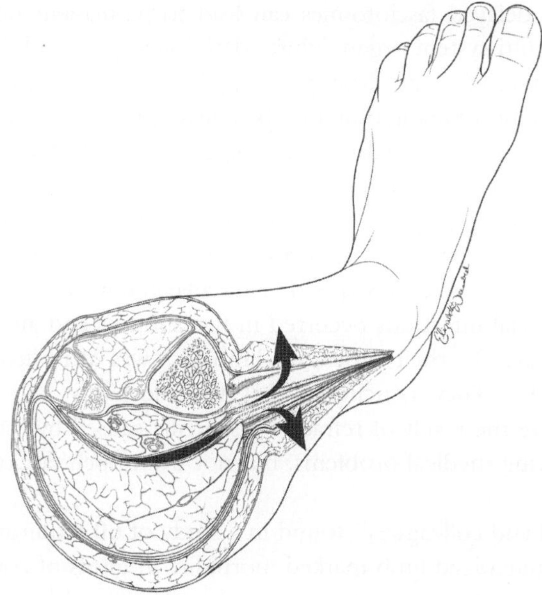

Fig. 15. Entry into and release of the deep posterior compartment requires separating both the gastrocnemius and soleus from the underside of the tibia. Identification of the neurovascular bundle confirms that the deep posterior compartment has been entered.

Device — ABRA® Surgical Skin Closure, Canica, Almonte, ON, Canada) for closure of fasciotomy incisions. A total of eleven consecutive subjects who had undergone two incision fasciotomies for CS were studied. Among them ten of the 11 subjects (91%) had their wounds closed in a delayed primary fashion after application of the wound-closure device. They found that the subjects benefited from the use of the device and avoided the need to create additional wounds in multiple-injury patients. However, long-term follow up of this small group was limited because of the rapid evacuation of soldiers to the United States and the expedient discharge from the hospital of host-nation soldiers.

Complications

In spite of numerous articles in the literature regarding fasciotomy, there is surprisingly little published about the complications of this procedure. Patients with open fasciotomy wounds are at risk for infection and incomplete or delayed fasciotomies can lead to permanent nerve damage, loss of limb, multi-system organ failure, rhabdomyolysis, and death. If muscle injury is extensive, either from prolonged ischemia or from direct crush, significant amounts of myoglobin may be released as the muscle is reperfused after fasciotomy. Early recognition and aggressive fasciotomy will help to minimize these adverse outcomes.

Rush and colleagues[16] reported on a retrospective series of 127 lower extremity fasciotomies performed for CS after acute ischemia and revascularization in subjects with either vascular trauma or arterial occlusive disease. Superficial infections occurred in five subjects and all resolved with local wound care. In their series, no limb loss was attributed to primary open fasciotomy. They concluded that the morbidity and mortality of fasciotomy were the result of refractory ischemia caused by associated injuries or underlying medical problems, but not from open fasciotomy wound complications.

Fitzgerald and colleagues[17] found in a study of 60 requiring open fasciotomy of a traumatized limb marked morbidity in terms of continued pain, altered sensation, and poor cosmetic result as perceived by the patients as well as ongoing wound morbidity. The majority of patients (95%) in this study suffered continued altered sensation within the affected limb postoperatively. However, this altered sensation was restricted to within the limits of the fasciotomy wound in 77% of patients. Furthermore, altered sensation was more marked in those whose wounds were split skin grafted rather than those where the wound was directly closed. Continuing pain existed in 55% of patients in the affected limbs. However, only 10% of patients had pain that could be solely attributed to their fasciotomy wounds. Much of the perceived pain was attributable to stiff joints that were relatively immobile for long periods of time. No patient in this study developed subsequent contracture or required amputation. The fasciotomy wounds were a considerable source of continuing morbidity.

Fasciotomy of Other Compartments

In both civilian and combat trauma,[3,9] the lower leg is the most likely location of CS requiring fasciotomy (68.5% and 51% respectively), followed by the forearm (14% and 22%), and the thigh (~8.5%). A detailed description of CS and the technique for fasciotomy of the forearm and thigh is beyond the scope of this chapter, but the highlights will be briefly covered.

CS and Fasciotomy of the Forearm and Hand

CS of the forearm may be associated with fractures, crush or blast injury, burns or vascular injury.[18] CS of the hand can occur from trauma but is more commonly associated with infiltration of intravenous fluids. As there are no sensory nerves in the hand compartments physical findings do not include sensory abnormalities, and the pressure threshold is much less than in the legs (15–20 mmHg is indication for release). The classic fasciotomy of the forearm is performed though a curvilinear incision on the volar surface (to release the anterior or volar and the lateral compartments) which is extended to the hand to release the carpal tunnel (Fig. 16). The dorsal or posterior compartment of the forearm is released through a linear dorsal incision, with two additional incisions on the dorsum of the hand to release the hand (Fig. 16).

CS and Fasciotomy of the Thigh

CS is uncommon in the thigh because of the large volume that the thigh requires to cause an increase in interstitial pressure. In addition, the compartments of the thigh blend anatomically with the hip allowing for extravasation of fluids outside the compartment. Risk factors for thigh CS include: severe

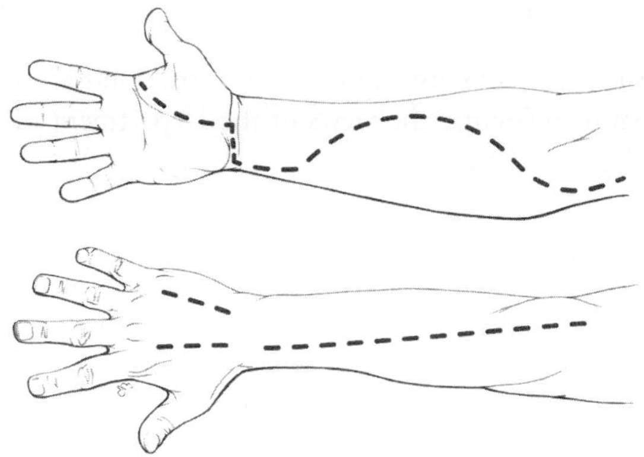

Fig. 16. The volar incision enables decompression of the anterior compartment of the forearm and is carried down onto the hand to release the carpal tunnel. The dorsal incision allows for decompression of the posterior compartment and the two dorsal hand incisions enable release of the intraosseous compartments.

femoral fractures, severe blunt trauma/crush or blast injury to thigh, vascular injury, iliofemoral deep venous thrombosis, and the use of military antishock trousers or other external compression of the thigh.[19] The thigh contains three compartments — anterior, posterior, and medial. If CS of the thigh exists, a lateral incision which decompresses both the anterior and posterior compartments, is often all that is needed.

CS of the hand and foot are much less frequently encountered, and optimal outcomes are achieved with appropriate subspecialty input.

Summary

CS must be suspected in all polytrauma patients with extremity injury. Additionally, patients in the intensive care unit are also at risk to develop CS from a variety of non-traumatic conditions — principally: sepsis, massive resuscitation, and reperfusion. It is essential that all clinicians caring for these patients have an intimate knowledge of the pathophysiology, etiology, and evaluation of CS. Additionally, all surgeons need to have a comprehensive knowledge of the relevant anatomy, and the techniques for performing a proper fasciotomy. A high index of suspicion must be maintained (especially in patients with altered levels of consciousness), and early and aggressive fasciotomy will minimize the morbidity and mortality associated with failure to adequately treat CS.

Disclaimer

The views expressed herein are those of the author and are not to be construed as official or reflecting the views of the Department of Defense. The author has nothing to disclose.

Acknowledgment

The author is grateful to Ms. Elisabeth Weissbrod, MA for her expert illustrations contained in this chapter.

References

1. Matsen FA. Compartment Syndrome: A unified concept. *Clin Orthop* 1975; 113: 8–14.
2. Frink M, Klaus A-K, Kuther G, Probst C, Gosling T, Kobbe P *et al.* Long term results of compartment syndrome of the lower limb in polytraumatised patients. *Injury* 2007; 38: 607–613.

3. Branco BC, Inaba K, Barmparas G, Schnüriger B, Lustenberger T, Talving P *et al.* Incidence and predictors for the need for fasciotomy after extremity trauma: A 10-year review in a mature level I trauma centre. *Injury* 2011; 42: 1157–1163.
4. Gourgiotis S, Villias C, Germanos S, Foukas A, Ridolfini MP. Acute limb compartment syndrome: A review. *J Surg Educ* 2007; 64: 178–186.
5. Feliciano D, Cruse P, Spjut-Patrinely V, Burch J, Mattox K. Fasciotomy after trauma to the extremities. *Am J Surg* 1988; 156: 533–536.
6. Bhattacharyya T, Vrahas MS. The medical-legal aspects of compartment syndrome. *J Bone Joint Surg* 2004; 86-A: 864–868.
7. Rush RJ, Arrington E, Hsu J. Management of complex extremity injuries: Touriquets, compartment syndrome detection, fasciotomy, and amputation care. *Surg Clin North Am* 2012; 92: 987–1007.
8. Bernot M, Gupta R, Dobrasz J, Chance B, Heppenstall RB, Sapega A. The effect of antecedent ischemia on the tolerance of skeletal muscle to increased interstitial pressure. *J Orthop Trauma* 1996; 10: 555–559.
9. Ritenour AE, Dorlac WC, Fang R *et al.* Complications after fasciotomy revision and delayed compartment release in combat patients. *J Trauma* 2008; 64: S153–S162.
10. Taylor RM, Sullivan MP, Mehta S. Acute compartment syndrome: Obtaining diagnosis, providing treatment, and minimizing medicolegal risk. *Curr Rev Musculoskelet Med* 2012; 5: 206–213.
11. Kirk KL, Hayda R. Compartment syndrome and lower-limb fasciotomies in the combat environment. *Foot Ankle Clin* 2010; 15(1): 41–61.
12. Whitesides TE, Haney TC, Morimoto K, Harada H. Tissue pressure measurements as a determinant for the need for fasciotomy. *Clin Orthop* 1975; 113: 43–51.
13. Shadgan B, Menon M, O'Brien PJ, Reid WD. Diagnostic techniques in acute compartment syndrome of the leg. *J Orthop Trauma* 2008; 22: 581–587.
14. Berman SS, Schilling JD, McIntyre KE, Hunter GC, Bernhard VM. Shoelace technique for delayed primary closure of fasciotomies. *Am J Surg* 1994; 167: 435–436.
15. Singh N, Bluman E, Starnes B, Andersen C. Delayed primary closure for decompressive leg fasciotomy wounds. *Am Surg* 2008; 74: 217–220.
16. Rush DS, Frame SB, Bell RM, Berg EE, Kerstein MD, Haynes JL. Does open fasciotomy contribute to morbidity and mortality after acute lower extremity ischemia and revascularization. *J Vasc Surg* 1989; 10: 343–350.
17. Fitzgerald A, Gaston P, Wilson Y, Quaba A, McQueen M. Long-term sequelae of fasciotomy wounds. *Br J Plast Surg* 2000; 53(8): 690–693.
18. Kalyani BS, Fisher BE, Roberts CS, Giannoudis PV. Compartment syndrome of the forearm: A systematic review. *J Hand Surg Am* 2011; 36: 535–543.
19. Ojike N, Roberts C, Giannoudis P. Compartment syndrome of the thigh: A systematic review. *Injury* 2010; 41: 133–136.

Chapter 23

Burns, Cold Injury and Electrical Injury

Karen M. Cross and Joel S. Fish

Chapter Overview

This chapter is an overview of the assessment and management of adult burn patients. The focus is on thermally injured patients with special considerations for chemical, cold injury and electrical burns. The management principles in the first 48 hours after burn injury until the patient can be transferred to a specialized burn care facility are highlighted. Burn care involves a multidisciplinary team of specialists and allied health professionals to manage both the medical and psychological impact of the injury.

Acute Burn Management

The initial management of the burn patient follows the Advanced Trauma Life Support Course as outlined by the American College of Surgeons. The American Burn Association has also designed its own Advanced Burn Support Life Course and specific differences in the two protocols will be outlined in this section.

Primary survey

Airway management of a burn patient is important for transport as well as the long-term management. The endotracheal tube needs to be of large bore to protect from the massive fluid shifts and edema that occur in the early burn period. Intubation for burns greater than 20% body surface area is prophylactic recognizing that the process of swelling and possibly large volumes of fluid will be required in the first 72 hours. Securing the airway with facial burns might require intraoral fixation to dentition or bone if dentition is absent.

High flow oxygen (FiO_2 100%) should be initiated for every patient and especially if carbon monoxide (CO) poisoning is suspected. Ventilation may be restricted with low tidal volumes and high airway pressures in the setting of inhalation injury and/or circumferential thorax and abdominal wounds. Escharotomies may be required to correct this abnormality.

Systemic and peripheral circulation is monitored. Peripheral IV access is preferentially obtained through non-burned tissue. In massive burn injury indwelling catheters through burned tissue are sometimes required. Burned extremities should be evaluated by Doppler examination if pulses cannot be palpated. Circumferential burns, especially full thickness injuries, will impair blood flow to the limbs by acting as a tourniquet. Escharotomies may be required to restore perfusion. Central access with multi-lumen catheters is required to manage the number and types of resuscitation fluids and medications, these patients require. Ringer's lactate fluid should be started and titrated to treat the degree of burn shock.

The burn patient may initially be awake and alert. If there is altered level of consciousness then consider CO poisoning, head injury, substance abuse, hypoxia or pre-existing medical conditions. Finally, the patient should be kept warm to avoid hypothermia. All clothing and jewelry should be removed and the patient covered with dry warming blankets. Intravenous and irrigation solutions should be warmed.

Secondary survey

History and physical exam

A thorough history, physical, and determining the etiology of the burn are important. Etiology is divided into flame, scald, electrical, chemical and contact burns. The environment where the patient was injured will give clues to further injuries or the degree of injury. If the patient was found in an enclosed space (e.g., house fire) then inhalation injury should be suspected. A patient in a MVA requiring extrication could be a multi-trauma patient with life threatening fractures, head injury or intra-abdominal injuries. The same is also true if there was an explosion or a "no-let-go" phenomenon from an electrical injury as the patient may have fallen from a height or been thrown away from the high-tension current. The "when, what, where, how, and who" details surrounding first aid should be determined. In all cases of thermal injury the history and the pattern of the burn seen must fit. If there is a discrepancy then noting this on the history can be very helpful much later on in cases of suspected neglect, abuse or even homicide (rare). A patient post electrical burn requiring cardiopulmonary resuscitation at the scene may have heart conduction defects requiring monitoring. A chemical burn may not be decontaminated adequately if first aid has not been applied appropriately. The burning process can continue and cause extension of the injury. The history should include Tetanus status.

A complete head to toe examination of the patient is important to determine the burn depth, burn size and other associated injuries that may have been missed in the primary survey. Posterior surfaces require inspection and are often missed with health care providers not familiar with thermal injury. The Rule of Nine's determines the burn severity for adults and the Lund Browder for pediatrics, see Fig. 1.[1] The Rule of Nine's gives each anatomic region a designation of 9%. For example, the chest as part of the anterior torso is 9% and in combination with the abdomen is 18%. In children, the head surface area represents a larger component of the total body surface area (TBSA). After the age of 12 months, 1% is taken off the head surface area for each year of age. A quick and practical method for determination of burn extent is to use the hand surface area (palm plus the fingers equals one percent of the body surface area) of the patient to represent the body surface area burned. This is particularly helpful in irregular or scattered surface area burns.

Treatment

All health care personnel involved with the resuscitation of the patient should take universal precautions. All patients requiring intubation should have a bronchoscopy performed as part of the initial workup. Not only will this provide quick evidence of proper ETT tube placement but also will add to the possible diagnosis of smoke inhalation injury grade and subsequent fluid requirements. Directed intravenous fluid resuscitation should occur for all patients with greater than 15–20% TBSA or larger. The Parkland Formula (4 mL/kg/%TBSA) should be calculated and utilized to guide resuscitative measures. TBSA calculations should utilize only partial thickness and full thickness injuries. The first half of the fluid volume is estimated to be given in the first 8 hours and the second half over the next 16 hours. The calculation is a guide and is modified to account for time from the burn and fluids that have already been received. Ringer's lactate is the crystalloid solution of choice for resuscitation. Urine output is monitored hourly with a goal output of 0.5–1cc/kg/ hour.

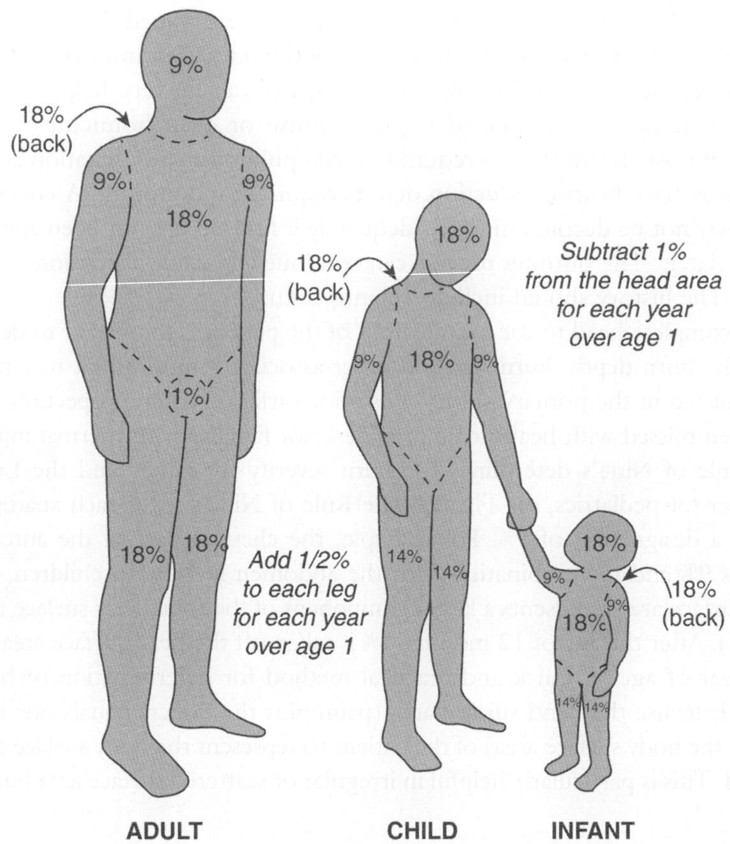

Fig. 1. TBSA calculation.

Under resuscitation could lead to renal failure and secondary effects of hypotension but over resuscitation can lead to extremity or abdominal compartment syndrome and cardiac failure. Extremity perfusion should be monitored hourly especially in patients with circumferential burns that are deep partial thickness or full thickness to determine the need for escharotomies. A high clinical suspicion for compartment syndrome should be maintained. Intra-abdominal pressure (IAP) by bladder transduction should be measured every 4 hours in high volume resuscitations.

Wound irrigation with copious amounts of warm water or saline is important but should not delay transfer to a health care facility. In the absence of sufficient water for cooling, patients should be promptly covered with warm dry towels or sheets to limit air currents circulating over the tissue causing pain and hypothermia. The treatment of chemical and electrical burns will be discussed in a separate section.

A gastric tube should be inserted for burns greater than 20% BSA to start early enteral feeding to meet the increased metabolic demands and prevent gastric dilatation in the patient. Laboratory investigations include CBC, electrolytes, BUN, CR, ABG, carboxyhemoglobin, glucose, ECG, and appropriate imaging. The patient should be continuously monitored and prepared for transfer to a specialized burn center.

Criteria for transfer to a burn unit and transport safety

The American Burn Association recommends that all patients with the following criteria should be transferred to a Burn Center (Table 1) (http://www.ameriburn.org/BurnCenterReferralCriteria.pdf)

Table 1. ABA burn center referral criteria.

1. Partial thickness burns greater than 10% TBSA.
2. Burns that involve the face, hands, feet, genitalia, perineum and major joints.
3. Third degree burns (full thickness) of any age group.
4. Electrical burns including lightening injury.
5. Chemical burns.
6. Inhalation injury.
7. Burn injury in patients with pre-existing medical disorders that could complicate management, prolong recovery, or affect mortality.
8. Any patient with burns and concomitant trauma (fractures) in which the burn injury poses the greatest risk of morbidity or mortality. In such cases, if the trauma poses the greater immediate risk, then the patient may be initially stabilized in a trauma center before transfer to a burn unit. Physician judgment is necessary in such situations and should be in concert with the regional medical control plan and triage protocols.
9. Burned children in hospitals without qualified personnel or equipment for the care of children.
10. Burn injury in patients who will require special social, emotional, or rehabilitative intervention.

Airway Management

Three major processes can affect oxygenation in a burn patient: CO poisoning, direct thermal injury to the airway above the glottis and an inhalation injury. Indications for intubation include the following factors:

- Smoke inhalation
- Large burns >20% TBSA
- Deep facial or neck burns
- Closed range explosion
- Steam Inhalation
- Respiratory distress, oxygenation failure or ventilation failure

Carbon Monoxide (CO)

CO Poisoning should be suspected in patients with decreased level of consciousness who were found in an enclosed space. CO impairs tissue oxygenation by preferentially binding to hemoglobin and displacing oxygen from the hemoglobin molecule. CO has an affinity for hemoglobin 240 times that of oxygen. CO also competitively inhibits the cells' P450 cytochrome system and depresses cellular oxidative metabolism resulting in a shift towards anaerobic metabolism. This shifts the oxygen dissociation curve to the left resulting in a decreased unloading of bound oxygen at the tissue level. Physical signs of CO poisoning include headache, cherry red lips (50% of patients), arrhythmias and seizures. Levels of CO above 10% are clinically significant. Treatment for CO poisoning is humidified oxygen at 100% FiO_2 by mask. The half-life of CO is 320 minutes on room air, and is reduced to 45 minutes on 100% O_2.

Direct thermal injury

Direct thermal injury to the airway usually occurs above the level of the glottis. Direct injury is rare in the lower airway because of the heat dissipating capacity of the oro/hypopharynx and the reflex closure of the glottis. The exception is steam inhalation as it has 4,000 times the heat carrying capacity of air. Upper airway obstruction can occur rapidly in a burn patient with pharyngeal edema or a direct thermal injury. Intubation is important to protect the airway and ensure airway patency for transfer to a burn center.

Inhalation injury

Inhalation injury is defined as a tracheobronchial mucosal injury secondary to inhaled toxins and particulate debris in smoke. These toxins include noxious chemicals such as aldehydes, sulfur oxides and phosphogens, which cause direct injury to the tracheobronchial mucosa. The presence of an inhalation injury is an independent risk factor for mortality in a burn patient. It has been shown to increase mortality by 30–40%.[2] In the 4–12 hours after exposure, the tracheobronchial mucosa has increased capillary permeability resulting in transudation of fluid and protein into the lungs. The bronchial mucosa sloughs resulting in obstruction of the bronchi and alveoli. Severe bronchospasm ensues and mucous production increases.

Inhalation injury should be considered if the flame burn occurred in a closed space, there was expectoration of carbonaceous sputum, greater than 10% carboxyhemoglobin, the patient was unconscious at the scene and with greater than 5 min of smoke exposure. On physical exam, singed nasal hairs, facial or oropharyngeal burns, hoarseness, decreased level of consciousness and signs of upper respiratory obstruction and distress are suggestive. A persistent metabolic acidosis despite what appears to be adequate fluid resuscitation is also suggestive of inhalation injury. Arterial blood gases may show a normal PaO_2 and early chest x-rays are generally normal and non-predictive of the degree of smoke inhalation injury. The gold standard test for the diagnosis of inhalation injury is a fiber optic bronchoscopy. Physical findings to confirm the diagnosis include vocal cord edema, charring, mucosal sloughing, plugging from casts, and edema of the hypopharynx and upper tracheal mucosa. The inhalation injury should be evaluated and graded according to the scale designed by Endorf and Gamelli, see Table 2.[3]

Table 2. Grading of inhalation injury.

Grade O	No inhalation injury	Absence of carbonaceous deposits, erythema, edema or bronchorrhea or obstruction.
Grade I	Mild Injury	Any or a combination of Minor or patchy areas of erythema, carbonaceous deposits in proximal and distal bronchi.
Grade II	Moderate Injury	Any or a combination of Moderate degree of erythema, carbonaceous deposits, bronchorrhea with or without compromise of the bronchi.
Grade III	Severe Injury	Any or a combination of Severe inflammation with friability, copious carbonaceous deposits, bronchorrhea, bronchial obstructions.

Lung ventilation protection strategies should be implemented to reduce the risk of barotrauma. The techniques for lung protection are important for stabilization and the long term care of the burn patient in the ICU setting and beyond the scope of emergency room care. β-2 agonists are used for bronchodilation and to decrease bronchospasm. Nebulized heparin and n-acetyl cysteine loosen and dissolve casts located in the airway promoting sloughed mucosal clearance. Aerosolized hypertonic saline reduces the amount of edema in the parenchyma.

Fluid Resuscitation and Edema Management

The goals of fluid resuscitation in a burn patient are to maintain tissue perfusion and organ function. In the early post burn period, hypovolemia is a result of decreased fluid in the intravascular space secondary to increased capillary permeability and an extravasation of protein and fluid into the interstitial space. Cardiac output is decreased secondary to myocardial depression and decreased pre-load. Hypotension and tachycardia are physical signs of burn shock that ensues.

The amount of edema formation post burn injury is dependent on the depth of burn injury, TBSA involvement, fluid resuscitation and the presence or absence of inhalation injury.[4] Edema forms rapidly in a burn patient with peak edema at 12 hours post injury and resorption dependent on the above features. Fluid accumulation occurs in burned and non-burned tissue along with the organs.[5] The accumulation of burn edema occurs in a biphasic pattern, as there is a rapid increase in interstitial fluid within the first hour post injury. Approximately 80% of total edema is present at 4 hours post injury. The second phase is marked by a gradual increase in fluid accumulation over the next 12–24 hours. Normally, fluid movement from the capillary to the interstitium is balanced by lymphatic clearance so that excess fluid does not accumulate. However, in burn injury the movement of fluid and protein into the extravascular space occurs rapidly and edema ensues.

The goals of resuscitation in a burn patient are to maintain tissue perfusion and organ function. Crystalloids (e.g., Ringer's Lactate) are the fluids of choice as it is balanced, buffered and nearly isotonic with plasma. The major disadvantage of using Ringer's Lactate alone is that one liter only achieves about 250cc of plasma volume and the rest ends up as interstitial fluid.

Immediate use of colloids for resuscitation is a controversial topic in the literature but there is evidence to suggest that colloids can decrease the crystalloid volume delivered, overall total fluid volume, and reduce the amount of edema formation. The institution of colloids might help prevent or minimize the devastating consequences of tissue edema. Colloid, 5% albumin, is generally given at 60–100ml/hour or 0.3–0.5ml/kg/%TBSA per hour. When used, colloid should be given within 8–12 hours post burn and in patients with > 50% TBSA or requiring more than 200mL/kg of resuscitation fluid. Albumin infusions can continue for 48 hours post burn injury. Serum albumin levels should be monitored beyond 48 hours and the albumin infusion titrated to these levels. Target serum albumin level is greater than 20g/L.

Hypertonic saline (3% TBSA) has been shown to have no survival advantage over crystalloid alone. The risk of hypernatremia is high and therefore this practice is not recommended for resuscitation.

Hexastarch and other starches are contra-indicated in burn resuscitation as the retained starch passes into the interstitium particularly the lung.

Resuscitation is monitored by systemic parameters such as urine output, blood pressure, and pulse and central venous pressure along with clinical examination of capillary refill, edema, and sensorium. Mean arterial pressure should be maintained above 60mmHg. Adult urine output should be maintained at 0.5 cc/kg/hour and children less than 30 kg at 1 cc/kg/hour. Base deficit can be utilized to determine the adequacy of resuscitation with levels less than 3 mmol/L considered adequate. Lactate is a measure of ischemia and levels should be maintained less than 2 mmol/L.

Over resuscitation results in excess edema accumulation, compromising local blood flow to tissue and organs. Patients with inhalation injuries, rhabdomyolysis, or large TBSA burns are at increased risk for large volume resuscitations (8 cc/kg/TBSA or 250 mL/kg). IAP monitoring is important in large volume resuscitation as fluid volume is directly proportional to IAP. IAP should be measured in high risk patients such as burn patients with circumferential burns to the torso, poor pulmonary compliance, BMI >30, prone position, associated trauma, and with a previous history of abdominal compartment syndrome. Intra-abdominal hypertension is defined as bladder pressures >12 mmHg (Normal 5–7 mmHg). Abdominal compartment syndrome is defined as elevation of IAP >20mmHg with new organ failure. New organ failure is defined but not limited to: Oliguria, mechanical ventilation or oxygenation failure (decrease in tidal volume and/or increase in airway pressures, hypoxemia), increased serum lactate, and hypotension. Abdominal compartment syndrome has a high mortality rate and should be treated aggressively. Sedation and paralysis of the patient, escharotomies of the chest and abdomen, close titration of IV fluids, and diuresis can improve end organ failure. If conservative strategies fail then an urgent decompressive laparotomy is performed.

The Parkland formula underestimates fluid resuscitation in children, electrical burns, inhalation injury, delayed resuscitation, alcoholics, and full thickness burns. Under resuscitation results in hypovolemia, ischemia to tissue and organs, shock, and multi-organ failure. Oliguria is one of the signs of under resuscitation; however, it is important to rule out other causes such as ACS or rhabdomyolysis. High voltage electrical injuries or patients with rhabdomyolysis are at increased risk of myoglobinuria. Myoglobin is directly cytotoxic to kidney tubules and cast formation occurs from epithelium sloughing in the distal convoluted tubule causing acute renal failure. Alkalinizing the urine with sodium bicarbonate (40 mEq/1L Ringer's lactate) to keep the pH around 6.5 is helpful in solubilization of myoglobin crystals in the tubules. Fluids should be increased to keep urine output 1–1.5 cc/kg/hour. Diuresis with mannitol or furosemide may be used as an adjunct to alkalinization and fluids.

Burn Wound Management

General

Burn wounds are classified according to the depth of injury. This classification is used to determine the treatment required for each of the burn types. Burn types are divided into superficial (1st degree), partial thickness (2nd degree) and full thickness injuries (3rd degree). Clinically, superficial wounds are pink, with brisk capillary refill, and hair follicles remain attached to the dermis. They tend to be dry and painful. Healing time is less than 7 days.

Partial Thickness injuries are divided into superficial or deep injuries. Superficial partial thickness burns are pink, form blisters, have brisk capillary refill, and hair follicles remain attached. They tend to be moist and painful and can regenerate in less than 3 weeks. Deep partial thickness injuries are mottled, pink-white in color, with sluggish cap refill. These wounds are moist, hair follicles are not viable and they detach from the dermis with minimal pain. These wounds are unlikely to regenerate in less than 3 weeks if at all. Full thickness injuries are white in color, with no capillary refill, dry, and leathery. The hair follicles detach and there is no pain. Fourth degree burns involve full necrosis of the skin, muscle, tendon and bone.[1]

In 1953, Jackson described the zones of injury within the burn wound. He was the first to suggest that the burn wound is more than an anatomic determination of depth but represented physiologic zones that were dynamic and could change over time. The zone of coagulation is a central area of necrosis. The zone of hyperemia is an area of vasodilation and increased blood flow. Between these two zones exists the zone of stasis or "progression" zone. This is a dynamic region with a mixture of patent and occluded vessels along with viable and non-viable cells .[6] Resuscitation efforts and antimicrobial dressings are designed to preserve the zone of stasis and prevent conversion to a zone of necrosis. If conversion occurs, then the zone of injury increases and adds to the TBSA that requires surgical excision and adds to patient mortality.

Wound management

Definitive wound management is not required if the patient is going to be transferred to a burn center in the first 24 hours. Clean sterile dry sheets should be placed over the burned regions and are adequate for transfer. A warm heating blanket and elevating the environmental room temperature will help prevent hypothermia. However, if there is a delay in transfer, burn wounds need to be cleaned and debrided in the early period. It is important to communicate with the accepting burn institution to determine the type of dressings they utilize for wound management. Silver based dressings are utilized for partial thickness and full thickness injuries. Silver sulfadiazine is recommended as the dressing of choice for burn wounds due to its capacity to penetrate burn eschar. Limitations of this dressing include the development of pseudo-eschar and the requirement to perform dressing changes twice daily. Advances have been made in silver based dressings with slow release silver that can penetrate eschar but do not need to be changed daily. Basic wound care involves providing complete pain relief and washing the open wounds with simple soap and water and providing a pain free dressing that can be replaced once they arrive at a burn center. Emergency rooms are ill equipped to dress a 30% BSA burn which will use up resources in the emergency room (dressing supplies and ointments) only to be removed immediately when they arrive for definitive care.

Specific wound treatments based on anatomic location

Facial burn will become edematous in the early period and airway protection should be considered. The head of the bed should be elevated at least 30° to promote venous and lymphatic drainage of interstitial fluid. Water or saline soaks should be used to clean the face twice daily and a petrolatum-based antimicrobial applied topically.

Corneal injury should be assessed using fluorescein dye or examination by an ophthalmologist. Lubrication for the eye is imperative. Frost sutures or eyelid taping can be considered if a Bell's phenomenon is not present or edema prevents eyelid closure and therefore protection of the globe.

Examination of the ears is important to rule out a ruptured tympanic membrane and/or otitis media. Burned ears need to be protected with pressure prevention, no occlusive dressings and mafenide acetate for cartilage penetration in order to prevent chondritis. Ear cartilage is relatively avascular and can become secondarily infected with ***Staphylococcus*** or ***Pseudomonas***. If this occurs then the ear should be drained appropriately and antibiotics instituted.

A neurovascular exam of the extremity is important in the acute period. Any compromise in circulation of the burned extremity should be recognized early. Circumferential burns may require early escharotomies to preserve blood flow to the digits. Monitoring can be performed with a Doppler monitoring of radial and ulnar arteries, palmar arch and digital perfusion. The extremity should be elevated above the level of the heart. Resting splints should be placed on the extremities in a position of safety and active/passive range of motion initiated to reduced joint stiffness and preserve muscle tone.

An indwelling catheter may be required to keep the urethra patent and to prevent urine contamination of burn sites in the region. Scrotal edema is common with fluid resuscitation and should be managed conservatively.

Emergency Surgical Procedures

Escharotomies versus fasciotomies

The most common cause of absent pulses in a burned extremity is hypovolemia with peripheral vasoconstriction. Increased tissue pressure from edema surrounded by a non-compliant circumferential burn occludes venous outflow first and then arterial inflow. Escharotomies can release this increased tissue pressure and could be performed under sterile conditions at the bedside with cautery or knife dissection as explained in Table 3.

Fasciotomies should be performed if pulses do not return with escharotomies and the patient meets the criteria for a compartment syndrome. This is discussed in a separate chapter.

Table 3. Escharotomy incisions.

Chest & abdomen	lateral longitudinal incisions ± "H" pattern ± more "criss-crosses" (checkerboard).
Neck	Mastoid, cross anterior to SCM, approach sternal notch.
Upper extremity	Medial and lateral.
Interossei	short longitudinal skin incisions over the 2nd 4th MC's thru inter-MC spaces carried down to the dorsal interossei.
Palm	incision along the palmar crease; at the wrist, continue the incision ulnarward to avoid the palmar cutaneous branch of the median nerve.
Digits/Toes	One or both sides nontactile surface: thumb/ D5 = radial; D2, D3, D4 = ulnar.
Leg	Midmedial & midlateral incisions.

Surgical excision

The details of the surgical management of burn injuries are beyond the scope of this text but should be performed at a burn center by burn surgeons. Tangential or fascial excision is performed at early time points to reduce the morbidity and mortality associated with burn injury. Definitive management involves skin grafting of the burned regions with donor skin from the same patient. If donor skin cannot cover the entire surface area burned then it is either meshed or temporary skin substitutes are utilized such as allograft (human cadaver skin). Skin grafts are classified as spilt thickness or full thickness grafts. A split thickness graft (STSG) is harvested with a dermatome and is based on the thickness of the dermis acquired. STSG have reliable graft take, the donor site heals faster (less than 2 weeks), can cover larger areas and the donor site can be harvested multiple times. Disadvantages of STSG are increased wound contraction, abnormal pigmentation, minimal eccrine glands and hair follicles. These grafts are also thin and not as durable as full thickness grafts. Full thickness skin grafts (FTSG) involve the entire surface area of the skin to the subcutaneous tissue. FTSG are advantageous in areas such as the face or hands because there is less scar contraction. The texture and pigment match is superior with eccrine glands and hair follicles can be transplanted. The disadvantage of using these grafts is the graft take is less reliable and the possible donor site size is small.

The recipient bed preparation is achieved by removing the necrotic burn eschar down to healthy viable tissue. Skin grafts can be applied to exposed muscle, fat and fascia. Periosteum, perichondrium and paratenon will also support a graft. Cortical bone if debrided, can promote granulation tissue and accept a skin graft. Failure of skin grafting is related to a loss of contact of the skin as occurs with hematoma, seroma, shearing and edema. A poorly vascularized wound bed, infection, malnutrition, systemic illness, and immunocompromised patients and pressure can impair skin graft take. Finally, technical error such as malposition of the skin graft, rough handling, inappropriate thickness and stabilization are additional risks of failure.

Skin grafts survive transplantation in the first 48 hours by plasmatic imbibition. The graft is nourished by the diffusion of plasma, oxygen and nutrients. The attachment to the recipient bed is by fibrin only. After 48 hours, inosculation and capillary ingrowth begin and create a fine vascular network in the fibrin layer. Capillary buds from the recipient bed blood vessels connect with the graft vessels and open channels are formed. After 6 days the revascularization process begins and the vascular channels differentiate into afferent and efferent vessels. Lymphatic drainage is established and collagen links begin to form between the graft and the wound bed. Dressings are not changed in the skin graft region for 5–7 days and the area is generally kept immobilized to allow neovascularization and preliminary adherence of the skin graft to the wound bed.

Other Considerations

Deep venous thrombosis/pulmonary embolism

Burn injured patients are at increased risk for deep venous thrombosis (DVT) and pulmonary embolism. These patients meet the three criteria of Virchow's triad as they are frequently immobilized, hypercoagulable, and have a vascular injury. DVT rates can be as high as 23% during their length of stay. DVT prophylaxis should be initiated on admission to the hospital. A low molecular weight heparin is appropriate and generally enoxaparin is the drug of choice. Prophylaxis should continue even if the patient is ambulatory. Some burn centers routinely perform Doppler investigations to assess for the presence of DVT in their patient population.

Sedation/analgesia

Medical management of pain in burn patients is important at all stages of burn injury and rehabilitation. General guidelines follow the World Health Organization consensus for pain. Initial management includes the utilization of a combination of NSAIDS (acetaminophen, ibuprofen or ketorolac), opioids (morphine, hydromorphone, or fentanyl) and anticonvulsant medication (gabapentin or pregabalin). Opioids should be both, long acting for continuous pain and given every 8 or 12 hours. Shorter acting intermittent narcotic medications are required for breakthrough pain. Intubated patients experience pain that should be treated at the time of burn resuscitation. Enteral analgesia should include acetaminophen and gabapentin in combination with an intravenous opioid. At the time of patient weaning from IV opioids, long acting oral agents should be initiated. Procedures, such as dressing changes, can be excruciatingly painful and pre-medication is required with opioids and possible anxiolytics in both awake and intubated patients.

Electrical Injury

Introduction

Electrical injuries are a global phenomenon and whilst only accounting for 5–8% of the total admissions to a burns unit, may be disproportionately devastating with respect to their size.[7] They usually occur in young, working men and are a common cause of work related trauma deaths.

Epidemiology and incidence

Electrical burns typically account for approximately 1.7–8% of all major burn unit admissions with 20–43% being low-voltage (<1000V) and 57–64% high-voltage (>1000V).[8,9]

The causes of domestic injury are electrical device misuse or malfunction, carelessness, inadequate education regarding safety and precautions and insufficient parental supervision.[8] Low-voltage injuries are usually caused by domestic appliances with 77% of these injuries involving children under 5 years, and are associated with electrical and extension cords (60–70% cases) and wall outlets (10–15% cases); 61% involving electrical contact with an extremity. Due to the attempted theft of copper, which has soared in price over the last 20 years and is a principal component in electrical distribution lines, there has been a rise in the number of high-voltage injuries, often in young males.

Definitions/etiology

Electrical burns may be classified by voltage, current type and injury mechanism. Arbitrarily electrical burns may be classified as low-voltage (<1000 volts) or high-voltage (≥1000 volts). Almost all electrical injuries occurring indoors, except for those in industrial locations, are low-voltage. An electrical current may be alternating current (AC), such as from an over-head high-voltage power line, or a direct current (DC), such as the electrified rail of an electrical train system.

Electrical injury may occur via one or combination of mechanisms: Direct contact, arc or flash burn. In direct contact, current flows through an individual from a contact point with dissipation into the tissues following the path of least resistance.[10] The current leaves the body wherever a potential difference exists to allow for an arc. This combination of arc burns plus current conduction may lead to far more extensive deep tissue destruction than can be realized externally.

Physics and pathophysiology

Pathophysiology

The principal determinant of tissue damage in electrical injury is voltage. Three major mechanisms are responsible for tissue injury: Direct tissue damage, conversion of electrical into thermal energy and mechanical injury. Electrical energy causes direct tissue damage by both altering cell membrane potentials and causing pores to develop in lipid bilayers. This results in a rapid influx of calcium into the cytoplasm causing cell apoptosis. Nerve and muscle are the most susceptible to supraphysiologic electric fields.[11] (Electrical to thermal energy conversion causes massive tissue destruction, coagulative necrosis and macromolecule denaturation. Thermal injury causes thrombosis, necrosis or epineural vessel hemorrhage thus impairing perineural vascularity and perfusion. In the extremities peripheral nerves are at risk of direct damage from localized thermal injury; influenced by the nerve's cross-sectional resistance or proximity to bone. Late fibrosis leads to delayed presentation of neurological symptoms is common. Mechanical injury with direct trauma may result from falls or violent muscle contractions.

Factors influencing electrical burn severity

Electrical injuries may arise directly and indirectly. Direct injury is due to the conversion of electrical to thermal energy or the deleterious effect of electric current on body tissues or cells as outlined above. Indirect injuries are usually due to current induced tetanic muscle contraction or the victim being

Table 4. Current intensity and its expected clinical manifestation.

Current intensity	Expected clinical manifestation
1 mA	Imperceptible, probable tingling sensation.
3–5 mA	"*Let go*" current for an average child.
6–8 mA	"*Let go*" current for an average woman.
7–9 mA	"*Let go*" current for an average man.
16 mA	Maximum current a person can grasp and "*let go*".
16–20 mA	Tetany of skeletal muscles.
20–50 mA	Paralysis of respiratory muscles (respiratory arrest).
50–100 mA	Threshold for ventricular fibrillation.
Greater than 2 A	Asystole.
15–30 A	Common household circuit breakers

thrown or falling from a height. Electrical burn severity depends on: Current type, amount of current, current pathway, voltage, resistance of body tissues, duration of contact and individual susceptibility.

The current type may be AC or DC. At low-voltages (<1000 volts) an AC is three times more dangerous than a direct current of the same voltage. At high-voltages (^{3}1000 volts) an AC is as dangerous as a DC. At low-voltages with an AC the "no let go" phenomenon may result in prolonged contact from muscle tetany (as forearm flexors are stronger than the extensors). Conversely, a DC tends to throw victims away from current sources.

The greater the current the greater the electrical burn severity. Unlike voltage, the current amount is often unknown. The current pathway through a victim of electrical injury and the entrance and exit points are unknown. Contact points, points of extreme energy transfer, may vary from none to many and some, or all, may be invisible. Consequently, there may be little external damage. Traditionally, literature discussed transverse current or "hand-to-hand" pathways and vertical or "hand-to-foot" pathways.

Voltage influences the electrical injury severity; the higher the voltage the greater the damage. Low-voltage burns are usually associated with localized injury. Due to the transformation of electrical into thermal energy, injuries range from simple erythema to full-thickness burns. Conversely, in high-voltage burns more extensive and deeper tissue destruction, similar to crush injuries, occurs.

Body tissue resistance

Externally, skin resistance is the principal factor impeding current flow. With greater resistance the more thermal energy (heat) is generated (Joule's Law). Skin resistance is extremely variable depending on, probably most importantly moisture, but additionally skin thickness and callosities. Consequently, exposure of a common household voltage to the thick, calloused adult laborer's palms, in which resistance may be greater than 100,000 Ohms, may create a barely perceptible 1–2 mA current. Conversely, an identical voltage applied to a newborn baby's thinner and high water content skin, probably results in serious damage.

Internally the body's resistance consists of all the remaining tissues and is approximately 500–1,000 Ohms. Although fat, tendon and bone, offer the highest resistance, they are unlikely contact points. Furthermore, given their intrinsic resistance, on exposure to a current, they tend to heat up and coagulate before conducting current. Conversely, nerves, evolved as conductors, and blood vessels, with high water content, are the best conductors. The traditional theory was these properties created a preferential pathway of least resistance allowing current conduction along neurovascular structures after entering the body. Thus electrical injury primarily affected the neurovascular structures and tissues with the highest resistance produced the most heat. However, this is now considered only to be true for low-voltage injuries. High-voltage current travels the most direct path between the contact point and the ground

The longer the duration of contact the greater the damage. The 'no let go' phenomenon associated with an AC, as opposed to the victim being 'thrown' away from a power source by a DC, may exacerbate this. Decreased consciousness, described in approximately half of those with high-voltage injuries, may prolong contact duration.[12] Contact pressure and individual susceptibility are important. It is unclear why victims exposed to the same electrical source have different injuries; this may be due to the degree of tissue resistance.

Management

At the scene

No attempt should be made to deliver medical care until either the victim has been safely removed from the current source with the use of correctly insulated equipment or the origin of the electrical current has been disconnected. If a victim of electrical injury remains in contact with the source of the current (as may occur with AC), they become a conductor that may electrocute any rescuer. Likewise, in high-voltage injuries, the ground, particularly if it is wet, may carry current to the rescuers. In contrast to popular belief, touching a lightning victim is safe and therefore, treatment should be initiated immediately.

Electrical injury to specific organs and tissues

Electrical injury may cause multisystem injuries and all organs are vulnerable. Injury to vital organs may ultimately result in the patient's demise. Intensive care and supportive therapies are often required.

Cardiac injury and monitoring

Cardiac arrhythmia and direct myocardial necrosis may occur, often rapidly, after low and high-voltage electrical injury, emphasizing that an ECG should be performed in all patients.[13,14] The amount of myocardial necrosis tends to be greater with higher voltage, and for any given voltage, more extensive with AC than with DC. Normal ECG is possible after cardiac injury and creatine kinase and MD-creatine kinase are not accurate markers OD myocardial damage. Inadequate data on troponin levels prevents guideline formation.[14]

It is challenging to formulate appropriate management guidelines regarding the required duration of cardiac monitoring post electrical injury as no studies have specifically investigated this. Several series documented 24 hours monitoring post-admission if there were no ECG abnormalities on admission or monitoring for 24 hours after following arrhythmia cessation. Arrowsmith *et al.* stated all arrhythmias dissipated within 48 hours of admission either spontaneously or with medical therapy.[15]

Myoglobinuria

Hemoglobinuria or myoglobinuria is the presence of hemoglobin or myoglobin in the urine. An electrical burns victim may suffer rhabdomyolysis (skeletal muscle breakdown), with myoglobin and hemoglobin released from damaged myocytes and erythrocytes. Consequently, the myoglobin and hemoglobin pigments are excreted into the urine resulting in myoglobulinuria or hemoglobinuria, demonstrable by progressive urinary darkening (darker than light pink). Treatment must be quickly instigated; the window of opportunity to avoid complications is a few hours post-injury and a 59% mortality rate is reported for patients with renal failure and electrical burns.[8]

Urine dipstick is overly sensitive and urinary assessment of hemochromogens is not an accurate guide to effective management.

Fluid resuscitation

Hidden injuries associated with electrical injuries may mean patients receive inadequate fluid if fluid resuscitation regimes are based on body surface area alone. Crystalloid fluids (Hartmann's / Ringer's lactate) should be used to achieve urine output of 0.5–1 mg/kg/hour (in the absence of macroscopic myo/hemoglobin) or 2 mg/kg/hour (in the presence of macroscopic myo/hemoglobinuria).

Traumatic Injuries

The rate of traumatic injuries (15%) in those with electrical injuries is almost double that of those seen in other burn victims. Consequently, all burns patients, including those with electrical injuries should undergo a careful history and examination to detect any traumatic injuries.

Diagnosis and tissue damage assessment

Assessment of tissue damage extent in electrical injury is notoriously imprecise. Furthermore, the outer TBSA burnt may substantially underestimate deeper tissue damage; small, insignificant marks may be all that is visible externally, despite serious underlying injury. Whilst there is general consensus regarding the need for early debridement, some have debated the rationale of aggressive and total burn excision and support delayed soft tissue coverage.

Compartment syndrome

Compartment syndrome results from raised pressure, greater than capillary pressure, within an unyielding osseo-fascial compartment reducing blood flow and ultimately resulting in muscle ischemia. If prolonged this can lead to muscle death, myoglobulinuria and acute renal failure, ischemic contracture and death. Limbs with high-voltage electrical injuries are susceptible to compartment syndrome, particularly in the immediate 48 hours electrical injury. A high degree of clinical suspicion and expeditious management is essential.

Lightning injury

Lighting comprises approximately 2% of electrical injuries and is the second leading cause of weather-related death in much of the world.[14] If the electrical difference between a thundercloud and the ground is greater than the insulating effects of the surrounding air lightening occurs as a form of direct current. The duration of a lightning strike is only 1–2 m/sec, with the current peaking within approximately 2 microseconds. The voltage of a lightning strike maybe greater than 1,000,000 volts and generate currents over 200,000 A. Whilst the conversion of this electrical energy into heat can generate temperatures as high as 25,000°C the extremely short duration of lightning prevents hit item from melting. Generally, four mechanisms of lightning injury are reported: Direct strike (the predominant current pathway is through the body); side flash (a direct strike to an object or a person is followed by a secondary discharge from the object/person to a nearby victim); stride potential (lightning hits the ground and subsequently enters the body via one foot and exits via the other foot; and flash-over phenomenon (electricity flows outside the body, often vaporizing surface water with a blast effect to clothing.[16] Often the morbidity is 5–10 times higher than other forms of electrical injury and maybe as high as 17.6%.[14]

A heterogeneous spectrum of injury severity is seen from minimal cutaneous burns to life-threatening burns of similar magnitude to industrial high-voltage injury. Significant skin injury is rare, as despite the huge energy and heat generation the short duration and flash-over effect are often protective. An exception is injury caused by associated flash/flame-burn following ignition of a nearby item (e.g., a carried bag of golf clubs). When they occur, burns may be of various categories, including partial-thickness linear (usually in areas of high sweat concentration), punctate (clusters of small, deep, circular burns), thermal (for example, from ignition of garments or contact with metallic objects), and feathering burns, known as Lichtenberg Flowers or Figures the latter is pathognomonic of a lightning strike and is a dendritic, fern-like branching erythematous pattern on the skin. This occurs within one hour post-injury and appears to be wheal and flare reaction and it is unclear whether they are an actual burn.[16]

Table 5. Comparison of the low-voltage, high-voltage and lightning induced electrical injuries.[17]

Lightning	Low-voltage	High-voltage
Voltage, V $>30\times10^6$	<1000 (typically 120–240)	>1000
Current, A >200000	<240	<1000
Duration Instantaneous	Prolonged	Brief
Current Type DC	Usually AC	DC or AC
Cardiac arrest (cause)	Ventricular fibrillation Asystole	Ventricular fibrillation
Respiratory arrest (cause)	Tetanic contractions of respiratory muscles	Indirect trauma or tetanic contraction of respiratory muscles
Muscle contraction	Tetanic	DC: Single; AC: Tetanic
Burns	Usually superficial Rare, superficial	Common, deep
Rhabdomyolysis	Common	Very common
Blunt injury (cause)	Fall (uncommon) Blast effect, shock wave Low	Muscle contraction, fall
Mortality (acute)	Very High	Moderate

Lightning may cause cardiac and respiratory arrest; cardiopulmonary resuscitation is especially effective if commenced quickly. Neurologic complications are relatively common manifesting over several days after injury. Keraunoparalysis describes the constellation of symptoms including unconsciousness, seizures, paresthesia and paralysis, which may have an insidious progression over a number of days post-injury. Vasomotor disorders may also occur. These lightning induced symptoms, usually resolve and have a good prognosis. However, vague neurological changes may remain. Altered levels of conscious may also suggest epidural, subdural or intracerebral hematomas. Otologic injuries are common, mostly involving ruptured tympanic membrane although middle and inner ear injuries occur. Post-traumatic stress disorder occurs in about 30% of patients after lightning.

Electrical injuries, particularly lightning, may produce multiple casualties; medical efforts are typically concentrated on those with signs of life and those considered to be already dead given the least priority.[16] Lightning victims are an exception as those hit by lightning may be apneic following respiratory control center paralysis, have fixed dilated pupils from autonomic dysfunction, and be pulseless following asystole. However, due to innate cardiac automaticity sinus rhythm may spontaneously return. Successful resuscitation is achievable with immediate and appropriate management as most lightning victims are usually previously healthy individuals and relatively young. Therefore, oxygen administration and bag and mask ventilation should be immediately commenced on a non-breathing patient. The airway should be expeditiously protected to minimize anoxia, a prime cause of death. This potential for successful recovery has propagated the myth, that lightning induces "suspended animation" from which a victim can recover almost unscathed.

Summary

Electrical injuries, are a global phenomenon, and may be arbitrarily divided into high-voltage (≥1000 V) and low-voltage (<1000 V) injuries and should be managed in a multi-disciplinary setting. Compared with thermal burns, they may be more devastating and complex manifesting as cardiorespiratory, neurologically, renal, gastrointestinal, ophthalmologic and psychiatric disturbances. Electrical injuries may result in deceptively large tissue destruction, potentially leading to limb amputation. Following resuscitation and management of any rhabdomyolysis, early debridement, necessary decompression of neurovascular structures, and early wound closure are essential to successful restoration of function. Extensive surgical procedures including free soft-tissue transfer may be required to gain wound closure, and to save and restore limb function.

Chemical Injuries

Chemical agents injure tissue by a chemical reaction rather than a thermal process. The amount and nature of the exposed tissue surface, duration of contact, and the concentration/quantity of the agent determine degree of tissue destruction. Damage continues until the agent is washed off or removed, neutralized or exhausted by a reaction with the tissues. According to the ABLS handbook, "the extent of chemical burn is directly related to the interval between injury and institution of appropriate medical therapy. Prompt recognition and timely treatment is essential". WHMIS or (Workplace Hazardous Materials Information System) or poison control should be contacted for treatment and clinical complications of exposure.

Chemical injuries are broadly classified according to the type of chemicals, acids, alkalis, or organic compounds. Acids produce free hydrogen ions, an exothermic reaction, cellular dehydration and protein precipitation. This results in a coagulation necrosis which limits the extent of the acid penetration in tissue. Examples of acids include, hydrochloric acid (HCl) (bathroom cleaners), oxalic acid and hydrofluoric acid (HF) (rust removers), along with sulfuric acid (industrial drain cleaners). Acids can produce severe and long lasting pain that does not disappear until the hydrogen ion is neutralized. Pain is used frequently as a marker of endpoints for decontamination in acid injured tissue. Alkalis include the caustic sodas of sodium, potassium, lithium, ammonium and calcium. They are found in oven cleaners, drain cleaners, fertilizers, cement and concrete. Alkali's cause injury via liquefaction necrosis and protein denaturation. This promotes a deeper and more extensive burn injury. Organic compounds, phenols and petroleum products produce contact burns and systemic toxicity. Tissue damage is caused by fat solvent action or delipidation, therefore, any part of the body which has fat or absorbs fat (e.g., Liver and kidney) is affected.

Management of chemical burns

Universal precautions should be observed with all patients with suspected chemical injuries to ensure that health care providers do not become victims. Management specific to chemical injuries includes removal of the chemical by removing the patient from the source, removing clothing and brushing dry particulate debris. Irrigation, NOT immersion, of the patient with copious amounts of tap water is important. Antidotes are generally avoided but there are exceptions to this rule as shown in Table 6. A poison control center or WHMIS should be contacted, as lists of complications and systemic toxicity will be available for the particular chemical. Chemical burns, otherwise, should be treated like a thermal injury.

Hydrofluoric acid

One of the more common chemical injuries seen in the emergency room are exposure to HF. HF is an inorganic acid commonly used in many domestic

Table 6. Treatment of chemical burns.

Compound	Atypical feature	Special measure
Sodium and lithium metals	Ignite on contact with water.	Cover burn with oil. Pieces must be excised.
Hydrofluoric acid	Requires neutralization of extremely toxic fluorideion Severe systemic toxicity.	Calcium gluconate preparations (topical, injected, intra-arterial).
Phenols	Poorly soluble in water, systemic toxicity.	Polyethylene glycol wipe.
White phosphorus	Ignites spontaneously on exposure to air.	Immerse in H_2O, Copper sulfate irrigation, debride particles.

and industrial settings, and also is a cause of chemical burns encountered in burn centers. At high concentrations (>20%), small quantities of HF can cause life threatening burns, and if the diagnosis is missed or treatment delayed the consequences may be devastating for the patient.

HF causes tissue destruction in two main ways. At concentrations above 50%, HF acidity increases dramatically and it then behaves like a strong acid. The hydrogen ion causes a corrosive burn similar to other acid burns. Liquefaction necrosis of deeper tissues is unique to HF acid since the acid is highly lipophilic and readily penetrates down to deep tissue. The molecule then wreaks havoc as it releases its acidic hydrogen ion and fluoride ion in the presence of cations such as calcium and magnesium. This often-delayed reaction is responsible for the 'pain out of proportion' to physical exam findings; a result thought to be related to the local hyperkalemia effect secondary to calcium binding.

Pain out of proportion to physical exam is a hallmark finding in HF burns. For all cutaneous HF burns, the clinician must include an assessment of any systemic effects. Late clinical manifestations of systemic toxicity include nausea, vomiting, abdominal pain, convulsions, hypotension, cardiac arrhythmias, and cardiac failure. These findings are often not present in the majority of cases with low concentration exposure. Patients are usually asymptomatic beyond the pain in the area of cutaneous exposure. In order to diagnose the systemic toxicity a high level of suspicion on the history is needed so that an appropriate treatment can be commenced. Immediate tap water skin surface irrigation should be initiated to remove acid from the skin and prevent rapid penetration by the extremely lipophilic HF acid. There is general consensus that lavage should take place immediately at the site of the accident for 15–30 minutes before proceeding to the medical department.

Topical gluconate gel is used to deactivate the free fluoride ions that have penetrated to deeper tissues. The calcium gluconate gel can be created in the ER department with a water-soluble lubricant such as K-Y jelly, added to calcium gluconate solution or calcium gluconate powder (75 ml K-Y jelly plus 25 ml of 10% calcium gluconate or 100 ml of K-Y jelly plus 2.5 g of calcium gluconate).

Infiltration of the tissues with Calcium Gluconate have widely adopted its use for HF burns, likely because it has been shown in humans to reliably reduce pain after injection. Indications for injection are a central hard gray area with surrounding erythema and throbbing severe pain despite management with irrigation and gel. Most authors agree that infiltration is unnecessary for burns with HF concentration less than 20%.

The use of a local anesthetic injection is controversial as some authors feel it either masks the pain — which is a valuable clinical indicator of treatment effectiveness or may also further increase tissue tension. The ability to use short term sedation such as propofol has allowed for repeated injections to occur and the masking effect of the local anesthetic is avoided.

Intra-arterial calcium infusion is reserved for patients with severe HF burns with unrelenting pain despite aggressive calcium gel therapy.

The technique was originally developed for high concentration HF digital burns where large numbers of fluoride ions needed to be neutralized but available tissue space was too limited to use the infiltration method safely. Intra-arterial infusion requires cannulation of the brachial artery caries high morbidity and requires ICU monitoring. Calcium gluconate can also be given intravenously with an above elbow cuff based on Bier's method. There is no consensus on indications for immediate surgical debridement, but in general immediate debridement is reserved for high concentration burns or those that show systemic toxicity despite more conservative management. In the large majority of cases, Surgery is delayed until wounds are well demarcated. HF readily passes through and around the nail plate causing severe damage to the delicate subungual tissues. Involvement of the nail bed poses a unique challenge in calcium gel delivery and removal of the fingernail is often required. One should not hesitate to remove the nail if there is severe pain. This requires local block or sedation and the finger pads can be injected at the same time.

Cold Injury

Cold injury is a spectrum of localized or systemic injuries resulting from a loss of heat. Frostbite is a specific type of cold injury that results from ice crystals formation leading to four distinct phases. Phase-I, the cooling and freezing phase, where cold exposure causes a peripheral vasoconstriction resulting in a decrease in skin temperature promoting intracellular and extracellular ice crystals formation. Extracellular, ice crystals cause an increase in interstitial osmolarity resulting in cellular dehydration. Direct intracellular injury from freezing causes a denaturation of cell membrane lipoproteins and cell death via mechanical disruption. The combination of vasospasm, cell destruction and red cell hemolysis causes skin ischemia. Phase-II occurs during the thawing and rewarming phase. As ice crystals melt, they cause an endothermic reaction. Capillary endothelium becomes permeable to fluid and protein causing edema. A reperfusion injury is mediated through oxygen free radicals promoting endothelial injury, cytokine production (thromboxane), vasoconstriction, and platelet aggregation. Phase-III, the progressive phase, prostaglandins within the blisters propagates the vasoconstriction and platelet aggregation causing further cellular injury and necrosis of the skin. The final phase is the resolution phase where the injury is fully declared and the zone of injury defined.

Frostbite is classified according to wound depth but treatment is the same for all types with adequate wound care and waiting for the eschar to fully delineate. Certain populations are at increased risk for frostbite and include persons with altered mental status, military personnel, outdoor enthusiasts, the homeless, the elderly, and persons with co-morbidities such as atherosclerosis or open wounds.

In order to determine the severity of the injury, it is important to ask about the environmental exposure of the patient. These questions should include the outdoor temperature including wind chill. The length of exposure and wetness of the clothing should be determined. Water conducts heat 25 times faster than air and frostbite can occur much more quickly in wet clothing. The presence of clothing or protection from the cold should also be determined. Contact with metal promotes conductive heat loss and may cause injury to other areas of the body. The host factors are also important as compromised circulation, such as peripheral vascular disease, smoking or tight clothing can increase the degree of injury. Patients who have had frostbite previously have a two times increased risk of recurrence. The lower extremity is most commonly involved but the entire surface area of the body should be examined for potential regions of exposure.

Early management of frostbite is to rewarm the region with a water bath of 40–42°C for 20–30 minutes while encouraging active range of motion. Blisters should be debrided in order to reduce the burden of thromboxane and prostaglandins in the fluid. Aloe Vera 10% every 6 hours in the first 7 days, inhibits thromboxane synthase reducing thromboxane production and helps to preserve the sub-dermal plexus. Ibuprofen, a cyclooxygenase inhibitor, reduces the formation of prostaglandins. The depth of injury should be determined once the wound is fully defined as these wounds are also dynamic and change over time. Daily wound care is important and a silver based product or iodine can be used to decrease bacterial load. Thrombolytic, such as tissue plasminogen activator, have been utilized in patients with a high risk for life altering amputation within 24 hours of injury. This evidence is retrospective in a small cohort of patients but the risk of digital amputation was reduced from 40% to 10%.[18]

Conclusions

Thermal, Electrical, Chemical and Cold injuries all have distinct pathophysiology leading to distinct complications. It is important in the acute period to manage these patients appropriately as resuscitation can impact morbidity and mortality. In a trauma setting or critical care unit with no specialized burn center, it is important to prepare the patient for safe transfer using the guidelines provided in this chapter.

References

1. Herndon D. *Total Burn Care*, 4th edition. London, England, Saunders, 2012.
2. Ryan CM *et al.* Objective estimates of the probability of death from burn injuries. *NEJM* 1998; 338: 362–366.
3. Endorf FW, Gamelli RL. Inhalation injury, pulmonary perturbations, and fluid resuscitation. *J Burn Care Res* 2007; 28(1): 80–83.
4. Lund T, Onarheim H, Reed RK. Pathogenesis of edema formation in burn injuries. *World J Surg* 1992; 16(1): 2–9.
5. Demling RH. The burn edema process: Current concepts. *J Burn Care Rehabil* 2005; 26(3): 207–227.
6. Jackson DM. The diagnosis of the depth of burning. *Brit J Surg* 1953; 40(164): 588–596.
7. Jain S, Bandi V. Electrical and lightning injuries. *Crit Care Clin* 1999; 15(2): 319–31.

8. Haberal MA. An eleven-year survey of electrical burn injuries. *J Burn Care Rehabil* 1995; 16(1): 43–48.
9. Tredget EE, Shankowsky HA, Tilley WA. Electrical injuries in Canadian burn care. Identification of unsolved problems. *Ann N Y Acad Sci* 1999; 888: 75–87.
10. Martinez JA, Nguyen T. Electrical injuries. *South Med J* 2000; 93(12): 1165–1168.
11. Lee RC, Canaday DJ, Doong H. A review of the biophysical basis for the clinical application of electric fields in soft-tissue repair. *J Burn Care Rehabil* 1993; 14(3): 319–335.
12. Grube BJ, Heimbach DM, Engrav LH *et al.* Neurologic consequences of electrical burns. *J Trauma* 1990; 30(3): 254–258.
13. Purdue GF, Hunt JL. Electrocardiographic monitoring after electrical injury: Necessity or luxury. *J Trauma* 1986; 26(2): 166–167.
14. Arnoldo B, Klein M, Gibran NS. Practice guidelines for the management of electrical injuries. *J Burn Care Res* 2006; 27(4): 439–447.
15. Arrowsmith J, Usgaocar RP, Dickson WA. Electrical injury and the frequency of cardiac complications. *Journal of the International Society for Burn Injuries* 1997; 23(7–8): 576–578.
16. Fahmy FS, Brinsden MD, Smith J *et al.* Lightning: The multisystem group injuries. *J Trauma* 1999; 46(5): 937–940.
17. Koumbourlis AC. Electrical injuries. *Crit Care Med* 2002; 30(11 Suppl): S424–S430.
18. Bruen KJ, Ballard JR, Morris SE *et al.* Reduction of the incidence of amputation in frostbite injury with thrombolytic therapy. *Arch Surg-Chicago* 2007; 142(6): 546–551; discussion 51–53.

Chapter 24

Multiorgan Dysfunction Syndrome in the Surgical Patient

P. Dhar and G. Papia

Chapter Overview

The most common cause of death in the critically ill surgical patient is multiple organ failure (MOF).[1] This concept was first described in the 1960s. As treatments evolved, so did morbidity and mortality, and increasingly patients survived long enough to develop MOF. In 1991, the American College of Chest Physicians and the Society for Critical Care Medicine held a consensus conference leading to more formal definitions of sepsis and multi organ failure. MOF was revised to multiple organ dysfunction syndrome (MODS), defined generally as altered function in at least two organ systems in the setting of acute illness that results in impaired homeostasis, requiring intervention.[2] This consensus statement attempted to standardize these terms for the purposes of investigation and prognostication. The subsequent publication of the MODS score in 1995 was the first objective scale to measure the severity of MODS as an outcome in critical illness.[3] This score is summarized in Table 1. While the MODS score is not considered a true prognostic score, the risk of intensive care unit (ICU) mortality increases with severity of organ dysfunction, both in the number of organs involved and the degree of dysfunction. Outcomes in MODS are summarized in Tables 2 and 3. The MODS score focuses on objective measures of physiologic dysfunction in six organ systems: respiratory, cardiac, renal, hepatic, neurologic and hematologic. These systems will form the basis of the following discussion of MODS

Table 1. MODS score.

Organ system	Measure	0	1	2	3	4
Respiratory	PaO_2/FiO_2	>300	226–300	151–225	76–150	≤75
Cardiovascular	PAR	≤10	10.1–15.0	15.1–20.0	20.1–30.0	>30.0
Hepatic	Bilirubin (mmol/L)	≤20	21–60	61–120	121–240	>240
Renal	creatinine (mmol/L)	≤100	101–200	201–350	351–500	>500
Neurologic	Glasgow Coma Score	15	13–14	10–12	7–9	≤6
Hematologic	platelet count ($\times 10^3$/mL)	>120	81–120	51–80	21–50	≤20

Table 2. Outcomes in MODS by score.

MODS score	ICU mortality (%)	Hospital mortality (%)
0	0	0
1–4	1–2	7
5–8	3–5	16
9–12	25	50
13–16	50	70
17–20	75	82
21–24	100	100

Table 3. Outcomes in MODS by organ system involvement.

Number of failing organ systems	Mortality (%)
0	<10
1	0–30
2	20–50
3	40–80
4	60–100
5+	>80

in the surgical patient. The discussion will hopefully increase the awareness of the intensivist to the likelihood of MODS in its earliest phases and prompt timely diagnostic and therapeutic interventions to improve outcome.

Respiratory

Respiratory failure manifests as impaired gas exchange, reflected as hypoxemia and hypercapnia. While multiple clinical syndromes can be grouped in this category, the following sections focus on what are, arguably, the most significant in the surgical population: acute respiratory distress syndrome (ARDS) including the related transfusion related acute lung injury (TRALI) and pulmonary embolus (PE).

ARDS

ARDS is a leading cause of postoperative respiratory failure. The most up to date definition of ARDS is described by the Berlin definition as outline in Table.[4] Several prediction models have been developed to identify patients at risk for the development of ARDS, including some that focus specifically on surgical populations. The surgical lung injury prediction (SLIP) score was designed for elective surgical procedures, and includes variables of surgical procedure (high risk cardiac, vascular and thoracic surgery), comorbid conditions (diabetes mellitus, chronic obstructive pulmonary disease,

Table 4. Berlin definition of acute respiratory distress syndrome.

TIMING	— Within 1 week of a known clinical insult or new/worsening clinical symptoms.
CHEST IMAGING	— Bilateral opacities not fully explained by effusions, lobar/lung collapse or nodules.
ORIGIN OF EDEMA	— Respiratory failure not fully explained by cardiac failure or fluid overload. — Requires objective assessment e.g., ECGO to rule out hydrostatic edema if no risk factor is present.
OXYGENATION*	
Mild	200 mmHg $< PaO_2/FiO_2 \leq$ 300 mmHg
Moderate	100 mmHg $< PaO_2/FiO_2 \leq$ 200 mmHg
Severe	$PaO_2/FiO_2 \leq$ 100 mmHg

*With PEEP or CPAP ≥ 5 cm H_2O.

Table 5. Slip model.

Predictor variables	**Slip points**
Surgical Procedure	
High risk vascular surgery	32
High risk cardiac surgery	19
High risk thoracic surgery	16
Comorbid conditions	
Diabetes mellitus	6
COPD	10
GERD	7
Modifying conditions	
Alcohol abuse	11

gastroesophageal reflux disease), and modifying conditions (alcohol abuse).[5] The recently updated SLIP-2 addresses more heterogeneous high risk surgical populations, including those presenting as emergencies. The SLIP-2 model is summarized in Table 5.[6] A number of algorithms have also been developed for the trauma population, the most recent of which was published in 2012.[7–9] This model incorporates variables including APACHE II, injury severity score, blunt mechanism of injury, pulmonary contusion, flail chest, massive transfusion and older age.

The ability to predict those surgical patients at high risk for the development of respiratory failure is helpful in studying potential interventions. The so-called magic bullet for ARDS in the general critical care population has yet to be identified.

Ventilation Strategies

Lung protective ventilation is one intervention which is regarded as both a preventative and treatment strategy for ARDS. It is based on the rationale that low tidal volume ventilation is less likely to cause alveolar injury from over distension. This ventilation strategy, targeting a tidal volume of 6 mL/kg of ideal body weight, has been shown to be of benefit in a number of trials demonstrating decreased mortality and days of mechanical ventilation.[10] High frequency oscillation (HFOV) is another ventilation strategy, incorporating the rationale for low tidal volume ventilation that has been studied in the treatment of ARDS. Recent randomized trials suggest that HFOV has no mortality benefit in ARDS, and may actually cause harm.[11,12] Despite these recent studies, HFOV is still considered potential rescue therapy in the management of ARDS.

Prone Positioning

Early randomized trials investigating the use of prone positioning in ARDS did not show a mortality benefit, and the management strategy fell out of favor in many centers. Based on the rationale of improved ventilation-perfusion matching in ARDS afflicted lungs, this technique was recently readdressed in the literature with the PROSEVA trial.[13] This study used a more prolonged period of prone positioning of 16 hours compared to previous trials. Patients categorized as severe ARDS (criteria PaO_2:FiO_2 <150 mmHg, FiO_2 ≥0.6, PEEP ≥ 5 cm H_2O) did actually show a mortality benefit, without an increase in complications.

Pharmacologic

Inhaled vasodilators have been investigated in the treatment of ARDS. Meta-analyses have shown that nitric oxide (NO) at least transiently improves oxygenation, without an improvement in mortality or duration of mechanical ventilation.[14] NO therapy is expensive, with a theoretical risk of methemoglobinemia, and a reported increased risk of renal impairment. At this time, the use of NO therapy in ARDS is limited to the setting of refractory hypoxemia.

The use of steroids in ARDS remains an area of controversy. Several meta-analyses have addressed the use of glucocorticoids in this setting, but the benefit remains unclear. There is a suggestion that steroids given early in the clinical course may be of some benefit, where as those patients treated after 14 days may actually have higher mortality.[15] This potential benefit has to be weighed against the morbidity of steroids in the critical care setting, including neuromuscular weakness and the potential for major fractures and potentiation of sepsis.

Extracorporeal Membrane Oxygenation (ECMO)

ECMO has been studied as salvage therapy in patients with hypoxemic respiratory failure refractory to conventional ventilatory management. In venovenous ECMO, a cannula is placed in a central vein which facilitates withdrawal of blood into an extracorporeal circuit that directly oxygenates and removes carbon dioxide from the blood. The oxygenated blood is returned to a central vein, bypassing the need for gas exchange at the level of the lung. It is important to note that patients must be anti-coagulated to maintain the ECMO circuit, and this must be taken into account in the surgical patient with ARDS. Current guidelines suggest that ECMO therapy should be considered for patients with a $PaO_2/FiO_2 < 150$ on $FiO_2 > 90\%$ and is indicated in those with a $PaO_2/FiO_2 < 100$ on $FiO_2 > 90\%$.[16] These guidelines also suggest that a decision to initiate ECMO should be made within seven days of mechanical ventilation at high settings (e.g., $FiO_2 > 90\%$ and plateau pressures greater than 30 cm H_2O).

PE

Pulmonary embolism is implicated in approximately 10% of hospital deaths.[17] The physiologic implications of PE involve multiple systems including cardiovascular (e.g., cardiogenic shock) and respiratory (e.g., pulmonary infarction, hypoxemic respiratory failure). The patients who develop symptomatic or clinically significant PE in the acute setting are vulnerable to developing multi-organ dysfunction, either as a precipitating event or as a complication of ICU admission. Even relatively small PEs may be tolerated poorly by the critically ill. There are multiple risk factors for PE in the surgical patient, including the type and duration of surgery, trauma, postoperative immobilization, previous venous thromboembolism (VTE), malignancy, and inherited or acquired hypercoaguable states. The current gold standard for diagnosis of pulmonary embolism is CT-angiography. When IV contrast cannot be administered, V/Q scanning and/or lower extremity doppler ultrasound can be obtained. If the patient is too unstable for these imaging techniques bedside echocardiography can be performed to identify secondary signs of pulmonary embolism (e.g., right ventricular systolic pressure [RVSP], evidence of right ventricular strain, septal flattening).[18] The approach to management of pulmonary embolism is divided into two arms: its prevention and its treatment. The American College of Chest Physicians (ACCP) publishes updated guidelines for both the prevention and treatment of VTE.[19]

Prevention

Several models of risk assessment for VTE in surgical patients have been developed. The 2012 guidelines use a modification of the Caprini risk assessment model which stratify patients into categories of very low risk, low, moderate and high risk for postoperative VTE with recommendations for perioperative thromboprophylaxis accordingly. These guidelines also differentiate between orthopedic and non-orthopedic surgical procedures, the former conferring higher risk of VTE. It is established that patients who have had surgery prior to ICU admission are at higher risk for VTE, but this risk is compounded in critical illness with its associated immobilization and increased risk of postoperative bleeding. Implementation of evidence-based care bundles in ICU patients has been shown to improve outcomes. VTE prophylaxis is included in the so-called ventilator bundle. Appropriate use of chemoprophylaxis, or alternatively mechanical VTE prophylaxis, in the critically ill is now used as a quality indicator in the ICU.

Treatment

Treatment of PE is determined by the patient's clinical stability, diagnostic certainty and any contraindications to anticoagulation. Cardio-respiratory compromise requires stabilization of airway and hemodynamics in the critical care setting. Patients with confirmed PE and persistent hypotension are appropriate candidates for systemic thrombolysis.[19] The risks of major bleeding are accepted for the patient in shock, but the role of thrombolysis — both systemic and catheter — directed — in patients who are hemodynamically stable but with evidence of right ventricular strain or extensive clot burden, is less clear. Patients who are hemodynamically stable are typically started on parenteral anticoagulation for initial management, with transition to oral agents once stabilized.[19] Those patients who are hemodynamically stable but have contraindications to anticoagulation are considered for inferior vena cava filter placement to prevent propagation of clot from the lower extremities, until they become candidates for full anticoagulation.

Cardiovascular

Cardiovascular (CV) dysfunction in multiorgan failure is an interesting problem because it has direct implications on every other organ system. The MODS score uses heart rate (HR), central venous pressure (CVP), and mean arterial pressure (MAP) to determine the pressure-adjusted heart rate (PAR) to measure degree of cardiac dysfunction. With this equation ($PAR = HR \times CVP/MAP$), higher values reflect worsening CV dysfunction and therefore

MODS scores. The practical clinical manifestation of CV dysfunction in this setting is essentially hypotension refractory to increasing preload.[20]

The discussion of primary CV dysfunction resulting in myocardial infarction, is beyond the scope of this discussion of MODS. The pathophysiology of secondary CV dysfunction in multiorgan failure is thought to involve a number of sequential and parallel steps:

1. Tissue injury/sepsis results in endothelial damage, neuroendocrine activation and release of inflammatory mediators.
2. Massive immune/inflammatory response results in:
   — Peripheral vasodilation mediated by NO;
   — Increased capillary permeability;
   — Microvascular stasis and thrombi causing arteriovenous shunting resulting in high mixed venous oxygen saturation.
3. Redistribution of regional blood flow results in selective tissue hypoperfusion.
4. Acidosis and impaired cellular function result in myocardial depression, and autonomic dysfunction.

The management of CV dysfunction in MODS is primarily supportive. Vasoactive medications including pressors and inotropes are used for hemodynamic support after a trial of fluid resuscitation. Determining fluid responsiveness in the critically ill population is an area of extensive study (see chapter on Shock and cardiovascular dynamics). At a physiologic level, responsiveness is measured as an increase in stroke volume with fluid challenge. Based on the Frank Starling curve, as preload increases, left ventricular stroke volume increases until optimal preload is achieved. After this point, stroke volume remains relatively constant and the patient is no longer fluid responsive and vasoactive medications should be considered. Guidelines for resuscitation, such as the Surviving Sepsis Campaign, identify end points of resuscitation such as central venous pressure, mean arterial pressure, urine output, normalization of lactate and mixed venous oxygen saturation although central venous pressure is no longer regarded as a reliable index of volume responsiveness.[21] These end points, while important for goal directed resuscitation, are not sufficient to assess volume responsiveness. Dynamic measures such as pulse pressure variation or inferior vena cava collapsibility on echocardiography have all been studied with reasonable results, but can only be used reliably in fully ventilated patients without cardiac dysrhythmias.[22]

Gastrointestinal (GI)/Hepatic

The GI system is considered by some to be both a culprit and a victim in the development of multi organ dysfunction. In steady-state physiology, the GI tract and its associated solid organs receive a significant percentage of cardiac output (for example, the liver alone receives 25% of output), but this is significantly curtailed at times of systemic stress as blood flow is preferentially directed to the cerebral and cardiac circulation. The resultant ischemia/reperfusion injury results in release of proinflammatory mediators which can exacerbate systemic stress. GI dysfunction in critical illness is difficult to quantify because there is no validated objective clinical measure that encompasses all of its manifestations. The MODS score uses serum bilirubin as a measure of GI function, with higher serum bilirubin corresponding to a higher MODS score. This measure of hepatic function, while objective and easy to obtain, does not incorporate the classically described stress related mucosal disease (SRMD) or the even more common GI dysmotility which manifests as feeding intolerance in the critically ill. There is limited data on association of hepatic dysfunction and mortality in critical illness, and so at this time the relationship between GI dysfunction and outcomes is considered a reflection of overall severity of illness.

Hepatic Dysfunction

Hepatic dysfunction in critical illness falls into two main categories: ischemic hepatopathy and cholestasis.

Ischemic Hepatopathy

Ischemic hepatopathy refers to a diffuse pattern of injury evolving from decreased blood flow to the liver, passive venous congestion, or hypoxemia from a different primary source (e.g., lung injury). Clinical diagnosis is based on abnormal liver tests that usually manifest within 24 to 48 hours of an ischemic insult. Aminotransferase levels can reach greater than 25 times the upper limit of normal but usually return to normal within 7 to 10 days of stabilized hemodynamics.[23] Hyperbilirubinemia may be present but rarely exceeds three to four times the upper limit of normal, and is generally the last abnormality to resolve. There is typically minimal evidence of dysfunction in synthesis as measured by INR and PTT. Management of ischemic hepatopathy focuses on restoring adequate cardiac output and addressing the underlying etiology of hemodynamic instability. Ischemic liver injury is typically self-limited when the underlying insult is reversed, and morbidity and mortality are usually related to underlying systemic disease. Fulminant hepatic failure is rare (2–5%) and generally occurs in patients with baseline cirrhosis.[23]

Cholestasis

Cholestasis is found in up to 40% of critically ill patients, and is the most common hepatic abnormality. In this patient population, the etiology is usually intrahepatic. Shock, sepsis, medications, and parenteral nutrition all have hepatotoxic effects leading to impairment in bile production and transport.[24] Cholestasis is defined by hyperbilirubinemia and elevated alkaline phosphatase (usually greater than three times the upper limit of normal) with only mild associated elevation in aminotransferases. INR may be elevated because of the effect on vitamin K-dependent coagulation factors. The management of ICU cholestasis addresses the underlying mechanism of injury. As in ischemic hepatopathy, restoring hemodynamic stability is crucial. Sepsis should be managed with antibiotics and adequate source control. When drug induced cholestasis is suspected, new medications in the past three months should be reviewed, and any offending agents removed. Medications implicated in cholestasis are summarized in Table 6. Management of

Table 6. Medications implicated in cholestasis.

Antimicrobials
Amoxicillin–clavulanate
Trimethoprim–sulfamethoxazole
Ketoconazole
Cardiac
Captopril
Amiodarone
Endocrine
Ezetimibe
Rosiglitazone
Estrogens
Anabolic steroids
Immunosuppression
Azathioprine
Infliximab

TPN-induced cholestasis requires adjustment of composition, and consideration of metronidazole for bacterial overgrowth.

Stress Related Muscosal Disease

Over 75% of critically ill patients have endoscopically-detectable mucosal erosions within 24 hours of ICU admission.[25] The most common complications of SRMD are bleeding and perforation. Clinically significant bleeding, requiring transfusion or causing hemodynamic instability, is associated with increased morbidity, mortality, and length of ICU stay.[26] As discussed earlier, this association with mortality is thought to be a reflection of illness severity (i.e., patients die from underlying illness) rather than GI bleeding. Patients who have clinically significant bleeding should be managed with standard resuscitative measures including intravenous fluids, transfusions and correction of underlying coagulopathy as appropriate. Intravenous proton pump inhibitors (PPI) should also be initiated until endoscopy can be performed. In the ICU setting, exclusive of acute bleeding, the treatment of SRMD is focused on prevention, primarily prophylactic acid suppression. Mechanical ventilation greater than 48 hours and coagulopathy are considered significant risk factors for clinically significant bleeding from SRMD. The surgical populations of burns, traumatic brain injuries and spinal cord injuries are also uniquely and specifically at risk of hyperacidity and warrant stress ulcer prophylaxis. The choice of acid suppression therapy generally falls into two categories: histamine-2 receptor antagonists (H2RAs) and PPI. Meta-analyses suggest that PPIs are associated with less bleeding than H2 blockers without affecting rates of nosocomial pneumonia or mortality.[27]

Dysmotility/Feeding Intolerance

GI dysmotility is a frequent occurrence in the critically ill population and is associated with feeding intolerance. The development of GI dysmotility is likely related to a combination of the patient's baseline medical issues (e.g., diabetes) and the superimposed hemodynamic liability, electrolyte disturbances and medications associated with critical illness. The implications of dysmotility for the ICU population include malnutrition and risk of aspiration with feeding intolerance. Gastric residual volume (GRV) though neither standardized nor validated, is often used as a surrogate for identifying feeding intolerance. Studies suggest there is no difference in rates of ventilator associated pneumonia, ICU length of stay and ICU mortality whether GRV is measured routinely or not.[28] Many trials have actually implicated measurement of GRV with severe underfeeding, since the practice is to hold feeds once a high GRV is detected. A reasonable approach to management of dysmotility manifesting as feeding intolerance is to rule out a mechanical distal obstruction, followed by the use of prokinetics. Domperidone and metoclopramide mediate their prokinetic effects on the GI system through their antidopaminergic activity, and in the case of metoclopramide, enhanced cholinergic transmission. Not all patients tolerate these prokinetics due to their side effects e.g., QT interval abnormality. There is reasonably good evidence for post pyloric feeding tubes in patients who manifest persistent feeding intolerance in terms of pneumonia rates and percentage of caloric intake.[29] In general post pyloric feeding tubes are well tolerated, but often require fluoroscopic placement.

Renal

Acute kidney injury (AKI) occurs in at least 30% of patients admitted to the ICU and contributes to multiorgan dysfunction.[30] The MODS score uses serum creatinine as a measure of renal function, with increasing creatinine values corresponding to a higher MODS value. Current definitions of AKI include the RIFLE (risk, injury, failure, loss of function, end stage renal disease) and AKIN (AKI network) criteria, which incorporate both serum creatinine and glomerular filtration rate with urine output to classify severity of AKI. Acute renal failure is an independent risk factor for mortality in the critically ill even after adjustment for demographics and severity of illness.[31]

Renal failure in the critical care setting is often multifactorial. Risk factors for AKI in the critically ill include sepsis, shock, burns, trauma, cardiopulmonary bypass, nephrotoxic medications and intravenous contrast agents. The impact of these risk factors is influenced by so-called susceptibility factors such as advanced age, diabetes, chronic renal dysfunction and cancer.[32] In the surgical critically ill subset, the pathophysiology of AKI is usually acute tubular necrosis (ATN), either ischemic or toxic.

Regardless of pathophysiology, the indications for supportive care in the form of renal replacement therapy (RRT) are unchanged from those of the general population and include: volume overload, refractory hyperkalemia, and refractory acidosis, uremia associated with encephalopathy or pericarditis and dialyzable toxins. Dialysis-dependent AKI patients in the critical care unit demonstrate higher mortality rates and ICU length of stay than those managed without RRT.[33] The various modes of RRT involve either diffusive or convective clearance and can be carried out in intermittent or continuous timelines. Although statistically the majority of critically ill patients are initiated on continuous RRT (CRRT), studies have suggested that if tolerated hemodynamically, intermittent hemodialysis (IHD) and CRRT are equivalent in terms of days on RRT, ventilatory days, length of ICU stay and short term survival.[34] The majority of survivors of AKI in the critical illness setting remain dialysis-dependent upon hospital discharge.

Most studies of AKI in the critically ill are directed towards management — mode, timing of initiation of therapy — rather than prevention. The use of low dose dopamine for its vasodilatory effects, while providing short term improvements in urine output and renal physiology does not reduce RRT requirements or mortality.[35] Prevention of contrast-induced nephropathy is centered on ensuring adequate hydration and maintenance of urine output. The use of N-acetylcysteine or isotonic bicarbonate hydration have been studied primarily in the outpatient population. These supplementary interventions may reduce the incidence in rise of serum creatinine, but it is unclear whether they actually decrease the need for RRT based on current data. Although the benefit in the ICU population has yet to be demonstrated, there is no increase adverse events with N-acetylcysteine. In combination with the relatively low cost, there is little disadvantage — though no proven benefit — in its use to prevent contrast induced nephropathy.[36,37]

Neurologic

The MODS uses the Glasgow coma scale (GCS) score (Table 7) as a measure of neurologic function. The GCS was originally developed to assess level of consciousness (LOC) after head injury but is now applied more broadly as part of the assessment of the central nervous system function in hospitalized patients, including those in intensive care. There are many possible causes of altered LOC in the ICU patient. These include, but are not limited to, traumatic brain injury, anoxic brain injury and ischemic and hemorrhagic stroke. Discussion of altered LOC as it relates to MODS, however, generally falls into the category of delirium. The incidence of delirium in the ICU ranges between 45 and 87%,[38] with incidence in the surgical, burn and trauma subset over 70%.[39] Recognition and treatment of delirium in the ICU population is important because this clinical diagnosis has significant implications for short term and 6-month mortality, hospital length of stay and long term cognitive outcomes.[39]

Table 7. Glasgow coma scale.

BEST EYE RESPONSE (E)	Spontaneous	4
	To Speech	3
	To Pain	2
	No response	1
BEST VERBAL RESPONSE (V)	Oriented	5
	Confused	4
	Inappropriate words	3
	Incomprehensible sounds	2
	No response	1
BEST MOTOR RESPONSE (M)	Obeys commands	6
	Localizes to pain	5
	Flexion to pain	4
	Decorticate posturing	3
	Decerebrate posturing	2
	No response	1

Detection of delirium in the ICU patient can be difficult because of unique factors such as mechanical ventilation and sedation requirements. The diagnosis is also challenging because delirium can be hyperactive, hypoactive or mixed in its clinical presentation. In order to address this issue, a number of standardized tools have been developed to screen for ICU delirium: in a systematic review published in 2007, six validated instruments were identified. The two most commonly studied screening tools are the Confusion Assessment Method for the ICU (CAM-ICU) and the Intensive Care Delirium Screening Checklist (ICDSC).[40] The routine use of a standardized screening method is more important than which specific method is used because studies have shown that without standardized evaluation, delirium is identified in less than one third of affected ICU patients.[40]

Management of delirium requires two parallel pathways: treatment of any reversible underlying medical conditions and the management of behavior disturbances. The former includes treatment of infections, management of underlying electrolyte and metabolic disturbances, as well as drug toxicity or withdrawal. Another factor to be addressed, and especially relevant to the surgical population, is management of postoperative pain. Management of behavior disturbances is challenging because of the varied clinical presentation and the broad range of risk factors for delirium making targeted prevention difficult.

Guidelines published by the Society of Critical Care Medicine (SCCM) in 2013 examine the baseline and acquired risk factors for ICU delirium.[41] Most studies included in systematic reviews of treatment of ICU delirium are limited to pilot studies. This is reflected in the limited recommendations in the 2013 clinical guidelines. These guidelines identify benzodiazepines as a possible risk factor, and also suggest that dexmetomidine infusions may be less deliriogenic than benzodiazepines. The only preventative measure for delirium in these guidelines recommends early mobilization of adult ICU patients. Preventative pharmacologic management is not recommended, including haloperidol and the atypical antipsychotics. Interestingly, one of the traditional mainstays of ICU delirium treatment, haloperidol, is highlighted for the lack of evidence that it reduces duration of ICU delirium. Atypical antipsychotics are mentioned as possibly reducing duration of ICU delirium, but caution is suggested with their use in patients with QT prolongation. The other significant treatment suggestion is the use of dexmetomidine infusions rather than benzodiazepines to reduce the duration of delirium. At this time, there are no specific recommendations for the treatment of hypoactive delirium, although there are case series describing the use of methylphenidate in this patient population.[41]

Hematologic

The marker designated as a measure of hematologic function in the MODS score is platelet count, with increasing scores assigned to lower platelet counts. Thrombocytopenia is the most common hemostatic disorder in the ICU, with a reported incidence of 20% to 50%.[42] Thrombocytopenia as a prognostic indicator in the critically ill has been studied in the literature, and has been associated with increased mortality, duration of ICU stay, duration of mechanical ventilation and transfusion requirements.[42,43]

Thrombocytopenia is defined as a platelet count less than 150,000/μL. Severe thrombocytopenia is defined as a platelet count less than 50,000/μL and is generally thought to be associated with a greater risk of bleeding, but the correlation between absolute platelet count and bleeding varies with the underlying etiology. Causes of thrombocytopenia can be classified as the following:

- Blood loss and/or hemodilution;
- Decreased production (e.g., infection, toxic medications, bone marrow suppression);

— Redistribution (e.g., portal hypertension, hypersplenism);
— Enhanced consumption (e.g., disseminated intravascular coagulation (DIC)).

Major risk factors for developing thrombocytopenia in the critically ill surgical patient include sepsis, blood transfusion, DI and severity of illness on admission to the ICU (measured in most studies by the APACHE II score).[43]

In addition to thorough history and physical exam, investigation of thrombocytopenia in the critically ill patient includes laboratory studies, medication review and an analysis of the time course of thrombocytopenia.

Labs

The initial laboratory studies for thrombocytopenia should include a CBC and peripheral blood smear. Combined abnormalities of the blood counts on CBC can help point to an etiology e.g., pancytopenia may suggest bone marrow suppression. The peripheral blood smear should be done to rule out spurious thrombocytopenia from platelet clumping, prior to any other extensive investigations. The remainder of laboratory studies should be guided by clinical context, keeping in mind that for the surgical ICU patient sepsis, blood transfusion requirements and DIC are frequent culprits. Cultures, coagulation and liver profiles may therefore also be included in the initial workup.

Medications

Drug-induced thrombocytopenia may be difficult to diagnose in the critically ill patient since this population is usually on multiple classes of medications. Commonly implicated medications include quinine, valproic acid and heparin. It is worth pointing out that heparin induced thrombocytopenia (HIT) is not a common cause of thrombocytopenia in the critical care population but should be ruled out if other workup for the more common etiologies is non-contributory. The American Society of Hematology (ASH) scoring system to determine probability of HIT incorporates "The 4Ts" of thrombocytopenia: timing of platelet fall, thrombosis or other sequelae, and no alternative cause of thrombocytopenia.[44] The detection of HIT antibodies on immunoassay alone is not sufficient to diagnose HIT. Clinical correlation is important, because certain populations including those requiring RRT and after cardiopulmonary bypass have higher heparin-induced antibody levels of uncertain clinical significance.[45] If HIT is suspected on clinical grounds, all sources of heparin (including low molecular weight heparin) should be stopped and a non-heparin anticoagulant e.g., danaparoid or argatroban started while awaiting the results of laboratory testing.

Timeline

Major surgery, including cardiopulmonary bypass, vascular and trauma can precipitate a temporary drop in platelet count. The platelet nadir is typically by postoperative day three to four in a range of 50 to 100×10^9/L, with an increase to levels above baseline by postoperative day seven. Platelet nadirs early in the postoperative course are usually a reflection of intraoperative blood loss or degree of tissue injury in trauma. Patients that are septic or suffer major blood loss requiring ongoing resuscitation can develop thrombocytopenia at any point in their ICU course. Development of HIT antibodies usually requires heparin exposure for at least four days.

Given the complexity of critically ill patients, the etiology of thrombocytopenia may be multifactorial. Management of thrombocytopenia should be determined by investigations and time course in the clinical context. Like any blood product, platelet transfusion is associated with a number of risks including transmission of bacterial or viral infection, transfusion associated lung injury, anaphylaxis and post transfusion purpura. The decision to transfuse a critically ill patient must therefore be based on not only absolute platelet count but also clinical context. The underlying cause of thrombocytopenia must be addressed in the treatment plan, and it is important to remember that for some underlying etiologies e.g., HIT, thrombotic thrombocytopenic purpura (TTP) platelet transfusion is not indicated. Table 8 below summarizes current recommendations regarding platelet transfusions in the surgical ICU patient.

Conclusion

Multi organ dysfunction in the critically ill population is associated with significant mortality. Various scoring systems have been developed that address the severity of deranged physiology in addition to the number of organ systems involved. The MODS score was the first objective scale to measure the

Table 8. Indications for platelet transfusion in the surgical ICU.

Platelet count ($\times 10^9$/L)	Clinical setting	Recommendation
ANY	— Platelet dysfunction and clinical bleeding e.g., post cardiopulmonary bypass, antiplatelet medications	— Transfuse 1 pool of platelets
<10	— Non-immune thrombocytopenia	— Transfuse 1 pool of platelets
<20	— Non-immune thrombocytopenia + $T > 38.5$°C or + coagulopathy	— Transfuse 1 pool of platelets
	— Procedures with low risk of blood loss e.g., bronchoscopy, endoscopy	— Transfuse 1 pool of platelets immediately before procedure
<50	— Epidural anesthesia — Lumbar puncture — Procedures with high risk of blood loss	— Transfuse 1 pool of platelets immediately before procedure
<100	— Neurosurgery — Traumatic brain injury	— Transfuse 1 pool of platelets

Source: Adapted from Ref. 46.

severity of organ dysfunction as an outcome in critical illness. The treatment of MODS in the surgical population involves supportive care in the critical care unit while attempting to address the inciting etiology. The most important aspect of patient management in this population, however, is to use available prophylactic measures to prevent the development of MODS, or complications of its treatment in the critical care setting.

References

1. Mayr VD *et al.* Causes of death and determinants of outcome in critically ill patients. *Crit Care* 2006; 10: R154.
2. Bone *et al.* Definitions for sepsis and organ failure and guidelines for the use of innovative therapies in sepsis. *Chest* 1992; 101(6): 1645.

3. Marshall JC, Cook DJ *et al.* Multiple organ dysfunction score: A reliable descriptor of a complex clinical outcome. *Crit Care Med* 1995; 23(10): 1638–1652.
4. Ferguson N, Fan E, Camporota L *et al.* The Berlin definition of ARDS: An expanded rationale, justification, and supplementary material. *Intens Care Med* 2012; 38: 1573–1582.
5. Kor DJ *et al.* Derivation and diagnostic accuracy of the surgical lung injury prediction model. *Anesthesiology* 2011; 115: 117–128.
6. Kor DJ *et al.* Predicting risk of postoperative lung injury in high-risk surgical patients: A multicenter cohort study. *Anesthesiology* 2014; 120(5): 1168–1181.
7. Miller PR, Croce MA, Kilgo PD *et al.* Acute respiratory distress syndrome in blunt trauma: Identification of independent risk factors. *Am Surg* 2002; 68(10): 845–850.
8. Navarrete-Navarro P, Rivera-Fernandez R, Rincon-Ferrari MD *et al.* Early markers of acute respiratory distress syndrome development in severe trauma patients. *J Crit Care* 2006; 21(3): 253–258.
9. Watkins TR *et al.* Acute respiratory distress syndrome after trauma: Development and validation of a predictive model. *Crit Care Med* 2012 Aug; 40(8): 2295–2303.
10. Ventilation with lower tidal volumes as compared with traditional tidal volumes for acute lung injury and the acute respiratory distress syndrome. The acute respiratory distress syndrome network. *N Engl J Med* 2000; 342(18): 1301.
11. Ferguson ND, Cook DJ, Guyatt GH, Mehta S, Hand L, Austin P, Zhou Q, Matté A, Walter SD, Lamontagne F, Granton JT, Arabi YM, Arroliga AC, Stewart TE, Slutsky AS, Meade MO. OSCILLATE trial investigators, Canadian critical care trials group: High-frequency oscillation in early acute respiratory distress syndrome. *N Engl J Med* 2013; 368: 795–805.
12. Young D, Lamb SE, Shah S, MacKenzie I, Tunnicliffe W, Lall R, Rowan K, Cuthbertson BH. OSCAR Study Group: High-frequency oscillation for acute respiratory distress syndrome. *N Engl J Med* 2013; 368: 806–813.
13. Guérin C, Reignier J, Richard JC *et al.* Prone positioning in severe acute respiratory distress syndrome. *N Engl J Med.* 2013; 368(23): 2159–2168.
14. Adhikari NK, Dellinger RP, Lundin S *et al.* Inhaled nitric oxide does not reduce mortality in patients with acute respiratory distress syndrome regardless of severity: Systematic review and meta-analysis. *Crit Care Med* 2014; 42(2): 404–412.
15. Steinberg KP, Hudson LD, Goodman RB *et al.* Efficacy and safety of corticosteroids for persistent acute respiratory distress syndrome. *N Eng J Med* 2006; 354(16): 1671–1684.
16. Extracorporeal life support organization guidelines. December 2013. Version 1.3. Available at https://www.elso.org/Portals/0/IGD/Archive/FileManager/989d4d4d14cusersshyerdocumentselsoguidelinesforadultrespiratoryfailure1.3.pdf [accessed on 14 December, 2014].
17. Konstantinides SV, Torbicki A, Agnelli G *et al.* 2014 ESC guidelines on the diagnosis and management of acute pulmonary embolism. *Eur Heart J* 2014; 35(43): 3033–3069.

18. Goldhaber S. Echocardiography in the Management of Pulmonary Embolism. *Ann Int Med* 2002; 136: 691–700.
19. Kearon C, Akl EA, Comerota AJ *et al.* Antithrombotic therapy for VTE disease: Antithrombotic therapy and prevention of thrombosis, 9th ed.: American College of Chest Physicians evidence-based clinical practice guidelines. *Chest* 2012 Feb; 141(2 Supply):e419S–e494S.
20. Marshall JC. The multiple organ dysfunction syndrome, in Holzheimer RG, Mannick JA (eds.). Surgical Treatment: Evidence-Based and Problem-Oriented. Munich, Zuckschwerdt, 2001.
21. Dellinger RP, Levy MM, Rhodes A *et al.* Surviving sepsis campaign: International guidelines for management of severe sepsis and septic shock: 2012. *Crit Care Med* 2013; 41(2): 580–637.
22. Marik PE, Monnet X, Teboul JL. Hemodynamic parameters to guide fluid therapy. *Ann Intensive Care* 2011; 1(1): 1.
23. Horvatits T, Trauner M, Fuhrmann V. Hypoxic liver injury and cholestasis in critically ill patients. *Curr Opin Crit Care* 2013; 19: 128–132.
24. Nesseler N, Launey Y, Aninat C, Morel F, Mallédant Y, Seguin P. Clinical review: The liver in sepsis. *Crit Care* 2012; 16(5): 235.
25. Mutlu GM, Mutlu EA, Factor P. GI complications in patients receiving mechanical ventilation. *Chest* 2001; 19(4): 1222.
26. Cook DJ, Fuller HD, Guyatt GH *et al.* Risk factors for GI bleeding in critically ill patients. *N Engl J Med* 1994; 330(6): 377.
27. Barkun AN, Bardou M, Pham CQ *et al.* PPI vs histamine 2 receptor antagonists for stress-related mucosal bleeding prophylaxis in critically ill patients: A meta-analysis. *Am J Gastroenterol* 2012; 107(4): 507.
28. Reignier J, Mercler E, Le Gouge A *et al.* Effect of not monitoring residual gastric volume on risk of ventilator-associated pneumonia in adults receiving mechanical ventilation and early enteral feeding: A randomized controlled trial. *JAMA* 2013; 309(3): 249–256.
29. Strategies to optimize deliver and minimize risks of enteral nutrition: Small bowel feeding vs gastric. *Canadian Clinical Practice Guidelines* 2013. [epub]
30. Palevsky PM, Zhang JH, O'Connor TZ *et al.* Intensity of renal support in critically ill patients with AKI. *N Engl J Med* 2008; 359: 7–20.
31. Cruz DN, Ronco C. AKI in the ICU: Current trends in incidence and outcome. *Crit Care* 2007; 11: 149.
32. Ricci A, Di Nardo M, Ronco C. Year in review 2013: Critical care — nephrology. *Crit Care* 2014; 18(5): 574.
33. Elseviers MM, Lins RL, Van der Niepen P *et al.* RRT is an independent risk factor for mortality in critically ill patients with AKI. *Crit Care* 2010; 14: R221.
34. Schenfold JC, von Haehling S, Pschowski R *et al.* the effect of continuous versus intermittent RRT on the outcome of critically ill patients with acute renal failure

(CONVINT): A prospective randomized controlled trial. *Crit Care* 2014; 18: R11.

35. Friedrich JO, Adhikari N, Herridge MS, Beyene J. Meta-analysis: Low-dose dopamine increased urine output but does not prevent renal dysfunction or death. *Ann Intern Med* 2005; 142(7): 510–524.
36. Gonzales DA, Norsworthy KJ, Kern SJ *et al.* A meta-analysis of N-acetylcysteine in contrast-induced nephrotoxicity: Unsupervised clustering to resolve heterogeneity. *BMC Med* 2007; 5: 32.
37. Kelly AM, Dwamena B, Cronin P *et al.* Meta-analysis: Effectiveness of drugs for preventing contrast-induced nephropathy. *Ann Intern Med* 2008; 148(4): 284–294.
38. Reade MC, Phil D, Finfer S. Sedation and delirium in the ICU. *NEJM* 2014; 370: 444–454.
39. Pandharipande P, Cotton BA, Shintani A *et al.* Prevalence and risk factors for development of delirium in surgical and trauma ICU patients. *J Trauma* 2008; 65(1): 34–41.
40. Cavallazzi R, Saad M, Marik PE. Delirium in the ICU: An overview. *Ann Intensive Care* 2012; 2: 49.
41. Barr J, Fraser GL, Puntillo K *et al.* Clinical practice guidelines for the management of pain, agitation, and delirium in adult patients in the ICU. *Crit Care Med* 2013; 41(1): 263–306.
42. Greinacher A, Selleng K. Thrombocytopenia in the ICU patient. *Hematology Am Soc Hematol Educ Program* 2010; 2010: 135–143.
43. Stephan F, de Montblanc J, Cheffi A, Bonnet F. Thrombocytopenia in critically ill surgical patients: A case-control study evaluating attributable mortality and transfusion requirements. *Crit Care* 1999; 3(6): 151–158.
44. Linkins LA, Dans AL, Moores LK *et al.* Treatment and prevention of heparin-induced thrombocytopenia: Antithrombotic Therapy and Prevention of Thrombosis, 9th ed.: American College of Chest Physicians Evidence-Based Clinical Practice Guidelines. *Chest* 2012; 141: E495S.
45. Selling S, Malowsky, Strobel U *et al.* Early-onset and persisting thrombocytopenia in post-cardiac surgery patients is rarely due to heparin-induced thrombocytopenia, even when antibody tests are positive. *J Thromb Haemost* 2010; 8(1): 30.
46. Callum JL, Lin Y, Pinkerton PH. Bloody easy 3: Blood transfusions, blood alternatives and transfusion reactions, a guide to transfusion medicine, 3rd ed. Canada: Ontario Regional Blood Coordinating Network; 2011.

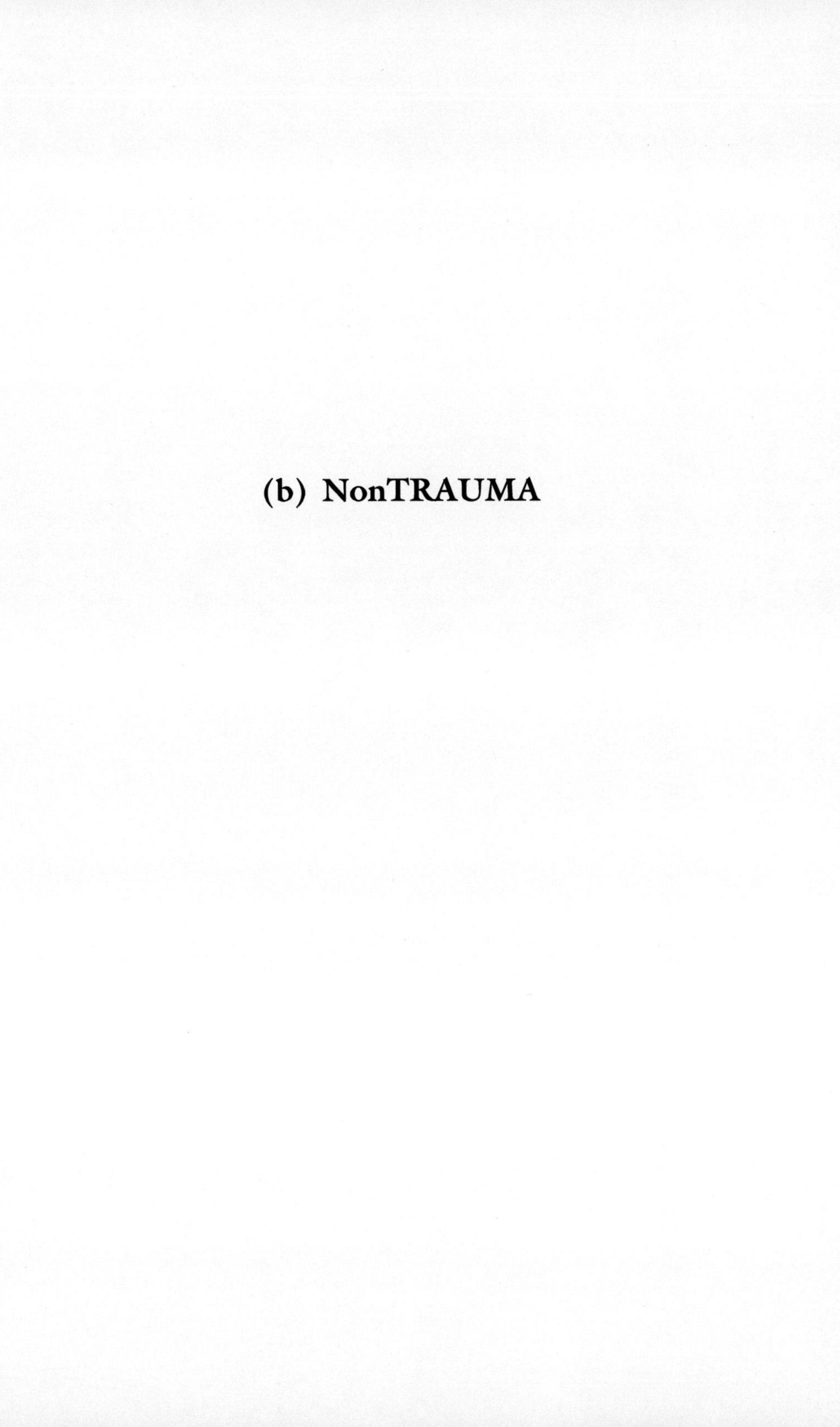

(b) NonTRAUMA

Chapter 25

Intra-abdominal Sepsis

Shuyin Liang and Joao B. de Rezende-Neto

Chapter Overview

Intra-abdominal sepsis (IAS) is a common condition in critically ill patients that frequently originates from localized or diffuse intra-abdominal infections (IAIs). In its most severe form, IAS can lead to severe sepsis and ultimately to multiple organ failure. Those conditions are the leading causes of death in patients admitted in non-cardiac intensive care units (ICUs).[1–4] The key elements in the management of patients with IAS are: early recognition of the problem, aggressive resuscitation, hemodynamic support, prompt administration of broad-spectrum antibiotics, and definitive source-control by means of surgical and/or non-surgical procedures.[5–8] Even though certain recommendations from published guidelines have led to improved survival in sepsis, the mortality rate of this condition remains extremely high.[2,9] A recent meta-analysis, compared 28-day mortality of severe sepsis in patients enrolled in multicenter randomized trials (1991–2009) to that of administrative data (1993–2009). Results showed a mortality rate of approximately 30%; Despite an annual mortality decline of 3.0–3.5%, respectively.[10]

The aim of this chapter is to review the clinical manifestations, microbiology, host defenses, and general principles of the management of IAS.

Epidemiology

Every year there are approximately 20 to 30 million cases of sepsis worldwide. A recent study in the United States showed an increase of approximately 71%

in the number of cases of severe sepsis from 415,280 cases in 2003 to 711 and 736 in 2007.[2] The infection site was located in the abdomen for roughly 19% of the patients with a statistically significant increase throughout the years ($p < 0.001$).[2] Approximately 1.3–2.5% of all ICU admissions for severe sepsis or septic shock result from IAIs.[4]

Severe sepsis is a frequent cause of mortality in surgical patients. A study with 200,000 septic patients from hospitals in seven different states of the United States showed that a surgical condition was present in approximately 30% of the cases.[11] Surgical patients admitted to ICUs also have several risk factors for sepsis. A recent study assessed prospective data from more than 1,300 surgical patients admitted to ICUs to determine preoperative, intra-operative and postoperative risk factors for sepsis. Patients with previous infections and those on antibiotics were excluded generating a final sample size 625 patients; 54% underwent neurosurgical or gastro-intestinal (GI) procedures.[12] Approximately 30% of the patients had an infectious complication, 13% had sepsis/severe sepsis and 11.5% presented septic shock; the mortality rate was 18%. An intra-abdominal source was found in 15% of the patients and approximately 50% had an infectious source in the lung. Multivariate analysis of the significant risk factors showed that urgent surgeries, mechanical ventilation, need for vasopressors/fluid resuscitation, and higher sepsis related organ failure assessment (SOFA). Scores at ICU admission were independent predictors for sepsis and septic complications.[12] Similar findings were reported in a study using data from the American College of Surgeons National Surgical Quality Improvement Project (NSQIP) on approximately 6,500 patients with sepsis or septic shock.[1] The authors report that in general surgery patients aged older than 60, emergency surgery, and presence of comorbid conditions were significant risk factors for death from sepsis and septic shock; Co-morbidities increased the risk of sepsis or septic shock by fivefold.[1] For the most part, these studies underscore the fact that an urgent abdominal operation to treat IAS in a patient with pre-existing clinical conditions sets the stage for poor prognosis. That is a timely concern, because the growing elderly population with pre-existing clinical conditions is prone to IAIs that frequently require urgent surgical interventions.

Definitions

To better understand IAIs and IAS, it is important to review the definitions of: Systemic inflammatory response syndrome (SIRS), sepsis, severe sepsis, and septic shock.[13] SIRS can be triggered by infectious and non-infectious sources. In general terms, a patient with more than one of the following clinical findings is deemed to have SIRS: temperature >38°C or <36°C, heart rate >90/min, respiratory rate >20/min or $PaCO_2$ <32 mmHg, white blood cell count >12,000/μL or <4,000/μL. In contrast to SIRS, sepsis is defined by the presence of both SIRS and infection. Septic shock is defined as the state of acute circulatory failure as a result of sepsis; it is characterized by persistent hypotension (systolic pressure <90 mmHg, MAP <60 mmHg or a reduction in systolic blood pressure of >40 mmHg from baseline) despite adequate volume resuscitation, in the absence of other causes of hypotension. Severe sepsis refers to sepsis complicated by organ dysfunction.[13] Pneumonia is the most common cause of severe sepsis, followed by IAIs and urinary tract infections.

IAIs arise from a wide variety of sources. If the infection extends beyond the wall of a hollow viscus into the abdominal or retro peritoneal cavity, it is considered a complicated intra-abdominal or retro peritoneal infectious process. Peritonitis and abscess are the most frequent forms of IAIs treated by surgeons.

Peritonitis is usually classified as primary, secondary and tertiary based on its presentation. Primary peritonitis presents without a breach the GI tract. The most common example is the spontaneous bacterial peritonitis (SBP) that occurs in patients with chronic ascites. In dwelling peritoneal catheters can result in a form of peritonitis that is sometimes considered in conjunction with primary peritonitis. Both diseases are microbiologically defined as mono-microbial infections treated with antibiotics, and only infrequently require major surgical intervention. Secondary peritonitis is the most common type of infectious processes in the abdominal cavity and the retro peritoneal space to require surgical treatment. It usually results from GI perforations and frequently presents as intra-abdominal or retro peritoneal abscess.[6] Abscess formation, is for the most part, an effective immune response that restricts the extension of intraperitoneal/retro peritoneal infections. Experimental data show that abscess formation is hampered in defective immune response where the productions of Tumor Necrosis Factor alpha (TNFα), Interleukin (IL-1), and Intercellular Adhesion Molecule-1 (ICAM-1) are blocked.[4] Similar findings are also observed in the absence of IL-6.[4] Aforementioned cytokines are required for adequate polymorphonuclear neutrophil (PMN) function and ultimately abscess formation. Tertiary peritonitis is sometimes considered a "chronic" form of primary or secondary peritonitis that fail to resolve completely.[16] Patients with tertiary peritonitis are severely sick, have pre-existing medical problems, and are incapable of mounting an adequate immune response. Those patients are frequently immuno-suppressed and develop persistent inflammatory response that ultimately leads multiple organ dysfunction[17,18]

Specific management strategies for common causes of IAIs will be discussed in separate chapters of this book.

Pathophysiology

The peritoneal cavity has roughly 50–100cc of peritoneal fluid that contains macrophages, mast cells, and lymphocytes. Inflammatory and infectious processes in the peritoneal cavity trigger the release of cytokines from the leukocytes of the peritoneal fluid, activate the coagulation cascade, and enhance the recruitment of circulating neutrophils and monocytes.[6] Localized peritonitis occurs when the activation of the coagulation cascade and the deposition of fibrin isolate the infection to form an abscess. Thus, shielding the rest of the peritoneal cavity from the infectious process.

The greater omentum also plays an important role in restricting the expansion of IAIs.[4] Leukocyte aggregates within the rich vascular supply of the omentum form what is referred to as "milky spots". Intra-peritoneal Inflammatory processes are directly exposed to post capillary venules through the "milky spots" facilitating PMN recruitment to the peritoneal cavity.[19] Moreover, the greater omentum is also capable of promoting rapid neovascularization and formation of fibrin and collagen, all important in the process of restricting IAIs.[20] Similarly, adhesions between bowel loops, mesentery, and the undersurface of the abdominal wall, also confine and temporarily seal GI perforations and contaminated fluids.

In contrast, generalized peritonitis occurs when local mechanisms are overwhelmed by rapid, or prolonged contamination and the peritoneal cavity becomes acutely inflamed. Bacteria and some particulate matter are carried by peritoneal fluid to the diaphragmatic stomata and removed from the peritoneum. Generalized peritonitis provokes significant fluid shifts (third spacing) that ultimately results in hypovolemic shock. The sympathetic nervous system is activated resulting in catecholamine release. This response leads to significant reduction in urinary output and hinders peristalsis.[6,15] The latter results in stasis of bowel content, promotes microbial overgrowth, and translocation across the bowel wall. Vasodilatation in response to systemic inflammation causes bowel wall edema and further compromise of the natural barrier formed by the gut lining. These processes interfere with intestinal perfusion and contribute to additional ischemic damage to the intestinal barrier.[6]

Microbiology

The microorganisms involved in IAIs generally originate from the resident GI flora. Therefore, when deciding on the antimicrobial usage it is important to consider the origin of the potential source of infection in the GI tract.[17,21,22] The upper jejunum and the stomach are usually populated by gram-positive cocci, mainly streptococci and lactobacilli. Given the low PH and rapid peristalsis in those areas the number of microorganisms is low, approximately 103–104 bacteria/mL of fluid content.[23] With decreased peristalsis and increase in PH the bacterial count in the more distal portions of the small bowel and terminal ileum, can reach up to 10^8 organisms per gram of contents.[23] A more diverse microflora is present in those areas, with aerobic and facultative anaerobic gram negative bacilli. The latter are particularly present in the terminal ileum.[23]

In the colon, slow motility and very low oxidation-reduction potentials create the perfect environment for bacterial proliferation. Making this section of the GI tract the most important site of microbial colonization in humans. Approximately 10^{10} to 10^{11} microorganisms are present per gram of contents and 99.9% are obligate anaerobic organisms.[23,24] Enterobacteriaceae species are the most common pathogens in SBP. This condition is treated with extended-spectrum cephalosporin and quinolone. However, in nosocomial-acquired SPB the resistance to cephalosporin and quinolone is very common (23–50%), and the prevalence of methicillin-resistant staphylococcus aureus (MRSA) is alarmingly high (27%).[25] This is a worrisome pattern of change, since patients with multidrug-resistant bacteria have four times higher risk of death than those without.[26] Moreover, approximately 5–15% of patients with SBP and infected ascites, have a perforated viscus as the source of the infection. Treatment of those patients with antibiotics alone, frequently results in 100% mortality. However, patients with SBP who undergo unnecessary laparotomy also have high mortality rates; approximately 80%. Therefore, precise indication for surgical intervention is of utmost importance in SBP patients.[27,28]

As expected, microorganisms from resident GI bacterial flora are involved in secondary peritonitis. Although stool cultures are usually polymicrobial, cultures from peritoneal collections of patients with IAIs from secondary peritonitis generate a predictable microbiological pattern. *Escherichia coli* and *Klebsiella pneumonia* are responsible for most community-acquired IAIs. *Pseudomonas aeruginosa* and *Acinetobacter baumannii* are the most common causative pathogens of hospital-acquired IAIs.[29] There is also a recent increase in prevalence of multidrug-resistant *Enterobacteriaceae* species that produce extended-spectrum *β*-lactamases (ESBL) and carbapenemases. Data from the study for monitoring Antimicrobial Resistance trends (SmARt) surveillance program showed that, in North America, 6.8% of *E. coli* and isolates from IAIs are ESBL-positive, but resistance to carbapenems is uncommon.[29] Intra-abdominal fluid cultures from septic ICU patients with GI tract perforation showed aerobic gram-negative bacteria in 52.9% of abdominal fluid samples, of which 45% were *E. coli*[22] In that study, the incidence of aerobic gram-negative bacteria was 68.8% in colorectal perforation and 77.8% in perforated acute appendicitis.[22] The incidence of anaerobic bacteria was the same in the latter. Candida was cultured in 20% of the patients with GI perforation. The prevalence of aerobic gram-negative bacteria decreased over time after surgical treatment and antibiotic therapy, from 52.9–6.7% in the first culture after 4 weeks. Whereas, the incidence of gram-positive bacteria increased from 42.5–86.7% in the same period.[22] Therefore, antimicrobial coverage should be modified over time to provide adequate coverage if patient improvement is not as evolving as expected, and surgical intervention may also be considered.

Clinical Manifestations and Physical Examination

Abdominal pain is the hallmark symptom of patients with IAIs, and was the main reason for 8 million emergency department visits in the United States in 2006; making it the most common complaint in that hospital setting.[30] Fever, tachycardia and tachypnea are frequently associated with IAIs. Non-specific findings, such as, loss of appetite, diarrhea, nausea, and abdominal distention are also common, and are reported in up to 30% of cases of IAIs. Underestimation of those complaints may lead to delay in diagnosis.[31] Clinical manifestations of IAIs can be obscure in the elderly, children, and in patients who cannot inform appropriately. Moreover, the effects of analgesia, and sedation also hinder the diagnosis, particularly in ICU patients.[4] Past medical history often provides valuable clues for the diagnosis. For example, primary peritonitis should be considered in a septic patient with known cirrhosis. History of recent abdominal surgery should prompt the suspicion for bowel obstruction, abscess, anastomotic leak, and less frequently, unrecognized bowel injury.[6] Undetected abdominal wall hernias can cause delayed diagnosis. A patient with multiple cardiovascular risk factors who rapidly deteriorates, despite adequate therapy may have intestinal ischemia, and the onset of new organ dysfunction is commonly linked to abdominal sepsis in that context. From a surgical perspective, acute abdomens are generally classified as —

1. Inflammatory
2. Perforated
3. Obstructive
4. Vascular
5. Hemorrhagic

Acute abdomens caused by inflammatory processes and GI perforations are most frequently associated with IAIs. However, prolonged time interval between the onset of the symptoms and the diagnosis will ultimately lead to IAIs regardless of the primary cause.[31,32] But for the most part, IAIs originated from acute abdominal conditions other than inflammatory processes and perforated viscus, are usually linked to delayed diagnosis resulting in sepsis and poor outcome. The most common sources of IAIs in inflammatory acute abdomens are appendicitis, cholecystitis, non-perforated diverticulitis, acute pancreatitis, and any condition that leads to intra-abdominal abscess formation. IAIs from GI perforations usually result from complications of diverticulitis and appendicitis, advanced GI cancer, and peptic ulcer disease.[32]

The most important elements in the assessment of pain caused by IAIs are —

1. Location
2. Nature
3. Triggering and alleviating factors

Infectious processes that cause pain in the left and right upper quadrants typically originate from the liver, biliary tract, and the kidneys. However, sub-phrenic abscess, a typical long ascending inflamed appendix, and intrathoracic conditions can present with pain in those regions.[31,32] Inflammatory processes located in the sub-phrenic areas can irritate the phrenic nerves and produce referred pain in the supraclavicular fossa (Kehr's sign).

Acute pancreatitis, perforated ulcers, and infectious processes of the biliary tract often lead to epigastric pain. IAIs as a result of appendicitis, diverticulitis, pelvic inflammatory disease, and complicated abdominal wall hernias manifest with pain in the left or the right lower quadrants. Peri-umbilical pain is frequently present in the initial phases of acute appendicitis. Pain in the supra-pubic region is common in gynecological, bladder, and pelvic infections. Diffuse abdominal pain is non-specific for intraperitoneal infections, except when triggered by diffuse peritonitis. Infections are located in the retro peritoneum usually because of pronounced systemic inflammation and back pain. That condition can also irritate the genito femoral nerves and cause referred pain in the testicles, labia or on the shaft of the penis.

Abdominal pain provoked by IAIs likely to require a surgical intervention, is usually localized and persistent in nature, and worsens with movement. Whereas, non-surgical conditions usually cause poorly localized pain generated by the visceral nervous system. Moreover, IAIs are not associated with pain of sudden onset, in which case there is not enough time for inflammation to occur. Peritoneal inflammation is usually present within the first 24–48 hours after the onset of the pain. For example, biliary colic pain has an average duration of 5–16 hours. In contrast, abdominal pain provoked by acute cholecystitis is persistent, lasts for a few days, and is frequently associated with right upper quadrant tenderness and a positive Murphy sign.[3,34] Migrating pain initiated at the peri-umbilical region, followed by rebound tenderness and rigidity in the right lower quadrant are strong discriminators of acute appendicitis.[35]

Peritoneal irritation caused by IAIs provokes unrelenting pain. Given the rich somatic innervation of the parietal peritoneum practically any movement can trigger significant pain. Therefore, patients usually adopt antalgic positions, frequently by keeping the knees flexed and bringing the thighs closer to the abdominal wall. Coughing also triggers significant pain and is used for the diagnosis of peritonitis.[36]

A thorough physical examination is important in the assessment of patients with IAIs. Among the elements of abdominal physical examination, i.e., inspection, auscultation, percussion and palpation, the last named is the cornerstone but requires careful technique. The main finding obtained by palpation is involuntary guarding reflex, indicating peritoneal inflammation. For the most part, involuntary guarding can only be appreciated by means of gentle palpation of the abdominal wall, since excessive pressure will not only obscure that physical finding but will also induce voluntary guarding. The full potential of abdominal wall palpation is often missed when checking for rebound tenderness by abruptly releasing pressure applied to the abdominal wall (Blumberg's sign). In that context, patients often manifest voluntary guarding interfering with the diagnostic accuracy of the technique. Therefore, the use of indirect methods to diagnose peritonitis prior to actually touching the patient's abdomen is appropriately indicated to prevent voluntary guarding; The coughing test is an important example. This method was investigated in 143 consecutive patients with abdominal pain from multiple causes.[36] The test was considered positive if the patient showed signs of flinching, grimacing, or hand movement towards the abdomen. When applying the coughing test, clinicians should not tell the patient that the objective is to detect abdominal pain, since previous warning may decrease the accuracy of this test. The accuracy of the coughing test in the detection of peritonitis was assessed by comparing the clinical findings with the final diagnosis. Results showed that the diagnostic value of the test was highly significant for the odds ratio 13:1 (95% confidence interval 5.8–28.9, $p < 0.001$). Sensitivity and specificity of the test were 0.78 and 0.79 respectively, and the positive predictive value was 76%.[36] Another prospective study investigated the coughing test in 60 patients with pain in the right iliac fossa and presumptive diagnosis of acute appendicitis.[37] In that study, all patients who tested positive underwent appendectomy, and those that tested negative were admitted for observation and re-assessment.[37] Only four of the 60 patients did not have appendicitis histologically confirmed. No patients with a persistently negative cough sign required an operation.

Clinical prediction rules are additional ancillary methods that can be used in the management of acute abdomens, and potentially increase the diagnostic accuracy. With respect to abdominal pain caused by IAIs, clinical prediction rules have been most extensively investigated in acute appendicitis and inflammatory pelvic disease.[38,39] The Alvarado score uses six clinical criteria and two laboratory measurements in the diagnosis of acute appendicitis; the maximum score is 10. A recent systematic search of 42 validation studies assessed the diagnostic accuracy of that method at two cut off points; score of 5 (1–4 versus 5–10) and score of 7 (1–6 versus 7–10), among men, women and children.[38] Results showed that the Alvarado score is a useful diagnostic "rule out" method at a cut point of 5. The method is well calibrated in men, but over-predicts appendicitis in women and is inconsistent in children.[38] Another study assessed a prediction rule to distinguish acute appendicitis from pelvic inflammatory disease.[39] In that study, the prediction method correctly ruled out appendicitis from pelvic inflammatory disease with sensitivity of 99% (95% CI, 94–100%) by three clinical criteria: no migration of pain, bilateral abdominal tenderness, and no nausea and vomiting.[39]

Finally, in addition to Blumberg's and Murphy's signs clinicians should also be mindful of other specific findings in patients with acute abdominal pain that can correlate with IAIs. Most importantly—

1. Cullen's sign: Tracking of retro peritoneal hemorrhagic fluid along the gastro-hepatic and the falciform ligament to the umbilicus. Even though this sign was originally described in a patient with a ruptured extra-uterine pregnancy it also correlates, in less than 3% of the cases, with severe acute pancreatitis.[40]
2. Grey Turner's sign: Tracking of retro peritoneal hemorrhagic fluid along the edges of the quadratus lomborum muscles through a defect in the transversalis fascia and subsequently to the subcutaneous tissue. This sign is detected in 1–3% of all cases of acute pancreatitis.[40]
3. Rovsing's sign: Referred pain in the right iliac fossa with palpation of the contralateral region. This sign is sometimes present in acute appendicitis, but the accuracy is unknown.
4. Psoas sign: This sign can be investigated in two ways. Having the patient raise the thigh from a supine position against resistance, or passively extending the hip with the patient laying on the contralateral. The psoas sign correlates with inflammatory process in the retro peritoneum that provoke irritation to the psoas muscle.
5. Obturador sign: The patient's right thigh is passively flexed towards the abdominal wall from supine position with the knee flexed at 90°. Afterwards the right hip is rotated internally. Pain in the area of the obturador internus indicates an inflammatory process next to that muscle, most frequently caused by pelvic inflammatory disease, retro cecal pelvic appendicitis, and complicated diverticulitis.

Diagnostic Tests

Laboratory studies include, but not limited to, complete blood count with differential, electrolytes, creatinine, urea, blood glucose, liver enzymes, amylase, lipase, cardiac enzymes, coagulation panel, lactate, and peripheral and central venous blood gases. Complete blood count often shows leukocytosis with a left-shift. Some patients may present with leucopenia from their sepsis overwhelming the bone marrow's synthetic capacity. Increased serum lactate and metabolic acidosis often correlate with advanced peritonitis, preoperative organ failure, and frequently determine worse prognosis. Delay in surgical intervention and the presence of multiorgan failure are significant risk factors associated with increased mortality.

Although overt peritonitis is essentially of clinical diagnosis, radiologic studies are frequently used in the investigation.[4,6] Plain radiographs of the abdomen can detect ileus, and air fluid levels. Chest radiograph can show pneumo-peritoneum in up to 80% of patients with duodenal perforation, albeit less accurate to demonstrate that finding in perforations of other segments of the GI tract. Ultrasonography is useful in the evaluation of intra-abdominal collections, infections of the liver, and the biliary tree. Moreover, that method is also used for percutaneous drainage of fluid collections at the bedside, this is particularly important in patients who are too unstable for a trip to the computed tomography (CT) scanner. However, ultrasonography is highly operator dependent, and visualization can be impaired by the patient's body habitus and overlying bowel gas. Therefore, CT scan is arguably the most commonly used method to determine the source of IAIs in stable patients who do not require immediate laparotomy.[5] Additionally, CT scan outperforms ultrasonography in patients with postoperative IAS, and should be used when IAIs are suspected in that context.[41] CT with oral and rectal contrast can reveal anastomotic leaks if the patient has recently undergone GI surgery. Furthermore, CT-guided percutaneous drainage of intra-abdominal and retro peritoneal abscesses is an effective strategy to definitively or temporarily manage those conditions.[41] Magnetic resonance imaging is rarely used and there is no clear advantage of MRI over CT for most indications in the setting of IAIs.[6]

Management

Successful management of IAIs requires timely resuscitation, early administration of antimicrobial agents, and adequate source control.[7,41,42] The recommendations of the Surviving Sepsis Campaign (2012) help guide the management of patients with severe sepsis and septic shock. A summary of those recommendations are depicted in Table 1.[7]

Securing adequate vascular access and aggressive fluid resuscitation are the first priority. Early goal-directed resuscitation has been shown to improve survival in septic shock.[7,43] The targets are CVP 8–12 mmHg, mean arterial pressure ≥65 mmHg, urine output ≥0.5 cc/kg/hour, central venous oxygen saturation ≥70% or mixed venous saturation ≥65%.[7] In order to achieve those targets, initial resuscitation requires rapid administration of crystalloid and colloid fluids; any advantage of one type of fluid over another remains debatable. The initial choices of vasopressors are norepinephrine and dopamine if the mean arterial pressure remains less than 65 mmHg after adequate fluid resuscitation.

Table 1. Recommendations published by the Surviving Sepsis Campaign guidelines committee. (Reproduced with permission).[7]

A. Initial Resuscitation

1. Protocolized, quantitative resuscitation ot patients with sepsis- induced tissue hypoperfusion (defined in this document as hypotension persisting after initial fluid challenge or blood lactate concentration ≥4 mmol/L). Goals during the first 6 hrs of resuscitation:

   a) Central venous pressure 8–12 mmHg
   b) Mean arterial pressure (MAP) ≥65 mmHg
   c) Urine output ≥0.5 mL/kg/hr
   d) Central venous (superior *vena cava*) or mixed venous oxygen saturation 70% or 65%, respectively (grade 1C).

2. In patients with elevated lactate levels targeting resuscitation to normalize lactate (grade 2C).

B. Screening for Sepsis and Performance Improvement

1. Routine screening of potentially infected seriously ill patients for severe sepsis to allow earlier implementation of therapy (grade IC).
2. Hospital–based performance improvement efforts in severe sepsis (UG).

C. Diagnosis

1. Cultures as clinically appropriate before antimicrobial therapy if no significant delay >45 mins) in the start of antimicrobial(s) (grade 1C). At least two sets of blood cultures (both aerobic and anaerobic bottles) be obtained before antimicrobial therapy with at least 1 drawn percutaneously and 1 drawn through each vascular access device, unless the device was recently (<48 hrs) inserted (grade 1C).
2. Use of the 1,3 beta-D-glucan assay (grade 2B), mannan and anti-mannan antibody assays (2C), if available and invasive candidiasis is in differential diagnosis of cause of infection.
3. Imaging studies performed promptly to confirm a potential source of infection (UG).

D. Antimicrobial Therapy

1. Administration of effective intravenous antimicrobials within the first hour of recognition of septic shock (grade 1B) and severe sepsis without septic shock (grade 1C) as the goal of therapy.

2a. Initial empiric ant-infective therapy of one or more drugs that have activity against all likely pathogens (bacterial and/or fungal or viral) and that penetrate in adequate concentrations into tissues presumed to be the source of sepsis (grade 1B).

(*Continued*)

2b. Antimicrobial regimen should be reassessed daily for potential deescalation (grade 1B).
3. Use of low procalcitonin levels or similar biomarkers to assist the clinician in the discontinuation of empiric antibiotics in patients who initially appeared septic, but have no subsequent evidence of infection (grade 2C).
4a. Combination empirical therapy for neutropenic patients with severe sepsis (grade 2B) and for patients with difficult-to-treat, multidrug-resistant bacterial pathogens such as *Acinetabacter* and *Pseudomonas* spp. (grade 2B). For patients with severe infections associated with respiratory failure and septic shock, combination therapy with an extended spectrum beta-lactam and either an aminoglycoside or a fluoroquinolone is for *P. aeruginosa* bacteremia (grade 2B). A combination of beta-lactam and macrolide for patients with septic shock from bacteremic *Streptococcus pneumoniae* infections (grade 2B).
4b. Empiric combination therapy should not be administered for more than 3–5 days. De-escalation to the most appropriate single therapy should be performed as soon as the susceptibility profile is known (grade 2B).
5. Duration of therapy typically 7–10 days; longer courses may be appropriate in patients who have a slow clinical response, undrainable foci of infection, bacteremia with *S. aureus*; some fungal and viral infections or immunologic deficiencies, including neutropenia (grade 2C).
6. Antiviral therapy initiated as early as possible in patients with severe sepsis or septic shock of viral origin (grade 2C).
7. Antimicrobial agents should not be used in patients with severe inflammatory states determined to be of noninfectious cause (UG).

E. Source Control

1. A specific anatomical diagnosis of infection requiring consideration for emergent source control be sought and diagnosed or excluded as rapidly as possible, and intervention be undertaken for source control within the first 12 hour after the diagnosis is made, if feasible (grade 1C).
2. When infected peripancreatic necrosis is identified as a potential source of infection, definitive intervention is best delayed until adequate demarcation of viable and nonviable tissues has occurred (grade 2B).
3. When source control in a severely septic patient is required, the effective intervention associated with the least physiologic insult should be used (e.g., percutaneous rather than surgical drainage of an abscess) (UG).

(*Continued*)

Table 1. (*Continued*)

4. If intravascular access devices are a possible source of severe sepsis or septic shock, they should be removed promptly after other vascular access has been established (UG).

F. Infection Prevention

1a. Selective oral decontamination and selective digestive decontamination should be introduced and investigated as a method to reduce the incidence of ventilator-associated pneumonia; This infection control measure can then be instituted in health care settings and regions where this methodology is found to be effective (grade 2B).

1b. Oral chlorhexidine gluconate be used as a form of oropharyngeal decontamination to reduce the risk of ventilator-associated pneumonia in ICU patients with severe sepsis (grade 2B).

After obtaining cultures, antimicrobial agents should be initiated within the first hour of recognition of septic shock. Each hour delay of antimicrobial is associated with a 7.6% decrease in survival.[44] The choice of empiric antimicrobial coverage for IAIs includes broad-spectrum activity against gram-negative bacilli and anaerobes. Depending on the suspected etiology, gram positive and fungal coverage may also be added. Prevalence of antimicrobial resistance in the local community or hospital should prompt coverage against those microorganisms as part of the empiric therapy. After identification of the pathogens in cultured specimens, antimicrobial therapy should be narrowed accordingly to reduce the risk of developing infections from antimicrobial-resistant organisms and super infections from Clostridium difficile. However, blood cultures can be negative in over 50% of cases of severe sepsis.[7] Therefore, the most appropriate clinical decisions regarding maintenance, narrowing or stopping antimicrobial therapy should be based on the overall clinical status of each patient.

BPIGS put together by University of Toronto's Division of General Surgery provides initial guidelines on choosing empiric antimicrobial therapy in patients with IAIs (Table 2).[45]

Those guidelines stratified the initial antimicrobial therapies by uncomplicated versus complicated IAIs, and community acquired versus health care-associated IAIs. Uncomplicated IAIs, such as non-perforated appendicitis, can be treated with first generation cephalosporin and metronidazole as

Table 2. BPIGS recommendations, University of Toronto — Division of general surgery. Guideline number 4 (Reproduced with permission).[45]

		Selection of antibiotics			
Type of IAI	**Examples**	**Spectrum of antimicrobial activity**	**Recommended antibiotics**	**PCN allergic patients**	**Duration**
Community Acquired IAI: Uncomplicated					
Uncomplicated IAI	Non-perforated appendicitis	Enteric gram- negative bacilli and anaerobes	Cefazolin and metronidazole	Gentamicin and metronidazole	Preoperatively only
Perforation without Established Infection	Perforations of stomach and duodenum and traumatic bowel perforations who are taken to the O.R. within 12–24 hours	Gram-positive cocci and aerobic/ facultative anaerobes +/− anaerobes	Cefazolin and metronidazole	Gentamicin and metronidazole	"Ultrashort" 24 hours only
Community Acquired IAI: Complicated					
Mild-to-Moderate Severity	Perforated appendicitis; perforated diverticulitis	Enteric gram-negative bacilli andanaerobes	Cefazolin (iv) or cephalexin (po) and metronidazole	Gentamicin and metronidazole	3–7 days (until clinical signs of resolution)

(*Continued*)

Table 2. (*Continued*)

Type of IAI	Examples	Selection of antibiotics: Spectrum of antimicrobial activity	Recommended antibiotics	PCN allergic patients	Duration
High severity	Shock; new organ failure; ICU patient	Enteric gram-negative bacilli and anaerobes; possibly enterococcus	Ceftriaxone and metronidazole, (may consider piperacillin-tazobactam)	Gentamicin and metronidazole	3–7 days (until clinical signs of resolution)
Other risk factors for treatment failure	Age >70; immunosuppression; poor nutrition; delayed/inadequate source control	Enteric gram-negative bacilli and anaerobes; possibly enterococcus in immunosuppressed	Ceftriaxone and metronidazole (may consider piperacillin-tazobactam)	Gentamicin and metronidazole	3–7 days (until clinical signs of resolution)
Health Care Associated cIAI					
Mild-to-Moderate	Hospitalized ≥5 days; anastomotic leak; postoperative abscess	Enterococcus, drug-resistant gram-negative bacilli	piperacillin tazobactam* (may consider ceftriaxone and metronidazole)	Vancomycin, gentamicin and metronidazole OR carbapenem** (meropenem or imipenem) and vancomycin	3–7 days (until clinical signs of resolution)

High severity	Hospitalized ≥5 days; anastomotic leak; postoperative abscess	Enterococcus, drug-resistant gram-negative bacilli	Piperacillin tazobactam*	vancomycin, gentamicin & metronidazole OR carbapenem** (meropenem or imipenem) and vancomycin	3–7 days (until clinical signs of resolution)
Other risk factors for Health-care Associated Infection	Nursing home; rehab facility; dialysis patient; recent antibiotics	Enterococcus, drug resistant gram negative bacilli	Piperacillin tazobactam* (may consider ceftriaxone and metronidazole)	vancomycin, gentamicin and metronidazole OR carbapenem** (meropenem or imipenem) and vancomycin	3–7 days (until clinical signs of resolution)
Biliary Tract					
Mild-to-Moderate	Ascending cholangitis; acute calculous cholecystitis	Enteric gram-negative bacilli	Cefazolin	Gentamicin	3–7 days (until clinical signs of resolution)
High severity	—	—	Ceftriaxone and ampicillin	Gentamicin and vancomycin	3–7 days until (until signs of resolution)

empiric therapy, and substitute the cephalosporin with an aminoglycoside such as gentamicin if patient is penicillin-allergic. For complicated community acquired IAIs and mild — moderate health care-associated IAI, it is recommended to use third-generation cephalosporin in addition to metronidazole, or piperacillin-tazobactam alone. For severe health care-associated IAIs, piperacillin-tazobactam is recommended; In penicillin-allergic patients, combination of vancomycin, gentamicin and metronidazole, or a carbapenem with vancomycin regimens can be considered.[45]

In addition to adequate resuscitation, administration of antibiotics, and identification of the etiology, physical measures are often necessary to effectively treat IAIs; this last action is referred to as source control.[46] Given that delayed surgical interventions can be disastrous, keen judgment is required to decide when to intervene and the most appropriate surgical procedure. Nevertheless, there is strong supporting evidence that unnecessary or premature surgical interventions can be equally catastrophic.[4] Moreover, it is important to consider minimally invasive options of source control. In several occasions that can be the sole intervention necessary for source control. For instance, abscess drainage can be achieved by percutaneous image-guided procedures, and cholangitis from obstructed common bile duct is preferably treated with endoscopic retrograde cholangiopancreatography (ERCP) and sphincterotomy with or without stone extraction or stenting. However, understanding the limitations of image guided and endoscopic procedures is very important. For example, multiple abscess, high residual after the procedure, and abscess not amenable to percutaneous drainage for anatomical reasons often require surgical exploration.[4,6] Additionally, early surgical interventions are lifesaving in the following settings: anatomical disruption of the GI tract, necrotic tissue from intestinal ischemia, intra-abdominal or retro peritoneal foreign bodies, and diffuse peritonitis. The main objectives of surgical management are

1. Debridement of non-viable tissue
2. Removal of foreign body
3. Elimination of fecal contamination
4. Reconstitute GI continuity or create a stoma
5. Ample drainage of abscesses

Even though those objectives are generally achieved during a single intervention, multiple operations are sometimes required. Studies showed that morbidity and mortality rates in scheduled relaparotomy were not significantly different from on-demand relaparotomy.[47] Nonetheless, the latter strategy resulted in shorter hospital and ICU lengths of stay.[47] Currently, the decision to manage IAIs with a single operation or alternatively a staged approach ultimately depends on the clinical condition of the patient and on the surgical findings.[4,48] Whether to perform definitive anastomosis or a stoma in patients with severe IAIs is open to debate. A recent study compared the outcomes of patients with deferred primary anastomosis to those with stoma formation in severe secondary peritonitis managed with staged laparotomies.[49] In the deferred primary anastomosis group, patients were subjected to GI resection with the ends left in discontinuity and "open abdomen". Results showed that surgeons were able to perform a definitive anastomosis in 80% of the patients that had initially undergone deferred primary anastomosis with similar fistula rates to those with a stoma formation, respectively 8.8% and 5.1%. In the latter, the majority of the fistulas were related to complications of the stoma.[49] Interestingly, the trauma surgeons at the institution tended to use the deferred primary anastomosis strategy, while the non-trauma general surgeons uniformly favored resection with stoma formation. For the most part, this study underscores two important points. First, it shows that a staged laparotomy approach doesn't necessarily implicate in creation of a stoma. Second, it calls attention to the challenges in performing stomas in patients with IAIs. Those patients frequently present with intestinal edema, mesenteric shortening, and are usually obese, all of which make it difficult to create an adequate stoma.[50]

Even though aforementioned interventions are critically important to improve survival, other factors contribute to poor outcomes. A review of 1,182 cases of complicated IAIs revealed that the following patient characteristics are predictive of in-hospital mortality: age ≥70, APACHEII score ≥15, ICU admission, maximum temperature ≥38.5°C, pre-existing cardiac and liver diseases, malignancy, solid organ transplantation, and chronic renal failure requiring renal replacement therapy.[42] The study also showed that in addition to aforementioned characteristics, poor nutritional status, delay in the initial surgical intervention (>24 hours), degree of peritoneal involvement (diffuse peritonitis), and inability to achieve adequate debridement or control of drainage were the most important clinical factors predicting failure of source control in IAI.[42] Patients with those high-risk characteristics are more likely to develop IAIs caused by resistant pathogens. Therefore, it is prudent to consider broadening the empiric antibiotic coverage. Given that the mortality rate for sepsis alone is approximately 5%, 15% with septic shock, and increases dramatically to 80–90% in severe sepsis and multi organ failure.[11,14]

Summary

IAS in critically ill patients remains a diagnostic and therapeutic challenge. Careful history and physical examination often raise the suspicion of IAS. Abdominal imaging, especially CT, is particularly important in establishing a diagnosis. Immediate resuscitation, early antibiotics and timely source control are crucial in successful multidisciplinary management of IAS.

References

1. Moore LJ, Moore FA, Jones SL *et al.* Sepsis in general surgery: A deadly complication. *Am J Surg* 2009; 198: 868–874.
2. Lagu T, Rothberg MB, Shieh MS *et al.* Hospitalizations, costs and outcomes of severe sepsis in the United States 2003–2007. *Crit Care Med* 2012; 40: 754–761.
3. Pieracci FM, Barie PS. Management of severe sepsis of abdominal origin. *Scand J Surg* 2007; 96: 184–196.
4. Rezende-Neto JB, Rotstein OD. Abdominal catastrophes in the intensive care unit setting. *Crit Care Clin* 2013; 29: 1017–1044.
5. Sartelli M, Viale P, Catena F *et al.* 2013 WSES guidelines for management of intra-abdominal infections. *World J Emerg Surg* 2013; 8(1): 3 doi 10.1186/1749792283.
6. Marshall JC. Intra-abdominal infections. *Microbes Infect* 2004; 6: 1015–1025.
7. Dellinger RP, Levy MM, Rhodes A *et al.* Surviving sepsis campaign: International guidelines for management of severe sepsis and septic shock: 2012; *Crit Care Med* 2013; 41: 580–637.
8. Dellinger RP, Levy MM, Carlet JM *et al.* Surviving Sepsis Campaign: International guidelines for management of severe sepsis and septic shock: 2008. *Crit Care Med* 2008; 36: 296–327.
9. Gaieski DF, Edwards JM, Kallan MJ *et al.* Benchmarking the incidence and mortality of severe sepsis in the United States. *Crit Care Med* 2013; 41: 1167–1174.
10. Stevenson EK, Rubenstein AR, Radin GT *et al.* Two decades of mortality trends among patients with severe sepsis: A comparative meta-analysis. *Crit Care Med* 2014; 42: 625–631.
11. Angus DC, Linde-Zwirble WT, Lidicker J *et al.* Epidemiology of severe sepsis in the United States: Analysis of incidence, outcome and associated costs of care. *Crit Care Med* 2001; 70: 672–680.
12. Elias ACGP, Matsuo T, Grion CMC *et al.* Incidence and risk factors for sepsis in surgical patients: A cohort study. *J Crit Care* 2012; 27: 159–166.
13. Levy, M.M *et al.* 2001 SCCM/ESICM/ACCP/ATS/SIS International Sepsis Definitions Conference. *Crit Care Med* 2003; 31(4): 1250–1256.

14. Angus, D.C. and T. van der Poll, Severe sepsis and septic shock. *N Engl J Med*, 2013; 369(9): 840–851.
15. Gibson III FC, Onderdonk AB, Kasper DL *et al.* Cellular mechanism of intra-abdominal abscess formation by Bacteroides Fragilis. *J Immunol* 1998; 160(10): 5000–5006.
16. Nathens AB, Rotstein OD, Marshall JC *et al.* Tertiary peritonitis: clinical features of a complex nosocomial infection. *World J Surg* 1998; 22(2): 158–163.
17. Cholongitas E. *et al.* Increasing frequency of Gram-positive bacteria in spontaneous bacterial peritonitis. *Liver Int* 2005; 25(1): 57–61.
18. Gentile LF, Cuenca AG, Efron PA, *et al.* Persistent inflammation and immunosuppression: A common syndrome and a new horizon for surgical intensive care. *J Trauma Acute Care Surg* 2012; 72(6): 1491–1501.
19. Doherty NS, Griffiths RJ, Hakkinen JP *et al.* Post-capillary venules in the "milky spots" of the greater omentum are the major site of plasma protein and leukocyte extravasation in rodent models of peritonitis. *Inflammation Res* 1995; 44: 167–177.
20. Konturek SJ, Brzozowski T, Majka I *et al.* Omentum and basic fibriblast growth factor in healing of chronic gastric ulcerations in rats. *Dig Dis Sci* 1994; 39: 1064–1071.
21. Chromik AM, *et al.*, Identification of patients at risk for development of tertiary peritonitis on a surgical intensive care unit. *J Gastrointest Surg* 2009; 13(7): 1358–1367.
22. De Ruiter J, Weel J, Manusama E *et al.* The epidemiology of intra-abdominal flora in critically ill patients with secondary and tertiary abdominal sepsis. *Infection* 2009; 37(6): 522–527.
23. Hao WL, Lee YK. Microflora of the gastro-intestinal tract: A review. *Methods Mol Biol* 2004; 268: 491–502.
24. Mackowiak PA. The normal microbial flora. *N Engl J Med* 1982; 307: 83–93.
25. Piroth L., *et al.*, Bacterial epidemiology and antimicrobial resistance in ascitic fluid: A 2 year retrospective study. *Scand J Infect Dis* 2009; 41(11–12): 847–851.
26. Chen YH, Hsueh PR. Changing bacteriology of abdominal and surgical sepsis. *Curr Opin Infect Dis* 2012; 25(5): 590–595.
27. Pinzello G, Simonetti RG, Craxi A *et al.* Spontaneous bacterial peritonitis: A prospective investigation in predominantely non-alcoholic cirrhotic patients. *Hepatology* 1983; 3: 545–549.
28. Garrison RN, Cryer HM, Howard DA *et al.* Clarification of risk factors for abdominal operations in patients with hepatic cirrhosis. *Ann Surg* 1984; 199: 648–655.
29. Hawser SP *et al.* Trending eight years of in vitro activity of ertapenem and comparators against Escherichia coli from intra-abdominal infections in North America—SMART 2002–2009. *J Chemother* 2011; 23(5): 266–272.

30. Pitts SR, Niska RW, Xu J *et al.* National hospital ambulatory medical care survey: 2006 emergency department summary. National health statistics report; no 7. Hyattsville, MD: National Center for Health Statistics; 2008; 6: 1–38
31. Flasar MH, Goldberg E. Acute abdominal pain. *Med Clin North Am* 2006; 90: 481–503.
32. Savassi Rocha PR, Andrade JI, Souza C. Abdomen agudo — diagnostico e tratamento. Rio de Janeiro: *Medsi*; 1993; 1, 13–22
33. Silen W. Method of diagnosis: The history. In Cope's Early Diagnsosis of the Acute Abdomen. New York, Oxford, 2010; 1: 18–27.
34. Silen W. Cholecystitis and other causes of acute pain in the right upper quadrant of the abdomen. In Cope's Early Diagnsosis of the Acute Abdomen. New York, Oxford, 2010; 1: 131–140.
35. Andersson REB. Meta-analysis of the clinical and laboratory diagnosis of appendicitis. *Br J Surg* 2004; 91: 29–37.
36. Bennett DH, Tambeur LJMT, Campbell WB. Use of coughing test to diagnose peritonitis. *BMJ* 1994; 308: 1336.
37. Jeddy TA, Vowles RH, Southam JA. "Cough sign": A reliable test in the diagnosis of intra-abdominal inflammation. *Br J Surg* 1994; 8281: 279.
38. Ohle R, O'Reilly F, O'Brien K *et al.* The Alvarado score for predicting acute appendictis: A systematic review. *BMC Medicine* 2011; 9: 139.
39. Morishita K, Gushimiyagi M, Hashiguchi M *et al.* Clinical prediction rule to distinguish pelvic inflammatory disease from acute appendicitis in women of childbearing age. *Am J Emerg Med* 2007; 25(2): 152–157.
40. Bosman M, Schreiner O, Galle PR. Coexistence of Cullen's and Grey Turner's signs in acute pancreatitis. *Am J Med* 2009; 122: 333–334.
41. Go H, Baarslaga H, Vermeulenb H *et al.* A comparative study to validate the use of ultrasonography and computed tomography in patients with post-operative intra-abdominal sepsis. *Eur J Radiol* 2005; 54(3): 383–387.
42. Swenson BR, *et al.* Choosing antibiotics for intra-abdominal infections: What do we mean by "high risk"? *Surg Infect* (*Larchmt*) 2009; 10(1): 29–39.
43. Rivers E *et al.* Early goal-directed therapy in the treatment of severe sepsis and septic shock. *N Engl J Med* 2001; 345(19): 1368–1377.
44. Kumar A *et al.* Duration of hypotension before initiation of effective antimicrobial therapy is the critical determinant of survival in human septic shock. *Crit Care Med* 2006; 34(6): 1589–1596.
45. Doyle J *et al.* Best practice in general surgery guideline #4: Management of intra-abdominal infections. 2012.
46. Schein M, Marshall J. Source control for surgical infections. *World J Surg* 2004; 28: 638–645.
47. Van Ruler O, Mahler CW, Boer KR *et al.* Comparison of on-demand versus planned relaparotomy strategy in patients with severe peritonitis: A randomized trial. *JAMA* 2007; 298: 865–872.

48. Hanisch E, Schmandra TC, Encke A. Surgical strategies — anastomosis or stoma, a second look — when and why? *Langenbecks Arch Surg* 1999; 384(3): 239–242.
49. Ordonez CA, Sanchez AL, Pineda JA *et al.* Deferred primary anastomosis versus diversion in patients with severe secondary peritonitis managed with staged laparotomies. *World J Surg* 2010; 34: 169–176.
50. Cataldo PA. Technical tips for stoma creation in the challenging patient. *Clin Colon Rectal Surg* 2008; 21(1): 17–22. doi: 10.1055/s-2008-1055317.

Chapter 26

Bowel Obstruction

Dave D. Paskar and Neil G. Parry

Overview

Most patients with bowel obstruction (BO) are not initially managed in the ICU. However, those with significant associated comorbidities (e.g., age, cardiorespiratory, metabolic and fluid derangements) or complications of BO (e.g., ischemia, fluid deficits, perforation or severe sepsis) should be treated in the ICU. The intensivist managing such patients must be familiar with the general principles of management, clinical features and complications of BO.

This chapter will discuss general features of BO and various ICU specific issues. BO occurs when the normal passage of enteric material through the gastro-intestinal (GI) tract is impaired by the mechanical blockage of the bowel lumen. In contrast, functional BO ("paralytic ileus") occurs when normal GI peristalsis ceases due to some physiologic disruption. Patients with BO present with varying degrees of abdominal pain, nausea, vomiting and obstipation depending on the cause, location, severity and duration of the BO. Physiologically, BO can result in hypovolemia, electrolyte deficiencies and acid–base imbalances which require urgent correction. BO classically describes blockage of the small or large intestine. The most common cause of small bowel obstruction (SBO) in adults is postoperative intra-abdominal adhesions, whereas the most common cause of large bowel obstruction (LBO) is malignancy (i.e., colorectal cancer). The diagnosis of BO is clinical; however, the use of radiographic imaging, especially computed tomography (CT), is very helpful in determining the underlying etiology of BO, as well as initial management (operative or nonoperative). Considerations for urgent surgery include hemodynamic instability, peritonitis, closed loop BO, concerns of bowel ischemia or perforation and low likelihood of nonoperative resolution.

Introduction

BO is a clinical state in which the normal anterograde passage of digestive materials along the GI tract is partially or completely interrupted by mechanical obstruction of the bowel lumen by a mechanical and/or anatomical phenomenon.[1,2] This is distinguished from ileus, in which effective GI transit is hampered by diminished intestinal peristalsis, typically due to more systemic or physiological factors (i.e., sepsis, electrolyte abnormalities).[2]

The management principles of BO depend to some degree on the underlying obstructive etiology. All cases mandate traditional management principles of: identifying and treating the underlying cause; prevention and correction, as necessary, of volume, electrolyte and acid–base disturbances; proximal decompression of the GI tract; and symptom relief of resultant pain, nausea and vomiting with analgesic and anti-emetic medications.[3,4] In some cases, parenteral nutritional support may be needed if there is a prolonged cessation of GI function. The role and timing of emergency surgery for BO depends on the overall patient status, etiology and severity of the obstruction, as well as the degree of concern for intestinal ischemia, perforation or peritonitis.

As such, critical care providers should be comfortable with the medical and surgical management principles for BO. Delay in diagnosing and appropriately managing BO will result in greater overall physiologic disruption, increased likelihood of requiring bowel resection, and overall increased morbidity and mortality.[7]

Epidemiology/Risk Factors

BO accounts for approximately 15% of all in-patient general surgery admissions and adhesive SBO (ASBO), which occur in up to 25% of patients following GI surgery, results in more than $1.3 billion (USD) in annual associated healthcare costs in the United States, alone.[5,6]

Globally, SBO is much more common than LBO, with their relative incidences occurring in a 4:1 ratio.[8] The most common causes of SBO in North American and Europe are post-surgical adhesions (65–75%), abdominal wall hernias (10–15%) and intraperitoneal malignancy (5–10%) (Table 1).[1,7] This contrasts with African and Asian populations, in which hernias are by far the most common cause of SBO.[7,8]

Table 1. Common causes of bowel obstruction.

Small Bowel Obstruction	Large Bowel Obstruction
Intra-abdominal adhesions — 65–75%	Colorectal cancer — 60–80%
Abdominal wall hernias — 10–15%	Diverticular strictures — 15–20%
Malignancy — 5–10%	Colonic volvulus — 5–10%
All other causes (i.e., gallstone ileus) — 5–10%	All other causes (i.e., non-GI cancer) — 1–5%

The risk of ASBO varies depending on the type of surgery. For instance, larger pelvic surgeries such as hysterectomy, abdominal-perineal resection and ileo-anal pouch formation are associated with lifetime rates of 25–38% for at least one ASBO episode. Prior laparotomy for acute perforation with notable peritoneal contamination and inflammation are also associated with more extensive adhesions.[10,11] These rates contrast with the lifetime BO incidence of 0.1–2% in individuals without prior intra-abdominal surgery.[8] Additionally, patients undergoing minimally-invasive surgery are much less likely to develop ASBO.[11]

The most common causes of LBO in Western nations are colorectal cancer (60–80%), diverticular strictures (15–20%) and colonic (cecal and sigmoid) volvulus (5–10%) (Table 1). Conversely, in Asia and Africa, volvulus is the most common cause of LBO (upwards of 40%) and colorectal cancer is much less common. Anatomically, the sigmoid colon is the most common site for LBO, and overall, malignant LBO episodes are more likely to be distal or left-sided.[2]

Diverticular disease tends to cause LBO via structuring and narrowing of the colonic lumen at sites of recurrent inflammation and subsequent scarring. Risk factors for colonic volvulus include congenital colonic abnormalities (i.e., non-fixation) and factors associated with underlying chronic constipation (which include narcotic use, institutionalization, increasing age and diet imbalances) leading to colonic redundancy.[8]

Pathophysiology

The common underlying pathophysiology of BO is a physical (or "mechanical") occlusion of the GI tract lumen that cannot be overcome by peristalsis, resulting in partial or complete blockage of anterograde flow of digestive contents beyond the point of obstruction. As a result, numerous pathophysiologic processes occur. These include changes in fluid volume distribution, electrolyte and acid–base disturbances, changes in the distribution of GI flora, malnutrition and in severe cases, decreased blood supply of the affected segment of intestine which may subsequently result in intestinal ischemia, infarction and finally perforation with resultant peritonitis and sepsis.[8]

The etiology of BO is classically organized by the location of the obstructing mechanism relative to the intestinal wall (Table 2). 'Extrinsic' processes compress or twist the lumen of the intestine and may cause pressure necrosis or restrict blood supply to the affected bowel, which can result in ischemia and subsequent perforation. 'Mural' phenomena that arise from the intestinal wall itself cause obstruction by narrowing or obliterating the

Table 2. Etiology of mechanical bowel obstruction.

Extrinsic	Mural	Intraluminal
Adhesions: postoperative, inflammatory, congenital	GI-primary neoplasia: malignant (i.e., adenocarcinoma), benign (i.e., leiomyoma)	Bezoars: vegetable matter (phyto-); ingested hair (tricho-); food boluses
Malignancy: Non-GI (i.e.,prostate), peritoneal carcinomatosis	Metastatic malignancy (i.e., melanoma)	Ingested foreign bodies, barium
Abdominal wall hernias: Inguinal, incisional	Intramural hematoma: iatrogenic, trauma	Gallstone ileus
Internal hernias, volvulus, malrotation	Stricture: Ischemic, inflammatory (i.e., Crohn's, diverticulitis), radiation	Intussusception (usually due to pathologic lead point in adults)
Non-malignant masses: Abscess, pseuocyst, endometriosis, benign neoplasia	Active inflammation: Infectious, Chron's, radiation enteritis	Stool impaction
	Congenital phenomena: Enteric duplication, webs, stenosis, atresia, Meckel's diverticulum	Polyps, exophytic lesions (i.e., GIST)

lumen at the involved location. Finally, 'intraluminal' causes physically occlude the lumen.[2,7]

Postoperative abdominal adhesions are by far the most common cause of BO in North American and Europe and are the result of deposition of fibrous tissue within the peritoneal cavity following intra-abdominal events such as surgery, sepsis or inflammation. While the mechanism of adhesion formation is not fully understood, it is thought to arise from a complex interplay of peritoneal tissue damage, inflammatory cascades, bleeding with subsequent coagulation and inhibition of fibrinolysis. In the case of post-operative adhesion formation, the processes of adhesiogenesis begin in the days following surgery.[8–10] Since postoperative adhesions are by far the most common cause of SBO in developed nations, a past history of surgery should always be sought.

Any type of abdominal wall hernia may cause bowel incarceration and subsequent obstruction, but the most common hernia types include groin (inguinal and femoral), umbilical and incisional ("ventral") hernias. Rare hernia types such as obturator and Spigelian hernias may also cause BO. However, they may not be as readily apparent on physical exam and as such often require cross-sectional imaging to diagnose. 'Internal hernia' refers to the passage of bowel through a peritoneal or mesenteric defect not associated with the abdominal wall proper, such as incarceration through Peterson's space following laparoscopic Roux-En-Y bariatric surgery.

Mechanical BO is contrasted with 'paralytic ileus' (small intestine) or colonic pseudo-obstruction (Ogilve's Syndrome) in which GI transit is impaired by diminished peristalsis in response to a systemic insult such as electrolyte abnormalities, infection (i.e., pneumonia) or abdominal surgery.[2] Distinguishing between mechanical and functional BO is important, as their management is very different.

Blockage of the GI tract by an obstructive mechanism results in the build-up of ingested elements and digestive secretions within the intestinal lumen proximal to the point of obstruction. This intraluminal fluid accumulation leads to distension of the bowel lumen, impairing absorption and paradoxically increasing secretion of water and electrolytes into the lumen, proximal to the point of blockage. This accumulation of fluid and ingested materials may decompress resulting in retrograde filling of the lumen with vomiting and further loss of water and electrolytes. Distension may also increase enteric wall tension which can impair local perfusion and respiratory function by decreasing lung volume due to elevation of the diaphragm.[2–3,8]

Acid–base imbalances may also occur. Prolonged vomiting may initially lead to metabolic alkalosis due to loss of acid secretions from the stomach as well as renin-angiotensin mediated effects on renal physiology ('contraction alkalosis'). Alternatively, if the patient is in shock due to hypovolemia or sepsis, then metabolic acidosis may be present due to global tissue hypoperfusion. Metabolic acidosis may also result from diminished bicarbonate absorption in the jejunum.[8]

Changes in the distribution of bacterial flora may also occur proximal to the level of the obstruction. In the unobstructed GI tract, the proximal small intestine contains minimal levels of bacteria (less than 10^4 organisms per milliliter) and those present are typically gram-positive aerobes (e.g., *Staphylococcus sp.*). In the colon, there are much higher levels (10^{11} organisms per mL) with a preponderance of anaerobes and gram-negative aerobes (e.g., *E. coli* and *Bacteroides*, respectively). The unobstructed terminal ileum usually functions as a transition zone, with low to moderate levels of colonic flora. It is thought that normal GI transit activity serves to maintain the stability of this distribution.[8] However, in the obstructed intestine this distribution changes with increasing levels of colonic-type bacteria proximal to the obstruction. The rise in bacteria levels also contributes to enteric distension, dehydration and worsening electrolyte abnormalities. Additionally, the combination of GI stasis, bacterial proliferation and potential intestinal wall compromise may result in translocation of intestinal flora in the systemic circulation, which will further contribute to the systemic inflammatory response syndrome.[3,8]

BO may be classified as (1) complicated/strangulated (with intestinal compromise or perforation); (2) simple/incarcerated (without compromise or perforation); (3) partial/incomplete (some liquid and gas can still pass site of obstruction); or (4) complete (collapsed distal bowel as point of obstruction impedes passage of all bowel contents). 'Closed loop' BO occurs when the bowel is obstructed at two separate locations (i.e., volvulus). The interceding portion of bowel then becomes a closed space in which proximal decompression is not possible. As a result, the affected intestinal loop's walls are subjected to exponentially increasing tension as the contents of the loop accumulate. Eventually, this process may result in impaired perfusion and/or mechanical failure of the bowel wall, resulting in perforation and release of contents into the peritoneal cavity.[2] Isolated cases of LBO may also behave as closed loop obstructions if the patient's ileocecal valve remains competent. As such, the cecum is at greatest risk of perforation as it has the largest diameter and thinnest wall of the colon.[8]

Non-mechanical BO, or paralytic ileus, is frequently seen in the ICU and in the postoperative patient. The main causes include electrolyte imbalances (i.e., hypokalemia, hyponatremia, hypomagnesemia), medications (i.e., narcotics), trauma (i.e., pelvic and spine fractures), infection/inflammation (i.e., pancreatitis, intra-abdominal sepsis), and various postoperative states (orthopaedic, cardiac, abdominal and retroperitoneal).

Finally, BO states can result in numerous nutritional deficiencies in addition to the loss of electrolytes and water (volume). This is often more evident with chronic, recurrent BO or when compounded by a postoperative ileus following surgical management of BO. Such deficiencies include both macronutrient (i.e., carbohydrate) and micronutrient (i.e., zinc, vitamin B12) losses which may mandate either replacement with parenteral nutritional support or oral supplementation upon BO resolution. The nutritional status of patients particularly when requiring surgery must be carefully assessed and preoperative parenteral nutrition may be necessary to optimize post-surgical healing and recovery.[2]

Diagnosis

The diagnosis and initial triage of BO is largely clinical. However, laboratory and imaging investigations are essential adjuncts especially in the ICU setting as they will help determine the cause of BO as well as delineate the severity of the physiologic derangements. Imaging (predominantly CT scan) will determine if the obstruction is (1) truly mechanical; (2) 'simple' or 'complicated'; (3) 'partial' or 'complete'; and (4) a closed loop.[2]

The classic features of BO include cramping, intermittent abdominal pain (colic), reduced or absent flatus and bowel movements (obstipation), abdominal bloating/distension, nausea, and vomiting.[1,8] Other pertinent elements in the patients history are time since the last flatus and/or bowel movement and extent of past surgical and medical history. The duration and frequency of vomiting may provide insight into how severe the patients resulting physiologic derangements may be. Patients with ileus usually have less pain, and when present it is often a constant dull discomfort from abdominal distension.

Pain that is described as more sharp and/or constant in nature is suggestive of underlying intestinal compromise and merits expedited investigation and management. Patients presenting early on in their obstructive course or with partial BO may still have feces and flatus downstream to the obstruction. Others with partial LBO may experience paradoxical 'overflow diarrhea' as the peristaltic function of the GI tract increases in an attempt to overcome the blockage which only allows liquid elements to pass (spurious diarrhea).

Physical examination for BO starts with an assessment of vital signs. Tachycardia and hypotension suggest hypovolemia from vomiting and bowel fluid sequestration. However, if profound and/or seen in combination with fever or marked abdominal findings, it may be due to intestinal ischemia infarction or impending perforation. Hypoxia in the setting of BO may be due to aspiration from vomiting or loss of lung volume due to elevation of the diaphragm from the distended abdomen and increased abdominal pressure. Decreased breath sounds over the lung bases suggest basilar atelectasis (or pneumonia) which can lead to shunt hypoxemia and respiratory alkalosis from the tachypnea.

Examination of the abdomen begins with visual assessment for abdominal distension and presence of masses in the groins or abdominal wall. Skin colour changes (erythema or ecchymosis) overlying hernias is a concerning factor for underlying bowel ischemia.

The abdomen is usually tympanitic to percussion. However, percussion tenderness in BO suggests peritonitis secondary to bowel ischemia, infarction, impending or frank perforation requiring urgent surgical intervention. Auscultation of bowel sounds is of minimal clinical utility given the poor sensitivity and specificity in distinguishing between ileus and SBO. Finally, a digital rectal examination is essential to evaluate the rectal vault for an obstructing lesion (i.e., rectal cancer) and to assess for the presence of stool or blood.

Laboratory investigations should be ordered for all patients presenting with BO. In hypovolemic patients, hemoglobin may be elevated due to hemoconcentration and serum creatinine may be elevated as result of decreased renal perfusion. A multitude of electrolyte abnormalities, in particular hypokalemia, hyponatremia and hypochloremia, may be seen depending on the stage of the BO. Mild leukocytosis usually results from the global stress state, with more profound leukocytosis associated with sepsis, intestinal compromise and peritonitis. Acidosis or alkalosis may be present depending on the predominant underlying process (early or late BO), and often a mixed picture is seen (i.e., contraction alkalosis followed by severe hypovolemia and anaerobic lactic acidosis).[1]

The acute abdominal X-ray series still has a role in the ICU. The supine and lateral decubitus abdominal views are used to assess for dilated bowel loops, air-fluid levels and free intra-peritoneal air. In the setting of complete BO, there will be a paucity of intraluminal gas distal to the point of obstruction, most reliably detected on X-ray in the rectum. Differentiating SBO from ileus on X-ray can be difficult. Patients with an ileus are more likely to have gas throughout the GI tract and tend to have more uniformly distended bowel loops with less profound air-fluid levels. Chest X-ray often reveals basilar atelectasis with diaphragmatic elevation and the lateral decubitus abdominal film or upright chest X-ray is a reliable method of demonstrating free intra-peritoneal air. However, the gold standard imaging for BO, especially in the ICU, is CT scan. It is typically performed with oral (or via NG) water-soluble contrast, IV contrast, as well as rectal contrast depending on the likelihood of LBO. Luminal contrast is used to determine the anatomic level (transition point) and degree of the obstruction, whereas IV contrast is used to assess the perfusion status of the involved viscus.

The absence of air distal to the transition point with profound proximal dilatation is indicative of a 'high-grade' BO (Fig. 1). These are more likely to require surgical decompression. Other high-grade features include proximal fecalization and free intra-peritoneal fluid. Findings suggestive of intestinal ischemia (non-enhanced bowel wall and/or pneumatosis intestinalis), perforation, closed-loop BO or non-ASBO such as malignant masses and internal hernia typically mandate urgent operative intervention.[9]

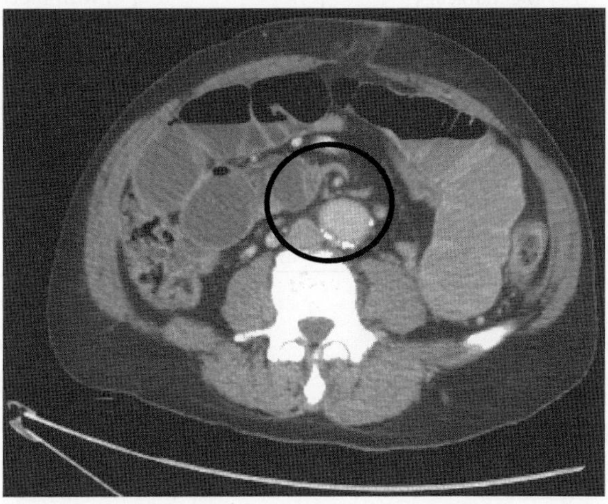

Fig. 1. High-grade adhesive small bowel obstruction on axial CT image.

Treatment

The management of patients with presumed BO should start with resuscitation occurring in parallel sequence with diagnostic work-up (Fig. 2). As in all unwell patients, a patent airway and adequate oxygenation/ventilation should be achieved early. Occasionally, tracheal intubation and mechanical ventilation may be necessary when there is increased work of breathing from the increased intra-abdominal pressure or when hypoxia does not respond to oxygen supplement alone. Patients presenting with signs of hypovolemia should be resuscitated with IV crystalloid fluid boluses after establishing IV access and this resuscitation should be directed by the patient's vital signs, repeated blood gas analysis and urine output.[1]In elderly patients with impaired cardiopulmonary reserve, fluid administration may require titrating with central hemodynamic monitoring (e.g., point of care ultrasound or central venous pressure). This is particularly important because the sequestrated third space volume cannot be measured in estimating fluid deficits. An NG tube should be placed with subsequent clinical or radiographic confirmation of placement, and connected to intermittent suction for proximal

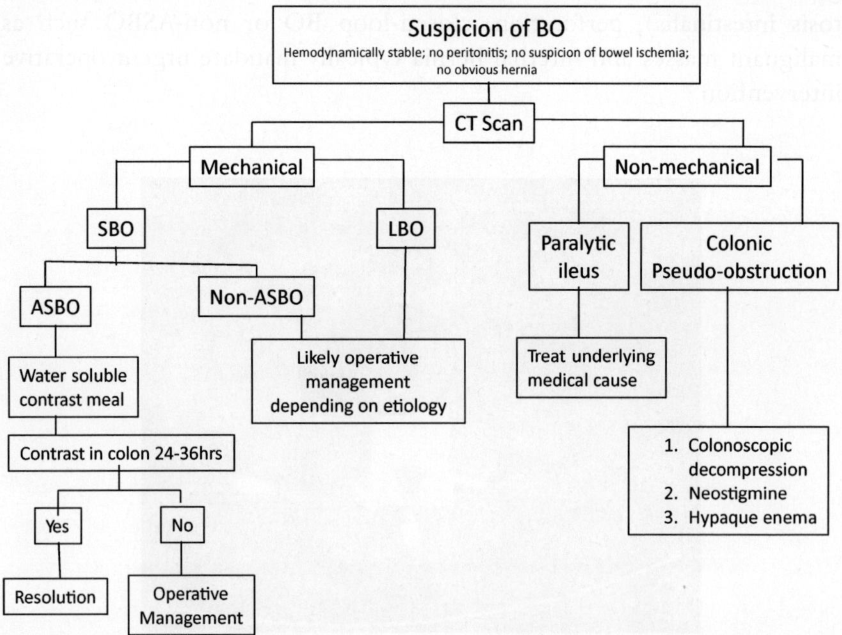

Fig. 2. Management of bowel obstruction in ICU.

decompression of the GI tract.[4] Patient comfort should be addressed with judicious administration of parenteral narcotics and anti-emetics. Routine use of antibiotics is not indicated. However, if the patient is septic, has an ileus secondary to an infection (i.e., UTI) or there are concerns of intestinal compromise, broad spectrum IV antibiotics should be administered.

Patients with peritonitis, intestinal ischemia, or confirmed mechanical LBO and non-ASBO etiologies require urgent surgery. Endoluminal stenting is an option for certain malignant BO (e.g., rectal cancer with diffuse metastatic disease). Patients presenting with BO due to external incarcerated hernia should undergo an attempt at reduction with adequate analgesia and/or sedation.[6] SBO secondary to acute Crohn's disease or radiation enteritis may respond to a trial of pulse glucocorticoids.

Patients with ileus should undergo a broad search for offending causes and they should be treated accordingly. Serial clinical examination and imaging is still very helpful to assess for intestinal ischemia which most often occurs in the caecum. Colonic pseudo-obstruction/Ogilve's Syndrome can be treated with colonoscopic decompression or Neostigmine. Hypaque enema can also be diagnostic and therapeutic in such cases. Although trials are still underway, prokinetic agents have not yet been shown to resolve ileus. However, early feeding and ambulation are important factors to help reduce postoperative ileus.

The majority (65–70%) of stable patients with presumed ASBO will resolve within 48–72 hours of hospital presentation with the nonoperative management. There are two well recognized guidelines on management of ASBO.[9,12] Although slightly different, both promote the use of CT scan as the imaging modality of choice and the use of water-soluble contrast meal performed within 48 hours of presentation. The presence of the contrast in the colon within 24 hours on repeat imaging is highly predictive of non-operative resolution, whereas a paucity of colonic contrast would suggest that surgical intervention is mandated. The value of administering luminal contrast extends beyond diagnostic benefit, as the osmotic effects also help to overcome simpler forms of ABSO.[9] There is now good evidence that delaying operative intervention beyond 72 hours for ASBO increases morbidity, mortality and length of stay. In patients requiring operative intervention for ASBO, there is strong evidence to support the use of initial laparoscopic exploration and attempts at adhesiolysis provided there is adequate surgical expertise and peritoneal domain for visualization. Caution should be exercised as the addition of pneumoperitoneum to facilitate laparoscopy may worsen respiratory and cardiac status.

Summary

BO is amongst the most common reasons for surgical in-patient admission. The diagnosis and assessment of BO is dependent on a thorough history and physical examination as well as laboratory and imaging adjuncts. All patients with BO are at risk of developing varying degrees of physiological disturbances which need to be considered and managed expeditiously. The potential causes of BO are variable and the methods for relieving obstruction are dependent on the underlying etiology as well as the clinical status of the patient and the level of concern regarding possible intestinal ischemia. All patients with BO should receive proximal GI decompression and resuscitation to euvolumia and, adequate urine output and normalization of pH and electrolytes. The majority of patients with adhesive SBO can be managed without surgery, whereas other causes of SBO and most forms of LBO will require procedural and/or operative intervention. While most of these patients do not require ICU treatment, specific situations may warrant care in the ICU.

Disclaimer

The authors do not have anything to disclose in regards to the content of this chapter.

References

1. Welch JP. Bowel obstruction: Differential diagnosis and clinical management. Philadelphia PA: WB Saunders Co; 1990: 3–27.
2. Soybel DI, Landman WB. Ileus and bowel obstruction. Greenfield's Surgery: Scientific Principles & Practice. 5th ed. Philadelphia PA, Lipincott Williams & Wilkins, 2011, 748–772.
3. Shields R. The absorption and secretion of fluid and electrolytes by the obstructed bowel. *Br J Surg* 1965; 52: 774–779.
4. Wangensteen OH, Paine JR. Treatment of acute intestinal obstruction by suction with a duodenal tube. *JAMA* 1933; 101: 1531–1539.
5. Ray NF *et al.* Abdominal adhesiolysis: Inpatient care and expenditures in the United States in 1994. *J Am Coll Surg* 1998; 186: 1–9.
6. Fevang BT *et al.* Delay in operative treatment among patients with small bowel obstruction. *Scand J Surg* 2003; 92(2): 131–137.
7. Miller G *et al.* Etiology of small bowel obstruction. *Am J Surg* 2000; 180: 33–36.

8. Ellis H. Intestinal obstruction. New York NY: Appleton-Century-Crofts; 1982; 1–68: 235–302.
9. Di Savero S *et al.* Bologna guidelines for diagnosis and management of adhesive small bowel obstruction (ASBO): 2013 update of the evidence-based guidelines from the world society of emergency surgery ASBO working group. *World J Emerg Surg* 2013; 8: 42.
10. Attard JP, MacLean AR. Adhesive bowel obstruction: Epidemiology, biology and prevention. *J Surg* 2005; 50(4): 291–300.
11. Angenete E *et al.* Effect of laparoscopy on the risk of small bowel obstruction: A population-based register study. *Arch Surg* 2012; 147(4): 359–365.
12. Maung AA, Johnson DC, Piper GL *et al.* Evaluation and management of small-bowel obstruction: An Eastern Association for the Surgery of Trauma practice management guideline. *J Trauma Acute Care Surg* 2012; 73: S362–S369

Chapter 27

Mesenteric Ischemia

John B. Kortbeek

Introduction

Mesenteric ischemia often presents as a sudden and catastrophic illness with a very high mortality rate despite medical and surgical therapy. Understanding the anatomy and pathophysiology provides the background for guiding diagnosis and management. The prevalence of mesenteric vascular disease as well as the clinical, laboratory, and radiologic features supporting prompt diagnosis will be presented. Evolving medical as well as open and endovascular surgical treatment will be reviewed.

Anatomy

The embryonic intestines grow more quickly than the body of the fetus. As a result they protrude through the umbilical ring. They are supplied primarily by the Vitelline artery, which will become the superior mesenteric artery (SMA). After the 6th week the intestines rotate counterclockwise 90° and the cranial limb, the future small intestine now lies to the right side. It elongates and forms a number of loops. The shorter left side caudal limb will become the large intestine. After 10 weeks the intestines return to the abdominal cavity and undergo a further counterclockwise rotation of 180°. The small intestine returns first followed by the large intestine which now forms its characteristic loop, lying anterior to the SMA.

The small intestine and right colon are supplied by the SMA. The celiac trunk supplies the duodenum as well as some potential collateral supply at the ligament of Treitz through the pancreatico-duodenal artery (via the right hepatic artery). The inferior mesenteric artery supplies the left colon. There is variable collateral supply to the transverse colon through the marginal artery of Drummond. The terminal branch of the inferior mesenteric artery supplies the proximal rectum. Distally the rectum is supplied by the inferior and middle rectal arteries, which originate from the Internal Iliac. Collateral supply between the superior and inferior rectal arteries is usually good. Both the superior and inferior mesenteric arteries fan out into arcades. Their terminal branches are the vasa recta. The mesenteric branches are short, the anti-mesenteric branches are long and as a result the anti-mesenteric side has a more tenuous blood supply.

The venous drainage parallels the arterial anatomy. The inferior mesenteric artery drains into the distal splenic artery. The superior mesenteric vein passes posterior to the head of the pancreas where it joins the splenic vein to form the portal vein. The only jejunal, ileal, and colonic direct venous drainage to the vena cava is via collaterals distally through the middle and inferior rectal veins.

The anatomy of the arterial and venous systems dictates the distribution of ischemia with arterial or venous disorders. The abrupt angled origin of the celiac artery protects it from most embolic events. Emboli are more likely to pass through the SMA, which, has a large orifice and has a wide proximal angle of takeoff from its origin at the aorta. A smaller orifice protects the inferior mesenteric artery and the left colon benefits from collateral supply via the inferior and middle rectal arteries. The venous drainage via the portal system results in thrombosis associated with diseases that affect hepatic drainage or predispose to hepatic and splenic vein thrombosis.

The development of atherosclerotic disease may promote development of collateral supply to the proximal small bowel and transverse colon via the celiac artery and its branches. More often however, collateral supply from the inferior rectal arteries as well as through the marginal artery of Drummond is compromised. The watershed area at the Arc of Riolan (splenic flexure) is particularly at risk.[1]

Epidemiology

Mesenteric ischemia is frequently encountered by busy emergency general, colorectal and vascular surgical services as well as critical care practitioners. Atherosclerosis increases with age and is prevalent in over 20% of patients aged 65 and greater. The majority of patients with atherosclerosis involving the mesenteric arteries are asymptomatic. A population study in Malmo, Sweden is illustrative. Over a 12-year period the hospital autopsy rate was over 80%. The incidence of mesenteric ischemia at surgery or autopsy was 12.9/100,000 person years. Two thirds had an acute SMA occlusion, nearly 1/3 were divided equally between mesenteric vein thrombosis and non-occlusive ischemia. The disease was distributed equally between men and women.[2]

In cases of SMA occlusion, thrombosis was four times as common as embolic occlusion. The thrombi were both more proximal and more extensive resulting in greater intestinal necrosis. Arterial emboli were frequently multiple and could be suggested by the presence of other solid organ infarcts on CT, at surgery or on autopsy.

Non-occlusive ischemia was associated with congestive heart failure, dysrhythmias and a history of recent surgery. These patients had a terrible prognosis reflecting their co-existent disease. Mesenteric thrombosis was associated with thrombophilia and thromboembolic disease.

Another large series from Leipzig, Germany summarized the characteristics of thrombotic intestinal ischemia (embolic and thrombotic) over a 6-year period. Arterial emboli, arterial thrombosis and venous thrombosis each were responsible for a third of the patient presentations. The overall mortality was 60%.[3]

Table 1 Demographics data and clinical presentations of patients

	Embolism, *n*=20 [*n* (%)]	Arterial thrombosis, *n*=19 [*n* (%)]	Venous thrombosis, *n*=21 [*n* (%)]	Total, *n*=60 [*n* (%)]
Sex				
Male	8 (40)	5 (26.3)	10 (47.6)	23 (38.3)
Female	12 (60)	14 (73.7)	11 (52.4)	37 (61.7)
Age				
Median	74	74	65	73
Range	61–96	47–91	43–85	43–96
ASA-classification				
Grade 2+3	8 (40)	9 (47.4)	12 (57.1)	29 (48.3)
Grade 4+5	12 (60)	10 (52.6)	9 (42.9)	31 (51.7)
Clinical presentation				
Pain	20 (100)	19 (100)	21 (100)	60 (100)
Nausea	19 (95)	18 (94.7)	19 (90.5)	56 (93.3)
Vomiting	17 (85)	15 (78.9)	16 (76.2)	48 (80)
Bloody diarrhea	8 (40)	12 (63.2)	9 (42.9)	29 (48.3)

Values in parentheses are percentages.

Fig. 1. Demographic and clinical features.

Source: Table 1, Demographics, mesenteric ischemia.[3]

Table 2 Laboratory test results at initial presentation

	Embolism (*n*=20)	Arterial thrombosis (*n*=19)	Venous thrombosis (*n*=21)
Lactate (mmol/l)[a]	6.57 ± 0.96	8.35 ± 1.39	4.46 ± 1.18
CRP (mg/l)	173.51 ± 28.90	121.31 ± 23.97	129.10 ± 14.20
WBC (gpt/l)	18.26 ± 1.36	18.16 ± 2.31	18.30 ± 1.90
Creatinine (umol/l)	87.60 ± 13.46	114.68 ± 32.06	108.52 ± 15.28
BUN (mmol/l)	9.40 ± 1.71	9.99 ± 1.60	11.70 ± 2.39

Values represent mean ± SEM.
CRP C-reactive protein, *WBC* white blood cell count, *BUN* blood urea nitrogen
[a]Values of lactate were available for 46 patients.

Fig. 2. Laboratory findings.
Source: Table 2, Demographics, mesenteric ischemia.[3]

Table 3 Associated conditions and risk factors found in patients with AII

	Embolism, *n*=20 (33.3)	Arterial thrombosis, *n*=19 (31.7)	Venous thrombosis, *n*=21 (35.0)	Total, 60 (100)
Associated conditions				
Cardiac disease	17 (85)	15 (78.9)	13 (61.9)	45 (75)
Atrial fibrillation	15 (75)	8 (42.1)	11 (52.4)	34 (56.7)
Atherosclerosis	18 (90)	17 (89.4)	13 (61.9)	48 (80)
Thromboembolic disorders	1 (5)	1 (5.2)	7 (33.3)*	9 (15)
Cerebrovascular disorders	3 (15)	9 (47.4)	3 (14.3)	15 (25)
History of myocardial infarction	4 (40)	3 (15.8)	1 (4.8)	8 (13.3)
History of thromboembolism	2 (20)	4 (21.1)	7 (33.3)	13 (21.7)
Chronic renal insufficiency	5 (25)	8 (42.1)	10 (47.6)	23 (38.3)
Risk factors				
Diabetes mellitus	12 (60)	9 (47.4)	7 (33.3)	28 (46.7)
Hypertension	17 (85)	13 (68.4)	14 (66.7)	44 (73.3)
Peptic ulcer disease	2 (10)	3 (15.8)	1 (4.8)	6 (10)
Chronic obstructive pulmonary disease	2 (10)	1 (5.3)	7 (33.3)****	10 (16.7)
Smoking	10 (50)	14 (73.7)***	6 (28.6)	30 (50)
Malignancy	1 (5)	4 (21.1)	5 (23.8)	10 (16.7)
Digitalis use	10 (50)	5 (26.3)	6 (28.6)	21 (35)
Overweight (BMI ≥25)	8 (40)	8 (42.1)	2 (9.5)**	16 (26.7)

Values in parentheses are percentages.
BMI Body mass index (kg/m^2)
*p=0.014 compared to embolism and arterial thrombosis
**p=0.043 compared to embolism and arterial thrombosis
***p=0.017 compared to embolism and venous thrombosis
****p=0.042 compared to embolism and arterial thrombosis

Fig. 3. Associated conditions and risk factors.
Source: Table 3, Demographics, mesenteric ischemia.[3]

Classification and Pathophysiology

Mesenteric Ischemia includes four distinct presentations:
Arterial emboli
Arterial thrombosis
Venous thrombosis
Non-occlusive mesenteric ischemia (acute and chronic)

The Intestines receive > 20% of cardiac output rising to > 30% in the postprandial state. Terminal arterioles and venules provide a rich supply to the mucosa and submucosa layers. The villi are supplied by parallel arterioles and venules with multiple connections providing a countercurrent loop. The terminal villous is metabolically active and at greatest risk of hypoxia and cell injury in states of impaired circulation or hypoxemia. Regardless of the etiology of mesenteric ischemia, (vessel occlusion, vasoconstriction or venous obstruction and thrombosis), the final common pathway involves cellular hypoxia. Anaerobic metabolism, acidosis, cell wall and endothelial permeability ensue. Leukocyte adhesion and platelet aggregation occur. Cytokines are released. Interstitial edema and progressive vascular occlusion occur. Intestinal permeability and bacterial translocation follow. Ischemia leads to infarction and septic shock. Multi-organ system failure and death may follow. The progressions from ischemia to infarction and septic shock may occur within 6–12 hours. In cases of SMA thrombosis the presentation may be subacute and occur over 24–72 hours due the presence of established collaterals.[4]

Arterial emboli are associated with cardiac dysrhythmias, most commonly atrial fibrillation, as well as ventricular thrombi and valvular heart disease. Arterial thrombosis is associated with advanced atherosclerosis and associated risk factors including diabetes, hypertension and smoking history. Chronic non-occlusive mesenteric ischemia is also seen in this patient population.

Mesenteric thrombosis is most commonly seen in hyper-thrombotic states with inherited or acquired thrombophilias. Pancreatitis and hepatic diseases resulting in splenic and portal vein thrombosis are also commonly seen in mesenteric thrombosis.

Acute non-occlusive ischemia is associated with any condition that results in compromised blood flow to the intestines, particularly shock and hypoxic respiratory failure. Surgery, which compromises or temporarily occludes the arterial or venous circulations, may also result in mesenteric ischemia or infarction. In younger patients midgut volvulus can result in small bowel ischemia and infarction.

Diagnosis

Acute mesenteric ischemia should be suspected in any patient presenting with severe abdominal pain. Typically the pain is central and diffuse and may be accompanied by nausea, vomiting, diarrhea, and melena or hematochezia. None of these features are constant. The patients are frequently elderly and may be immuno-compromised, so fever is not constant and systemic inflammatory response (SIRS) criteria may be muted. Intestinal ischemia should be suspected in patients who present with SIRS or septic shock.

Laboratory studies may reveal a leukocytosis, a left shift (bandemia) and hemo-concentration. C-reactive Protein may be elevated. In advanced stages an elevated lactate, base deficit and metabolic acidosis will be present.

Physical examination may reveal tenderness and abdominal distention. Peritonitis with guarding and rebound are late findings that suggest infarction and/or perforation.

Plain images including three views of the abdomen may demonstrate an ileus with thickened loops of small bowel. Air visible in the portal venous system is virtually pathognomonic. The three views may identify the presence of a mechanical obstruction. Free air is a very late sign indicating progression of infarction to perforation. Ultrasound is usually non-diagnostic and may be challenging once dilated air filled loops of bowel are present.[5] CT has become the gold standard for diagnosis. Common CT findings are bowel wall thickening (>3mm) mesenteric haziness and visible thrombus (SMV).

CT criteria most predictive of transmural ischemia are[6]:

Homogeneous enhancement
Decreased enhancement
Indistinct outer margins
Ascites
Maximal luminal diameter >20mm
Pneumatosis intestinalis
Extraluminal air
Portal venous air
Splenic infarcts

Criteria predictive of non-transmural infarction are:

Layered enhancement
Maximal luminal diameter <10mm

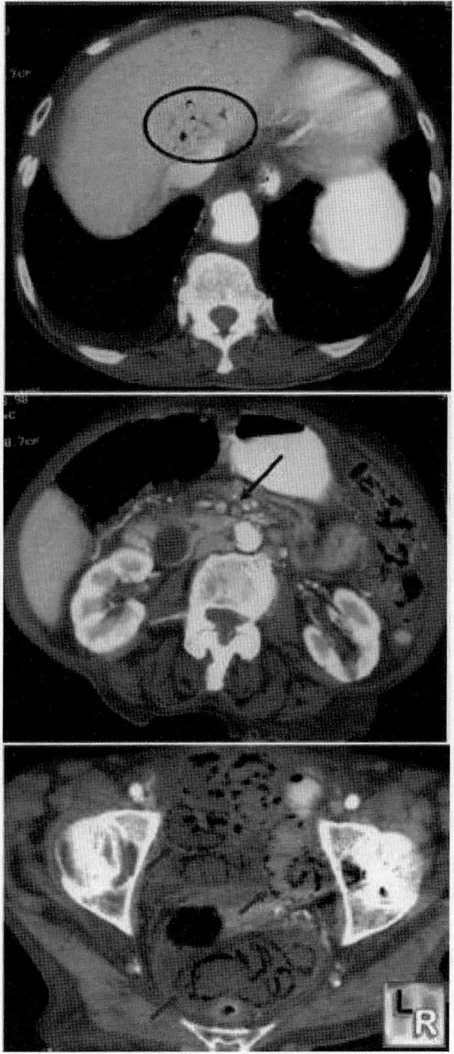

Fig. 4. CT findings.

Source: CT findings in mesenteric ischemia.[5]

Note: Computed tomography angiography (CTA) demonstrating hepatic venous air (top, blue circle). The superior mesenteric artery (SMA) is occluded (middle image, blue arrow). There is extensive colonic pneumatosis and atscites, (bottom image, red arrows). Available at: http://www.learningradiology.com/notes/ginotes/mesentericischemiapage.htm.

In patients with non-transmural infarction (or indeterminate findings) CT angiography will define the vascular anatomy and areas of thrombosis and obstruction and has replaced celiac and SMA angiography. This is critical in guiding efforts at revascularization.

Chronic mesenteric ischemia presents in patients who typically have the associated risk factors or an established diagnosis of atherosclerosis. They typically present with episodic abdominal pain, which is often postprandial. They are usually thin and may appear malnourished. The vast majority have a smoking history. High resolution Contrast CT angiography has become the gold standard for diagnosis.

Management

Diagnosis of acute mesenteric ischemia should prompt emergency open or endovascular surgery (or both). The mortality for these conditions remains very high even with prompt diagnosis and management. Oxygen and resuscitation with crystalloids as well as prompt broad-spectrum antibiotics should be administered and the patient prepared for the operating room. Central venous access, monitoring and restoration of perfusion pressure with pressors may be required. Intubation and mechanical ventilation are required for patients presenting in septic shock or with severely reduced level of consciousness.[7]

During surgery the bowel should be identified and areas of irreversible necrosis resected. In patients with reversible or non-transmural ischemia revascularization offers the ability to salvage and preserve intestinal function and reduce mortality. Traditional operative techniques have relied on supraceliac aorta-mesenteric bypass or iliac-mesenteric bypass. In the event of a simple arterial embolus the SMA can be approached at the base of the transverse mesocolon through a transverse arteriotomy. Systemic heparinization and embolectomy with a 4Fr (or smaller) Fogerty catheter is performed.[8]

If a bypass is performed then the duodenum is typical mobilized and the peritoneum opened lateral to the mesentery, exposing the proximal SMA, the aorta and the iliac artery. A vein, or 6–8 mm Dacron graft is used for the bypass depending on the degree of fecal contamination. The anatomic location of the bypass is dependent on patient factors but typically an Iliac — SMA graft has the most advantageous lie and avoids aortic cross clamping and supra-celiac dissection.

More recent advances in endovascular technology and stents have changed the interventions for SMA occlusion. Pure endovascular techniques have limited applicability when acute mesenteric ischemia occurs, as bowel viability cannot be established. However, hybrid approaches are now being

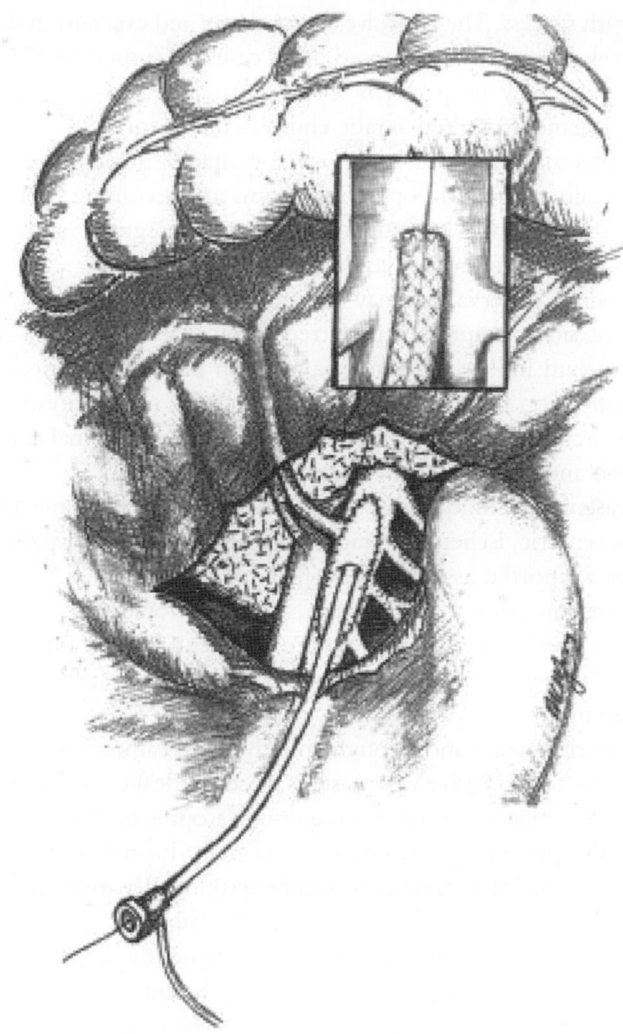

Fig. 5. Retrograde open mesenteric endovascular stent.

Source: Retrograde open mesenteric stent.[5]

Note: Retrograde open mesenteric stent schematic with long 6Fr sheath placement through the patched superior mesenteric artery (SMA). The inset illustrates a stent deployed in the proximal SMA.

published with success. These involve a laparotomy and exposure and inspection of the bowel. The SMA is exposed as in cases of suspected SMA emboli. Endarterectomy may be performed and a patch graft is placed providing access for placement of a retrograde endovascular stent.

Restenosis may occur but can now be managed through primary endovascular techniques. Hybrid operating rooms are becoming more prevalent and offer the potential of supporting both antegrade and retrograde approaches and techniques as required.[9]

A period of observation may be required to confirm bowel viability. Erring on the side of caution is preferred. Temporary abdominal closure has facilitated second look laparotomies and often provides the necessary window of observation to maximize preservation of as much intestine as possible. It also circumvents the immediate risk of intra-abdominal compartment hypertension and abdominal compartment syndrome.[5,10]

Endovascular techniques are also becoming the first line therapy for chronic mesenteric ischemia. Traditional open surgical bypass for these patients has a reported associated mortality of 5–20%.[11,12]

Administration of systemic heparin, ASA and clopidrogel or similar antiplatelet agents will be determined by the intervention (endarterectomy, balloon angioplasty or endovascular stenting) weighed against the immediate risk of bleeding.

Intra-arterial papaverine through an indwelling catheter has been used in isolated cases when extensive vasospasm is present. Ideally these patients would be hemodynamically stable and not requiring vasopressors for septic shock.[13]

In cases of mesenteric or portal-splenic vein thrombosis without transmural ischemia the initial treatment will be systemic heparinization and close observation. Experience with intravenous thrombolysis is limited and the co-existent risk of partial intestinal ischemia frequently precludes its use.[14,15]

Use of retrograde endovascular hybrid techniques has been associated with impressively low mortality rates of 20% in selected patients. This offers significant promise in a disease with historic mortality rates of 60–90%.

Summary

Mesenteric ischemia may follow embolism, thrombosis or result from conditions associated with diminished blood pressure, flow and oxygen delivery. Bowel ischemia continues to result in very high mortality rates however the advent of high resolution CT and CT angiography has facilitated both diagnosis and preoperative mapping of the vascular anatomy. The development of standardized resuscitation for patients with severe sepsis or SIRS has increased survival or patients with septic shock. The advent of hybrid operative and endovascular interventions has provided new options and improved the care and outcomes for patients with mesenteric ischemia.

References

1. Debus ES, Müller-Hülsbeck S, Kölbel T, Larena-Avellaneda A. Intestinal ischemia. *Int J Color Dis* 2011; 26(9):1087–1097. Available at http://www.ncbi.nlm.nih.gov/pubmed/21541663.
2. Acosta S. Epidemiology of mesenteric vascular disease: clinical implications. *Semin Vasc Surg* (Elsevier Inc.) 2010; 23(1): 4–8. Available at http://www.ncbi.nlm.nih.gov/pubmed/20298944 (accessed on 18 December 2014).
3. Kassahun WT, Schulz T, Richter O, Hauss J. Unchanged high mortality rates from acute occlusive intestinal ischemia: Six year review. *Langenbecks Arch Surg* 2008; 393(2):163–171. Available at http://www.ncbi.nlm.nih.gov/pubmed/18172675 (accessed on 18 December 2014).
4. Vollmar B, Menger MD. Intestinal ischemia/reperfusion: Microcirculatory pathology and functional consequences. *Langenbecks Arch Surg* 2011; 396(1):13–29. Available at http://www.ncbi.nlm.nih.gov/pubmed/21088974 (accessed on 18 December 2014).
5. Wyers MC. Acute mesenteric ischemia: diagnostic approach and surgical treatment. *Semin Vasc Surg* (Elsevier Inc.) 2010; 23(1): 9–20. Available at http://www.ncbi.nlm.nih.gov/pubmed/20298945 (accessed on 18 December 2014).
6. Lee SS, Ha HK, Park SH, Choi EK, Kim AY, Kim JC *et al.* Usefulness of computed tomography in differentiating transmural infarction from nontransmural ischemia of the small intestine in patients with acute mesenteric venous thrombosis. *J Comput Assist Tomogr* 2008; 32(5): 730–737. Available at http://www.ncbi.nlm.nih.gov/pubmed/18830102.
7. Renner P, Kienle K, Dahlke MH, Heiss P, Pfister K, Stroszczynski C *et al.* Intestinal ischemia: Current treatment concepts. *Langenbecks Arch Surg* 2011; 396(1): 3–11. Available at http://www.ncbi.nlm.nih.gov/pubmed/21072535 (accessed on 4 December 2014).
8. Endean ED, Barnes SL, Kwolek CJ, Minion DJ, Schwarcz TH, Mentzer RM. Surgical management of thrombotic acute intestinal ischemia. *Ann Surg* 2001; 233(6): 801–808. Available at http://content.wkhealth.com/linkback/openurl?sid=WKPTLP:landingpage&an=00000658-200106000-00010.
9. Arthurs ZM, Titus J, Bannazadeh M, Eagleton MJ, Srivastava S, Sarac TP *et al.* A comparison of endovascular revascularization with traditional therapy for the treatment of acute mesenteric ischemia. *J Vasc Surg* (Elsevier Inc.) 2011; 53(3): 698–704; discussion 704–705. Available at http://www.ncbi.nlm.nih.gov/pubmed/21236616 (accessed on 18 December 2014).

10. Resch TA, Acosta S, Sonesson B. Endovascular techniques in acute arterial mesenteric ischemia. *Semin Vasc Surg* (Elsevier Inc.) 2010; 23(1): 29–35. Available at http://www.ncbi.nlm.nih.gov/pubmed/20298947 (accessed on 18 December 2014).
11. Chandra A, Quinones-Baldrich WJ. Chronic mesenteric ischemia: How to select patients for invasive treatment. *Semin Vasc Surg* (Elsevier Inc.) 2010; 23(1): 21–28. Available at http://www.ncbi.nlm.nih.gov/pubmed/20298946 (accessed on 18 December 2014).
12. Schoch DM, LeSar CJ, Joels CS, Erdoes LS, Sprouse LR, Fugate MW *et al.* Management of chronic mesenteric vascular insufficiency: an endovascular approach. *J Am Coll Surg* (Elsevier Inc.) 2011; 212(4): 668–675; discussion 675–677. Available at http://www.ncbi.nlm.nih.gov/pubmed/21463809 (accessed on 18 December 2014).
13. Björck M, Wanhainen A. Nonocclusive mesenteric hypoperfusion syndromes: Recognition and treatment. *Semin Vasc Surg* (Elsevier Inc.) 2010; 23(1): 54–64. Available at http://www.ncbi.nlm.nih.gov/pubmed/20298950 (accessed on 18 December 2014).
14. Acosta S, Ogren M, Sternby N-H, Bergqvist D, Björck M. Mesenteric venous thrombosis with transmural intestinal infarction: a population-based study. *J Vasc Surg* 2005; 41(1): 59–63. Available at http://www.ncbi.nlm.nih.gov/pubmed/15696045 (accessed on 18 December 2014).
15. Singal AK, Kamath PS, Tefferi A. Mesenteric venous thrombosis. *Mayo Clin Proc* (Mayo Foundation for Medical Education and Research) 2013; 88(3): 285–294. Available at http://www.ncbi.nlm.nih.gov/pubmed/23489453 (accessed on 18 December 2014).

Chapter 28

Upper GI Hemorrhage

Brad S. Moffat, Sarah Knowles and Neil G. Parry

Overview

Gastrointestinal (GI) bleeding can be a very challenging problem in the critically ill patient. Unlike many other sources of bleeding, the GI tract source is not readily compressible. It is not surprising, therefore, that patients who present in hemorrhagic shock or require ICU admission from upper GI bleeding have a mortality rate of up to 30%.[1,2]

GI bleeding is a unique issue in the ICU patient because it can not only be the primary reason for ICU admission, but it can also present as a common complication in critically ill patients. This chapter will discuss both the patient who presents with massive upper GI hemorrhage requiring ICU admission, as well as the patient already admitted to ICU who develops an acute upper GI bleed as a complication of their stay. While the pathogenesis differs, the management is essentially the same. In this chapter, special aspects of Upper GI hemorrhage are presented to enhance the intensivist's capability in managing these cases.

Introduction

GI bleeding is classified by the anatomic source of hemorrhage. Upper GI bleeding refers to a source in the foregut, proximal to the ligament of Treitz. The three main structures in the foregut are the esophagus, stomach, and duodenum; Each having its own blood supply and causes for bleeding.

Bleeding from the upper GI tract can present along a spectrum from very slow, intermittent bleeding with mild anemia, to brisk life-threatening exsanguination. Most are managed medically or endoscopically by gastroenterology and/or general surgery. A small minority will present with massive bleeding requiring ICU admission.

Patients with hemodynamic derangements secondary to GI bleeding should be admitted to the ICU for close monitoring and aggressive resuscitation. Early involvement of a surgeon and a gastroenterologist is mandatory.

Epidemiology

The incidence of GI bleeding requiring hospitalization, in the USA, is approximately 170 cases per 100,000 adults per year and accounts for 1–2% of all acute admissions.[3] An upper GI source is the cause in 80% of cases.[2] The majority of hospitalized GI bleeds will stop spontaneously or return to normal after minimal transfusion. About 15% of cases will continue to bleed despite initial resuscitative measures and may require admission to ICU.[4]

Admission to the ICU is also an independent risk factor for developing an upper GI bleed. Various factors contribute to a process known as stress ulceration in the stomach. Since the advent of acid suppression therapy, the overall risk of upper GI bleeding secondary to stress ulcers is relatively low at about 1 in 1,000. However, ventilation for greater than 48 hours with concomitant coagulopathy increases that risk to 3%, even with acid suppression therapy.[5,6]

Risk Factors

Several factors have been associated with increased risk of upper GI bleeding and certain risk factors predispose specific sites to bleeding. The most pervasive risk factor in the general population is the use of non-steroidal anti-inflammatory medications. They inhibit endogenous prostaglandins, primarily in the stomach, which predispose the gastric mucosa to acid injury and consequent ulceration and bleeding. The risk increases substantially with prolonged usage and at high doses.

Helicobacter pylori infection is another common risk factor. *H. pylori* infection significantly increases the risk for ulceration thereby increasing the risk of associated bleeding as compared to the non-infected population. This tends to result in duodenal ulceration but can also affect the distal stomach (antrum).

Several scoring systems have been devised to predict the risk of rebleeding following intervention and the subsequent associated mortality. They have also been used to predict high risk patients who likely need ICU admission. The AIMS65 score uses five criteria (albumin, INR, mental status, hypotension, age > 65) to estimate mortality. This scoring system precedes the age of ubiquitous endoscopy and has been well validated.[7] If all five risk factors are present, the mortality rate is 25%. More recent scoring systems, such as Rockall and Blatchford incorporate biochemistry, comorbidities, and endoscopic findings to predict mortality and rebleed rates.[8]

A less common but important risk factor for upper GI bleeding is gastroesophageal varices. They tend to form around the gastroesophageal junction and when they bleed, they can be very difficult to control. Variceal bleeding occurs in 25–40% of patients with cirrhosis.[2] The variceal location, size, and severity of liver disease are all predictors of bleeding risk.

Pathophysiology

Upper GI bleeding emanates from the foregut which consists of the esophagus, stomach, and duodenum. Each of these structures has unique physiology which can contribute to different patterns of bleeding (Table 1).

Table 1. Common causes of upper gastrointestinal bleeding.

Esophagus	Esophageal varices Reflux esophagitis Infectious (fungal, viral) Neoplasms
Stomach	Peptic ulcer disease Gastroesophageal varices Mallory-Weiss tear Stress gastritis Portal gastropathy Gastric antral vascular ectasia Dieulafoy ulcer Arteriovenous malformation Neoplasms
Duodenum	Peptic ulcer disease Arteriovenous malformation Neoplasms Dieulafoy ulcer Aortoduodenal fistula Diverticula
Hepatobiliary/pancreatic	Hemobilia Pancreatitis-induced pseudoaneurysm

Esophagus

The most common source of major bleeding in the esophagus is variceal.[2] Esophageal varices form at the lower end of the esophagus, typically within 5–10 centimeters of the gastro esophageal junction. While they can develop throughout the GI tract, they are most prone to bleeding in the esophagus due to their close proximity to the mucosal surface and repeated minor trauma (food boluses and acid reflux). Less common causes of esophageal bleeding include: esophageal tears (Mallory–Weiss tears), mucosal bleeding from acid reflux and neoplasms.

Stomach

The most common cause of bleeding in the stomach is peptic ulcer disease.[9] A peptic ulcer forms when the normal mucosal physiology is disrupted and acid in the stomach is allowed to penetrate into the submucosal and muscular layers resulting in an ulcer. Peptic ulcers in the duodenum form more readily as it lacks the normal defenses of the stomach. However, peptic ulcers that form in the stomach are more prone to bleeding so the rates of bleeding from each are about equal accounting for up to 40% of all upper GI bleeding.[2]

NSAIDs inhibit prostaglandins, which play a key role in mucous secretion, and thus chronic NSAID use disrupts the normal protective layer of the stomach which predisposes to peptic ulceration.

Any insult which causes inflammation (e.g., *H. Pylori*) of the stomach can lead to peptic ulceration. *H. pylori* infection is implicated in 60% of gastric peptic ulcers.[2] *H. pylori* colonize the mucosa below the mucous layer and lead to chronic inflammation and gastric ulceration. The chronic inflammation also leads to increased production of gastrin which also increases acid production. Other causes of bleeding from the stomach include: arterial or venous malformations (Dieulefoy lesion, gastric varices, gastric antral vascular ectasia) and neoplasms.

Duodenum

Like the stomach, the most common cause of bleeding in the duodenum is from peptic ulceration. The mucosa of the duodenum is more susceptible to acid injury than the stomach. Conditions which increase the acid load in the duodenum, such as chronic gastritis or *H. pylori* infection can easily lead to ulceration. *H. pylori* is responsible for approximately 90% of duodenal ulcers.

Due to its fixed location in the retroperitoneum, ulcers in the duodenum are at higher risk for eroding directly into surrounding blood vessels, most commonly, the gastroduodenal artery. Bleeding from this artery can be brisk and result in life threatening hemorrhage. Other causes of bleeding from the duodenum include: biliary or pancreatic sources (hemobilia, hemosuccus pancreaticus), aortoenteric fistula (a complication of aortic aneurysm repair) or neoplasms.

Stress ulceration

Stress ulceration is a unique entity and is considered separately from peptic ulcer disease. It is thought to be primarily the consequence of a low flow state to the stomach mucosa and is caused by an imbalance between increased acid production and impaired mucosal protection in the setting of reduced gastric blood flow, mucosal ischemia and reperfusion injury.

The systemic inflammatory response exhibited by critically ill patients appears to increase acid production and impair mucous secretion in the stomach. This was first observed in the 1970's with specific patterns of stress ulcer formation among head injured (Cushing's ulcers) and burn patients (Curling's ulcers). The stomach lining also appears to be susceptible to mucosal ischemia during shock states and exhibits early mottling and microcirculatory insufficiency which further predisposes it to acid damage.

Acid suppression therapy is recommended for all patients admitted to the ICU and typically consists of H2 blockers or proton pump inhibitors. This gut prophylaxis has resulted in a dramatic decrease in stress ulcer complications, principally bleeding. Two major risk factors have repeatedly been shown to increase the risk of stress ulceration and bleeding in the ICU patient: Prolonged mechanical ventilation, and coagulopathy (Table 2). Patients with these risk factors should be closely monitored for signs of upper GI hemorrhage.

Clinical Presentation

The majority of patients presenting to hospital with GI bleeding can be managed on the ward. These patients may only exhibit clinical symptoms of anemia or overt signs of GI bleeding such as melena, blood per rectum, or hematemesis.

Table 2. Risk factors for stress ulcer bleeding.[5,6]

Risk Factor	Odds Ratio/Relative Risk of Bleeding
Respiratory Failure (Mechanical Ventilation > 48 hours)	OR = 15.6 ($P < 0.001$)
Coagulopathy	OR = 4.3 ($P < 0.001$)
Renal Failure	RR = 1.16 ($P = 0.023$)
Hypotension	3.7 ++
Sepsis	2.0 ++
Hepatic Failure	1.6 ++
Enteral Nutrition **	RR = 0.30 ($P = 0.004$)
Stress Ulcer Prophylaxis with Ranitidine **	RR = 0.39 ($P = 0.024$)

** Protective against stress ulcers.

++ Not statistically significant with multivariable regression.

Upper and lower GI bleeding can usually be distinguished based on clinical history. Blood in emesis is indicative of a bleeding source proximal to the ligament of Treitz. It is typically a dark red or black color which appears as dense flecks in the vomitus ("coffee ground emesis"). Blood which has time to sit in the stomach and oxidize usually suggests that the bleeding rate is slower. Frank red blood in the emesis is referred to as hematemesis and can occur if the stomach is filling rapidly with blood.

Melena stool is fairly specific to an upper GI source of hemorrhage. However, up to 10% of melena can be traced to the small bowel or right colon.[2] Lower GI bleeding from the hindgut almost always presents as bright red blood per rectum; However, a rapid upper GI bleed can present with bright red blood per rectum as well.

A nasogastric (NG) tube is a helpful adjunct in upper GI bleeding. For a patient with excessive vomiting, an NG tube can also reduce the risk of aspiration. If melena is the only clinical symptom and there is question about an upper or lower source, frank blood or coffee ground material from an NG tube is diagnostic of an upper GI source. Gastric decompression is mandatory in the unstable or ventilated patient.

Hemoglobin and hematocrit are part of the standard bloodwork which should be obtained for the bleeding patient. Acute GI bleeding typically presents as a normocytic anemia with a normal hematocrit. A normal hemoglobin does not rule out bleeding and in fact can be an ominous sign with rapid acute blood loss. Blood in the GI tract is digested and reabsorbed resulting in increased blood urea nitrogen levels. Coagulation indices including INR, PTT, platelets, and fibrinogen should be assessed and corrected, especially in variceal bleeding where liver dysfunction often results in hematologic and clotting derangements.

Patients with severe massive upper GI bleeding can present in hemorrhagic shock. "Massive" upper GI bleeding is typically defined as bleeding that requires greater than six units of red blood cells in a 24 hour period or, the more clinically relevant, bleeding to the extent of hemodynamic instability. They may be also show signs of end-organ dysfunction including altered mental status, oliguria, cardiac abnormalities, and skin mottling. Any patient presenting in shock from a presumed upper GI source requires urgent transfer to the ICU and early, aggressive resuscitation and therapy with involvement of the surgeon.

Initial Resuscitation

The initial resuscitation of patients presenting to the ICU with upper GI bleeding must focus on attempts to rapidly restore blood volume and provide supportive care as the resources for definitive management are mobilized (Fig. 1). In patients with massive upper GI bleeding, endotracheal intubation may be required to prevent airway compromise and aspiration.

Concurrently, rapid establishment of large-bore IV access is required. A large bore single lumen catheter, such as a Cordis, should be placed if central venous access is required.

Once appropriate venous access has been established, volume replacement should be undertaken. While initial volume replacement with readily accessible crystalloids is often the first step, it is important to recognize that these patients are bleeding, and therefore the mainstay of resuscitation should be blood and blood products. Early transfusion of uncross-matched blood should be transitioned as soon as possible to cross-matched blood. A significant number of patients presenting to the ICU with severe upper GI bleeding will have laboratory evidence of coagulopathy with an elevated INR on admission. Given this, balanced resuscitation with red blood cells, plasma, and platelets is advisable in the vast majority of patients. Many centers have a massive transfusion protocol designed to aid staff in providing blood products in a balanced, rapid fashion and activation of this protocol should be considered early in the course of patients presenting with massive upper GI bleeding. In addition, cryoprecipitate should be considered for patients with

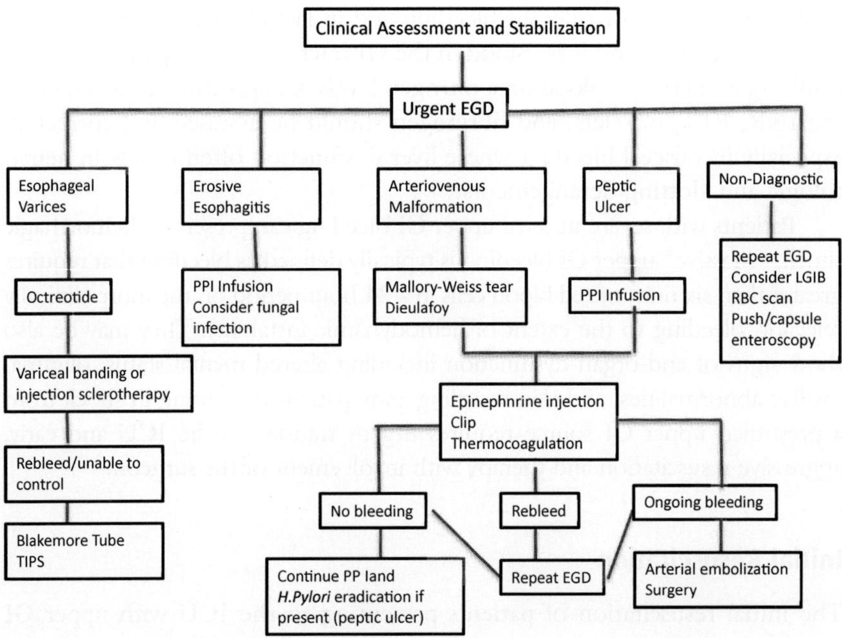

Fig. 1. Initial assessment and management of UGI bleed.

low fibrinogen (see section on Massive transfusion protocol). Recent data also suggest that there may be a benefit to the use of tranexamic acid in patients with upper gastrointestinal bleeding.[10]

For patients on therapeutic anticoagulation prior to presentation, the effects of these medications should be reversed, whenever possible, with the use of prothrombin complex concentrates or plasma. For patients taking aspirin or clopidigrel, platelets should be considered even in the presence of a normal platelet count. Unfortunately, few options exist for patients taking newer anticoagulants as many do not have antidotes. Early consultation with a hematologist may be warranted in these cases (see section on the bleeding anticoagulated patient).

Empiric therapy for upper GI bleeding should consist of high dose proton pump inhibitors to treat presumed ulcer bleeding and octreotide to treat presumed variceal bleeding. There are minimal risks associated with these therapies which can be stopped if diagnostic evaluation reveals another cause for bleeding.

Finally, fluid warmers such as the Level I transfusers should be used from the outset and patients should be kept warm with the aid of blankets or other warming devices to prevent worsening of any coagulopathy associated with hypothermia.

Diagnostic Evaluation

The first step in the diagnostic evaluation of patients with suspected upper GI bleeding is to ensure that the source of the bleeding is indeed from the upper GI tract. For patients in whom the source of GI bleeding is unclear, such as the patient presenting with melena stools or bright red blood per rectum, the insertion of an NG tube should be the first step. The return of bilious contents suggests an alternate source of bleeding, and focus should shift to a lower GI source. The return of blood however, confirms an upper GI source.

The initial diagnostic, and often therapeutic investigation is esophagogastroduodenoscopy (EGD). Performed by general surgeons and gastroenterologists in most centers, it provides invaluable information by localizing the bleeding source as well as providing therapeutic options. For those rare lesions not amenable to endoscopic treatment (i.e., hemobilia, aortoenteric fistula), diagnosis will allow rapid mobilization of the physicians and resources required for definitive treatment. Ideally, the endoscopy is conducted in the special fully equipped endoscopy suite outside the ICU, but the patient's condition may not allow safe transport. As such, many centers have protocols and are equipped with portable systems for safe conduct of endoscopy, including therapeutic interventions in the ICU itself.

Rarely, flexible endoscopy will be unable to diagnose the source of bleeding. If this occurs because a large volume of blood in the upper gastrointestinal tract cannot be adequately removed, early consultation with a surgeon is advised, as diagnosis may not be possible without operative exploration. If the patient is hemodynamically normal and the source of bleeding remains elusive, CT angiography or catheter-based angiography may aid in the diagnosis as well as afford the option of angio embolization where appropriate. Nuclear medicine tests (tagged Red Blood Cell or Meckel's scans) may be helpful in diagnosing occult GI bleeds but they tend to be more useful for lower GI bleeding.

Treatment

The first step in treatment of upper GI bleeding is to restore the blood volume and reverse any coagulopathy present. For patients with exsanguinating hemorrhage, the end-point of transfusion should be restoration of hemodynamics to normal values, and/or definitive hemorrhage control. For patients presenting without exsanguinating hemorrhage and without significant cardiovascular compromise, a more restrictive transfusion target (hemoglobin 70 g/L) has recently been shown to be associated with improved survival and a lower rate of rebleeding.[11]

In the vast majority of patients with upper GI bleeding, upper endoscopy will facilitate definitive therapy for the bleeding source. The importance of this diagnostic and therapeutic intervention is underscored by the finding in some studies that a delay to endoscopy is associated with an increase in mortality.[1] Therapeutic options for the endoscopist can be categorized broadly into three approaches: injection, thermal, and mechanical. Injection of saline, dilute epinephrine, and/or other products to induce sclerosis of the vessel have all been shown to be successful at controlling upper GI bleeding. Thermal treatments typically involve a probe placed through the endoscope, and are often used in conjunction with injection therapies. Mechanical methods typically involve the placement of one or more endoscopic clips or bands to occlude a visible vessel. For patients in whom endoscopic methods successfully control bleeding from a peptic ulcer, patients should be continued on high dose proton pump inhibitor therapy for a total of 72 hours to reduce the risk of rebleeding.[9]

For patients with an ongoing significant upper GI bleed, those who are not a candidate for initial endoscopic management, and/or those who fail initial endoscopic management, urgent consultation with a surgeon is imperative. In consultation, the surgeon can help to decide if the patient warrants additional attempts at endoscopic therapy, an attempt at arterial embolization, or if the patient would be better served in the operating room. Recent data suggests that arterial embolization is a good option for management in select cases of upper GI bleeding such as bleeding from difficult to access vessels, or those at extremely high operative risk.[12] Data suggests this method may be as effective as surgery for control of bleeding from the gastroduodenal artery eroding in to a duodenal ulcer.

Despite advances in endoscopic and interventional techniques, the role of the surgeon in the management of severe upper GI bleeding is paramount. For patients in extremis, or those in whom less invasive attempts have failed, operative intervention for hemorrhage control may be required. While historically anti-ulcer procedures, such as partial gastrectomies and vagotomies, were routinely performed if the patient's condition would allow, advances in proton pump inhibitor therapy and treatment for *H. pylori* have significantly reduced the need for such procedures. In fact, the surgical tenants for ulcer bleeding now suggest performing the minimum surgery possible to control hemorrhage and confirm the diagnosis.

For patients with variceal bleeding, additional medical therapies should be considered. These include somatostatin analogues (such as octreotide) and vasopressin analogues (such as terlipressin) to induce splanchnic vasoconstriction. Endoscopic therapies for variceal hemorrhage include banding and injection sclerotherapy. However in some patients, massive variceal bleeding will not be controlled with endoscopic and pharmacologic means alone. These patients may require temporary balloon occlusion (e.g., Blakemore tube) and/or a trans jugular intrahepatic porto systemic shunt (TIPS). While surgical options for the management of severe variceal bleeding do exist, they are rarely employed, and are associated with extremely high morbidity and mortality rates. Prophylaxis against spontaneous bacterial peritonitis should also be started in cirrhotic patients with variceal bleeding.

Outcomes and Complications

The mortality from major upper GI hemorrhage has declined significantly since the advent of gut prophylaxis and endoscopy. However, while the overall mortality rate associated with upper GI bleeding is reported to be approximately 15%,[2,3] patients who require admission to the ICU have a significantly higher risk of mortality at nearly double that.[2,5]

An important factor when considering management of upper GI bleed patients is the risk of rebleeding following initial therapy. The Forest classification is used to describe the rebleeding risk of peptic ulcers based on their endoscopic appearance (Table 3). A visible vessel in the ulcer base confers a 50% rebleed risk while a visibly spurting vessel has a rebleed risk of upwards of 85%. Endoscopic management of variceal bleeding is successful 70–90% of the time.[2]

If initial endoscopy fails, a repeat attempt is almost always warranted before moving on to secondary management strategies unless bleeding is profuse and/or the patient is unstable.

Rapid and effective intervention in massive GI bleeding is critical to minimize shock and limit the amount of blood products required for resuscitation. Massive transfusion carries a significant risk of subsequent development of adult respiratory distress syndrome (ARDS) and transfusion associated lung injury (TRALI). Furthermore, significant transfusion carries a theoretical risk of blood borne pathogen transmission (HIV, Hepatitis, etc.)

Table 3. Forrest classification — Prediction of rebleeding based on endoscopic appearance.[13]

Grade	Endoscopic Picture	Risk of Rebleeding
I	Active hemorrhage	—
Ia	Spurting	90%
Ib	Oozing without visible vessel	10–20%
II	Signs of recent hemorrhage	—
IIa	Non-bleeding visible vessel	50%
IIb	Adherent clot	25–30%
IIc	Haematin covered flat spot	7–10%
III	No hemorrhage — clean ulcer base	3–5%

Summary

Upper GI bleeding emanates from the esophagus, stomach, or duodenum and carries a significant mortality rate, especially among those patients who require ICU admission. GI bleeding is a common reason for admission to the ICU but can also be a complication of ICU stay. The treatment approach for both scenarios is similar. Aggressive resuscitation with blood products in the ICU is mandatory for all patients presenting with massive and/or unstable bleeding. The majority of upper GI bleeding can be managed endoscopically. Early endoscopy should accompany aggressive resuscitation while attempting to localize and treat the source of bleeding. Early involvement of general surgery and interventional radiology are also crucial in the management of massive upper GI bleed. An integrated team approach with involvement of the intensivist, endoscopist, surgeon, interventional radiologist and anesthetist is essential for successful outcome.

References

1. Wysocki JD, Srivastav S, Winstead NS. A nationwide analysis of risk factors for mortality and time to endoscopy in upper gastrointestinal haemorrhage. *Aliment Pharmacol Ther* 2012; 36(1): 30–36.
2. Townsend C, Beauchamp R, Evers B, Mattox K. Sabiston Textbook of Surgery: The Biological Basis of Modern Surgical Practice. 19th ed. Philadelphia, Elsevier, 2012.

3. Rockey DC. Gastrointestinal bleeding. *Gastroenterol Clin North Am* 2005; 34(4): 581–588.
4. Dulai GS, Gralnek IM, Oei TT, Chang D, Alofaituli G, Gornbein J *et al.* Utilization of health care resources for low-risk patients with acute, nonvariceal upper GI hemorrhage: A historical cohort study. *Gastrointest Endosc* 2002; 55(3): 321–327.
5. Cook D, Heyland D, Griffith L, Cook R, Marshall J, Pagliarello J. Risk factors for clinically important upper gastrointestinal bleeding in patients requiring mechanical ventilation. Canadian Critical Care Trials Group. *Crit Care Med* 1999; 27(12): 2812–2817.
6. Cook DJ, Fuller HD, Guyatt GH, Marshall JC, Leasa D, Hall R *et al.* Risk factors for gastrointestinal bleeding in critically ill patients. Canadian Critical Care Trials Group. *N Engl J Med* 1994; 330(6): 377–381.
7. Saltzman JR, Tabak YP, Hyett BH, Sun X, Travis AC, Johannes RS. A simple risk score accurately predicts in-hospital mortality, length of stay, and cost in acute upper GI bleeding. *Gastrointest Endosc* 2011; 74(6): 1215–1224.
8. Church NI, Dallal HJ, Masson J, Mowat NA, Johnston DA, Radin E *et al.* Validity of the Rockall scoring system after endoscopic therapy for bleeding peptic ulcer: A prospective cohort study. *Gastrointest Endosc* 2006; 63(4): 606–612.
9. Park T, Wassef W. Nonvariceal upper gastrointestinal bleeding. *Curr Opin Gastroenterol* 2014; 30(6): 603–608.
10. Bennett C, Klingenberg SL, Langholz E, Gluud LL. Tranexamic acid for upper gastrointestinal bleeding. *Cochrane Database Syst Rev* 2014; 11.
11. Villanueva C, Colomo A, Bosch A, Concepcion M, Hernandez-Gea V, Aracil C *et al.* Transfusion strategies for acute upper gastrointestinal bleeding. *N Engl J Med* 2013; 368(1): 11–21.
12. Lu Y, Loffroy R, Lau JY, Barkun A. Multidisciplinary management strategies for acute non-variceal upper gastrointestinal bleeding. *Br J Surg* 2014; 101(1): e34–e50.
13. Katschinski B, Logan R, Davies J, Faulkner G, Pearson J, Langman M. Prognostic factors in upper gastrointestinal bleeding. *Dig Dis Sci* 1994; 39(4): 706–712.

Chapter 29

Lower Gastrointestinal (GI) Hemorrhage

Jonathan Hong and Marcus Burnstein

Introduction and Chapter Overview

Lower gastrointestinal (GI) bleeding is defined as bleeding within the GI tract, originating distal to the ligament of Treitz.

The majority of lower GI bleeding is self-limited and does not require intervention. However, patients in a critical care unit frequently have comorbidities, particularly coagulopathy,[1] that can make the management of lower GI bleeding more challenging and urgent. The patient with poor cardiopulmonary reserve is more prone to develop complications such as coronary ischemia and its sequelae from the hemorrhage and its resulting state of hypo-perfusion. Knowledge about the clinical presentation and diagnostic techniques as well therapeutic options as discussed in this chapter will prompt early diagnosis and management of the disorders and hopefully prevent these complications which could prolong intensive care unit (ICU) care and increase the incidence of further complications such as respiratory and hemodynamic compromise in the ICU patient. This chapter will focus on the pathophysiology and current management of moderate to severe lower GI bleeding with an emphasis on the causes of lower GI bleeding that are more common in critical care patients.

Table. 1. Lower gastrointestinal causes of bleeding.

Diverticular disease
Ateriovenous malformation/Angiodysplasia
Ischemic colitis
Benign anorectal conditions e.g., Hemorrhoids, anal fissure
Inflammatory bowel disease
Neoplasia
Infectious colitis e.g., *Clostridium difficle*
Coagulopathy
Small bowel e.g., Meckels diverticulum, carcinoid, Gastrointestinal Stromal Tumor (GIST), adenocarcinoma

Epidemiology

The estimated annual incidence of lower GI bleeding is 20–30 per 100,000 persons but there is a range of severity from occult blood in the stool to life-threatening lower GI bleeding.[2] The majority of lower GI bleeding is self-limited and requires only close observation, supportive treatment, and outpatient investigation. Massive lower GI bleeding is arbitrarily defined as bleeding associated with a systolic blood pressure less than 100 mm Hg, and/or a hematocrit drop of greater than 20%, and/or a need for more than two units of packed red cells in a 24-hour period. The possible causes are listed in Table 1.

Pathophysiology and Clinical Features

Diverticular disease

Diverticular disease is estimated to have an incidence of 65% by age 85. Diverticula can be found throughout the colon but are more common in the sigmoid colon. Interestingly, bleeding originating from diverticula often originates from the right side of the colon.[3] Bleeding diverticula are thought to be the cause of lower GI bleeding in approximately 30% of cases.[4]

The vast majority of colonic diverticula are false or pseudodiverticula, the wall of the diverticula consisting only of the mucosal layer. Mucosal out-pouchings form at weak points where the circular muscle of the colonic wall is penetrated by blood vessels (vasa recta). The pathophysiology of colonic diverticulosis is disputed but the geographical distribution implicates a Western low fiber diet resulting in high intra-colonic colonic pressures and "pulsion" diverticula. Others have suggested that a connective tissue disorder may play a role. The increasing prevalence with increasing age suggests that this is also a risk factor.

The vasa recta are separated from the bowel lumen only by the diverticular mucosa and it is thought that recurrent injury leads to thinning of the media of the vessel, predisposing to rupture.

Approximately 17% of patients with diverticulosis with develop significant bleeding. Typically these episodes are not associated with pain. The majority of diverticular bleeding stops spontaneously but in up to 20% of cases the bleeding is more severe and requires intervention.[5]

Ischemic colitis

This condition results when blood flow is inadequate to meet the tissue demands for oxygen, which results in injury to the colon. The severity ranges from a reversible, transient mild colitis to colonic infarction.

The colon is particularly susceptible to ischemia as it receives less blood flow than the rest of the GI tract and the microvascular plexus of the colon is less well developed than in the small bowel.[6] As a result, colonic blood flow is strongly affected by mesenteric vasoconstriction.

Both ischemia and reperfusion play a role in injury to the colon. The earliest changes are seen in the mucosa, which eventually sloughs, resulting in ulceration. As hypo-perfusion resolves, the ulcerated areas can bleed.

The splenic flexure is the most vulnerable segment of colon due to its "watershed" anatomy, but the sigmoid and right colon may also be affected. About 2–3% of patients undergoing aortic repair will develop clinically significant ischemic colitis.[6]

The spectrum of ischemic colitis (IC) has been classified into the following types.[7]

1. Reversible ischemic colonopathy } ~50%
2. Transient IC }
3. Chronic ulcerative IC (20–25%)
4. Ischemic colon stricture (10–15%)
5. Colonic gangrene (15%)
6. Fulminant universal (1%)

This condition is particularly relevant in the critical care setting where hypotension, hemorrhage, or shock can precipitate an event and where coagulopathy can result in severe bleeding. Furthermore, the use of vasopressors can exacerbate low-flow states and contribute to mesenteric shunting, which may contribute to colonic ischemia.

In the non-intubated and awake patient the typical symptoms are left sided abdominal pain and bloody diarrhea. However, in intubated and sedated patients, bleeding may be the only feature. Laboratory tests, such lactate, are not reliable for diagnosis. A Computed Tomography (CT) scan enhanced with arterial phase intravenous contrast is a very useful modality to identify colitis and exclude arterial occlusion. The CT findings suggestive of colitis are bowel wall thickening and pericolonic stranding. Edema in the submucosa, which may occur after reperfusion, may result in a double halo sign.

Angiodysplasia

Angiodyplasia are acquired, vascular lesions found in the mucosa and submucosa. They are comprised of thin walled vessels, which are more common in the right colon and thought to be associated with aging. There is an association with aortic stenosis (Heyde syndrome), and lesions have been reported to resolve following valve replacement.

These lesions are best diagnosed endoscopically but are easily obscured by poor preparation. In addition, opiate sedation and anemia have been reported to make recognition of angiodysplasia more difficult. Argon beam coagulation is the preferred method of endoscopic therapy. Larger lesions can be lifted with saline to minimize the risk of perforation associated with coagulation.

Octreotide has been reported to reduce the incidence of recurrent bleeding from GI angiodysplasia. This effect is thought to relate to the reduction of portal and mesenteric blood flow.[8]

Infectious colitis

Salmonella, Shigella, *Campylobacter jejuni*, *Escherichia coli*, and *Clostridium difficile* are the commonest bacteria to produce colitis associated with bloody diarrhea. Campylobacter,[9] Salmonella, and Shigella[10] directly invade the colonic wall, which causes acute inflammation. *E. coli* and *C. difficile* produce a toxin which lyses the colonic mucosal cells.

Cytomegalovirus (CMV) has been reported to cause severe lower GI bleeding secondary to colitis.[11] Immunosuppressed patients, for example transplant recipients, and patients with IBD or AIDS, are particularly susceptible to CMV colitis.

Similar to ischemic colitis, the bleeding caused by infectious colitis tends to be self-limited. However, in critical care patients, other comorbidities may make the treatment of bleeding secondary to infectious colitis more difficult.

Benign anorectal conditions

These conditions have less relevance in the critical care patient population, and will not be discussed here, but the most common benign anorectal conditions responsible for lower GI bleeding are hemorrhoids and anal fissures.

Neoplasia

Adenocarcinoma and polyps of the colon and rectum are more likely to present with chronic gradual blood loss. They are a rare cause of severe lower GI bleeding but are an important consideration.

Post polypectomy bleeding occurs in up to 3.8% of patients and may occur in an immediate or delayed fashion. Delayed bleeding occurs most commonly three days post procedure but may occur after an interval of 9 days.[12] The risk factors for delayed bleeding are piecemeal resection, polyps size greater than 2 cm, intra-procedural bleeding and concurrent diverticulosis.

Investigations and Initial Treatment

In the event of massive lower GI bleeding, the first priority should be large bore intravenous access and resuscitation.

Localization and intervention

A large upper GI bleed should always be considered in patients who are hemodynamically unstable with bright bleeding per rectum. A nasogastric tube (NGT) can be helpful to exclude a gastric bleed but may miss duodenal bleeding and endoscopy is required to definitively exclude an upper GI source.

The next step in management is dictated by the rate of bleeding, the patient's comorbidities and clinical status, and the likely cause and site of bleeding. In patients presenting to an emergency department, it can be anticipated that massive lower GI bleeding will stop spontaneously in about 80% and only 20% will require urgent intervention.[13] The risk factors for persistent bleeding can be seen in Table 2. Critical care patients may be at

Table 2. Risk factors for ongoing bleeding.[14]

Risk factor	Likelihood of ongoing bleeding
HR ≥100	More than 3 risk factors = 60% risk of ongoing bleeding
Sys BP ≤115	
Age	
Comorbid illness	
Painless	1–3 risk factors = 43% risk of ongoing bleeding
History of diverticular disease or angiodysplasia	
Overt bleeding (within 4h)	0 risk factors = 6–9% risk of ongoing bleeding
ASA, anticoagulated	

higher risk of ongoing bleeding, as some of these features are more common in these patients.

Colonoscopy

Currently, colonoscopy is the first line therapy in many centers and has been reported to have a diagnostic yield of 80%, but it should be noted that a bowel preparation is generally required to achieve rates this high.[15]

Colonoscopy is particularly successful in controlling bleeding from a single site such as diverticular hemorrhage. Retrospective studies of colonoscopic treatment of diverticular hemorrhage have shown reduced rates of angiography and surgery.[4] Bowel preparation, Carbon dioxide (CO_2) insufflation, water jet irrigation, and CAP visualization are all useful adjuncts to optimize colonoscopic treatment of diverticular hemorrhage. The techniques employed to achieve hemostasis include epinephrine injection, bipolar probe, clipping, or rubber band. Tattoo marking of the bleeding site is useful if re-bleeding does occur. In a recent study, the rate of re-bleeding was 11.1% and surgery or angiography was required in only 5.5% of cases.[16]

Colonoscopy does have some limitations; it may not be possible and is less useful in patients with severe bleeding who cannot be stabilized or have a bowel preparation, which may be more likely in the critical care patient population. Furthermore, colonoscopy is only useful for very distal small bowel bleeding sites.

CT angiography (CT and selective catheter)[17]

Contrast-enhanced Multidetector Row Helical Computed Tomography (MDCT) scanning has a high sensitivity, specificity and accuracy in the detection and localization of lower GI bleeding. Arterial phase MDCT scan can detect bleeding as low as 0.3–0.5 ml/min, and may be used prior to catheter angiography to confirm ongoing bleeding and guide vessel selection (see the following section). Accurate localization also permits segmental resection in cases where surgery is required. CT angiography is relatively contraindicated in patients with renal impairment, as most widely available contrast agents are nephrotoxic.

Selective catheter angiography and embolization

Selective catheter angiography allows detection and treatment of GI bleeding if the rate of bleeding is ≥0.5 mL/min. There are three transcatheter options for control of lower GI bleeding[17]:

1. Pharmacologic control with vasopressin
2. Selective angio-embolization
3. Catheter-induced vasospam

Pharmacologic control with use of vasopressin

In this technique, the SMA or IMA is catheterized and vasopressin infused through the catheter. Initially, the rate of infusion of vasopressin is 0.2 U/min for 20 minutes. If bleeding continues then the rate is increased to 0.3 U/min and then 0.4 U/min. The effect is assessed over a 20 minute waiting period. If bleeding is controlled then the infusion is continued at this rate for 12–24 hours. The vasopressin is then switched to saline solution for 6–12 hours.

The effectiveness of this technique is limited by atherosclerotic arteries, which do not vasoconstrict, and by coagulopathy. Successful hemostasis has been reported in 60–90% of cases but recurrent bleeding may be as high as 71%.

Catheter related complications include pseudoaneurysm, infection, thrombosis, dissection, and catheter dislodgement into a non-target artery. Vasopressin related systemic complications include arrhythmias, hypotension, angina, and cardiac arrest. Regional complications include bowel infarction, mesenteric artery thrombosis, and spontaneous bacterial peritonitis.

Embolization

This technique involves identification of the bleeding vessel and superselective occlusion of the culprit vessel, preserving the collateral circulation to prevent bowel infarction. The catheter must be advanced to the mesenteric border of the colon to permit embolization. There are many materials available for embolization but microcoils have the advantage of being radiopaque and can be precisely deployed to prevent collateral occlusion. In cases where vessel tortuosity prevents safe embolization vasopressin may be used.

Pre-procedure CT angiography is desirable as it assists with identification of the site of bleeding, which permits faster catheterization of the bleeding vessel and decreases contrast and radiation exposure during arterial angiography. Moreover, if bleeding is not identified on CT angiography, then the patient may be closely monitored and angiography and embolization deferred.

General anesthesia is recommended to assist with hemodynamic control and reduction of motion artifacts during digital subtraction angiography.

The rate of successful arrest of hemorrhage ranges from 76–100%[18] but the rate of re-bleeding is 7–24%. Re-embolization can be attempted if re-bleeding occurs but this may be associated with a high rate of bowel ischemia and surgery.

Nuclear scintigraphy

The main advantage of Technetium-99m-(Tc-99m-) labeled red blood cell scan or Tc-99m sulfur colloid scintigraphy is the ability to detect bleeding even as slow as 0.04 mL/min. Precise anatomic localization of bleeding site may not be possible. This investigation is rarely used as CT angiography is readily available.

Surgical intervention

Historically, the recommended treatment of non-localized and uncontrolled lower GI bleeding was total abdominal colectomy. Using the previously described investigations and therapies to localize bleeding, a directed segmental colonic resection can be used to treat severe lower GI bleeding. The recurrence rate after total abdominal colectomy has been reported to be approximately 1%, compared to a directed segmental resection, which has a recurrence rate up to 14%.[19]

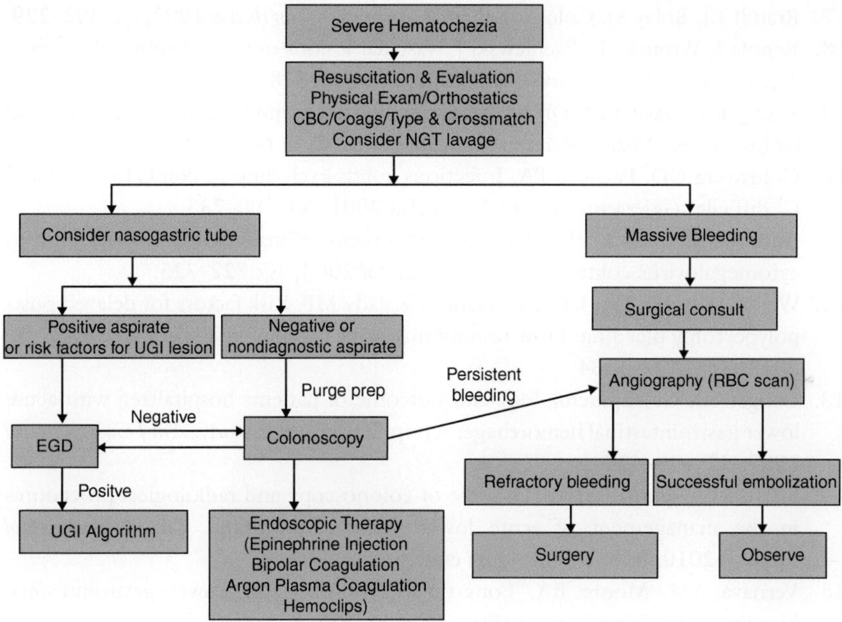

Fig. 1. ASGE suggested protocol for treatment of lower GI bleeding.[20]

References

1. Walsh TS, Stanworth SJ, Prescott RJ, Lee RJ, Watson DM, Wyncoll D. Prevalence, management, and outcomes of critically ill patients with prothrombin time prolongation in United Kingdom intensive care units. *Crit Care Med* 2010; 38: 1939–1946.
2. Talley NJ, Jones M. Self-reported rectal bleeding in a United States community: Prevalence, risk factors, and health care seeking. *Am J Gastroenterol* 1998; 93: 2179–2183.
3. Faucheron JL, Roblin X, Bichard P, Heluwaert F. The prevalence of right-sided colonic diverticulosis and diverticular haemorrhage. *Colorectal Dis* 2013; 15: e266–e270.
4. Ghassemi KA, Jensen DM. Lower GI bleeding: Epidemiology and management. *Curr Gastroenterol Rep* 2013; 15: 333.
5. Zuccaro G. Epidemiology of lower gastrointestinal bleeding. *Best Pract Res Clin Gastroenterol* 2008; 22: 225–232.
6. Theodoropoulou A, Koutroubakis IE. Ischemic colitis: Clinical practice in diagnosis and treatment. *World J Gastroenterol* 2008; 14: 7302–7308.

7. Brandt LJ, Boley SJ. Colonic ischemia. *Surg Clin North Am* 1992; 72: 203–229.
8. Regula J, Wronska E, Pachlewski J. Vascular lesions of the gastrointestinal tract. *Best Pract Res Clin Gastroenterol* 2008; 22: 313–328.
9. Young KT, Davis LM, DiRita VJ. Campylobacter jejuni: Molecular biology and pathogenesis. *Nature Reviews Microbiology* 2007; 5: 665–679.
10. Goldsweig CD, Pacheco PA. Infectious colitis excluding E. coli O157: H7 and C. difficile. *Gastroenterol Clin North Am* 2001; 30: 709–733.
11. Andrews CN, Beck PL. Octreotide treatment of massive hemorrhage due to cytomegalovirus colitis. *Can J Gastroenterol* 2003; 17: 722–725.
12. Wu XR, Church JM, Jarrar A, Liang J, Kalady MF. Risk factors for delayed post-polypectomy bleeding: How to minimize your patients' risk. *Int J Colorectal Dis* 2013; 28: 1127–1134.
13. Longstreth GF. Epidemiology and outcome of patients hospitalized with acute lower gastrointestinal hemorrhage: A population-based study. *Am J Gastroenterol* 1997; 92: 419–424.
14. Strate LL, Naumann CR. The role of colonoscopy and radiological procedures in the management of acute lower intestinal bleeding. *Clin Gastroenterol Hepatol* 2010; 8: 333–343; Quiz e44.
15. Vernava AM, Moore BA, Longo WE, Johnson FE. Lower gastrointestinal bleeding. *Dis Colon Rectum* 1997; 40: 846–858.
16. Jensen DM, Ohning GV, Kovacs TOG *et al.* How to find, diagnose and treat definitive diverticular hemorrhage during urgent colonoscopy in patients with severe hematochezia: Results and outcomes of a large prospective study. *Gastrointestinal Endoscopy* 2012; 75: AB179.
17. Cherian MP, Mehta P, Kalyanpur TM, Hedgire SS, Narsinghpura KS. Arterial Interventions in Gastrointestinal Bleeding. *Seminars in Interventional Radiology* 2009; 26: 184–195.
18. Tan KK, Strong DH, Shore T, Ahmad MR, Waugh R, Young CJ. The safety and efficacy of mesenteric embolization in the management of acute lower gastrointestinal hemorrhage. *Ann Coloproctol* 2013; 29: 205–208.
19. Hoeddema RE, Luchtefeld MA. The management of lower gastrointestinal hemorrhage. *Diseases of the Colon and Rectum* 2005; 48: 2010–2014.
20. Pasha SF, Shergill A, Acosta RD *et al.* The role of endoscopy in the patient with lower GI bleeding. *Gastrointestinal Endoscopy* 2014; 79: 875–885.

Chapter 30

Acute Pancreatitis

John B. Kortbeek

Chapter Overview

Acute pancreatitis is a common and life threatening condition. It is estimated that there are over a quarter of a million admissions in the USA per annum alone. Understanding of the pathophysiology and natural progression of acute pancreatitis has improved dramatically over the past century. Classification of acute pancreatitis has evolved and is now a useful guide to management. Early acute pancreatitis management focuses on resuscitation while late disease management focuses on complications. Improvements in resuscitation along with a staged approach in applying drainage and surgical intervention have improved the morbidity and mortality associated with acute pancreatitis.

This chapter discusses factors relevant to understanding of acute pancreatitis. Practical principles of management are introduced to guide assessment, monitoring, and therapeutic approaches in the ICU patient with acute pancreatitis.

Significance and History

Pancreatitis is a common disorder with significant morbidity and mortality. Pancreas is derived from its Greek origins *pan kreas*, meaning all flesh. Classical scholars felt its role was to protect the great vessels and stomach. Vesalius (Italy) and Wirsung (Germany) (15th century) outlined the anatomy and the drainage of the ducts into the duodenum. Understanding of the nature and pathophysiology has progressed significantly over the last two centuries. Reginald Fitz, an American 19th century pathologist described the clinical presentation of pancreatitis as well as proposed important subtypes (hemorrhagic, gangrenous, and suppurative) based on his observations. Chiari (Germany) soon after described the concept of autodigestion. Bernard (France) identified the ability of pancreatic secretions to digest fat, carbohydrate, and protein. Pavlov (Russia) received the Nobel Prize in 1904 for demonstrating that both physical (food) and psychic (neural) stimuli were responsible for the release of gastric and pancreatic enzymes.[1]

In the 20th century, Banting, Best, Collip, and McLeod (Canada) isolated insulin. Starling (UK) introduced the world to Hormones and began the field of endocrinology. By mid century, Comfort had described chronic pancreatitis. The advent of nutritional and organ support resulted in patients surviving with severe pancreatitis and led to classification and prognostic systems (e.g., Ranson's criteria) as well as evolving strategies to manage the complications associated with pancreatitis. Genetic models and advances in the sciences of immunology and inflammation have further advanced our knowledge of pancreatitis.[2]

Anatomy, Etiology, and Pathophysiology

The pancreas is located in the retroperitoneum and abuts the posterior abdominal wall, kidneys, and diaphragm as well as the stomach, the duodenum, and spleen. It is supplied by the pancreatico-duodenal and splenic arteries. Venous drainage is via the inferior and superior mesenteric and splenic veins. The confluence of the latter two forms the portal vein. The uncinate process encircles the superior mesenteric vessels (artery and vein). There is typically an accessory venous and arterial arcade lying along the posterior-inferior border and running parallel to the main splenic artery and vein.

The main pancreatic duct of Wirsung and a smaller accessory duct of Santorini open separately into the duodenum approximately 60% of the time. In 30%, the accessory duct ends blindly before reaching the duodenum. In 10%, the accessory duct drains most of the pancreas (pancreas divisum).[3]

The bulk of the pancreas is comprised of exocrine cells in clusters called acini and their related ducts. Embedded within these are numerous Islets of Langerhans, which are responsible for the production of endocrine hormones (primarily insulin and glucagon).

Autodigestion of the pancreas and surrounding tissues by excessive production or leakage of proteases may be precipitated in several ways. Hereditary pancreatitis appears to stem from alterations in genes resulting in increased production of proteases or decreased production of their inhibitors.[4]

Scorpion bites result in excessive acetylcholine and stimulation of exocrine cellular receptors. Exposure to certain insecticides containing acetylcholinesterase inhibitors can also result in excessive stimulation.

Caerulin is a peptide similar to cholecystokinin which when administered can result in secretagogue induced pancreatitis in animal models.

Gallstones are commonly associated with pancreatitis. The primary mechanism appears to be transient pancreatic duct obstruction. Pancreatic duct obstruction results in activation of lysosomal proteases (such as cathepsin) and subsequent release of intracellular calcium and induction of the cytokine inflammatory cascade with acinar and ductal cell wall disruption. The role of bile acid reflux in pancreatitis is less clear in recent studies. Alteration of ductal pH may also affect duct wall tight junctions and permeability. This may be important following endoscopic retrograde cholangiopancreatography (ERCP).[5]

Excessive alcohol consumption is also commonly associated with pancreatitis. These patients may have excessive lipopolysaccharide (LPS) production. LPS is a potent inducer of cytokines and inflammation.

Certain viral infections (coxsachie, mumps) may also induce pancreatitis. The virus is cleared from the pancreas though native immune response. Alcohol feeding and immunosuppressive therapy both potentiate pancreatitis in animal models.

This wide variety of pathologic mechanisms ultimately leads to inflammation of the pancreas and surrounding tissues, compounded by release of proteases and necrosis and the development of systemic inflammatory response syndrome (SIRS). If unchecked multiple organ dysfunction, failure, and death may ensue.

The two leading causes of pancreatitis are gallstones and alcohol. The relative incidence of these conditions will depend on the local prevalence of alcohol consumption. Less commonly hypertriglyceridemia, hypercalcemia, autoimmune, and drug induced acute pancreatitis may occur. Rarely arachnid bites that induce increased acetylcholine stimulation may be identified.

Diagnosis and Classification

The diagnosis of pancreatitis should be suspected in any patient presenting with generalized, central, or epigastric abdominal pain. A history of excessive or binge alcohol use or known cholelithiasis are suggestive. It should also be excluded in patients presenting with clinical SIRS.

SIRS can be diagnosed when two or more of the following criteria are present:

Tachycardia greater than 90 beats per minute.
Tachypnea greater than 20 breaths per minute of $PaCO_2 < 32$.
Fever greater than 38°C (100.4°F) or less than 36°C (96.8°F).
Leukocytosis greater than 12×10^9 cells/L or less than 4×10^9 cells/L.
Bandemia (immature neutrophils) greater than 3%.

Serum lipase or amylase should be measured and is greater than three times the upper limit of normal. Serum lipase elevation is more specific for pancreatitis and may be the preferred test. Depending on the age of the patient and clinical condition, Ultrasound or CT with intravenous contrast should be the initial imaging. Ultrasound may be preferable in mild disease to identify cholelithiasis as a potential causal agent. In younger patients, the risks and benefits of CT with its inherent radiation exposure should be considered against disease severity and the need to exclude other diagnoses. In severe pancreatitis, CT with intravenous contrast is the study of choice in order to identify the extent of pancreatic inflammation and necrosis, the extent of peripancreatic fluid and to identify vascular complications.

The Atlanta classification system has been updated since its introduction in 1991. The Classification of Pancreatitis 2012 reflects not only disease severity but recognizes that acute pancreatitis has two distinct phases. Acutely the degree of inflammation determines the systemic effects. Management is primarily resuscitation and support for organ failure. By the end of the first week the inflammation tends to resolve and the edema subsides or the disease progresses to necrosis and local complications included peripancreatic fluid collections, pseudocysts, infected necrosis, splenic, portal or mesenteric vein thrombosis, colonic infarction, gastric outlet obstruction, and pseudoaneurysm formation. Nutritional support may be challenging and superimposed fungal infections may occur. The first phase of acute pancreatits is best described by clinical parameters while the second phase is characterized by morphologic findings.[6]

Classification of acute pancreatitis

Mild pancreatitis

No systemic complications or organ failure.

Moderate pancreatitis

Organ failure resolving within 48 h

or

Local or systemic complications without organ failure.

Severe pancreatitis

Persistent organ failure (one or more) (Marshall and sequential organ failure assessment, SOFA).

Morphologic criteria

Interstitial edema
Necrosis
Acute peripancreatic fluid collections
Pseudocyst
Acute necrotic collection
Walled off necrosis

In the first week, differentiating pancreatic necrosis from edema in severe disease can be difficult, time is often required for certainty.

Medical Management and Outcomes

Early management is determined by the severity of pancreatitis. Patients may present with findings indistinguishable from early sepsis or septic shock. These patients should be managed in accordance with early goal directed therapy and sepsis bundles until the diagnosis is established. Treatments including airway management and supplemental oxygen, ventilator support if required, intravenous fluid resuscitation with crystalloid initially administering 1–2 L would be needed. If sepsis is suspected then administration of antibiotics within the first hour as well as collection of blood, sputum, and urine cultures should be performed. If adequate perfusion is not achieved with initial crystalloid infusion then a central line should be inserted to provide access for central venous pressure monitoring, additional fluids and pressors as required. Initial intravenous solutions are ideally isotonic and avoid exacerbation of acidosis.[7]

Ringer's lactate and plasmalyte offer advantages over normal saline if hyperkalemia and hypercalcemia do not preclude their use as they avoid hyperchloremic acidosis. There is no evidence that the early use of colloids, particularly albumin in critically ill patients offers improved outcomes and the use of starch solutions is associated with an increased incidence of acute kidney injury and mortality.

Patients should be monitored closely with hourly urine output initially in moderate and severe cases as IV rates of 250 to 300 cc per hour may be required to maintain urine output of >0.5cc/kg/h. Over-resuscitation should be avoided as it can exacerbate acute lung injury and lead to intra-abdominal hypertension and compartment syndrome.

Admission to a unit capable of close monitoring of critically ill patients and treatment by teams familiar with the management of acute pancreatitis and using standardized protocols have been associated with reductions in morbidity and mortality.[8]

Acute pancreatitis is a hypercatabolic state with insulin resistance. Recent evidence suggests that starting nutrition as early as possible enhances recovery and reduces morbidity. Enteral nutrition is preferable by the nasogastric or trans pyloric duodenal/jejunal routes. Enteral nutrition reduces the risks associated with parenteral nutrition, particularly thrombotic complications as well as bacterial and fungal sepsis. Functional gastric outlet obstruction frequently necessitates trans pyloric feeding via a tube placed at the bedside, fluoroscopically and endoscopically. If the patient has severe ileus or has suffered enteric necrosis or ischemia then parenteral nutrition will be required. Interestingly the pancreas does not respond to enteric nutrition in producing increased amounts of the protease trypsin, refuting the historical rationale for withholding feeding and resting the pancreas. Enteral nutrition promotes gut villous growth factors and may reduce bacterial translocation as a potential source of sepsis. There is currently insufficient evidence to recommend specialized nutritional formulas or probiotics in the management of acute pancreatitis.

Prophylactic antibiotics do not offer any benefit. Their use should be restricted to initial resuscitation when a diagnosis of sepsis or septic shock is being excluded or once infectious complications such as infected pancreatic necrosis occur. Fungal infections are associated with prolonged hospital and

ICU stays and with the use of broad spectrum antibiotics, another reason for avoiding their use prophylactically.[9–11]

Early ERCP in biliary pancreatitis has not been proven to be beneficial and its use should be restricted to patients with evidence of cholangitis or persistent choledocholithiasis.[12]

Surgery and Interventional Procedures

Necrosis leading to multi-organ system failure occurs in up to 10% of admissions for acute pancreatitis and in up to 30% of patients with severe pancreatitis. Almost half of patients with necrosis will have pancreatic ductal disruption leading to extrapancreatic fluid collections, peripancreatic necrosis and local complications including fistulas. Some of these patients develop infected pancreatic necrosis and have mortality rates approaching 30%. Traditionally patients with extensive and infected pancreatic necrosis were treated with laparotomy and open necrosectomy. Serial debridement, prolonged hospital stays, and high rates of morbidity and mortality were expected.

Pancreatic debridement is associated with the following complication rates:

Pancreatic fistula	45%
Enteric fistula	10%
Diabetes	16%
Exocrine insufficiency	20%
Hemorrhage	10%
Mortality >	20%

Recent experience with multidisciplinary management in high volume centers has suggested a staged approach. Ideally necrosectomy and debridement should be deferred until liquefaction is present and the necrosis is walled off by inflammatory tissue. A staged approach has also been demonstrated to reduce morbidity. This involves initial management of fluid collections, relief of abdominal hypertension, and control of infection using percutaneous drainage. Infection is rare in the first week. Subsequently it should be suspected with CT findings of extraluminal gas or determined by culture positive needle aspirate or percutaneous drainage. Clinical deterioration and positive blood cultures are suggestive. Debridement of infected or extensive necrosis may then occur using less invasive approaches such as trans gastric endoscopic necrosectomy or retroperitoneal small incision or video assisted necrosectomy. Using this approach a third of patients may be managed with percutaneous drainage alone.[13,14]

When surgery is required the anatomic area containing necrosis will determine the approach and whether adjunctive procedures are required (e.g., cholecystectomy or cholecystostomy). Collections confined to the lesser sac may be ideal for trans gastric drainage (endoscopic or open). When open trans peritoneal necrosectony and debridement is required either temporary closure or closure with placement of multiple large drains with serial irrigation may be performed. Intra-abdominal pressures with closure, the extent of necrosis, and whether there are significant intra-abdominal intestinal or vascular complications will determine the choice. The presence of these factors may preclude closure and drainage and require temporary abdominal closure.[15–18]

Pseudocysts

Pseudocysts occur in approximately 10% of cases of acute pancreatitis. Half of all pseudocysts will resolve independent of size. Drainage of pseudocysts should be performed if they are symptomatic, infected, or progressively increasing in size on serial assessment. Interventions are performed at least six weeks after onset of symptoms and frequently much later to determine if they will involute spontaneously. Asymptomatic pseudocysts may be monitored indefinitely if there is a clear association with onset after acute pancreatitis and a cystic neoplasm is not suspected.

Internal drainage is preferred in the absence of infection to avoid the risk of pancreatic cutaneous infection. Endoscopic drainage with papillotomy and stent placement may be ideal if there is documented duct disruption. Endoscopic ultrasound is a valuable adjunct in determining the final anatomic approach and guiding the procedure. Other options include endoscopic trans gastric or trans duodenal drainage, percutaneous trans gastric drainage, and laparoscopic or open trans gastric drainage. Recurrence rates are typically <20% and reported complication rates range from 12% to 25%.[19]

Conclusion

Acute pancreatitis is a common disorder presenting with various degrees of severity. The most serious manifestations, severe pancreatitis and infected pancreatic necrosis, frequently require management in an ICU setting. Understanding the etiology, clinical presentation, investigative and management approaches as well as close monitoring and appropriate, timely intervention are required to improve outcome.

References

1. Williams J. The nobel pancreas: A historical perspective. *Gastroenterology* 2013; 144(6):1166–1169.
2. Rustgi AK. A historical perspective on clinical advances in pancreatic diseases. *Gastroenterology* 2013; 144(6):1249–1251.
3. DiMagno MJ, Wamsteker EJ. Pancreas divisum. *Curr Gastroenterol Reports* 2011; 13(2):150–156.
4. Simeone DM, Pandol SJ. The pancreas: Biology, diseases, and therapy. *Gastroenterology* 2013; 144(6):1163–1165.
5. Lerch MM, Gorelick FS. (2013). Models of acute and chronic pancreatitis. *Gastroenterology* 2013; 144(6):1180–1193.
6. Sarr MG, Banks PA, Bollen TL, Dervenis C, Gooszen HG, Johnson CD, Swaroop Vege S. The new revised classification of acute pancreatitis 2012. *The Surg Clin North Am* 2013; 93(3):549–562.
7. Wu BU, Banks PA. Clinical management of patients with acute pancreatitis. *Gastroenterology* 2013; 144(6):1272–1281.
8. Talukdar R, Swaroop Vege S. Early management of severe acute pancreatitis. *Curr Gastroenterol Reports* 2011; 13(2):123–130.
9. Villatoro E, Mulla M, Larvin M. Antibiotic therapy for prophylaxis against infection of pancreatic necrosis in acute pancreatitis. *The Cochrane Database Syst Rev* 2010; Issue 5, Art No.CD 002941. DOI: 10.1002/14651858.CD002941.pub3. (5):1–49.
10. Jiang K, Huang W, Yang XN, Xia Q. Present and future of prophylactic antibiotics for severe acute pancreatitis. *World J Gastroenterol* 2012; 18(3):279–284.
11. Kochhar R, Noor MT, Wig J. Fungal infections in severe acute pancreatitis. *J Gastroenterol Hepatol* 2011; 26(6):952–959.
12. Tse F, Yuan Y. Early routine endoscopic retrograde cholangiopancreatography strategy versus early conservative management strategy in acute gallstone pancreatitis. *The Cochrane Database Syst Rev* 2012; Issue 5. Art No.CD 009779. DOI:10.1002/14651858. CD009879.pub2. (5):1–94.
13. Nieuwenhuijs VB, Timmer R. A step-up approach or open necrosectomy for necrotizing pancreatitis. *The New Engl J Med* 2010; 362(16):1491–1502.
14. Hart PA, Baron TH. What is the role of noninvasive treatment for infected pancreatic necrosis: Still an unanswered question. *Gastroenterology* 2013; 144(7):1574–1575.

15. Warshaw AL. Improving the treatment of necrotizing pancreatitis — A step up. *The New Engl J Med* 2010; 362(16):1535–1537.
16. Martin RF, Hein AR. Operative management of acute pancreatitis. *The Surg Clin North Am* 2013; 93(3):595–610.
17. Gooszen HG, Besselink MGH, van Santvoort HC, Bollen TL. Surgical treatment of acute pancreatitis. *Langenbeck's Arch Surg* 2013; 398(6):799–806.
18. Bahr MH, Davis BR, Vitale GC. Endoscopic management of acute pancreatitis. *The Surg Clin North Am* 2013; 93(3):563–584.
19. Blatnik JA, Hardacre JM. Management of pancreatic fistulas. *The Surg Clin North Am* 2013; 93(3):611–617.

Chapter 31

Colorectal Disorders

Jonathan Hong, D. Kagedan and Marcus Burnstein

Chapter Overview

Patients who require critical care may develop the same array of colorectal disorders as the general population. The disorders discussed in this chapter are those commonly encountered in patients requiring critical care, or conditions that may necessitate admission to a critical care unit. The patient may require ICU admission because of associated comorbidities, complications, or unusual presentations of the colorectal disorder. Information contained in this chapter will allow the intensivist to recognize the clinical presentation, and to understand the principles of management. Prompt management of disorders such as bowel obstruction, *Clostridium difficile* enterocolitis, and acute pseudo-obstruction improves patient outcomes, including reduction of the need for duration of mechanical ventilation.

Colon and Rectal Trauma

Introduction

Anatomically, the colon frames the abdomen, with the ascending and descending colon fixed to the retroperitoneum.[1] This makes the colon especially vulnerable to penetrating injury, with colonic injuries relatively rare in blunt trauma. Conversely, the rectum is contained within the bony pelvis, protecting it from external penetrating injury, but rendering it vulnerable to injuries associated with blunt pelvic trauma. Major controversies persist in the management of colon and rectal injuries, including the indications for primary repair, resection and anastomosis, and fecal diversion.

Epidemiology

Traumatic colon injury is relatively rare, occurring in less than 1% of all trauma patients.[2,3] The majority of colon trauma is caused by penetrating injury (56–71%), predominantly gunshots. In combat, colon injuries are frequent, occurring in up to 5% of trauma patients. In the combat setting, penetrating injuries are the most frequent mechanism of colon trauma with blast injuries the second most common, accounting for 35% of cases.[4] In the civilian population, colon injury occurs in 0.1–0.5% of blunt trauma cases.[3] The majority of these injuries occur among young males, ages 19–28.

Traumatic rectal injury is far less frequent, occurring in less than 0.1% of trauma patients.[3] Blunt trauma is the more frequent mechanism of rectal injury, and motor vehicle accidents are the most common cause (39%). Isolated injuries to the rectum are very rare, usually occurring secondary to foreign bodies. In blunt trauma, rectal injury often occurs in combination with bony, urological, and/or vascular injury, and it is associated with high mortality (21.2%).[3]

Mechanisms and patterns of injury

Blunt injuries to the colon and its mesentery tend to occur at points of transition from intraperitoneal to retroperitoneal, such as the ileocecal region, and the sigmoid colon, where the mobile colon becomes fixed. Penetrating colorectal injuries should be suspected based on the path of the instrument or projectile. Blast injuries should raise suspicion for devascularization, which may present as a delayed perforation. Rectal injury is often associated with pelvic fractures. Based on their close anatomic relationship, injury to the sigmoid colon and rectum may be associated with genitourinary tract injuries.

Historically, traumatic colorectal injuries have been associated with mortality rates of 60–75%,[2] both due to associated injuries and to secondary intra-abdominal sepsis.

Presentation

Most traumatic colorectal injuries are diagnosed either during the initial evaluation, imaging studies, or intra-operatively during exploratory laparotomy.

Findings of peritonitis, feculent abdominal discharge from a penetrating wound, or blood on digital rectal examination should raise suspicion for an injury to the intra-abdominal gastrointestinal tract. Signs of hemorrhagic shock may accompany a mesenteric injury. Evolving intra-abdominal sepsis should raise suspicion for an occult colorectal injury. At laparotomy, the anatomic location of the colon may obscure injuries, necessitating complete mobilization to permit inspection of the entire circumference of the colon and its mesentery to exclude a colon injury.

Diagnosis

The primary and secondary Advanced Trauma Life Support (ATLS) surveys have a low sensitivity for detecting injuries to the colon and rectum. If Digital Rectal Exam (DRE) reveals blood, foreign objects, or bony protrusions, a rigid proctoscope may be used to examine the rectal mucosa for damage or defects.[5] Unfortunately, the combined sensitivity of these two methods is approximately 33% for rectal injuries and 5% for any bowel injury. While non-specific for colorectal injury, an upright chest X-ray or Focused Assessment with Sonography for Trauma (FAST) ultrasound may reveal free air consistent with hollow viscus perforation.[5]

Triple contrast helical Computed Tomography (CT) scan has been shown to have 100% sensitivity, 96% specificity, 100% negative predictive value, and 97% accuracy in detecting peritoneal violation, colonic, major vascular, or genitourinary tract injuries following penetrating trauma.[6] The indications for diagnostic peritoneal lavage have decreased dramatically with the increasing availability of CT scans; DPL has a sensitivity for intestinal injury between 84–97%, and is particularly useful in the combat setting.[2] Additionally, DPL can distinguish blood from enteric contents, which may not be possible with CT scan. Diagnostic laparoscopy can also be used to evaluate colorectal injuries in stable patients with equivocal imaging findings.

The American Association for the Surgery of Trauma (AAST) Organ Injury Scale provides a classification scheme for injuries of the colon and rectum. Injuries may be subdivided into "non-destructive," involving <50% circumference of the bowel wall with no associated devascularization, and "destructive," involving >50% of the bowel wall or with segmental devascularization. Destructive lesions correspond to AAST grades 3–5, and non-destructive lesions grades 1–2.

Colon:

Grade I — contusion or hematoma; partial-thickness laceration
Grade II — full-thickness laceration <50% of circumference
Grade III — full-thickness laceration ≥50% of circumference
Grade IV — transection
Grade V — transection with tissue loss; devascularized segment

Rectum and rectosigmoid colon:

Grade I — contusion or hematoma; partial-thickness laceration
Grade II — full-thickness laceration <50% of circumference
Grade III — full-thickness laceration ≥50% of circumference
Grade IV — full-thickness laceration with perineal extension
Grade V — devascularized segment

Treatment

Traditionally, colon trauma was treated with fecal diversion, either by exteriorizing the injured segment of colon or creating a proximal colostomy to defunction the injured segment. In 1979, Stone and Fabian published a prospective randomized trial comparing primary repair with diversion, and found equivalent rates of infection (48% versus 57%, $p > 0.05$) and mortality (1.5% versus 1.4%, $p > 0.05$).[7] This study excluded patients with blood loss >1 L, hypotension, more than 2 intra-abdominal organs injured, significant peritoneal contamination, delay >8 hours following injury, destructive colon wounds, or major loss of abdominal wall; patients with any of these characteristics were treated with a colostomy. A 1991 trial randomized *all* patients with penetrating colonic trauma to either diversion or primary repair (simple closure or resection and anastomosis).[8] No anastomotic leaks were reported in the primary repair group, and septic complications were not significantly different between those who were diverted and those who were not. Further studies in the 1990s confirmed that there is no benefit to diversion even among patients with large destructive colon injuries, fecal contamination, systemic hypotension, or excessive blood loss.

In 1998, the Eastern Association for the Surgery of Trauma published guidelines recommending diversion only for patients with destructive colon injuries (AAST Grade 3 or higher) who also had any of: hemodynamic instability; significant comorbidities; or a penetrating abdominal trauma index (PATI) >25.[9] EAST guidelines recommended primary repair for all non-destructive (AAST Grade 2 or less) colon wounds in the absence of peritonitis.

In 2003, a *Cochrane Review* found no difference in mortality comparing primary repair to diversion.[10] Moreover, total complications, abdominal infections, wound complications, and dehiscence all significantly favored primary repair over diversion. While some authors have concluded based on level I data that primary repair without diversion may be performed independent of risk factors, this remains a contentious topic, with some experts advocating colostomy in select cases based on the surgeon's judgment.

The decision to perform a primary suture repair or a segmental colon resection with anastomosis is based on the degree of injury and state of the bowel wall. As a general rule, patients with destructive injuries of the colon (AAST grade 3–5) require resection and anastomosis, whereas non-destructive injuries may be amenable to primary suture repair. No major differences in outcome have been found comparing hand-sewn versus stapled anastomoses, or injuries to the right colon versus the left colon. In critically ill patients undergoing damage control surgery, injured segments should be stapled off and the decision to perform an anastomosis or stoma delayed until hypothermia, coagulopathy and acidosis is corrected. If a temporary stoma must be fashioned in an open abdomen, the stoma should be sited as laterally as possible to maximize medial mobility of the abdominal wall for closure. As colon injuries are high-risk for infectious complications, interventions such as debridement of necrotic tissue, early administration of intravenous antibiotics, and leaving the skin open or partially open, decrease the risk of infectious complications.

Historically, rectal trauma was managed according to the "4 Ds" of proximal diversion, pre-sacral drainage, direct repair, and distal rectal washout.[5] The evidence on this topic is limited, but current data supports treating intraperitoneal rectal injuries in a similar fashion to colonic injuries. Extraperitoneal injuries should usually be diverted proximally and, if feasible, repaired directly, although limited data suggests that direct repair is unnecessary if the fecal stream is diverted proximally, and the injury is allowed to heal by secondary intention. Distal rectal washout and presacral drainage have not been shown to improve outcomes, and current literature questions their usage, instead recommending they be used on a case-by-case basis at the discretion of the surgeon.

Mechanical Large Bowel Obstruction (LBO)

Introduction

Mechanical large bowel obstruction is defined as a physical blockage of the colon or rectum that prevents transit of the products of digestion.

Epidemiology

LBO is most commonly caused by malignancy (60%), diverticular strictures (20%), or colonic volvulus (5–15%). Infrequent causes include inflammatory bowel disease, radiation induced stricture, fecal impaction, intussusceptions, or extrinsic compression.[11]

Malignant large bowel obstruction occurs in up to 29% of patients with colorectal cancer.[12] Right-sided lesions cause obstruction only when large as the contents of this side of the colon are liquid and the caliber of the bowel is greater than the left.

The most common type of volvulus involves the sigmoid colon.[13] The archetypal group of patient is an elderly nursing home resident, with limited mobility and multiple co-morbidities. Patients raised in Africa, the Middle East, India, or Russia (the volvulus belt) are also at risk of volvulus but tend to present aged 40–50 years.

Diverticular strictures predominantly affect the sigmoid colon.[14] As with diverticular disease in general, patients are more likely to be older than 60 years.

Pathophysiology

Large bowel obstruction causes distension and increased secretions in the proximal bowel.[12] This damages the intestinal mucosa and impairs venous return, which leads to edema and ischemia. The resulting increase in bowel wall permeability can permit bacterial translocation and systemic toxicity. Continued ischemia will lead to bowel perforation. Consistent with Laplace's law, the cecum is particularly vulnerable if there is a competent ileo-caecal valve.

Presentation

Typical symptoms of LBO include abdominal distension and abdominal pain.[12] Obstipation, vomiting, and nausea may be present. The duration of symptoms may give an indication of etiology. Rapid onset is more likely to be volvulus but gradual onset and use of laxatives suggest diverticular stricture or carcinoma.

Physical examination reveals a distended, tympanic abdomen, and bowel sounds can be tinkling, increased, reduced, or absent.[12]

Diagnosis

An erect chest X-ray is used excluding pneumoperitoneum. An abdominal X-ray may be sufficient to diagnose sigmoid volvulus but the characteristic coffee bean sign in the right upper quadrant is not always present and markedly distended sigmoid colon due to stricture or neoplasm can have a similar appearance.[12] In the case of an axial caecal volvulus, the coffee bean sign points to the left upper quadrant.

A contrast enhanced CT scan of the abdomen and pelvis provides information on the site and nature of the obstruction and can help to confirm colorectal cancer but may not be necessary in volvulus.[13]

Water-soluble contrast enema can be used to diagnose and detort a sigmoid volvulus but should not be performed if there is localized lower abdominal peritonism suggestive of colonic ischemia.[13]

Treatment

Ensure adequate resuscitation and correction of electrolyte abnormalities. Surgery is indicated if a perforation is confirmed.

Colonic volvulus

A sigmoid volvulus may be treated in the emergency room using a rigid sigmoidoscope and a rectal tube to decompress the colon.[13] Decompression is confirmed clinically (with expulsion of gas and fecal material) and radiologically with abdominal X-ray. Flexible sigmoidoscopy and rectal tube can be used if this is unsuccessful. The rectal tube is left in place for 24–72 hours. Endoscopic decompression is successful in the majority of patients. Caecal volvulus may be decompressed endoscopically but the success rates are low and operation is recommended.

The recurrence rate of sigmoid volvulus following decompression is in the range of 70% and definitive treatment involves surgery.[13] However, the comorbidities of this group of patients often prohibit surgical intervention. Surgery involves resection of the redundant colon, with or without anastomosis. Sigmoidopexy is not recommended due to high recurrence rates. There are case series that show good results using mesosigmoidoplasty, using mesenteric flaps to widen the sigmoid colon mesentery, but this is not widely practiced.

The surgical treatment of caecal volvulus is resection and primary anastomosis.[13]

Neoplastic lesions

Resection and primary anastomosis are considered safe for right-sided obstructing colonic lesions.[12] A more extensive resection with primary anastomosis of the ileum to the colon may be applied for obstructing lesions in the transverse colon and descending colon, but the patient's bowel habits and continence must be considered. A subtotal colectomy with ileorectal anastomosis is used very selectively.

The treatment options for diverticular and left-sided colonic carcinoma are similar as both conditions are more common in the sigmoid colon.[12] Historically, the favored surgical option was resection of the obstructing lesion and creation of an end colostomy (Hartmann's procedure). More recently, resection with or without on-table colonic lavage and primary anastomosis, with or without diverting loop ileostomy has been promoted.

Loop ileostomy closure is a far less morbid procedure than Hartmann's reversal. These options have not been subject to randomized trials and the decision depends on surgeon preference and experience, and patient comorbidities. Postoperative morbidity and mortality are similar in comparison studies but the stoma was not reversed in 25% of patients undergoing Hartmann's procedure.[15]

Stents

Expandable metal stent placement is being used increasingly in management of malignant large bowel obstruction. Stents can be utilized in one of two ways: as a bridge-to-surgery or as a palliative procedure in patients whose prognosis is less than 3–6 months.

Left-sided colonic lesions are generally more suitable for treatment with stenting, but any lesion situated from 5 cm proximal to the anal verge to the right colon can be considered. Stents are appropriate for use in stable patients without signs of systemic toxicity or perforation.

When used as a temporizing measure, clinical success rates (clinical relief of obstruction) of up to 92% have been achieved. Patients may then undergo bowel preparation and be optimized for surgery. Studies suggest that this approach is more cost-effective[16] than emergency surgery.[17] A *Cochrane Review* found no significant difference in morbidity and mortality when emergency stenting was compared to surgery for the treatment of acute malignant large bowel obstruction. Stenting is associated with shorter hospital stay, less blood loss, and shorter procedure time than surgery.

Stenting may also be used to palliate patients whose medical comorbidities preclude surgery with up to 75% success rates. The duration of stent patency is 3–6 months, which suggests that patients with a prognosis greater than 6 months may be best treated with resection.[18]

Covered stents have a theoretical benefit in the reduction of tissue ingrowth; they also have an increased tendency to migrate, and studies comparing covered and uncovered stents have not found a significant difference in clinical success rates.[19]

Complications of stent placement include perforation (5%), stent migration (11%), and bleeding. Rates of perforation increase to 15% in patients receiving bevacizumab chemotherapy. Re-obstruction occurs in 12% of patients and approximately 20% of patients require some sort of re-intervention.[20] Low residue diet may minimize the rates of stent obstruction.

Colonic stenting has been used to treat benign disease, most commonly diverticular strictures but long-term patency is not known and the bridge-to-surgery approach should also be used for benign lesions.

In the critical care population, where medical comorbidities are common, colon stents have the potential to avoid emergency surgery in many patients with large bowel obstructions. However, careful selection of appropriate candidates for stenting is necessary, and stents should not be substituted for surgery in an unstable patient or one whose critical illness is secondary to the bowel obstruction itself.

Intestinal Acute Pseudo-Obstruction (APO)

Definition

APO is a disorder characterized by abdominal distension and pain in the absence of any occlusive gut lesion. In the critical care setting the acute form of this disease is more common and the chronic entity will not be discussed.

Epidemiology

The incidence of APO is not known. It is relatively common in the critical care setting. The morbidity rate is up to 30%, which probably relates to multiple comorbidities and delayed diagnosis.[21]

Table 1. Factors associated with developing colonic pseudo-obstruction.

Patients groups at risk for pseudo-obstruction	*Orthopaedic*: Particularly post pelvic or lower limb trauma or joint replacement (occurs in ~1% of lower limb joint replacements and spinal operations [22])
	Drug related: Opiates, anti-depressants, anti-cholinergics, anti-parkinsonisan agents, clonidine, benzodiazepines, Ca-channel blockers
	Obstetric: Pregnancy and post delivery (both vaginal or caesarian)
	Critical care: Patients with significant trauma, sepsis and/or cardiac disease

Pathophysiology

APO is a disorder of gut motility. The original report (by Ogilvie) described malignant invasion of the paravertebral ganglia causing "sympathetic deprivation". Additional mechanisms have been proposed[23]:

- Reflex motor inhibition through splanchnic afferents in response to noxious stimuli reduces intestinal tone;
- Excess sympathetic input inhibits gut contraction;
- Excess parasympathetic input prevents gut relaxation;
- Decreased parasympathetic input prevents gut contraction;
- Excess stimulation of opiate receptors;
- Inhibition of nitric oxide release from inhibitory motor neurons prevents gut relaxation;

Clinical features

APO presents with abdominal distension, pain, nausea, and/or vomiting. The abdomen will be distended and tympanic, usually non-tender, with high pitched, tinkling, or absent bowel sounds. The findings of pain and peritonism is concerning for ischemia-related perforation. It is difficult to clinically distinguish APO from a mechanical obstruction but the condition is commonly precipitated by an underlying illness or postoperative recovery (Table 1).

Differential diagnoses include mechanical obstruction, toxic megacolon (e.g., due to severe *C. difficile* infection), and colonic volvulus.

Investigations

Plain X-rays are useful to exclude free gas from perforation and assess the degree of colonic distension, particularly of the caecum, which is the most likely site of perforation in APO.

The next step in investigation should aim to exclude a mechanical obstruction. Colonoscopy may be therapeutic as well as diagnostic.

The multi detector CT scan has become more widely used to assess large bowel obstruction. This modality has the added advantage of assessing the regional lymph nodes and liver if malignancy is shown to be the cause.[24] We recommend rectal contrast be used to clearly delineate the level of obstruction.

Treatment

Initial treatment involves insertion of nasogastric and rectal tubes, correction of electrolyte abnormalities, minimizing use of precipitant medications where possible, encouraging mobility and arranging the appropriate investigations to exclude mechanical obstruction.

Pharmacologic

Intravenous neostigmine has been the subject of several placebo-controlled trials, which have demonstrated its effectiveness. Published success rates are approximately 80%, and the rate of recurrence is approximately 27%.[25] Patients require cardiac monitoring during administration as side effects include bradycardia and hypotension. Contraindications include myocardial infarction, acidosis, chronic obstructive pulmonary, bradycardia, peptic ulcer disease, renal insufficiency, and treatment with β blockers. These contraindications may limit the use of neostigmine in the critical care setting.

The use of neostigmine infusion (0.4–0.8 mg/h over 24h), or starting with a 1mg bolus, may reduce the risk of bradycardia.[25]

Osmotic laxatives (e.g., lactulose) are not recommended as they can worsen gaseous distension due to colonic bacterial fermentation.

Polyethylene glycol has been effectively used to prevent recurrence after decompression (using neostigmine or colonoscopy).[26]

Radiologic

Water-soluble contrast (e.g., gastrograffin) enema (WSCE) has been used to both exclude mechanical obstruction and treat pseudo-obstruction.[27]

The recurrence rate in this small series was 11% and a similar proportion required surgical intervention. The technique does require patients to change positions on fluoroscopy table to permit filling of the colon with contrast. However, the procedure is less technically demanding than a colonoscopy in unprepared and distended colon. The use of WSCE minimizes the risk of colonic perforation.

Endoscopic

Colonoscopy is an effective treatment for APO, with a reported success rate after the first colonoscopy of 82%.[28] The recurrence rate is approximately 22%.[21] The overall success rate can be improved to 88% after additional colonoscopy. However, the risk of colonic perforation is up to 2%.[25]

Colonoscopy in this group of patients, who are unable to be given bowel preparation, is challenging and should be performed by experienced endoscopists. Further colonic dilatation can be minimized by using carbon dioxide, or as little air, insufflation as possible.

The recurrence rate is reduced by endoscopically placing a guidewire, over which a rectal tube can be inserted with fluoroscopic guidance. The success rate is similar to neostigmine but the procedure may need to be repeated.

Surgical

More invasive decompressive procedures include percutaneous endoscopic colostomy or cecostomy. Decompression using percutaneous CT-guided caecostomy has also been reported. Laparotomy should be reserved for ischemia or perforation.

A management algorithm can be seen in Fig. 1.

***Clostridium difficile* Colitis**

Introduction

Clostridium difficile is a toxin producing gram positive spore-forming anaerobic bacillus, which causes pseudomembranous colitis. *Clostridium difficile* Infection (CDI) is commonly associated with antibiotic usage, and the spectrum of disease ranges from asymptomatic to toxic megacolon. CDI most frequently manifests in the colon, but it has been reported in patients who

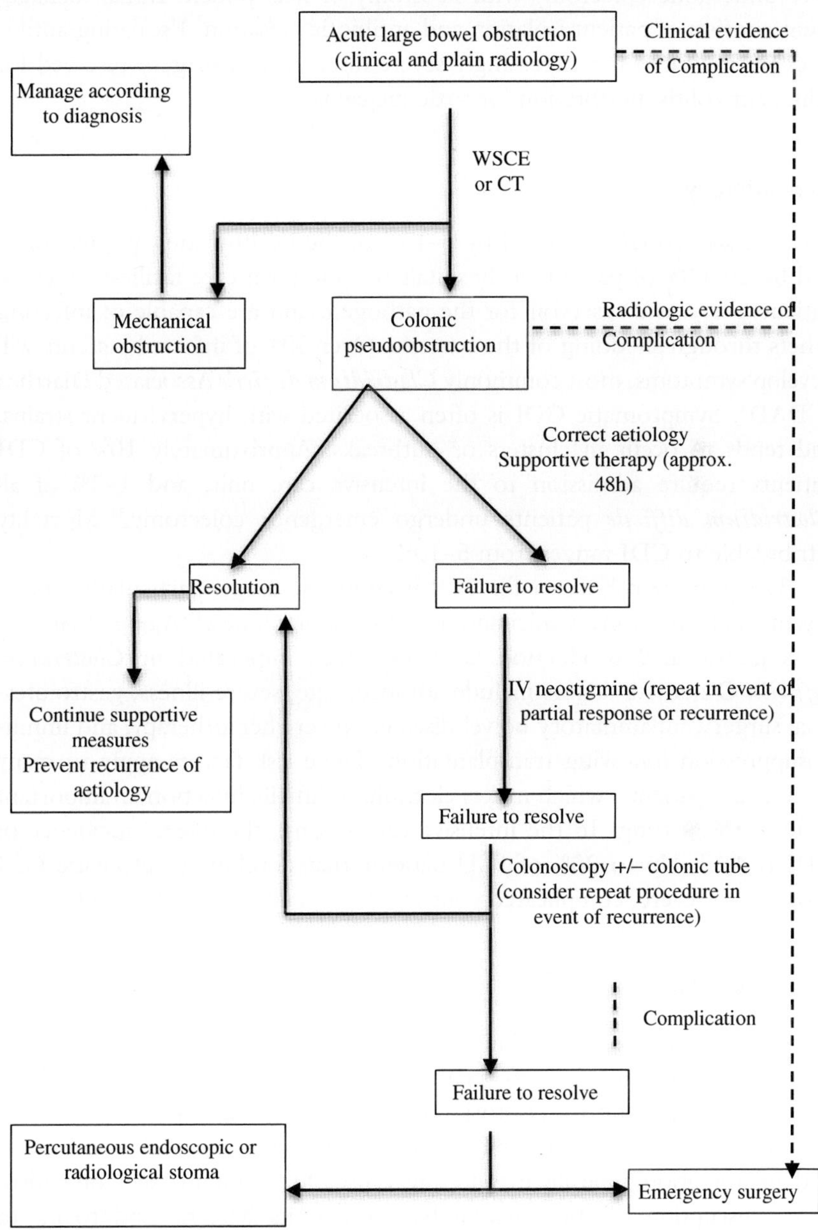

Fig. 1. Suggested management algorithm for acute colonic pseudo obstruction.[25]

have undergone colectomy with ileostomy or ileal pouch. Initial management consists of patient isolation and antibiotic cessation. Escalating antibiotics are indicated for increasingly severe disease, with surgery reserved for fulminant colitis, perforation, or toxic megacolon.

Epidemiology

Clostridium difficile is carried by 6–15% of the healthy adult population,[29] and by 20–50% of patients in hospitals or long-term care facilities.[30] These patients serve as a reservoir for the pathogen, and are capable of infecting others through shedding of the bacteria. Over 30% of infected patients will develop symptoms, most commonly *Clostridium difficile* Associated Diarrhea (CDAD). Symptomatic CDI is often associated with hypervirulent strains, and tends to occur in clusters or outbreaks. Approximately 10% of CDI patients require admission to the intensive care unit, and 1–2% of all *Clostridium difficile* patients undergo emergency colectomy.[31] Mortality attributable to CDI ranges from 5–10%.

The primary risk factor for CDI is antibiotic usage, particularly clindamycin, cephalosporins, penicillins, and fluoroquinolones.[31] Agents that suppress gastric acid production have also been implicated in *Clostridium difficile.* Other risk factors include advanced age, severe illness, gastrointestinal surgery, inflammatory bowel disease, cancer chemotherapy, and immunosuppression following transplantation. These risk factors apply to many critical care patients, which makes clotridium difficile infection an important issue in this setting. In the intensive care setting, the overall incidence of CDI is 4%.[32] Up to 20% of ICU patients that develop symptomatic CDI progress to severe, complicated colitis with mortality approaching 60%.

Pathophysiology

Clostridium difficile causes clinical disease by secreting two exotoxins, toxin A (enterotoxin), and toxin B (cytotoxin). These toxins act intra-cellularly, causing cell retraction, apoptosis, and disrupting tight junctions.[33] This causes mucosal damage, ulceration, neutrophil activation and recruitment, and inflammation, typically manifesting as pseudomembranes seen on endoscopy. Disruption of the mucosal barrier permits bacteria and toxins to enter the portal circulation, giving rise to a systemic sepsis. While CDI is thought to be due to decreased numbers of normal colonic flora, facilitating colonization with pathogenic *Clostridium difficile*, asymptomatic carriers of *Clostridium difficile* have lower rates of CDAD than patients who are naïve to *Clostridium difficile.*

A hypervirulent strain, NAP1/B1/027 has been implicated in multiple outbreaks in the last two decades, and is associated with lower cure rates and increased recurrence.[33] In addition to producing larger quantities of toxins A and B, NAP1/B1/027 elaborates binary toxin, which is thought to enhance the toxicity of *Clostridium difficile.*

Presentation

The hallmark of symptomatic CDI is profuse watery diarrhea (90–95%).[33] CDAD is rarely bloody, and hematochezia should prompt a workup for other potential causes. Other common symptoms include cramping abdominal pain (80–90%), anorexia, malaise, and fever. In some cases, an ileus may be present. Severe CDI may manifest with hemodynamic instability.[33] Physical findings depend on the severity of the infection, and can range from unremarkable, in mild disease, to peritonitis in fulminant disease.

Diagnosis

The diagnosis of *Clostridium difficile* colitis is confirmed by either a stool test positive for *Clostridium difficile* or its associated toxins, or endoscopic, or histologic demonstration of pseudomembranous colitis.[34] Laboratory tests for *Clostridium difficile* include Polymerase Chain Reaction (PCR), enzyme immunoassays for *Clostridium difficile* toxins A and B or glutamate dehydrogenase, cell culture cytotoxicity assay, and selective anaerobic culture. Some diagnostic algorithms utilize an initial enzyme immunoassay with a confirmatory PCR; others utilize PCR alone, as it is highly sensitive and specific.[34] Testing for cure is not indicated, as up to 50% of patients have positive stool samples 6 weeks after completion of therapy.

Endoscopic evaluation of the colon via sigmoidoscopy or colonoscopy is indicated in the setting of diagnostic uncertainty, such as high clinical suspicion with negative laboratory tests, failure of response to antibiotic therapy, or the need for urgent diagnosis. Visualization of pseudomembranes (raised yellow plaques scattered over the colorectal mucosa) is pathognomonic for CDI. Furthermore, the bowel wall may appear edematous, erythematous, friable, and inflamed. If pseudomembranes are not observed, biopsy is useful for diagnosis of CDI. If performed, an abdominal CT scan may reveal non-specific thickening of the colonic wall.

Treatment

Upon diagnosis of CDI, infection control measures should be instituted to contain the spread of infection. In addition, cessation of antibiotics associated with CDI, adequate replacement of fluids and electrolytes, avoidance of anti-motility medications, and reviewing the need for proton pump inhibitors are all recommended.[34]

Patients with CDI may be subdivided into those with mild/moderate CDI, and those with severe CDI; the latter includes patients with either a white blood cell count >15,000 cells/µL or a serum creatinine>1.5 times the baseline level. Patients with mild/moderate CDI may be managed with oral metronidazole (500 mg thrice daily or 250 mg four times daily, for 10–14 days) or oral vancomycin (125 mg four times daily) but this is usually reserved for severe cases. Intravenous vancomycin is ineffective in the treatment of ***Clostridium difficile***. Fidaxomicin is a macrocyclic antibiotic with activity against ***Clostridium difficile***, and a narrower spectrum of antimicrobial activity than metronidazole or vancomycin. A phase 3 randomized trial of fidaxomicin versus vancomycin demonstrated non-inferiority of fidaxomicin, as well as lower ecurrence following fidaxomicin treatment for non-NAP1 strains.[35] Mixed evidence exists for the use of probiotics, monoclonal antibodies, and toxin-binding polymers, and their administration is not recommended at this time.[34]

Severe CDI should be treated with oral vancomycin, between 125–500 mg four times daily. In patients unable to tolerate oral antibiotics, or in those with an ileus, vancomycin enemas may be combined with intravenous metronidazole.[34]

Surgery is indicated in patients with systemic toxicity unresponsive to medical management, peritonitis, toxic megacolon, or bowel perforation.[34] The recommended operation for CDI consists of a subtotal colectomy with end ileostomy. Recently, an alternative surgical approach involving formation of a diverting loop ileostomy and antegrade colonic lavage through the efferent ileostomy limb with postoperative vancomycin flushes has shown promise in reducing mortality while preserving the colon. When Neal *et al.* compared this approach to a traditional colectomy, diverting ileostomy, and lavage reduced mortality and successfully preserved colons in a population of severe, complicated CDI patients.[36]

The optimal timing of operative intervention is controversial, but operation is generally recommended when the white blood cell count is >20,000 cells/microL and/or the plasma lactate is 2.2–4.9 meq/L. Mortality following emergency surgery for severe complicated CDI ranges from 19–71%, with independent risk factors including: hypotension requiring vasopressors, increased serum lactate (>5 meq/L), mental status changes, end-organ dysfunction, renal failure, and preoperative intubation, or ventilatory support.[34]

References

1. Sakorafas GH, Zouros E, Peros G. Applied vascular anatomy of the colon and rectum: Clinical implications for the surgical oncologist. *Surg Oncol* 2006; 15: 243–255.
2. Causey MW, Rivadeneira DE, Steele SR. Historical and current trends in colon trauma. *Clin Colon Rectal Surg* 2012; 25: 189–199.
3. Brady RR, O'Neill S, Berry O, Kerssens JJ, Yalamarthi S, Parks RW. Traumatic injury to the colon and rectum in Scotland: Demographics and outcome. *Colorectal Dis* 2012; 14: e16–e22.
4. Glasgow SC, Steele SR, Duncan JE, Rasmussen TE. Epidemiology of modern battlefield colorectal trauma: A review of 977 coalition casualties. *J Trauma Acute Care Surg* 2012; 73: S503–S508.
5. Steele SR, Maykel JA, Johnson EK. Traumatic injury of the colon and rectum: The evidence versus dogma. *Dis Colon Rectum* 2011; 54: 1184–1201.
6. Shanmuganathan K, Mirvis SE, Chiu WC, Killeen KL, Scalea TM. Triple-contrast helical CT in penetrating torso trauma: A prospective study to determine peritoneal violation and the need for laparotomy. *AJR Am J Roentgenol* 2001; 177: 1247–1256.
7. Stone HH, Fabian TC. Management of perforating colon trauma randomization between primary closure and exteriorization. *Annals of Surgery* 1979; 190: 430–436.
8. Chappuis CW, Frey DJ, Dietzen CD, Panetta TP, Buechter KJ, Cohn I. Management of penetrating colon injuries a prospective randomized trial. *Annals of Surgery* 1991; 213: 492.
9. Pasquale M, Fabian TC. Practice management guidelines for trauma from the eastern association for the surgery of trauma. *The Journal of Trauma: Injury, Infection, and Critical Care* 1998; 44: 941–956.
10. Nelson R, Singer M. Primary repair for penetrating colon injuries. *Cochrane Review* 2003; 3: CD002247.
11. Kahi CJ, Rex DK. Bowel obstruction and pseudo-obstruction. *Gastroenterology Clinics of North America* 2003; 32: 1229–1247.

12. Sawai RJ. Management of colonic obstruction: A review. *Clinical Colon and Rectal Surgery* 2012; 25: 200–203.
13. Gingold D, Murrell Z. Management of colonic volvulus. *Clinical Colon and Rectal Surgery* 2012; 25: 236–244.
14. Fernhead NS, Mortensen NJ. Clinical features and differential diagnosis of diverticular disease. *Best Pract Res Clin Gastroenterol* 2002; 16: 577–593.
15. Allen-Mersh TG. Should primary anastomosis and on-table colonic lavage be standard treatment for left colon emergencies? *Ann R Coll Surg Engl* 1993; 75: 195–198.
16. Targownik LE, Spiegel BM, Sack J *et al.* Colonic stent versus emergency surgery for management of acute left-sided malignant colonic obstruction: A decision analysis. *Gastrointestinal Endoscopy* 2004; 60: 865.
17. Sagar J. Colorectal stents for the management of malignant colonic obstructions. *Cochrane Database of Systematic Reviews* 2011, Nov 9: (11): CD 007378
18. Zhang Y, Shi J, Shi B, Song CY, Xie WF, Chen YX. Comparison of efficacy between uncovered and covered self-expanding metallic stents in malignant large bowel obstruction: A systematic review and meta-analysis. *Colorectal Disease* 2012; 14: e367–e374.
19. Park S, Cheon JH, Park JJ *et al.* Comparison of efficacies between stents for malignant colorectal obstruction: A randomized, prospective study. *Gastrointestinal Endoscopy* 2010; 72: 304.
20. Watt AM, Faragher IG, Griffin TT, Rieger NA, Maddern, GJ. Self-expanding metallic stents for relieving malignant colorectal obstruction: A systematic review. *Annals of Surgery* 2007; 246: 24.
21. Vanek VW, Al-Salti M. Acute pseudo-obstruction of the colon (Ogilvie's syndrome): An analysis of 400 cases. *Dis Colon Rectum* 1986; 29: 203–210.
22. Norwood MG, Lykostratis H, Garcea G, Berry DP. Acute colonic pseudo-obstruction following major orthopaedic surgery. *Colorectal Dis* 2005; 7: 496–499.
23. Delgado-Aros S, Camilleri M. Pseudo-obstruction in the critically ill. *Best Pract Res Clin Gastroenterol* 2003; 17: 427–444.
24. Jacob SE, Lee SH, Hill J. The demise of the instant/unprepared contrast enema in large bowel obstruction. *Colorectal Dis* 2008; 10: 729–731.
25. De Giorgio R, Knowles CH. Acute colonic pseudo-obstruction. *British Journal of Surgery* 2009; 96: 229–239.
26. Sgouros SN, Vlachogiannakos J, Vassiliadis K *et al.* Effect of polyethylene glycol electrolyte balanced solution on patients with acute colonic pseudo obstruction after resolution of colonic dilation: A prospective, randomised, placebo controlled trial. *Gut* 2006; 55: 638–642.
27. Schermer CR, Hanosh JJ, Davis M, Pitcher D. Ogilvie's syndrome in the surgical patient: A new therapeutic modality. *J Gastrointestinal Surg* 1999; 3: 173–177.

28. Geller A, Petersen BT, Gostout CJ. Endoscopic decompression for acute colonic pseudo-obstruction. *Gastrointestinal Endoscopy* 1996; 44: 144–150.
29. Galdys AL, Nelson JS, Shutt KA *et al.* Prevalence and duration of asymptomatic clostridium difficile carriage among healthy subjects in Pittsburgh, Pennsylvania. *J Clinical Microbiology* 2014; 52: 2406–2409.
30. McFarland LV, Mulligan ME, Kwok RY, Stamm WE. Nosocomial acquisition of Clostridium difficile infection. *New England Journal of Medicine* 1989; 320: 204–210.
31. Honda H, Dubberke ER. The changing epidemiology of clostridium difficile infection. *Current Opinion in Gastroenterology* 2014; 30: 54–62.
32. Riddle DJ, Dubberke ER. Clostridium difficile infection in the intensive care unit. *Infectious Disease Clinics of North America* 2009; 23: 727–743.
33. Trudel JL. Clostridium difficle colitis. *Clinical Colon and Rectal Surgery* 2007; 20: 13–17.
34. Debast SB, Bauer MP, Kuijper EJ. European society of clinical microbiology and infectious diseases: Update of the treatment guidance document for clostridium difficile infection. *Clinical Microbiology Infect* 2014; 20 Supplement 2: 1–26.
35. Louie TJ, Miller MA, Mullane KM *et al.* Fidaxomicin versus vancomycin for clostridium difficile infection. *N Engl J Med* 2011; 364: 422–431.
36. Neal MD, Alverdy JC, Hall DE, Simmons RL, Zuckerbraun BS. Diverting loop ileostomy and colonic lavage: An alternative to total abdominal colectomy for the treatment of severe, complicated clostridium difficile associated disease. *Ann Surg* 2011; 254: 423–427; Discussion 427.

Chapter 32

The Bariatric Surgical Patient

Andrew Smith, Jameel Ali and Timothy D. Jackson

Chapter Overview

In discussing management of the bariatric surgery patient two major sets of issues must be addressed: first, the morbid obesity state itself and secondly the bariatric surgical procedures and their effects. Much progress has been made in both these areas to make bariatric surgery relatively safe.[1] Most bariatric surgery patients do not require care in the intensive care unit (ICU) but because of the unpredictable course in individual patients, availability of ICU facilities is essential for successful outcome in complicated cases. In this chapter we discuss; (1) general considerations in the morbidly obese which could impact outcome and ICU care and (2) bariatric surgical procedures themselves which carry their own risks. Understanding these concepts should promote better care for these patients if and when this care needs to be provided in the ICU.

General considerations in the morbidly obese that could impact ICU care

Obesity is an independent risk factor for heart disease, hypertension, diabetes mellitus, and obstructive sleep apnea,[2] all of which could impact on the perioperative care of the bariatric surgery patient. To minimize the effects of these factors, optimize overall care and limit complications. The patient requires a multi-disciplined approach which is an integral part of the bariatric surgical program. Nutritionists, psychologists, dedicated anesthetists, internists (endocrinologists), pulmonologists, gastroenterologists are all part of the care team.[3]

Laboratory investigations includes complete blood count, coagulation and metabolic profile, thyroid function tests and assessment of vitamin levels such as vitamin B12, fat soluble vitamins, and ferritin levels with preoperative correction of identified deficits including glycemic control and preparation for care of the frequently associated diabetes as well as preparation for continued support in the perioperative period to improve outcome.

Cardiorespiratory evaluation includes electrocradiography, stress test to identify occult coronary artery disease, chest X-ray, arterial blood gases, and pulmonary function tests. Sleep apnea is diagnosed by sleep study and where indicated preoperative continuous positive airway pressure (CPAP) is recommended.

If gastric pathology is suspected, upper endoscopy is conducted and *Helicobacter pylori* (*H. pylori*) infection is treated, if identified. Liver function is assessed by laboratory tests as well as ultrasound and if cirrhosis is a possibility, liver biopsy may be indicated. If gall stones are detected the surgeon may discuss concomitant cholecystectomy as an option.

Key elements in preventing perioperative complications and optimizing care of the bariatric surgery patient both in general and specifically in the ICU are anticipation of problems and being prepared to deal with these challenges.

Airway control, maintenance of ventilation, cardiovascular, and fluid dynamics as well as pharmacodynamics are areas that require close attention for optimal care of these patients.

Airway management

Being prepared for difficult intubation is always wise in the obese patient and this requires having appropriate medications available as well as regular and more invasive devices including Gum Elastic Bougie, Laryngeal Mask Airway (LMA), fiberoscopic bronchoscope, and the option of a surgical airway.

The large tongue, enlarged endopharyngeal mass, limitation of neck movement, and excessive presternal fat limit movement of the laryngoscope, making direct laryngoscopy extremely difficult for intubation. Careful assessment of these factors to determine ease of intubation is necessary, allowing a decision to proceed with general anesthesia induction and intubation or alternatively awake intubation. Fortunately, in most circumstances, general anesthesia induction followed by intubation is possible by using such techniques as the Head Elevated Laryngoscopy Position (HELP).[4] In the awake intubation technique, topical anesthesia may be used in the cooperative patient with premedication followed by direct laryngoscopy and intubation, or more commonly by fiberoptic bronchoscopy. The LMA is a good back-up temporary device to allow ventilation until a more definitive airway technique is used.

During prolonged attempts at intubation attention must be directed at maintenance of oxygenation by interruption of the intubation attempts to allow bag valve mask ventilation. In some circumstances the technique of apneic oxygenation[5] may be helpful to maintain oxygenation through passive means by way of continuous oxygen delivery using an LMA, bronchoscope, or nasal cannula.

The morbidly obese patient is generally considered to be at greater risk for aspiration of gastric contents because of increased abdominal pressure, increased incidence of gastro-esophageal reflux with or without hiatus hernia, and generally have a higher gastric residual after fasting. These factors together with the increased ventilator pressures and difficult mask ventilation predispose to regurgitation from gastric insufflation. Because of these factors many anesthetists use prokinetic agents, H_2 receptor antagonists, or proton pump inhibitors to minimize the effect of aspirated contents. If rapid sequence intubation appears safe this technique could minimize the chance of aspiration by decreasing the induction time.

Ventilatory management

Decreased chest wall compliance from the excessively fatty chest and abdominal wall tissue, decreased lung compliance from increased pulmonary blood flow, and viscosity all make ventilation difficult. The decreased functional residual capacity (FRC) which is worsened in the supine position may become lower than the closing volume (see chapter on Perioperative Respiratory Dysfunction) leading to airway closure and hypoxemia. These factors together with the increased oxygen demand from the increased metabolic needs of the obese patient lead to arterial desaturation not only in the operating room but also in the ICU. Based on the aforementioned considerations, techniques for optimizing gas exchange in the obese patient includes head up position, larger tidal volumes, positive end expiratory pressure (PEEP), and high inspired oxygen concentrations, recognizing the potential deleterious hemodynamic effects particularly on cardiac output of these maneuvers.[6,7]

As mentioned in the preceding paragraphs, many morbidly obese patients suffer from obstructive sleep apnea and these patients could desaturate particularly in the immediate post intubation period when residual anesthetic and analgesia decrease the respiratory drive leading to hypoventilation and adverse events including cardiac arrest. It is recommended that these patients bring their CPAP device to the hospital and that CPAP is available in the recovery room as a standby to deal with this possibility.[8]

Cardiovascular factors

As indicated earlier, morbid obesity is a high risk factor for coronary artery disease and its sequelae including myocardial ischemic events and cardiac dysrhythmia. Close cardiac monitoring and preoperative cardiac investigation, as well as preparedness to deal with these events in the perioperative setting including the ICU are essential elements in the care of the bariatric surgery patient. The obese patient develops cardiac dysfunction from a multitude of causes[9] including chronic ventricular stress from the increased circulating blood volume and metabolic demands, and later pulmonary hypertension. Patients deemed at greater risk based on assessment are ideally managed in an ICU setting where close monitoring and timely intervention including pharmacologic support is immediately available.

Pharmacokinetics

The obese patient metabolizes most drugs differently from the non-obese patient making drug management very challenging. There is increased sensitivity to respiratory depressant effects of sedatives such as benzodiazepines. Drug dosing based on total body weight results in over dosing and prolonged effects which could be very serious in respiratory depressant and myocardial depressant drugs.[10] Soluble inhalation agents accumulate in adipose tissue leading to longer clearance time and prolonged effects in the obese patient. Analgesia regimens can also prove very challenging in the obese patients because of increased sensitivity to the sedative effects of opioids. For open procedures, epidural analgesia supplemented by Non-steroidal Anti-inflammatory Drugs (NSAIDs) avoid the side effects of opioids. Other useful techniques include local anesthetic delivery through wound catheters and intravenous patient-controlled analgesia in a monitored setting.

Miscellaneous factors

The bariatric surgery patient has increased risk for thromboembolic complications and thromboembolic prophylactic measures as described elsewhere in this text are important considerations in their management.

Most of the surgical procedures are conducted laporoscopically with documented advantages in pain control, and other outcome parameters. Pneumoperitoneum itself predisposes to atelectasis and hypoxemia with decrease in FRC and increased compliance but there is no difference in the hemodynamic and partial pressure of carbon dioxide (PCO_2) effects between the obese and non-obese patients.[11,12] However, the uniform drop in renal and hepatic perfusion with pneumoperitoneum should be considered in the bariatric surgery patient some of whom may have borderline hepatic or renal dysfunction, emphasizing the need for maintaining adequate circulating blood volume.

Despite the many challenges presented by the bariatric surgery patients, anesthesia and surgery can be performed safely in these patients particularly with normal cardiac, pulmonary, renal, and hepatic function. In the patients with significant associated morbidity, outcome can still be very good if careful attention is directed at preoperative assessment and perioperative care based on appropriate preparation and monitoring.

Bariatric Surgery Procedures

Obesity is an epidemic that is replacing more traditional public health concerns such as under-a nutrition and infectious diseases.[1] Since 1980, the worldwide prevalence of obesity has doubled.[13] In North America, the prevalence of obesity is alarmingly high with 24.1% of Canadians and 34.4% of Americans having a body mass index (BMI) over 30 kg/m^2.[13,14] With the obesity epidemic, there has been a rise in the prevalence of obesity-related co-morbidities such as type 2 diabetes, coronary heart disease, hyperlipidemia, and hypertension.[15] In addition to increasing morbidity, obesity in and of itself leads to increased mortality by markedly lessening life expectancy.[16–18]

Although diet, exercise, and medical therapy have been attempted, bariatric surgery appears to be the only effective and durable treatment for obesity and its weight-related comorbidities.[19,20] In the Swedish Obese Subjects (SOS) trial, Sjostrom and colleagues have demonstrated that when compared to conventional therapy, bariatric surgery results in long-term weight loss, improved lifestyle, and amelioration of obesity-related comorbidities.[21] Follow-up to this prospective cohort study demonstrates that bariatric surgery not only leads to long-term weight loss and improvement of obesity-related comorbidities but also leads to decreased overall mortality.[22]

Classification of Obesity and Criteria for Surgery

BMI is an index of weight-for-height that is used to classify obesity. It is defined as weight in kilograms divided by the square of height in meters (kg/m^2). Obese individuals have a BMI over 30 kg/m^2.

Obesity is further classified into three categories; Class I obesity is defined as a BMI between 30.00 kg/m^2 and 34.99 kg/m^2, Class II obesity is defined as a BMI between 35.00 kg/m^2 and 39.99 kg/m^2, and Class III obesity is defined as a BMI over 40.00 kg/m^2.

Eligibility for bariatric surgery continues to be determined by the 1991 National Institutes of Health (NIH) consensus conference on gastrointestinal surgery for severe obesity. According to the NIH consensus, individuals are candidates for bariatric surgery if they are morbidly obese (BMI > 40 kg/m^2 or BMI > 35 kg/m^2 with obesity-related comorbidities), have failed numerous attempts at diet and exercise, are motivated and well-informed, and are free of significant psychological disease.[12]

Evolution of Bariatric Surgery

Operations to alter the gastrointestinal tract to induce weight loss have been in practice for over 60 years. Bariatric procedures are classified as purely malabsorptive, purely restrictive, or a combination of the two.

Following early animal studies by Kremen in 1954, jejunoileal bypass was introduced as one of the first procedures to address the surgical management of obesity.[13] This purely malabsorptive bariatric procedure fell out of favor due to severe complications related to bacterial overgrowth and hepatic failure.[14] In an effort to enhance the malabsorptive benefits of bariatric surgery while minimizing its complications, biliopancreatic diversion (BPD), was introduced by Scopinaro in 1979 as an alternative to jejunoileal bypass.[15] Several modifications ensued including the addition of the duodenal switch (DS) by Hess and Hess and the replacement of a distal gastrectomy with the creation of a sleeve gastrectomy by Marceau and colleagues.[16] Selected bariatric centers continue to employ BPD–DS in the surgical management of morbid obesity.

In the early 1970's, Printen and Mason introduced the gastroplasty.[17] This purely restrictive bariatric procedure was later modified to include a vertical banded gastroplasty (VBG)[18] and then ultimately developed into the laparoscopic VBG in the 1990's.[19] Due to long-term failures and high rates of revisional surgery, procedures involving gastroplasty have fallen out of favor. As an alternative to gastroplasty, Wilkinson described the use of a non-adjustable prosthetic material wrapped around the proximal stomach over a Nissen fundoplication in the early 1980's.[20] This purely restrictive procedure was later modified by Kuzmak and colleagues in the early 1990's to include the placement of an inflatable silicone gastric band.[21] In 1993, Belachew and colleagues were the first to place this silicone gastric band laparoscopically thus championing the laparoscopic adjustable gastric band (LAGB).[22] LAGB continues to be employed by selected centers in the surgical management of morbid obesity.

Mason and Ito are credited as the first to employ the gastric bypass as a surgical procedure for morbid obesity.[23] While initially utilizing a loop gastrojejunostomy and a significantly larger gastric pouch, these two surgeons were able to demonstrate the effectiveness of this bariatric procedure. Two critical modifications to the Roux-en-Y gastric bypass (RYGB) during the subsequent four decades include the replacement of a loop gastrojejunostomy with a Roux-en-Y by Griffen and colleagues[24] and the laparoscopic approach (LRYGB) championed by Wittgrove and colleagues.[25] With over 90% of bariatric procedures being performed laparoscopically, the LRYGB has emerged as the gold standard in the treatment of morbid obesity in North America.[26]

A more recent addition to the surgical management of morbid obesity is the laparoscopic sleeve gastrectomy (LSG). LSG was first developed by Marceau and colleagues as a component of BPD–DS.[16] Due to challenges associated with higher morbidity, mortality, and long-term weight loss failure in the super obese, Regan and colleagues proposed LSG as a first stage procedure in a two-stage approach to LRYGB.[27] Given the favorable outcomes of this first stage procedure, Baltasar and colleagues suggested that LSG is reasonable as a stand-alone procedure.[28] Although long-term outcomes of this bariatric procedure are not fully known, LSG remains a viable option in the surgical management of morbid obesity.

Bariatric Procedures

Laparoscopic Adjustable Gastric Band (LAGB)

LAGB involves placing an inflatable silicone band around the proximal portion of the stomach to achieve weight loss via a purely restrictive mechanism

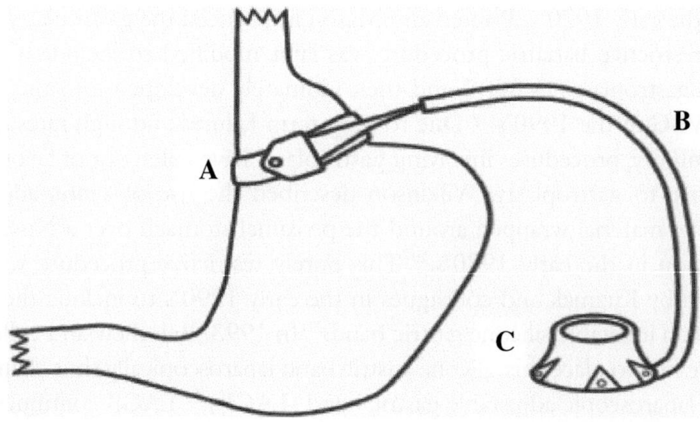

Fig. 1. LAGB.
A — Inflatable silicone band; B — Tube connecting band to port; C — External port.

(Fig. 1). This bariatric procedure is accomplished with minimal dissection. A retrogastric tunnel is created between the pars flaccida and right crus medially, and the phrenoesophageal ligament laterally. By placing a blunt instrument through this passage, the band is grasped and passed through the retrogastric tunnel. Once the band is in position, the tubing is passed through the buckle of the band and fastened. An anterior gastric tunnel is created so as to prevent band prolapse. This is achieved by placing anterior gastrogastric sutures from the greater curvature of the stomach to the lesser curvature of the stomach. Finally, the tubing is externalized and connected to an external port that is placed in the subcutaneous tissues.

Laparoscopic Sleeve Gastrectomy (LSG)

LSG involves removing the greater curvature of the stomach and fashioning a "sleeve" so as to achieve weight loss via a restrictive mechanism (Fig. 2). The gastrocolic ligament and greater omentum is separated from the greater curvature of the stomach beginning at a point approximately 3–5 cm from the pylorus. This dissection is continued proximally to the angle of His and includes division of the gastrosplenic ligament and intervening short gastric vessels. A 32– to 34– French bougie is passed down the oropharynx and esophagus and advanced along the lesser curvature of the stomach. The stomach is then divided using endoscopic linear staplers with the bougie in

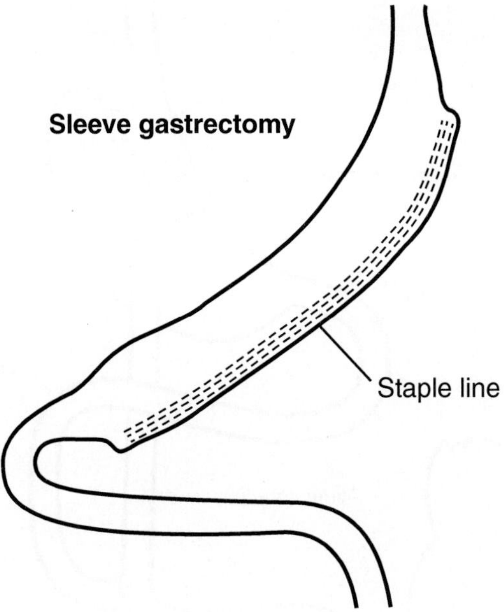

Fig. 2. LSG.
A — Gastric sleeve; B — Staple line.

place. Division of the stomach occurs from a point 3–5 cm from the pylorus and extends to the angle of His. The gastric remnant is removed from the abdomen via one of the laparoscopic trocar sites.

Laparoscopic Roux-en-Y Gastric Bypass (LRYGB)

LRYGB involves creating a small gastric pouch and two gastrointestinal anastomoses so as to achieve weight loss via a combined restrictive and malabsorptive mechanism (Fig. 3). A small gastric pouch between 15 and 30 mL fashioned around the lesser curvature of the stomach is created using endoscopic linear staplers. The proximal jejunum is divided approximately 50 cm from the ligament of Treitz (Lig. of Treitz) whereby the proximal stump is the biliopancreatic limb and the distal stump the alimentary limb. The alimentary limb is brought up to the gastric pouch and a gastrojejunostomy is created using either a linear stapler or a circular stapler. The defect created by the stapler is either oversewn intracorporally with absorbable suture or

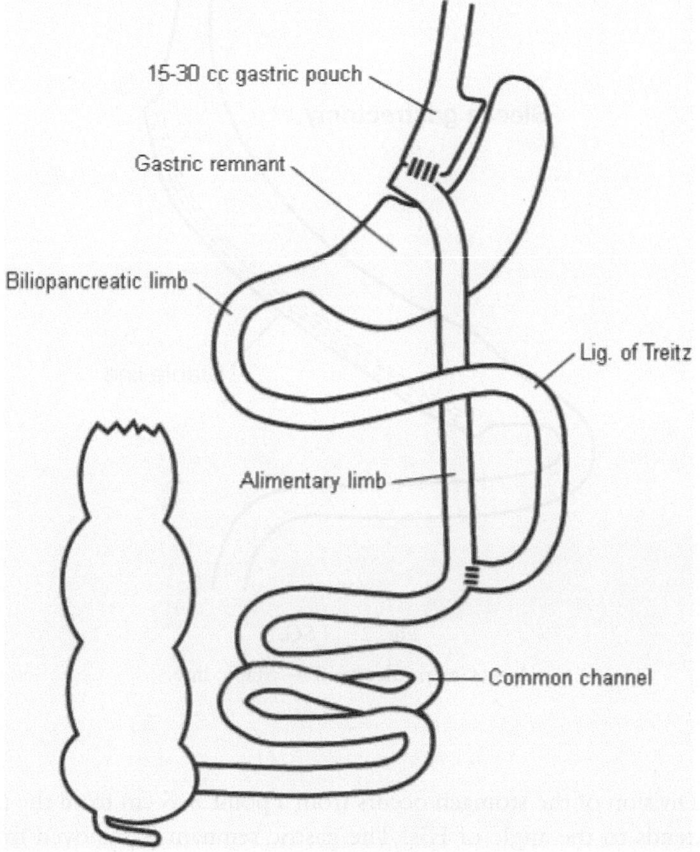

Fig. 3. LRYGB.

stapled with a linear stapler. The biliopancreatic limb is then anastomosed to the alimentary limb approximately 75–150 cm distal to gastrojejunostomy. The enteroenterostomy is created using a linear stapler. The enterostomy from the stapler is either oversewn intracorporally with absorbable suture or stapled with a linear stapler.

Outcomes

Outcomes of bariatric surgery can be measured by reduction in BMI and amelioration or resolution of obesity-related comorbidities. Two meta-analyses, one extensive evidence-based review, and one prospective, multi-institutional, observational study using the American College of Surgeons Bariatric Surgery Center Network database (ACS BSCN) provide reasonable evidence as to the effectiveness of LAGB, LSG, and LRYGB.[14,29,31]

Absolute reduction in BMI by procedure type is shown in Table 1. This table demonstrates that LSG is positioned between LRYGB and LAGB with regards to reduction in BMI.

Similar to its effectiveness in reducing BMI, LSG is positioned between LAGB and LRYGB with regards to improvement and resolution of obesity-related comorbidities. Table 2 outlines the improvement or resolution of obesity-related comorbidities for LAGB, LSG, and LRYGB.

Complications

Overall, the risk of death after bariatric surgery remains relatively low. Operative mortality for LAGB, LSG, and LRYGB is 0.05–0.4%,[29,31,32] 0.11–0.19%,[31,33] and 0.14–1.0%[29,31,34] respectively. Complications related to bariatric surgery can be broadly classified into perioperative complications, short-term complications, and long-term complications.

Table 1. Reduction in BMI.[31]

	LAGB	LSG	LRYGB
30-Day Reduction BMI (kg/m^2)	2.45	3.36	3.76
6-Month Reduction BMI (kg/m^2)	5.02	8.75	10.82
1-Year Reduction BMI (kg/m^2)	7.05	11.87	15.34

Table 2. Improvement or resolution of obesity-related comorbidities at 1-year.[31]

	LAGB	LSG	LRYGB
Diabetes Resolved or Improved (%)	44	55	83
Hypertension Resolved or Improved (%)	44	68	79
Hyperlipidemia Resolved or Improved (%)	33	35	66
Obstructive Sleep Apnea Resolved or Improved (%)	38	62	66
GERD Resolved or Improved (%)	64	50	70

Perioperative complications

Perhaps the most feared perioperative complication associated with bariatric surgery is related to anastomotic or staple line leaks. Given that there is minimal dissection and no bowel anastomoses, gastrointestinal leak is virtually non-existent with LAGB. The incidence of anastomotic or staple-line leak associated with LSG and LRYGB is approximately 0.3–5.2%.[35–43] Patients typically manifest symptoms within 48–72 hours following surgery. Anastomotic or staple line leak is a clinical diagnosis whereby patients exhibit objective signs of fever and tachycardia and subjective symptoms of abdominal pain. Once the clinical diagnosis is established, immediate arrangements should be made for laparoscopic exploration by a bariatric surgeon. At the time of surgery, the principles of surgical management include resuscitation with crystalloid fluid, source control and drainage with closed suction drains, identification of an anastomotic or staple line leak and definitive repair. If definitive repair of a leak is not feasible due to friability of the tissue, wide drainage with closed suction drains and placement of a feeding tube distal to the leak are reasonable options. If the leak is confined to the gastrojejunostomy, in addition to wide drainage, a feeding gastrostomy tube can be placed in the gastric remnant for decompression and future enteral nutrition. Nasogastric tubes may be employed to assist in drainage of the gastric pouch. These nasogastric tubes should be placed at the time of surgery rather than on the ward or the ICU due to the presence of a fresh anastomosis. Depending on their clinical status, patients may require short-course critical care observation for resuscitation and hemodynamic monitoring.

Postoperative hemorrhage is yet another major perioperative complication with potential devastating consequences. Rates of postoperative hemorrhage associated with LAGB are low given the minimal dissection and lack of anastomoses associated with this bariatric procedure. The incidence of postoperative hemorrhage associated with LSG and LRYGB is approximately 0.7–4.4%.[35,36,42–48] Similar to anastomotic or staple line leak, postoperative hemorrhage is a clinical diagnosis commonly occurring 48–72 hours following surgery. Patients typically exhibit objective signs and symptoms of tachycardia, melena, or hematemesis and subjective pre-syncopal symptoms. Bloodwork will commonly reveal a drop in hemoglobin with decreased hematocrit. Once the clinical diagnosis is made, management of the bariatric patient with postoperative hemorrhage is dictated by the patient's clinical status. Patients who remain hemodynamically stable with minimal symptoms can be managed on the ward with fluid resuscitation, cessation of anticoagulation, and serial bloodwork to monitor hemoglobin and hematocrit. Blood transfusions may be required for symptoms or hemoglobin values below 70 g/L. Patients who are hemodynamically stable with ongoing transfusion requirements may benefit from endoscopic injection of epinephrine if the source of the bleed is presumed to be from the gastrojejunostomy.[42] Emergent surgical exploration by a bariatric surgeon is necessary for any patient who is hemodynamically unstable, has significant symptoms, or has ongoing transfusion requirements where the origin of bleed is thought to be extraluminal or at the enteroenterostomy. Extraluminal bleeding, most commonly from the staple line, is best managed with laparoscopic evacuation of the hematoma, hemostatic measures such as clips, sealants, or suturing to arrest bleeding, and abdominal washout. Intraluminal bleeding at the enteroenterostomy can be more challenging to manage. In these situations, both the alimentary and biliopancreatic limbs are dilated with clot and gastric contents. The ensuing clot at the enteroenterostomy blocks the secretions of the biliopancreatic limb that in turn causes dilatation of the gastric remnant. Optimal surgical management of bleeding at the enteroenterostomy includes resuscitation of the patient with crystalloid fluid and blood products as needed, placement of a gastrostomy tube in the gastric remnant for decompression, and revision of the enteroenterostomy with subsequent evacuation of the clots located in the alimentary and biliopancreatic limbs. Similar to patients with anastomotic or staple line leaks, bariatric patients with postoperative hemorrhage may require short-course critical care observation for resuscitation and hemodynamic monitoring.

Short-term complications

Short-term complications unique to LAGB include gastric prolapse, also referred to as "band slippage", pouch dilattion, and port malfunction. These complications occur with an incidence of 1.62–31.0%, 3.9–12.0%, and 5.0–11.2% respectively.[30,32,49–56]

Gastric prolapse occurs following LAGB whereby either the anterior or posterior gastric fundus migrates cephalad through the band. Patients typically present with inability to swallow liquids and may have difficulties with their own secretions. Patients may also have episodes of emesis and associated nighttime reflux. A water-soluble upper gastrointestinal contrast study commonly depicts a mal-positioned band whereby the axis of the band is horizontal. Initial management of patients presenting with gastric prolapse in the setting of LAGB include fluid resuscitation and removal of fluid via the port using a blunt-tipped Huber needle. Laparoscopic surgical exploration by a bariatric surgeon is usually necessary for band repositioning or removal.

Pouch dilattion occurs when the portion of the stomach proximal to the band concentrically dilates. Patients typically present with frequent heartburn and reflux. A water-soluble upper gastrointestinal contrast study demonstrates a concentric enlargement of the stomach proximal to the band without a change in the band axis. Unlike gastric prolapse that commonly requires surgical intervention, management of pouch dilattion involves removal of fluid via the port using a blunt-tipped Huber needle and institution of a clear fluid diet. Patients should be instructed to follow-up with their bariatric centre for monitored re-inflation of the band following repeat water-soluble upper gastrointestinal contrast studies.

Port malfunctions include a myriad of complications ranging from port site infections to tube disruption and leakage, to port rotation. Port infections are the most serious complication associated with port malfunctions. Patients typically present with fever and erythema over the port site. If severe, patients may have clinical symptoms of peritonitis. Patients with port infections require emergent laparoscopic exploration by a bariatric surgeon. The band, tubing, and port should be removed and sent for culture and sensitivity. At the time of surgery, the stomach should be tested to rule out a gastrointestinal leak.

Anastomotic stricture at the gastrojejunostomy is one of the most common short-term complications following LRYGB. The incidence of stricturing at the proximal anastomosis is approximately 1.42–15.7%.[30,31,43,57–60] This incidence is affected by the method used for creation of the gastrojejunostomy. Patients typically present with an inability to tolerate solids and symptoms of retrosternal chest pain with meals that is relieved by vomiting. A water-soluble upper gastrointestinal contrast study may demonstrate stenosis at the gastrojejunostomy. Esophagogastroduodenoscopy (EGD) is both diagnostic and therapeutic. Patients should undergo endoscopy by an endoscopist who is familiar with bariatric surgical procedures. Dilation, either via pneumatic dilation or Savary–Gilliard bougies, is often effective. Repeat dilations may be required in certain circumstances.

In addition to anastomotic strictures, marginal ulceration at the gastrojejunostomy is another common short-term complication following LRYGB. The incidence of marginal ulceration is approximately 0.47–12.3%.[31,43,61–65] Certain factors such as NSAIDs, tobacco, *H. pylori*, infection, alcohol, foreign body reaction from staples or non-absorable sutures, or gastrogastric fistulas predispose patients to marginal ulceration post LRYGB.

Patients typically present with symptoms of pain, nausea, and dysphagia all of which are aggravated by eating. EGD by an endoscopist who is familiar with bariatric surgical procedures is used to confirm the diagnosis of marginal ulceration; a water-soluble upper gastrointestinal contrast may be helpful in ruling out additional pathology such as gastrogastric fistula but does little in way of diagnosis of marginal ulceration. Management of marginal ulceration includes limiting aggravating factors, ruling out *H. pylori* infection, and treatment with proton pump inhibitors and sucralfate. Repeat endoscopy may be helpful to evaluate treatment success or failure. Recalcitrant marginal ulcers may require revisional surgery by an experienced bariatric surgeon once aggravating factors have been eliminated and maximal medical therapy is fully exhausted.

Long-term complications

Perhaps the most dreaded complication of LAGB is band erosion. The incidence of band erosion is approximately 0.6–6.8%.[49,51,54,56] Patients typically present with weight regain despite adequate fluid adjustments. Alternatively, patients may present with a chronic port site infection. Although a water-soluble upper gastrointestinal contrast study may demonstrate band erosion, EGD provides definitive diagnosis. Once band erosion has been confirmed, patients should undergo laparoscopic exploration by a bariatric surgeon. The principles of surgical management include resuscitation with crystalloid fluid, source control and removal of the gastric band, localization of the gastric erosion and closure if feasible, and wide drainage with closed suction drains. If definitive repair of the gastric erosion is not feasible, placement of closed suction drains and a distal feeding tube for enteral nutrition is a reasonable option. Depending on their clinical status, patients may require short-course critical care observation for resuscitation and hemodynamic monitoring.

Intestinal obstruction is a long-term complication following any intra-abdominal surgery. Unique to LRYGB is the creation of potential spaces whereby small bowel can herniate leading to internal hernias. The overall incidence of intestinal obstruction due to internal hernia following LRYGB is approximately 0.84–2.54%.[66–71] Patients with an internal hernia typically present with a history of intermittent, vague abdominal pain. In situations where there is acute bowel obstruction with ischemic bowel, patients may present with clinical signs and symptoms of fever, tachycardia, and peritonitis. Computed tomography (CT) may reveal characteristic radiographic findings such as a mesenteric swirl[72] (Fig. 4).

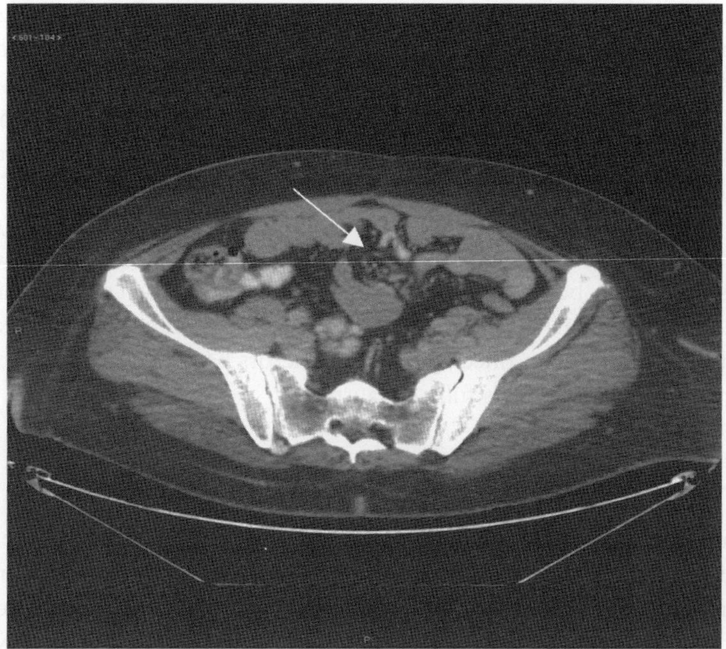

Fig. 4. Internal hernia — tip of arrow shows swirl through mesenteric defect.

If a CT scan is ordered in the work-up of a bariatric patient with suspected internal hernia, the volume of oral contrast required for post-bariatric surgery patients is less than that required for regular oral contrast protocols. Regardless of CT findings, any bariatric patient post LRYGB with a clinical history suspicious for internal hernia or signs and symptoms suggestive of acute bowel incarceration should undergo laparoscopic exploration by a bariatric surgeon. Internal hernias can occur at the enteroenterostomy mesenteric defect or between the alimentary limb and transverse mesocolon, a space commonly referred to as Peterson's space. Once the internal hernia has been reduced, the mesenteric defects should be closed so as to prevent future obstruction. Patients with compromised bowel in the setting of an internal hernia may require short-course critical care observation for resuscitation and hemodynamic monitoring especially if bowel resection was needed.

Aside from bowel obstructions, long-term complications of bariatric surgery are primarily associated with malasborptive procedures and revolve around macronutrient deficiencies such as protein-calorie malnutrition and fat malabsorption and micronutrient deficiencies such as vitamin B12, iron, folate, calcium, and thiamine.[84] Correction of these nutritional deficiencies requires involvement of a nutritionist and gastroenterologist as part of the management team.

Summary

Obesity and obesity-related comorbidities are a leading public health challenge. Bariatric surgery remains the only effective and durable treatment for obesity and its weight-related comorbidities. LAGB, LSG, and LRYGB are three common bariatric surgical procedures performed in North America. Although the complication rate of these bariatric procedures is relatively low, patients undergoing LAGB, LSG, or LRYGB may experience perioperative, short-term, or long-term complications that necessitate short-course critical care observation for resuscitation and hemodynamic monitoring. An understanding of the basic principles of bariatric surgery and the unique challenges of the morbidly obese patient as discussed in this chapter will assist the intensivist in managing these patients when admitted to the ICU. Optimal care of the bariatric patient incorporates a multidisciplinary approach involving the bariatric surgeon, intensivist, endocrinologist, psychiatrist, dietitian, and nursing staff.

References

1. World Health Organization (WHO). Obesity: Preventing and managing the global epidemic. *World Health Organ Tech Rep Ser* 2000; 894(i–xii): 1–253.
2. Sjostrom L, Lendroos A, Peltonen M *et al.* Lifestyle, diabetes and cardiovascular risk factors 10 years after bariatric surgery. *N Eng J Med* 2004; 351(26): 2683–2693.
3. Shirmer B, Jones DB. The American college of surgeons bariatric surgery center network: Establishing standards. *Bull Am Coll Surg* 2007; 92(8): 21–27.
4. Levita RM, Mechem CC, Ochroch EA, Shofer FS, Hollander JE. Head-elevated laryngoscopy position: Improving laryngeal exposure during laryngoscopy by increasing head elevation. *Ann Emerg Med.* 2003; 41(3): 322–330.
5. Ramachandran SK, Cosnowski A, Shanks A, Turner CR. Apneic oxygenation during prolonged laryngoscopy in obese patients: A randomized, controlled atrial of nasal oxygenation administration. *J Clin Anesth* 2010; 22(3): 164–168.
6. Malo J, Ali J, Wood LDH. How does positive end expiratory pressure reduce intra-pulmonary shunt in canine pulmonary edema. *J Appl Physiol* 1984; 57(4): 1002–1010.

7. Perili V, Sollazi L, Modesti C *et al.* Comparison of positive end-expiratory pressure with reverse Trendelenburg position in morbidly obese patients undergoing bariatric surgery: Effects on hemodynamics and pulmonary gas exchange. *Obes Surg* 2003; 13(4): 605–609.
8. Gross JB, Bachenberg KL, Benumof JL *et al.* American Society of Anesthesiologists Task Force on Perioperative Management Practice guidelines for the perioperative management of patients with obstructive sleep apnea: A report by the American Society of Anesthesiologists Task Force on Perioperative Management of patients with obstructive sleep apnea. *Anesthesiology* 2006; 104(5): 1081–1093. Quiz 1117–1118.
9. Frumin MJ, Epstein RM, Cohen G. Apneic oxygenation in man. *Anesthesiology* 1959; 20: 789–798.
10. Ingrande J, Lemmens HJ. Dose adjustment of anesthetics in the morbidly obese. *British Journal of Anaesth* 2010; 105(Supplement): i16–i23.
11. Nguyen NT, Anderson JT, Budd M *et al.* Effects of pneumoperitoneum on intraoperative pulmonary mechanics and gas exchange during laparoscopic gastric bypass. *Surg Endosc* 2004; 18(18)(1): 64–71.
12. Nguyen NT, Wolfe BM. The physiologic effects of pneumoperitoneum in the morbidly obese. *Ann Surg* 2005; 241(2): 219–226.
13. Obesity and overweight. World Health Organization. Available online http://www.who.int/mediacentre/factsheets/fs311/en/index.html [accessed on December 27th, 2013].
14. Shields M, Carroll M, Odgen C. Adult obesity prevalence in Canada and the United States. *NCHS Data Brief* No 56, 2011; 56: 1–8.
15. Must A, Spadano J, Coakley EH *et al.* The disease burden associated with overweight and obesity. *JAMA* 1999; 282(16): 1523–1529.
16. Manson JE, Walter MD, Willett MD *et al.* Body weight and mortality among women. *N Engl J Med* 1995; 333: 677–685.
17. Calle EE, Thun MJ, Petrelli JM *et al.* Body-mass index and mortality in a prospective cohort of U.S. adults. *N Engl J Med* 1999; 341: 1097–1105.
18. Fontaine KR, Redden DT, Wang C *et al.* Years of life lost due to obesity. *JAMA* 2003; 289: 187–193.
19. Buchwald H, Avidor Y, Braunwald E *et al.* Bariatric surgery: A systematic review and meta-analysis. *JAMA* 2004; 292(14): 1724–1737.
20. Steinbrook R. Surgery for severe obesity. *N Engl J Med* 2004; 350: 1075–1079.
21. Sjostrom L, Lindroos AK, Peltonen M *et al.* Lifestyle, diabetes, and cardiovascular risk factors 10 years after baritaric surgery. *N Engl J Med* 2004; 351: 2683–2693.
22. Sjostrom L, Narbro K, Sjostrom D *et al.* Effects of bariatric surgery on mortality in Swedish obese subjects. *N Engl J Med* 2007; 357: 741–752.
23. Consensus Development Conference Panel. Gastrointestinal surgery for severe obesity: Consensus development conference statement. *Ann Intern Med* 1991; 115: 956–961.

24. Kremen AJ, Linner LH, Nelson CH. An experimental evaluation of the nutritional importance of proximal and distal small intestine. *Ann Surg* 1954; 140: 439–448.
25. Buchwald H, Rucker RD (1987) The rise and fall of jejunoileal bypass. In: Nelson RL, Nyhus LM (eds.) Surgery of the small intestine. Appleton Century Crofts, Norwalk, CT, pp. 529–541.
26. Hess DS, Hess DW. Biliopancreatic diversion with duodenal switch. *Obes Surg* 1988; 8: 267–282.
27. Marceau P, Biron S, Bourque RA *et al.* Biliopancreatic diversion with a new type of gastrectomy. *Obes Surg* 1993; 3: 29–35.
28. Printen KJ, Mason EE. Gastric surgery for relief of morbid obesity. *Arch Surg* 1973; 106: 428–431.
29. Mason EE. Vertical banded gastroplasty for obesity. *Arch Surg* 1982; 117: 701–706.
30. Chua TY, Mendiola RM. Laparoscopic vertical banded gastroplasty: The Milwaukee experience. *Obes Surg* 1995; 5: 77–80.
31. Wilkinson LH, Peoloso OA. Gastric (reservoir) reduction for morbid obesity. *Arch Surg* 1981; 116: 602–605.
32. Kuzmak LI, Yap IS, McGuire L *et al.* Surgery for morbid obesity: Using an inflatable gastric band. *AORN J* 1990; 51: 1307–1324.
33. Belachew M, Legrand MJ, Defechereux TH *et al.* Laparoscopic adjustable silicone gastric banding in the treatment of morbid obesity. *Surg Endosc* 1994; 8: 1354–1356.
34. Mason EE, Ito C. Gastric bypass in obesity. *Surg Clin North Am* 1967; 47: 1345–1352.
35. Griffen WO, Young VL, Stevenson CC. A prospective comparison of gastric and jejunoileal bypass procedures for morbid obesity. *Ann Surg* 1977; 186(4): 500–507.
36. Wittgrove AC, Clark GW, Tremblay LF. Laparoscopic gastric bypass, Roux-en-Y: Preliminary report of five cases. *Obes Surg* 1994; 4: 353–357.
37. Buchwald H, Oien DM. Metabolic/bariatric surgery worldwide 2008. *Obes Surg* 2009; 19: 1605–1611.
38. Regan JP, Inabnet WB, Gagner M *et al.* Early experience with two-stage laparoscopic Roux-en-Y gastric bypass as an alternative in the super-super obese patient. *Obes Surg* 2003; 13: 861–864.
39. Baltasar A, Serra C, Perez N *et al.* A Multi-purpose bariatric operation. *Obes Surg* 2005 15: 1124–1128.
40. Maggard MA, Shugarman LR, Suttorp M *et al.* Meta-analysis: Surgical treatment of obesity. *Ann Intern Med* 2005; 142: 547–559.
41. Farrell TM, Haggerty SP, Overby DW. Clinical application of laparoscopic bariatric surgery: An evidence-based review. *Surg Endosc* 2009; 23: 930–949.
42. Hutter MM, Schirmer BD, Jones DB *et al.* First report from the American college of surgeons bariatric center network: Laparoscopic sleeve gastrectomy has morbidity and effectiveness between the band and the bypass. *Ann Surg* 2011 254: 410–422.

43. Chapman AAE, Kiroff G, Game P. Laparoscopic adjustable gastric banding in the treatment of obesity: A systematic literatures review. *Surgery* 2004; 135: 326–351.
44. Brethauer SA, Hammel JP, Schauer PR. Systematic review of sleeve gastrectomy as staging and primary bariatric procedure. *Surg Obes Relat Dis* 2009; 5: 469–475.
45. The Longitudinal Assessment of Bariatric (LABS) Consortium. Perioperative Safety in the Longitudinal Assessment of Bariatric Surgery. *N Engl J Med* 2009; 361: 445–454.
46. Himpens J, Dobbeleir J, Peeters G. Long-term results of laparoscopic sleeve gastrectomy. *Ann Surg* 2010; 252(2): 319–324.
47. Weiner RA, El-Sayes IS, Theodoridou S *et al.* Early postoperative complications: Incidence, management and impact on length of hospital stay. A retrospective comparison between laparoscopic gastric bypass and sleeve gastrectomy. *Obes Surg* 2013; 23: 2004–2012.
48. Ballesta C, Berindoague R, Cabrera M *et al.* Management of anastomotic leaks after laparoscopic Roux-en-Y gastric bypass. *Obes Surg* 2008; 18: 623–630.
49. Bellorin O, Adbemur A, Sucandy I *et al.* Understanding the significance, reasons and patterns of abnormal vital signs after gastric bypass for morbid obesity. *Obes Surg* 2011; 21: 707–713.
50. Fullum TM, Aluka KJ, Turner PL. Decreasing anastomotic and staple line leaks after laparoscopic Roux-en-Y gastric bypass. *Surg Endosc* 2009; 23(6): 1403–1408.
51. Gonzalez R, Haines K, Gallagher SF *et al.* Does experience preclude leaks in laparoscopic gastric bypass? *Surg Endosc* 2006; 20: 1687–1692.
52. Marshall JS, Srivastava A, Gupta SK *et al.* Roux-en-Y gastric bypass leak complications. *Arch Surg* 2003; 138: 520–524.
53. Papasavas PK, Caushaj PF, McCormick JT *et al.* Laparoscopic management of complications following laparoscopic Roux-en-Y gastric bypass for morbid obesity. *Surg Endosc* 2003; 17: 610–614.
54. Schauer PR, Ikramuddin S, Gourash W *et al.* Outcomes After Laparoscopic Roux-en-Y Gastric Bypass for Morbid Obesity. *Ann Surg* 2000; 232: 515–529.
55. Bakhos C, Alkhoury F, Kyriakides T *et al.* Early postoperative hemorrhage after open and laparoscopic Roux-en-Y gastric bypass. *Obes Surg* 2009; 19: 153–157.
56. Dick A, Byrne TK, Baker M *et al.* Gastrointestinal bleeding after gastric bypass surgery: nuisance or catastrophe? *Surg Obes Relat Dis* 2010; 6: 643–647.
57. Mehran A, Szomstein S, Zundel N *et al.* management of acute bleeding after laparoscopic Roux-en-Y gastric bypass. *Obes Surg* 2003; 13: 842–847.
58. Nguyen NT, Rivers R, Wolfe BM. Early gastrointestinal hemorrhage after laparoscopic gastric bypass. *Obes Surg* 2003; 13: 62–65.
59. Rabl C, Peeva S, Prado KI. Early and late abdominal bleeding after Roux-en-Y gastric bypass: Sources and tailored therapeutic strategies. *Obes Surg* 2011; 21: 413–420.

60. Bsoschi S, Fogli L, Berta RD *et al.* Avoiding complications after laparoscopic esophago-gastric banding: Experience with 400 consecutive patients. *Obes Surg* 2006; 16: 1166–1170.
61. Chevalier JM, Zinzindohoue F, Douard R *et al.* Complications after laparoscopic adjustable gastric banding for morbid obesity: Experience with 1000 patients over 7 years. *Obes Surg* 2004; 14: 407–414.
62. Favretti F, Segato G, Ashton D *et al.* Laparoscopic adjustable gastric banding in 1791 consecutive obese patients: 12-year results. *Obes Surg* 2007; 17: 168–175.
63. Lyass S, Cunneen SA, Hagiike M *et al.* Device-related reoperations after laparosopic adjustable gastric banding. *Am Surg* 2005; 71(9): 738–743.
64. Moser F, Gorodner MV, Galvani A *et al.* Pouch enlargement and band slippage: Two different entities. *Surg Endosc* 2006; 20: 1021–1029.
65. O'Brien PE, Dixon JB. Laparoscopic adjustable gastric banding in the treatment of morbid obesity. *Arch Surg* 2003; 138: 376–382.
66. Singhal R, Bryant C, Kitchen M *et al.* Band slippage and erosion after laparoscopic gastric banding: A meta-analysis. *Surg Endosc* 2010; 24: 2980–2986.
67. Suter M, Giusti V, Heraief E *et al.* Band erosion after laparoscopic gastric banding: Occurrence and results after conversion to Roux-en-Y gastric bypass. *Obesity Surgery* 2004; 14: 381–386.
68. Escalona A, Devaud N, Boza C *et al.* Gastrojejunal anastomotic stricture after Roux-en-Y gastric bypass: Ambulatory management with the Savary–Gilliard dilator. *Surg Endosc* 2007; 21: 765–768.
69. Goitein D, Papasavas PK, Gagne D *et al.* Gastrojejunal strictures following laparoscopic Roux-en-Y gastric bypass for morbid obesity. *Surg Endosc* 2005; 19: 628–632.
70. Nguyen NT, Stevens CM, Wolfe BM. Incidence and outcome of anastomotic stricture after laparoscopic gastric bypass. *J Gastrointest Surg* 2003; 7: 997–1003.
71. Takata MC, Ciovica R, Cello JP *et al.* Predictors, treatment, and outcomes of gastrojejunostomy stricture after gastric bypass for morbid obesity. *Obes Surg* 2007; 17: 878–884.
72. Csendes A, Burgos AM, Altuve J *et al.* Incidence of marginal ulcer 1 month and 1 to 2 years after gastric bypass: A prospective consecutive endoscopic evaluation of 442 patients with morbid obesity. *Obes Surg* 2009; 19: 135–138.
73. Gumbs AA, Duffy AJ, Bell RL. Incidence and management of marginal ulceration after laparoscopic Roux-Y gastric bypass. *Surg Obes Relat Dis* 2006; 2: 460–463.
74. Rasmussen JJ, Fuller W, Ali MR. Marginal ulceration after laparoscopic gastric bypass: An analysis of predisposing factors in 260 patients. *Surg Endosc* 2007; 21: 1090–1094.
75. Sacks BC, Mattar SG, Qureshi FG *et al.* Incidence of marginal ulcers and the use of absorbable anastomotic sutures in laparoscopic Roux-en-Y gastric bypass. *Surg Obes Relat Dis* 2006; 2: 11–16.

76. Schrimer B, Erenoglu C, Miller A. Flexible endoscopy in the management of patients undergoing Roux-en-Y gastric bypass. *Obes Surg* 2002; 12: 634–638.
77. Carmody B, DeMaria EJ, Jamal M *et al.* Internal hernia after laparoscopic Roux-en-Y gastric bypass. *Surg Obes Relat Dis* 2005; 1: 543–548.
78. Champion JK, Williams M. Small bowel obstruction and internal hernias after laparoscopic Roux-en-Y gastric bypass. *Obes Surg* 2003; 13: 596–600.
79. Hwang RF, Swartz DE, Felix EL. Causes of small bowel obstruction after laparoscopic bypass. *Surg Endosc* 2004; 18: 1631–1635.
80. Iannelli A, Facchiano E, Gugenheim J. Internal hernia after laparoscopic Roux-en-Y gastric bypass for morbid obesity. *Obes Surg* 2006; 1265–1271.
81. Nelson LG, Gonzalez R, Haines K *et al.* Spectrum and treatment of small bowel obstruction after Roux-en-Y gastric bypass. *Surg Obes Relat Dis* 2006; 2: 377–383.
82. Nguyen NT, Huerta S, Gelfand D *et al.* Bowel obstruction after laparoscopic Roux-en-Y gastric bypass. *Obes Surg* 2004; 190–196.
83. Lockhart ME, Tessler FN, Canon CL *et al.* Internal hernia after gastric bypass: Sensitivity and specificity of seven CT signs with surgical correlation and controls. *AJR* 2007; 188(3): 745–750.
84. Malinowski SS. Nutritional and metabolic complications of bariatric surgery. *Am J Med Sci* 2006; 331(4): 219–225.

Chapter 33

The Transplant Patient

Andrew S. Barbas and Anand Ghanekar

Chapter Overview

Perioperative critical care of the transplant recipient can be challenging, with multiple considerations across several organ systems that require management simultaneously. The principles of managing organ transplant recipients specifically include optimizing hemodynamic and metabolic parameters to ensure satisfactory graft perfusion, monitoring graft function and managing graft dysfunction, and preventing or managing potential complications of the underlying disease, transplant surgery and immunosuppression. This chapter will focus primarily on critical care of the liver transplant recipient, as these patients are the most commonly encountered transplant recipients in a typical surgical intensive care unit (ICU) and serve to illustrate many important considerations typical of recipients of other types of solid organ transplants.

As a field, liver transplantation has progressed dramatically since its origin in the 1960s. Advances in surgical technique, anesthetic management, perioperative critical care, and immunosuppression have led to consistently safe performance of liver transplantation in the modern era.

Currently over 20,000 liver transplants are performed annually worldwide for a variety of indications. The perioperative mortality in experienced centers is less than 5%, with expected 1 year and 5 year survival of 90% and 75%, respectively. The primary indications for liver transplantation are decompensated liver disease with an expected survival of less than one year, or hepatocellular carcinoma limited to the liver. Contraindications for liver transplantation include severe cardiopulmonary disease, active sepsis, and extrahepatic malignancy.

General considerations in the preoperative transplant evaluation include general medical condition, nutritional status, and psychosocial factors. The evaluation process is carried out by a multidisciplinary team including physicians, nurses, social workers, and other allied health professionals. In North America, patients are prioritized for liver transplantation by Model for End-Stage Liver Disease (MELD) score, a calculated score ranging from 6–40 based on bilirubin, international normalized ratio (INR), and creatinine that is predictive of 3 month waitlist mortality.

Patients with end-stage liver disease on the transplant waitlist frequently have derangements in multiple organ systems that must be managed simultaneously in the perioperative period. In the following discussion, we will approach the pertinent considerations for ICU care of the liver transplant patient using an organ system-based structure.

Neurologic

Several neurologic issues may affect liver transplant patients. Perhaps the most important is hepatic encephalopathy. Prior to transplantation, hepatic encephalopathy is common, with nearly 50% of cirrhotic patients displaying some degree of impairment. The degree of encephalopathy is graded on a scale from 1–4 (Table 1). The biochemical mechanisms responsible for the development of hepatic encephalopathy are not fully elucidated, but it is hypothesized that the failing liver is unable to appropriately clear ammonia and other metabolic byproducts that alter neurotransmitter activity in the brain. Hepatic encephalopathy is often triggered by specific events, such as the development of an infection, gastrointestinal (GI) bleed, or placement of transjugular intrahepatic portosystemic shunt (TIPS).[3] Closely related to hepatic encephalopathy is the development of cerebral edema, almost

Table 1. Severity of hepatic encephalopathy.

Grade	Clinical manifestations
1	Changes in behavior, mild confusion, slurred speech, disordered sleep
2	Lethargy, moderate confusion
3	Marked confusion (stupor), incoherent speech, sleeping but arousable
4	Coma, unresponsive to painful stimuli

exclusively seen in the setting of acute liver failure with high grade encephalopathy (grade 3–4). Ammonia and other chemical mediators are associated with neuronal and astrocyte swelling, contributing to the development of cerebral edema.[1] Additionally, the failure of cerebral blood flow autoregulation mechanisms may contribute to the pathogenesis. In its most severe form, cerebral edema ultimately progresses to coma, brainstem herniation, and death.

The treatment of mild hepatic encephalopathy includes reduction of dietary protein intake in order to limit the generation of ammonia and metabolic byproducts, administration of lactulose to acidify GI tract contents and reduce GI absorption of ammonia, and treatment with rifaximin targeting gut bacteria that produce ammonia. In severe (grade 3 or 4 hepatic encephalopathy) with associated cerebral edema, treatment strategies aimed at managing elevated intracranial pressure (ICP) are also necessary. The central principle in managing patients with elevated ICP is maintenance of adequate cerebral perfusion pressure (CPP). Cerebral perfusion pressure is calculated as the difference between mean arterial pressure (MAP) and ICP (CPP = MAP – ICP). Goals of treatment are to maintain CPP at 60–70 mmHg. Several interventions can be used to optimize CPP. Generally, patients in this state require intubation and mechanical ventilation to secure their airway and ensure appropriate gas exchange. Maneuvers to reduce elevated ICP include elevation of the head of bed to 30°, hyperventilation to achieve a PCO_2 of 35 mmHg (temporary measure), and administration of mannitol and hypertonic saline to draw interstitial fluid from the brain. In severe cases, invasive ICP monitoring may be necessary, which also may allow drainage of cerebrospinal fluid to lower ICP.[6]

Postoperatively, normal graft function is expected to facilitate rapid recovery of pre-existing hepatic encephalopathy. Close attention must be paid to the recipient's mental status, as failure of normalization can be indicative of impaired graft function. Additionally, patients recovering in the ICU following liver transplantation are also vulnerable to the common postoperative neurologic issues that affect the entire ICU population such as delirium and critical illness polyneuropathy. Treatments for these conditions are similar to those employed for non-transplant patients and discussed elsewhere in this text. A unique consideration in post-transplant patients is the potential for Central Nervous System (CNS) side effects of calcineurin inhibitors. Although, tacrolimus is more commonly used in the current era, both cyclosporine and tacrolimus have several potential associated neurotoxicities. Symptoms can include the development of tremors, headaches, seizures, focal neurologic deficits, and in rare cases the development of posterior reversible encephalopathy syndrome (PRES).[4] PRES is characterized by a constellation of symptoms that include severe headache, altered level of consciousness, visual disturbances, and seizures. Neuro-imaging typically demonstrates findings of symmetrical white matter edema in the posterior cerebral hemispheres, particularly the parietal and occipital lobes. Neurologic side effects from calcineurin inhibitors can generally be ameliorated by dose reduction or the substitution of alternative agents.

Cardiovascular

Liver transplantation imparts a significant physiological stress on the cardiovascular system. In general, patients are only activated on the transplant waitlist after undergoing careful preoperative assessment of their cardiac function, including cardiac catheterization if necessary. Severe underlying cardiovascular pathologies such as extensive coronary artery disease, valvular abnormalities, and congestive heart failure are absolute contraindications to proceeding with liver transplantation. Despite careful preoperative evaluation, occult cardiac abnormalities may be unmasked by the significant physiologic stress associated with liver transplantation. From an abdominal surgery perspective, there are few procedures as physiologically taxing as liver transplantation. Operations are commonly long in duration with significant blood loss. Additionally, in the classic surgical technique, the inferior vena cava (IVC) is fully clamped in the anhepatic phase, and cardiac preload is completely dependent on venous return from the upper body. Many patients require significant vasopressor support and fluid administration to maintain adequate blood pressure during this period. Another particularly challenging phase of the operation from a physiologic perspective occurs during reperfusion of the transplanted liver. Following completion of the IVC and portal vein anastomoses, these vessels are unclamped and the transplanted liver is reperfused. This imparts a sudden increase in venous return to the right heart, and the initial blood return is significantly cooler than body temperature and rich in potassium and lactate from the preservation solution. The sudden bolus of cold, potassium rich blood can lead to acute right heart dysfunction and potentially lethal arrythmias. Extreme vigilance on the part of the anesthesia and surgical teams is critical during this phase of the operation. These significant physiologic demands can also induce cardiac ischemia and subsequent myocardial infarction.

Large volume shifts and third spacing of fluids is typical in the early postoperative period, and aggressive fluid resuscitation is frequently necessary to maintain sufficient circulating volume and graft perfusion. When possible, rapid weaning of vasopressor agents is important to reduce the risk of hepatic artery thrombosis. While significant fluid administration is commonly required early, as recovery progresses, careful attention should be paid to avoid volume overload with elevations of central venous pressure, which may lead to liver congestion and graft dysfunction. Maintenance of electrolyte equilibrium and euvolemia are also essential for avoiding the development of atrial fibrillation. These considerations become even more important considering the increasingly elderly patient population undergoing liver transplantation.

In addition to the physiologic stress of the procedure itself, there are specific pathophysiologic changes from end stage liver disease and cirrhosis that affect the cardiovascular system and have implications for postoperative management. Patients with advanced liver disease and cirrhosis commonly exhibit decreased systemic vascular resistance (SVR) secondary to neurohormonal changes affecting the central, splanchnic, and peripheral vascular beds. Consequently, cirrhotic patients frequently exhibit a lower baseline mean arterial pressure, which should be taken into account when managing vasoactive medications in this population. The decreased SVR induces hyperdynamic circulatory physiology, and management of this high cardiac output state may require invasive monitoring including pulmonary artery catheterization. Additionally, approximately 50% of cirrhotic patients exhibit a constellation of abnormalities in cardiac function collectively termed cirrhotic cardiomyopathy. This is characterized by systolic dysfunction and abnormal diastolic relaxation, exacerbated during times of physiologic stress. Additional features include prolongation of the QT interval and elevated brain natriuretic peptide (BNP). The mechanisms underlying this phenomenon are related to altered function of ion channels and beta adrenergic receptors as well as alterations in myocyte morphology and function.[5,13] In addition, the specific disease process that has led to liver failure may also have systemic manifestations which include cardiovascular pathology. Wilson's disease, hemochromatosis, amyloidosis, and alcoholic cirrhosis are all characterized by concomitant non-ischemic cardiomyopathy which must be carefully managed in the perioperative period.

Pulmonary

There are several important pulmonary considerations relevant to postoperative care of the liver transplant recipient. Co-existing pulmonary pathology is common in patients with liver disease and ranges in severity from relatively benign to life threatening. Patients with large volume ascites from portal hypertension also commonly have accompanying pleural effusions, also known as hepatic hydrothorax. This is generally caused by the translocation of ascites from the abdomen into the chest through pores in the diaphragm. If pleural effusions reach sufficient size they may impair pulmonary function and require drainage in the perioperative setting.

Patients with advanced cirrhosis are also at risk for the development of specific abnormalities in the pulmonary circulation due to the systemic neurohormonal derangements affecting the vasculature throughout the body. **Hepatopulmonary syndrome** is characterized by abnormal dilatation of pulmonary capillary beds, leading to intrapulmonary shunting and subsequent hypoxemia, and can be found in up to 30% of patients undergoing liver transplantation. This may also be accompanied by the development of direct arteriovenous communications within in the lung, which further contribute to hypoxemia. Overproduction of pulmonary nitric oxide is thought to be an important contributor to the pathophysiology, although the mechanisms are not fully elucidated. Clinical manifestations of hepatopulmonary syndrome may include dyspnea on exertion or at rest, digital clubbing, and orthodeoxia: The drop in partial pressure of oxygen (PO_2) in arterial blood when changing positions from supine to upright. The primary diagnostic study to help establish the diagnosis is transthoracic echocardiography (ECHO) with micro-bubble examination. In this study, agitated saline with microbubbles is administered through a peripheral vein, and the appearance of these bubbles in the left heart after 3–6 beats is indicative of a right to left shunt through abnormally dilated pulmonary capillaries. The severity of hepatopulmonary syndrome is characterized on a range from mild to very severe, based on the partial pressure of oxygen in arterial blood gas (Table 2). There are no effective medical therapies to reverse this phenomenon preoperatively, and management consists primarily of supportive care and administration of oxygen. Fortunately, liver transplantation frequently leads to resolution over weeks to months.[9]

Portopulmonary hypertension is another important derangement in pulmonary circulation associated with liver disease, although the pathophysiology differs significantly from hepatopulmonary syndrome. Portopulmonary hypertension is characterized by increased pulmonary vascular resistance and elevated pulmonary artery pressure in the setting of portal hypertension. It is formally defined by a mean pulmonary arterial pressure ≥ 25 mmHg,

Table 2. Clinical features and grading of hepatopulmonary syndrome and portopulmonary hypertension.

	Hepatopulmonary syndrome	**Portopulmonary hypertension**
Distinguishing features	Abnormal dilatation of pulmonary capillaries and right to left AV shunting	Increased pulmonary artery pressure and pulmonary vascular resistance
Grade	Mild: $PO_2 \geq 80$ mmHg Moderate: PO_2 60–80 mmHg Severe: PO_2 50–60 mmHg Very severe: $PO_2 < 50$ mmHg	Mild: MPAP 25–35 mmHg Moderate: MPAP 35–45 mmHg Severe: MPAP ≥ 45 mmHg

pulmonary vascular resistance > 240 dyn-sec-cm^{-5}, and pulmonary capillary wedge pressure < 15 mmHg. It is a relatively rare complication, affecting 6–8% of cirrhotic patients, and does not seem to be related to the etiology or severity of the underlying liver disease. Portopulmonary hypertension is categorized as mild, moderate, or severe based on the mean pulmonary artery pressure by right heart catheterization (Table 2). The biologic mechanisms contributing to portopulmonary hypertension have not been fully elucidated but the development is thought to be related to aberrations of circulatory mediators and cytokines including endothelin-1 and IL-6. Clinical manifestation ranges from completely asymptomatic to dyspnea on exertion, and screening echocardiography generally demonstrates an elevated right ventricular systolic pressure. Formal diagnosis requires right heart catheterization to measure mean pulmonary artery pressure and pulmonary vascular resistance. Liver transplantation is considered unsafe in patients with moderate and severe portopulmonary hypertension due to prohibitively high morbidity and mortality rates. The goal of medical management of these patients is to reduce pulmonary artery pressure to a safe range. Many agents have demonstrated efficacy in improving pulmonary artery pressures including inhaled or infusional prostaglandin therapy, phosphodiesterase inhibitors such as sildenafil, and endothelin receptor antagonists. Liver transplantation has been shown to be safe in patients in whom pulmonary hypertension can be medically managed, and in many cases is curative of this process.[10]

In liver transplant recipients with either hepatopulmonary syndrome or portopulmonary hypertension, a more difficult postoperative recovery can be expected with potential for prolonged need for mechanical ventilation. However, in typical recipients who are otherwise stable clinically, many intensive care units have adopted a policy of early ventilator weaning and extubation. In many of these units, a protocol based weaning approach executed by respiratory therapists and the bedside nursing staff have been used to achieve effective rapid weaning and extubation following liver transplantation. Overall, these programs have been shown to decrease duration of mechanical ventilation, complication rate, and costs of ICU care.[8]

Renal

Pre-existing renal dysfunction is common in patients with advanced liver disease, and acute kidney injury is common in the perioperative period following liver transplantation, creating significant challenges in the management of volume status, electrolytes, and acid–base status postoperatively.

A significant percentage of patients have pre-existing renal dysfunction prior to liver transplantation. This can be multifactorial, but one of the primary contributors is the development of **hepatorenal syndrome (HRS)**, which is a functional renal failure specific to patients with end stage liver disease or fulminant hepatic failure, characterized by acute kidney injury without obvious parenchymal pathology (Table 3). The pathophysiology underlying HRS is characterized by vasodilation of the splanchnic circulation, mediated in part by abnormally high levels of nitric oxide. In turn, this sequestration of blood volume in the splanchnic circulation leads to a diminished effective circulating volume, thus initiating several compensatory mechanisms. These include the activation of the renin–angiotensin–aldosterone system (RAAS), sympathetic nervous system, and increased

Table 3. Clinical features of HRS.

Clinical features of HRS
Acute or chronic liver disease with portal hypertension
Serum creatinine >1.5 mg/dL
Absence of other apparent causes of AKI:
Shock
Nephrotoxic drugs
Parenchymal renal disease (proteinuria > 500 mg/day or > 50 RBCs/hpf)
Outflow obstruction

production of anti-diuretic hormone (ADH)/vasopressin. These compensatory mechanisms are similar to those initiated by pre-renal causes of kidney failure, and over time lead to renal vasoconstriction, acute kidney injury, and diminished glomerular filtration rate (GFR). Consistent with this pre-renal physiology, urine sodium is usually low in HRS (< 10 mEq/L), distinguishing it from acute tubular necrosis (ATN). Two variants of HRS are described in the literature, with significantly different clinical implications. HRS type 1 is characterized by a relatively acute deterioration in kidney function with a doubling of serum creatinine to a level > 2.5 mg/dL within a two week time frame. It is usually initiated by a precipitating insult such as an infection, and subsequent multisystem organ failure is common. Prognosis in HRS type 1 is poor, with only a 10% survival at 3 months. HRS type 2 follows a more gradual deterioration in renal function and usually is associated with the development of ascites. Median survival of patients with HRS type 2 is 6 months.

Management strategies for HRS are based on improving effective circulating volume by administration of albumin solution and administration of vasopressin analogues to induce vasoconstriction of the dilated splanchnic vascular system. Patients who experience worsening renal function and ultimately require renal replacement therapy prior to liver transplantation may become candidates for combined liver-kidney transplantation. Predicting the likelihood of renal recoveSry following liver transplantation is often difficult, and factors that are considered in the decision regarding whether to proceed with combined liver-kidney transplantation instead of liver transplant alone are the duration, severity, and etiology of renal failure. In general, the longer a patient has required renal replacement therapy prior to transplant, the lower the likelihood of recovery of native renal function. Fortunately, in the majority of cases, HRS is reversible following liver transplantation.[12]

Even patients with normal renal function are at significant risk for acute kidney injury following liver transplantation, due to the magnitude of the physiologic stress and significant fluid-volume shifts inherent to the procedure. Intraoperative hypotension is quite common, particularly during the anhepatic phase when the IVC is clamped, and may lead to renal hypoperfusion and postoperative ATN. Ongoing hemodynamic instability following surgery from causes ranging from bleeding complications to cardiovascular dysfunction may further exacerbate acute kidney injury. Furthermore, the initiation of immunosuppression with calcineurin inhibitors may have deleterious effects on kidney function and compound injury incurred from other causes as outlined.[8]

It is estimated that about 10% of patients undergoing liver transplant will ultimately develop renal failure requiring renal replacement therapy. In the perioperative period, triggers for initiating dialysis include significant electrolyte abnormalities, volume overload, and acid–base imbalance. Peritoneal dialysis is not an option early after liver transplantation, so most commonly patients are maintained on hemodialysis. If patients are hemodynamically labile, continuous veno-venous hemodialysis is generally better tolerated than intermittent hemodialysis.

Gastrointestinal

Graft function

The primary driver of the pace of postoperative recovery following liver transplantation is the performance of the graft. Due to the ongoing shortage of donor organs, transplant units are more frequently utilizing grafts from marginal donors (advanced age and comorbidities), leading to increased risk for postoperative graft dysfunction or primary non-function. From a biochemical standpoint, normal graft function is characterized by a trend of rapid normalization of aspartate tranaminase (AST), alanine transaminase (ALT), alkaline phosphatase (ALP), INR, bilirubin, lactic acid, and blood glucose over the first 24–48 hours after transplantation. Normal graft function is also indicated by global improvements in other organ systems including neurologic function, cardiovascular function, and renal function (Table 4). Primary non-function of the graft is characterized by opposite trends: Marked rise and persistent elevation of biochemical parameters, persistence or development of encephalopathy, cardiovascular instability and vasopressor requirement, and persistence or development of renal failure.

Frequently, the clinical picture is not completely clear and patients fall somewhere in between these two ends of the spectrum. In these cases, it is paramount to efficiently conduct a work-up that will determine if there are any technical factors responsible for graft dysfunction. The primary initial diagnostic study used is duplex ultrasound of the graft, with special attention to blood flow in the hepatic artery and portal vein. Hepatic artery thrombosis occurs in approximately 2–5% of adult cases and is graft threatening, requiring immediate return to the operating room for thrombectomy and revision of the anastomosis if possible. If this cannot be technically achieved, patients must urgently be listed for re-transplantation. Portal vein thrombosis is a less frequent complication, with an incidence of approximately 1% or

Table 4. Clinical indicators of optimal graft function after liver transplantation.

Clinical indicators of graft function
Normalization of biochemical markers
AST/ALT
INR
Bilirubin
Lactic acid
Glucose
Neurologic function
Resolution of hepatic encephalopathy
Maintenance of normal mental status
Cardiovascular function
Ability to wean vasopressors/inotropes
Maintenance of BP and sinus rhythm
Renal function
Adequate urinary output
Normalization of creatinine

less, but also requires immediate surgical correction to avoid graft failure. In both situations, adjunctive systemic anticoagulation with heparin following surgical intervention is usually initiated to prevent re-thrombosis.

If there is no obvious technical complication found on workup, graft dysfunction is likely multifactorial in nature and attributed to injury incurred in the ischemia-reperfusion process. To minimize the risk of this type of injury, it is paramount to select liver grafts with minimal steatosis, ensure fundamentally sound retrieval techniques including adequate flushing with preservation solution, and limit both cold and warm ischemic times as much as possible.[8]

GI function/nutrition

Following successful liver transplantation, gastrointestinal function generally returns to normal within a few days. Nasogastric tube decompression is commonly discontinued the first postoperative day, and patients are initiated on enteral feeds as soon as possible. In cases when a direct anastomosis between donor and recipient bile duct is not possible, a roux-en-Y hepaticojejunostomy is performed to achieve biliary drainage of the transplanted liver. This type of reconstruction requires division of the jejunum and a downstream bowel anastomosis, which may contribute to delayed return of bowel function.

The majority of patients undergoing liver transplantation exhibit some degree of protein-calorie malnutrition, characterized by muscle wasting and loss of subcutaneous fat. The prevalence of preoperative malnutrition combined with the significant physiological stress associated with liver transplantation makes nutritional support of paramount importance for optimizing recovery. The early postoperative period is characterized by a global state of catabolism induced by the neurohormonal stress response. Caloric requirements are increased and goal intake should be approximately 1.2–1.3 times the calculated basal energy expenditure. Optimal daily protein intake should be 1.5 –2 g/kg to account for the marked protein catabolism following surgery. In patients who are unable to progress to oral feeds due to issues such as neurologic dysfunction or the requirement for mechanical ventilation, enteral tube feeds should be initiated as early as feasible. Total parental nutrition (TPN) is generally reserved for patients with a non-functioning GI tract due to specific surgical complications.[11]

Biliary complications

Biliary complications following liver transplantation can generally be categorized as either biliary leak or stricture. Most pertinent in the early postoperative course is the occurrence of biliary leak. In general, this is due to a technical complication from the biliary anastomosis, most frequently caused by inadequate blood supply to the bile duct. In cases where operative drains are in place, this may be indicated by bilious drain output with high bilirubin content. In cases where no operative drains are present, biliary leak may be manifested by the development of postoperative fevers and leukocytosis, with a postoperative fluid collection demonstrated on cross sectional imaging. Bile leaks can also be detected by hepatic iminodiacetic acid (HIDA) scan, which demonstrates pooling of radiotracer outside of the GI tract. Bile leaks are most frequently managed by percutaneous drainage of the fluid collection, followed by the placement of a transampullary biliary stent by Endoscopic Retrograde Cholangiopancreatography (ERCP) if the donor bile duct was anastomosed to the recipient's native bile duct. Over time, this allows healing of the defect in the bile duct and resolution of the leak. Alternatively, a bile leak from a duct-to-duct anastomosis may be managed by open surgical drainage and conversion of the anastomosis to a roux-en-y choledochojejunostomy.

Biliary stricture is most often a late complication following liver transplantation, and this may be manifested by an elevation of liver tests in a cholestatic pattern (primarily bilirubin and ALP). Stricture is most commonly managed by balloon dilation and stent placement via ERCP or percutaneous transhepatic cholangiography (PTC), and less commonly by surgical revision of the biliary anastomosis.

Hematologic

Advanced liver disease is characterized by impaired liver synthesis of several coagulation factors including factors II, V, VII, IX, X, and XI, leading to marked abnormalities in laboratory measures of coagulation, specifically prothrombin time (PT), INR, and partial thromboplastin time (PTT). However, it must be noted that these traditional measures of coagulation may not truly reflect bleeding tendency, as deficiencies in procoagulant factors are commonly counterbalanced by a similar deficiency in anticoagulant factors such as protein C. Evidence for a state of balanced deficiency in both procoagulant and anticoagulant factors is supported by the low incidence of spontaneous bleeding in patients with advanced liver disease in comparison to patients with severe factor deficiencies like hemophilia. Point of care testing such as thromboelastography, which uses whole blood to measure the time required for clot formation and clot strength, may better reflect the true balance of hemostatic and fibrinolytic systems.[7]

In addition to the abnormalities in both procoagulant and anticoagulant factors described earlier, patients with advanced liver disease and portal hypertension also frequently exhibit thrombocytopenia due to sequestration of platelets in an enlarged spleen. Platelet deficiency can be a significant contributor to postoperative coagulopathy following liver transplantation and a balanced transfusion strategy must take this into account.

Postoperative blood product transfusion is frequently necessary following liver transplantation. In practice, a hemoglobin of 7 g/dL is commonly used as a trigger for transfusion of packed red blood cells, but should be evaluated in the context of the overall clinical condition. In the early postoperative period, the combination of thrombocytopenia and clotting factor deficiency can lead to the development of an intra-abdominal hematoma, which may require reoperation for evacuation in conjunction with a thorough examination for surgical sources of bleeding. Transfusion of fresh frozen plasma (FFP) should generally be reserved for situations in which there is an elevated INR and clinical evidence of ongoing bleeding. Patients who are clinically stable do not require FFP transfusion solely for correction of an elevated INR, as this interferes with the ability to use INR to gauge graft function.

Infectious Disease

Infectious complications are the most significant source of morbidity and mortality following liver transplantation. Liver transplant recipients are at increased risk for the development of infection due to several factors, including high dose immunosuppression used in the early postoperative period and frequent need for mechanical ventilation and invasive monitoring with indwelling vascular catheters.

The types of infections encountered in the postoperative period differ depending on the time frame. In the first postoperative month, most infections in liver transplant recipients are similar in nature to those experienced by non-transplant surgical patients. These include surgical site and deep space infections, urinary tract infections, central line associated bloodstream infections, pneumonia, and *Clostridium difficile* colitis. Pathogens involved in these infections are those typical for non-transplant patients. Management of these infections is also generally consistent with non-transplant patients, with some important caveats. In transplant recipients, a high index of suspicion should be maintained along with a lower threshold for initiating an infectious workup, commonly triggered by a fever of 38°C or above. It is particularly critical in transplant patients to avoid undue delay in initiating empiric therapy, and appropriate antibiotic selection should take into account the hospital antibiogram profile. Empiric therapy can subsequently be narrowed based on culture data. The occurrence of an early infection frequently leads to prolonged hospitalization, putting the patient at risk for the development of subsequent infections and initiating a vicious cycle that can be difficult to break.[2,8]

Starting from the second month after transplant, patients are at risk for the development of opportunistic infections that are not commonly encountered in typical surgical patients. The most common of these is cytomegalovirus (CMV) infection. Patients who are initially seronegative for CMV and receive organs from CMV positive donors are at increased risk. CMV infection is frequently characterized by fever and bone marrow suppression, but multiple organ systems can be affected, leading to a variety of possible clinical manifestations. From a pulmonary standpoint, CMV pneumonia can be particularly life threatening and generally requires ICU management. Chest X-ray findings are characterized by a diffuse pattern of interstitial involvement. From a GI perspective, CMV can involve any portion of the gastrointestinal tract causing ulcerative lesions that are manifested by abdominal pain, nausea and diarrhea. CMV hepatitis is characterized by abnormalities in liver function, which can be difficult to distinguish from rejection. Diagnosis is commonly made by CMV–PCR blood testing to establish the presence of viremia. First line treatment of CMV infection is with intravenous (IV) ganciclovir, which is commonly transitioned to oral valganciclovir after documentation of treatment response.

Fungal infections represent the other major cause of opportunistic infection in this time period. Transplant recipients are at risk for several different fungal infections affecting various organ systems. This includes urinary tract and bloodstream infections from Candida species, pulmonary infections from aspergillosis, pneumocystis, and histoplasma, and CNS infection from Cryptococcus. Treatment is typically initiated with intravenous antifungal agents and then tailored to specific pathogens isolated from culture.[8]

Due to the serious consequences of these opportunistic infections, antibiotic prophylaxis is commonly administered in high risk transplant patients. This practice varies by transplant center but can include valganciclovir for CMV prophylaxis, fluconazole for candidal prophylaxis, and trimethoprim-sulfamethoxazole for pneumocystis pneumonia (PCP) prophylaxis.

Immunosuppression

Management of immunosuppression after liver transplantation is best achieved by a multidisciplinary team including physicians, nurses, and transplant pharmacists. In the current era, there are multiple immunosuppressive regimens in use, and practice patterns can differ significantly by center. The following discussion describes the general practice in our program and the clinical factors that affect choices in therapy.

In the first few days after transplant, patients are generally administered a high dose IV corticosteroid taper. The most common clinically relevant effects include development of hyperglycemia and mood lability. Frequent point of care blood glucose monitoring is essential even in non-diabetic patients, with use of insulin therapy as necessary to establish optimal blood sugar control. As the steroid taper finishes, most patients are able to initiate oral medications. In patients with normal neurologic and renal function, our center commonly employs a three medication regimen, initiating a calcineurin inhibitor (most commonly tacrolimus) in conjunction with an anti-proliferative agent (mycophenalate mofetil or mycophenolic acid), and oral steroids (prednisone). However, there are some commonly encountered clinical scenarios that require alternative immunosuppression regimens. As discussed previously, a significant percentage of patients exhibit renal dysfunction following liver transplantation. In these patients, calcineurin inhibition is not initiated in the early postoperative course due to the significant risk of nephrotoxicity. Instead, these patients are treated with basiliximab (an antibody inhibitor of the IL-2 receptor) or anti-thymocyte globulin (ATG). Renal function is monitored closely postoperatively and calcineurin inhibition is started when creatinine begins to normalize and the patient exhibits satisfactory urinary output. Another subset of patients in which calcineurin inhibitors are withheld in the early postoperative course are those with ongoing encephalopathy or other neurologic dysfunction, owing to the possible neurotoxicity of these agents. These patients are also generally treated with basiliximab or ATG and calcineurin inhibitors are only started when neurologic status normalizes.

Rejection

Despite advances in modern immunosuppression, rejection following liver transplantation remains a significant cause of morbidity. The most common and relevant type of rejection in the early postoperative course is acute cellular rejection (ACR). ACR occurs most commonly in the first 90 days following transplant, and is mediated by T-cells that become sensitized to the graft. Clinical manifestations are generally non-specific and can include fever, abdominal pain, and hepatomegaly. From a biochemical perspective, ACR is indicated by abnormalities in liver tests, with elevation of serum transaminases, ALP, and bilirubin most commonly seen. Definitive diagnosis of ACR is made by liver biopsy, with demonstration of an infiltrate of inflammatory cells in the portal triad. Initial treatment generally entails a pulse of high dose IV corticosteroids over 3 days and ongoing monitoring of liver function tests. If improvement does not occur, the intensity of immunosuppression is increased, most commonly with a treatment course of anti-thymocyte globulin.

Other Transplant Patients

The foregoing discussion was primarily focused on the liver transplant recipient, but several concepts are applicable to transplant patients in general. Table 5 summarizes some organ specific differences in kidney, pancreas, intestine, heart, and lung transplant recipients.

Table 5. Clinical considerations in kidney, pancreas, intestine, heart, and lung transplant recipients.

Organ	Indicators of optimal graft function	Clinical management strategy	Common post-transplant complications	Common postoperative investigations
Kidney	• Adequate urinary output • Electrolyte and acid-base homeostasis • Maintenance of euvolemia • Normalization of serum creatinine and urea	• Close monitoring of urine output • Fluid administration to maintain CVP 8–12 mmHg • Maintenance of MAP 70–90 mmHg to optimize renal perfusion	• Delayed graft function • Postoperative fluid collection around graft (hematoma or lymphocele) • Renal artery or vein thrombosis • Urine leak • Ureteric stricture • Rejection	• Renal transplant ultrasound to assess vascular patency and fluid collections • Renal graft biopsy to assess rejection
Pancreas	• Normoglycemia without insulin • Return of normal bowel function	• Serial blood glucose measurement • Fluid administration to maintain pancreas perfusion	• Postoperative hematoma • Graft pancreatitis • Graft artery or venous thrombosis • Graft duodenal leak • Rejection	• Computed tomography (CT) to assess vascular patency and possible duodenal leak • Pancreas graft biopsy to assess rejection

(*Continued*)

Table 5. (*Continued*)

Organ	Indicators of optimal graft function	Clinical management strategy	Common post-transplant complications	Common postoperative investigations
Intestine	• Resumption of bowel motility • Maintenance of adequate nutrition and fluid balance without parenteral support	• Close monitoring of ostomy output • Fluid administration to maintain intestine perfusion in light of significant third space fluid losses	• Postoperative fluid collection • Chylous ascites/lymph leak • Graft artery or venous thrombosis • Rejection • Sepsis • Graft versus host disease	• CT to assess vascular patency and fluid collections • Graft endoscopy to assess for rejection and biopsy
Heart	• Normalization of hemodynamics • Ability to wean inotropic and vasopressor support	• Close hemodynamic monitoring with pulmonary artery catheter • Rapid weaning of inotropes and vasopressors as tolerated	• Postoperative hemothorax • Arrythmias • Diastolic dysfunction • Valvular dysfunction • Rejection	• ECHO • Myocardial biopsy to assess rejection
Lung	• Adequate oxygenation and ventilation • Ability to wean ventilator support	• Serial blood gas measurements • Rapid weaning of fraction of inspired oxygen (FIO_2) and ventilator support as tolerated • Restricted fluid administration	• Postoperative hemopneumothorax • Ischemia-reperfusion injury causing graft dysfunction • Graft pneumonia • Rejection	• Chest X-ray (CXR) • CT • Bronchoscopy with transbronchial biopsy to assess rejection

Conclusion

Optimal intensive care of the transplant patient is best achieved by a comprehensive, systems-based approach. The postoperative care of these complex patients can pose significant challenges, but with a logical and orderly approach, transplant patients can be expected to have favorable clinical outcomes.

References

1. Bernal W, Wendon J. Acute liver failure. *N Engl J Med* 2013; 369(26): 2525–2534.
2. DellaVolpe JD, Garavaglia JM, Huang DT. Management of complications of end-stage liver disease in the intensive care unit. *J Intensive Care Med* 2014 (online) doi: 10.1177/0885066614551144.
3. Felipo V. Hepatic encephalopathy: Effects of liver failure on brain function. *Nat Rev Neurosci* 2013; 14(12): 851–858.
4. Hinchey J, Chaves C, Appignani B *et al.* A reversible posterior leukoencephalopathy syndrome. *N Engl J Med* 1996; 334(8): 494–500.
5. McGilvray ID, Greig PD. Critical care of the liver transplant patient: an update. *Curr Opin Crit Care* 2002; 8(2): 178–182.
6. Mohsenin V. Assessment and management of cerebral edema and intracranial hypertension in acute liver failure. *J Crit Care* 2013; 28(5): 783–791.
7. Northup PG, Caldwell SH. Coagulation in liver disease: A guide for the clinician. *Clin Gastroenterol Hepatol* 2013; 11(9): 1064–1074.
8. Razonable RR, Findlay JY, A. O'Riordan A *et al.* Critical care issues in patients after liver transplantation. *Liver Transpl* 2011; 17(5): 511–527.
9. Rodriguez-Roisin R, Krowka MJ. Hepatopulmonary syndrome — A liver-induced lung vascular disorder. *N Engl J Med* 2008; 358(22): 2378–2387.
10. Safdar Z, Bartolome S, Sussman N. Portopulmonary hypertension: An update. *Liver Transpl* 2012; 18(8): 881–891.
11. Sanchez AJ, Aranda-Michel J. Nutrition for the liver transplant patient. *Liver Transpl* 2006; 12(9): 1310–1316.
12. Wadei HM, Gonwa TA. Hepatorenal syndrome in the intensive care unit. *J Intensive Care Med* 2013; 28(2): 79–92.
13. Wiese S, Hove JD, Bendtsen F *et al.* Cirrhotic cardiomyopathy: Pathogenesis and clinical relevance. *Nat Rev Gastroenterol Hepatol* 2014; 11(3): 177–186.

Chapter 34

Soft Tissue Infection in Critical Care

Sami Alissa, Nawaf Al-Otaibi and James Mahoney

Overview

Soft tissue infection present as the primary cause requiring critical care but also can be present as a complication after injury, surgical procedures or other interventions. These infections can involve the skin, subcutaneous tissue and can extend to other tissues with extension into adjacent tissue planes. The spectrum of patients presenting with infection as the primary cause covers a broad area of different types of presentation and severity. The most severe is necrotizing soft tissue infection (NSTI) a rapidly progressive infection that may affect the skin, subcutaneous tissue and muscle with necrosis. Associated systemic sepsis may require critical care.

In this chapter, the etiology, pathophysiology of these infections as well as principles of management are presented to guide the intensivist in understanding, diagnosing and participating in the care of these patients in conjunction with the soft tissue specialist surgeon and infectious disease expert as part of the care team.

Incidence

Soft tissue infection is common and a non-life threatening form may be seen in patients in the critical care setting. Any break in the skin barrier offers the portal of entry for bacteria. Surgical procedures are associated with a 5% infection complication rate. However, many are localized and will be managed in a non-critical care setting following the principles of antibiotics, drainage and immobilization. Similarly, other form of infection such as those following trauma will be managed using the same principles. A variety of factors contribute to the incidence such as the type of trauma, the severity, contamination, age and patient associated risk factors. Some of these patients will be in a critical care setting related to their initial trauma when the infection develops. Guidelines are present to help the management of different types of trauma, emphasizing the surgical management and to help minimize the development of infection as well as to facilitate treatment of different types. Procedures to drain collections are very important and should be performed as soon as the collections are identified.

More invasive infection, implying the development of systemic signs such as fever and chills are previously would be admitted to hospital. Many of these patients are now managed with appropriate drainage, initial wound management in an ambulatory setting and subsequently with intravenous antibiotics and appropriate wound management in a home care setting. Severe infection, however, implying additional systemic findings such as tachycardia, persistent elevated temperature, and confusion and associated laboratory abnormalities requiring critical care support is less common. The most alarming is a severe primary form of NSTI. There are about 1,000 cases per year in the United States. The mortality rate can be as high as 25% and the outcome is related to the timing of diagnosis and intervention.[1] When soft tissue infection is associated with generalized organ failure, as in NSTF, mortality rate is as high as 70%.

Pathophysiology

It is generally agreed that bacterial invasion of the subcutaneous tissues occurs either through external trauma or direct spread from a perforated viscus (most commonly colon or rectum) or urogenital organ. Bacteria then spread through subcutaneous planes producing endo- and exotoxins that cause tissue ischemia, liquefactive necrosis, and often systemic illness.[3–4]

Skin necrosis is secondary to vascular occlusion and because of the rich collateral vascular networks within the skin, the overlying skin changes usually does not reflect the magnitude of the underlying tissue necrosis.[3] In addition, superficial nerves in the subcutaneous planes can be affected by the ischemic changes, which eventually lead to decrease sensation in the area. Infection can spread as fast as 1 inch per hour depending on the virulence of

Table 1. Risk factors for soft tissue infection.

Host factors	**Wound factors**
Alcohol abuse	Blunt or penetrating injury
Peripheral vascular disease	Devitalized tissue
Liver disease	Foreign body
Renal calculi or failure	Inadequate debridement
Incarcerated hernias	Gross contamination
Odontogenic infection strep throat	Compound fractures
Drug abuser	Burns
Old age	
Obesity	
Smoking	
Immunocompromised states, such as AIDS, diabetes mellitus, and malignancy	

Table 2. Classification of soft tissue infection.

Classification according to:	**Depth**	Necrotizing adipositis	
		Fasciitis	
		Myositis	
	Microbes	*Clostridial*	Gas gangrene
			Necrotizing fasciitis (NF)
		Non-*clostridial*	*Streptococcal* toxic shock like Syndrome (Flesh-eating disease)

Note: Modified from Sarani.[3]

the bacteria and the host immunity.[18] A variety of risk factors are associated with NSTF and these are listed in Table 1.

Classification

NSTI can be classified according to depth of tissue involvement, anatomical area involved, or microbiology. The most popular classification is the one based on microbes. These are summarized in Table 2.

***Clostridial* Infections (Gas gangrene):** These are caused by *Clostridial* species, which are gram positive, spore forming, and anaerobic bacteria. These bacteria are found in the human body as gastrointestinal flora (*C. septicum*) and in the soil (*C. perfringens*). Severe soft tissue infection associated with clostridia is associated with three clinical scenarios. The most common scenario is direct contamination of a traumatic wound. Other presentations can involve postoperative wound infection especially gastrointestinal and biliary surgery as well as a secondary infection, in the setting of colonic malignancies. The incubation period varies from hours to days with death reported as early as 12 hours following the development of clinical infection. It can have a fulminant rapidly progressive course of infection with spread of infection and necrosis as fast as 1 inch/hour. The common and important isolated organism is *C. perfringens*, which is known for its lethal exotoxins. It produces an Alpha toxin; a lecithinase which destroys cell membranes: Theta toxin; a hemolysin also a cardiotoxin: Kappa toxin; a collagenase: Mu toxin; a hyaluronidase which facilitates spread as well as Nu toxin a deoxyribonuclease. The classic presentation is severe pain disproportionate to physical findings often early within several days of the traumatic event, followed by edema and bronze skin discoloration. Hemorrhagic skin blebs associated with dermal necrosis, a brawny foul smelling seropurulent discharge can be seen. Early systemic signs include low-grade fever, tachycardia, fever, CNS findings (usually lethargy and indifference), with rapid progression to cardiovascular collapse and multi-organ failure. Palpable wound crepitus may not present till late (if at all). When associated with traumatic injury, examination of all wounds whether traumatic or associated with surgical findings is very important, as these are usually the portals of entry for the infection.

Non-*clostridial* infections are classified into two groups, polymicrobial infection and monomicrobial infections (one organism) and are characterized in Table 3. Polymicrobial infections are more common and frequently aerobic and anaerobic organisms are cultured in the same wound. Polymicrobial infection usually develops more slowly, usually over days. The perineum, lower extremity (foot infections in diabetes) as well as postoperative wound sites are seen with this type of infection. Crepitus on palpation and gas in soft tissue on X-ray can be seen due to the presence of gas producing bacteria.

Monomicrobial infection has created considerable controversy with its diagnosis and treatment due to the rapidly progressive (<24 hours) presentation of a previously well person to someone with a life threatening infection in intensive care. They often require mutilating surgery and are at risk of limb loss. The usual organism associated with these severe infections is Group-A beta hemolytic *streptococcus*. However, in our experience *Staphylococcus aureus* and methicillin resistant *Staphylococcus aureus* (MRSA) infection can also present in a similar fashion. There may be a history of trauma to the

Table 3. Non-*clostridial* NSTI (Necrotizing Fasciitis or NF).

	Organism	Characteristic
Type I	Polymicrobial	• Most common type of NTSI and responsible up to 75% or more of infections. • Average of four or more organisms are isolated from the wound, and usually include a mix of aerobic and anaerobic bacteria. • May show a shift from facultative aerobes early on to fastidious anaerobes later as the O_2 tension is reduced. • Incubation period generally longer than type II (average 4–7 days). • Crepitus occurs in around 30% but typically late. • It is typically located in the trunk, abdominal wall, perianal and groin areas, postoperative wounds and diabetic associated lower extremity wounds. • Fournier's gangrene (perineal type 1 NF), Ludwig's angina (cerivcofacial type 1 NF) and meleney's gangrene are also examples for this type.
Type II	Monomicrobial	• Tends to occur in otherwise healthy, young, immunocompetent hosts. • Rapid fulminant infection caused by Group-A (beta hemolytic) *Streptococci.* • Infection initially confined to the superficial fascia spreading to the deep fascia and muscles. • Classically located on the extremities, although truncal involvement is reported. • Frequently, there is a history of recent trauma or operation on the area. • Short incubation period. (1–3 d).
Type III	*Vibrio vulnificus* (Marine *vibrios*)	• Not universal agreed. • Occurs after exposure to salt water following minor injuries. • Least common type.[19] • Associated with a fulminant course that can cause multi-organ failure if not treated within 24 hours.[5]

area: However, this is not always present. The infection starts superficially and preferentially involves the deep fascia and in this plane can rapidly spread. Toxins produced by ***streptococcus*** bacteria include a hyaluronidase, which facilitates spread as well as exotoxins creating systemic toxicity. Infection with ***streptococcus*** has a unique virulent characteristic related to the bacterial surface proteins, M-1 and M-3. These M proteins help the bacteria to escape phagocytosis by neutrophils by increasing bacterial adherence to body tissues. In addition, ***streptococcal*** and ***staphylococcal*** exotoxins A and B damage the endothelium and cause loss of microvascular integrity resulting in tissue edema and impaired blood flow at the capillary level.[3] Together M-proteins and some exotoxins exhibit "superantigen activity" which is responsible for a massive pro-inflammatory cytokine release, 2 to 3 orders of magnitude greater than that seen with an ordinary antigen which helps explain the overwhelming inflammatory response, septic shock and multi-organ failure seen in ***Streptococcal*** infection. There is clinical variation in the presentation with some patients demonstrating less in the way of systemic findings with significant local infection whereas others present early with life threatening findings (***Streptococcal*** toxic shock syndrome). The Infection associated with ***Vibrio*** is related to marine exposure and although very serious, are less common.[19]

Presentation

All types of NSTI have the same presentation initially and these are summarized in Table 4. The most common presentations are pain, erythema and swelling that may precede skin change such as bullae or discoloration. The key finding is pain out of proportion to what would be expected based on the physical findings extending beyond the erythematous area. Palpation elicits tenderness. These findings are rapidly progressive. The initial redness and swelling is followed by hypoesthesia, skin changes such as bullae, ***purpura*** or necrosis. These occur late as they are due to blood vessel thrombosis.[6] Crepitus related to gas production by bacteria can occur in 30% of the patients with NSTI.[3]

Shock, fever, and altered mental status typically develop during the first 24 to 48 hours of disease progression but are often absent at the time of initial presentation.[7] In the unconscious patient with systemic sepsis the skin findings are diagnostic. It is difficult to detect erythema in patients with dark skin and increased suspicion with more reliance on the other findings is necessary.

Table 4. Presentation NSTI.

	Local	Systemic
Early	Skin trauma Erythema Edema Hotness Tenderness	Pain out of proportion Fever Tachycardia
Late	Bullae Purple/blue skin color Hypoesthesia Crepitus Skin necrosis	Hypotension Mental confusion Multi-organ failure

Note: Modified from Lancerotto *et al.*[2]

Diagnosis

The diagnosis is mainly clinical and it remains one of the challenges because the symptoms are not specific and may mimic other diseases such as cellulitis or abscess. Laboratory tests, histopathology, and radiographic studies can aid in the diagnosis of NSTF.

Laboratory findings are non-specific. Multiple scoring systems utilizing laboratory findings have been suggested to aid in the diagnosis. The most common one is the Laboratory Risk Indicator for Necrotizing Fasciitis (LRINEC) score based on C-reactive protein, WBC, Hb, serum sodium, creatinine, and glucose levels, which classifies patients in low, intermediate, and high-risk categories of NF (Table 5).[8] However LRINEC score alone is not useful for the early recognition of NF.[9]

Biopsy for tissue diagnosis is critical. Percutaneous needle aspiration followed by Gram stain and culture for a rapid bacteriologic diagnosis has been used. Alternatively, the "finger-test" associated with tissue biopsy for Gram stain and rapid-frozen section biopsy is diagnostic. The area of concern is first infiltrated with local anesthesia. A 2 cm incision is made in the skin down to the deep fascia. Lack of bleeding is a sign of necrotizing fasciitis. A gentle probing maneuver with the finger is performed at the level of the deep fascia. If the tissues dissect with minimal resistance, the "finger test" is positive.[10] A watery edema like fluid is seen in this space. Adjacent subcutaneous tissue and fascia is sent for immediate Gram stain and pathology. If bacteria are identified this is diagnostic.

Table 5. Laboratory findings in necotizing fasciitis.

Variable	Value	Points
C-reactive protein (mg/dl)	<150	0
	>150	4
WBC (10*9/L)	<15	0
	12–15	1
	>25	2
Hb (g/dl)	>13.5	0
	11–13.5	1
	<11	2
Sodium (mmol/L)	≥135	0
	<135	2
Creatinine (mg/dl)	≤1.6	0
	>1.6	2
Glucose (mg/dl)	≤180	0
	>180	1
Risk Category	**Points**	**Probability**
Low	≤5	<50%
Intermediate	6–7	50%–75%
High	≥8	>75%

Note: Modified from Lancerotto *et al.*[2]

X-ray can show foreign body and subcutaneous gas. CT scan is sensitive and will show soft tissue inflammation and collection but the findings are not specific for NSTI. MRI can differentiate some necrotizing from non-necrotizing infections, however, its low sensitivity (80%–90%) and specificity (50%–55%), and the time required to complete a magnetic resonance imaging study tend to limit its usefulness.[1]

Radiographic imaging studies should not delay surgical intervention.

Treatment

The treatment of NSTI consists of two parts.

1. Medical treatment

The need for fluid resuscitation and correction of electrolyte abnormalities is immediate. The goal is to restore the intravascular volume that is depleted because of the systemic response to NSTI. This will maintain organ and tissue perfusion that can help to reduce the likelihood of the multi-organ failure. Crystalloids are the most common fluid. The most common electrolyte disturbances are hyponatremia, hypocalcaemia, and hyperglycemia. Blood products may be considered in the case of anemia due to hemolysis or diffuse intravascular coagulation.

Empirical antibiotic coverage should be given as soon as NSTI is diagnosed. It should be broad-spectrum, including activity against gram-positive, gram-negative, and anaerobic organisms. Special consideration for Group-A *streptococcus* and *Clostridium* species should be given when suspected.

Acceptable regimens include administration of a carbapenem or beta-lactamase inhibitor, together with clindamycin and drugs with activity against MRSA (such as Vancomycin, daptomycin, and linezolid). In cases where infection with *Vibrio* species is suspected, doxycycline plus ceftazidine is recommended. Ciprofloxacin is also considered as a reasonable alternative in the setting of age less than 8 years, allergy, or drug intolerance.[24]

Antibiotic should be tailored to the culture and sensitivity when the results are available.[1] These are summarized in Table 6.

2. Surgical treatment

Surgical treatment is the mainstay for NSTI treatment and should not be delayed once the diagnosis has been established. If surgical debridement is delayed >24 hours, mortality rate increase significantly.[11] The goal of the initial surgery is to expose all involved tissue planes and remove all necrotic tissue. Unlike other types of infection, there may be no abscess or collection to drain initially. It is important to recognize the infection extension and involvement of the fascia and at times deeper tissue planes. The findings at surgery can vary from actual frank necrosis to the more watery fluid

Table 6. List of recommended empirical antibiotic agents with their rational.

Antibiotic	Rational
Carbapenem	Coverage against Gram-positive, Gram-negative bacteria, and anaerobes.
Clindamycin	Decreases *clostridial* α-toxin, *Streptococcal* superantigens and suppress TNF α production by monocytes.[21–23]
Vancomycin, daptomycin and linezolid	Coverage against MRSA.

associated with loss of the integrity of the fascia only. The severity of the infection becomes evident later in the process with the progression of the development of more obvious tissue necrosis. At this stage exposure to healthy and bleeding tissue is required with removal of any non-viable tissue. Initial incisions should extend beyond the indurated and erythematous skin. Due to difficulty is assessing the extent of involvement, additional surgical procedures should be planned at 12–36 hour intervals until there is no clinical evidence of progression if the infection (necrosis, extension along tissue planes).[12] These procedures can be associated with additional significant systemic compromise and blood loss requiring additional supportive therapies further compromising the patient.

The necrotic tissue should be sent for culture and sensitivity. These infections not only involve the superficial fascia but also can involve deeper tissues such as muscle. In cases involving the perineum, temporary diverting colostomy may be indicated. Early amputation may need to be considered in extremity infections where there is extensive soft tissue (skin and muscle) necrosis where the limb may be so extensively involved that it is not salvageable. Once debridement is complete and there is no evidence of progression of the infection wound care becomes a new priority. Negative Pressure Wound Therapy can be used if the wound is clean to prepare it for definitive reconstruction. Wound reconstruction (skin graft or Flap) can be considered once the wound culture is negative.[2]

Other Therapies

Intravenous Immunoglobulin G (IVIG)

This can be given intravenously at the time of diagnosis. Its potential benefit is to act as a neutralizing antibodies binding exotoxins produced by *staphylococcus*, *streptococcus* and *clostridia* and thereby limits systemic inflammatory response.[10,13–15] The use of high-dose IVIG (up to 2g/kg) appears to be beneficial in severe infections caused by Group-A *streptococcus*, although there is not enough evidence to support its general use.[25–26]

Hyperbaric oxygen (HBO)

It can be used as an adjunct to the surgical and medical treatment.

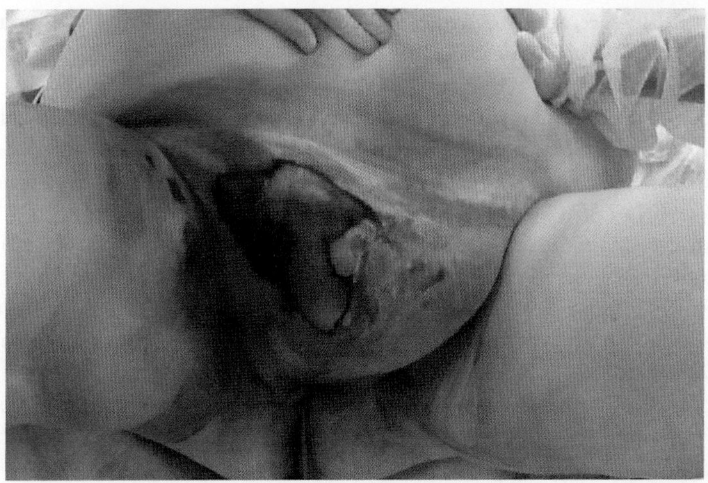

Fig. 1. Acute presentation of septic 45 year obese female with polymicrobial soft tissue infection. Necrotic skin involving pannus, thigh, perineum and buttock. Required 3 operations 24 hours apart, extensive soft tissue necrosis extending beyond the skin findings at surgery.

Administration of 100% oxygen at 2–3 atm absolute (ATA) has shown to increase tissue oxygen tension resulting in improved WBCs phagocytic and killing mechanisms. It has an independent bactericidal effect on anaerobes.[27]

Beyond the initial stages of infection, HBO therapy may also improve wound healing, which could lead to reductions in the number of debridement sessions.[16]

Hyperbaric oxygen therapy does not significantly decrease the mortality or amputation rate in patients with NSTI.[17]

References

1. Ustin J, Malangoni M. Necrotizing soft-tissue infections. *Crit Care Med* 2011; 39(9):2156–2162.
2. Lancerotto L, Tocco I, Salmaso R, Vindigni V, Bassetto F. Necrotizing fasciitis: Classification, diagnosis, and management. *J Trauma Acute Care Surg* 2012; 72(3):560–566.
3. Sarani B, Strong M, Pascual J, Schwab CW. Necrotizing fasciitis: Current concepts and review of the literature. *Journal of the American College of Surgeons* 2009; 208(2):279–288.

4. Salcido R. Necrotizing fasciitis: Reviewing the causes and treatment strategies. *Adv Skin Wound Care* 2007; 20(5): 288.
5. Tsai Y-H, Huang T-J, Hsu R, Weng Y-J, Hsu W-H, Huang K-C, *et al.* Necrotizing soft-tissue infections and primary sepsis caused by Vibrio vulnificus and Vibrio cholerae non-O1. *J Trauma* 2009; 66(3):899–905.
6. Rajan S. Skin and soft-tissue infections: Classifying and treating a spectrum. *Cleve Clin J Med* 2012; 79(1): 57–66.
7. Jamal N, Teach S. Necrotizing fasciitis. *Pediatr Emerg Care* 2011; 27(12):1195.
8. Chin-Ho W, Lay-Wai K, Kien-Seng H, Kok-Chai T, Cheng-Ooi L. The LRINEC (Laboratory Risk Indicator for Necrotizing Fasciitis) score: A tool for distinguishing necrotizing fasciitis from other soft tissue infections. *Crit Care Med* 2004; 32.
9. Chun IL, Yi-Kung L, Yung-Cheng S, Chin-Hsiang C, Chun-Hing W. Validation of the laboratory risk indicator for necrotizing fasciitis (LRINEC) score for early diagnosis of necrotizing fasciitis. *Tzu Chi Medical Journal* 2012; 24.
10. Edlich R, Cross C, Dahlstrom J, Long W. Modern concepts of the diagnosis and treatment of necrotizing fasciitis. *J Emerg Med* 2010; 39(2): 261–265.
11. Wong CH, Haw-Chong C, Shanker P, *et al.* Necrotizing fascitis: Clinical presentation, microbiology, and determinants of mortality. *J Bone Joint Surg Am* 2003; 85:1454–1460.
12. Voros D, Pissiotis C, Georgantas D, Katsaragakis S, Antoniou S, Papadimitriou J. Role of early and aggressive surgery in the treatment of severe necrotizing soft tissue infections. *Br J Surg* 1993; 80(9): 1190–1191.
13. Takei S, Arora Y, Walker S. Intravenous immunoglobulin contains specific antibodies inhibitory to activation of T-cells by staphylococcal toxin superantigens. *J ClinInvest* 1993; 91: 602–607.
14. Norrby-Teglund A, Kaul R, Low D. Plasma from patients with severe invasive group A streptococcal infections treated with normal polyspecific IgG inhibits streptococcal superantigen induced Tcell proliferation and cytokine production. *J Immunol* 1996; 156: 3057–3064.
15. Hakkarainen Timo W, Kopari Nicole M, Pham Tam N, Evans Heather L. Necrotizing soft tissue infections: Review and current concepts in treatment, systems of care, and outcomes. *Curr Probl Surg* 2014; 51(8): 344.
16. Zamboni WA, Wong HP, Stephenson LL. Effect of hyperbaric Oxygen on neutrophil concentration and pulmonary sequestration in reperfusion injury. *Arch Surg* 1996; 131: 756.
17. Massey Paul R, Sakran Joseph V, Mills Angela M, Babak Sarani, Aufhauser David D, Sims Carrie A, Pascual Jose L, Kelz Rachel R, Holena Daniel N. Hyperbaric oxygen therapy in necrotizing soft tissue infections. *J Surg Res* 2012; 177(1): 146–151.
18. Shiroff Adam M, Herlitz Georg N, Gracias, Vicente H. Necrotizing Soft Tissue Infections. *J Intensiv Care Med* 2014; 29(3): 138–144.

19. Howard R , Pessa M, Brennaman B, Ramphal R. Necrotizing soft tissue infections caused by marine vibrios. *Surg* 1985; 98(1): 126–130. 27.
20. Goodel K, Jordan M, Graham R, Cassidy C, Nasraway S.Rapidly advancing necrotizing fasciitis caused by Phytobacterium (Vibrio) damsela: A hyper aggressive variant. *Crit Care Med* 2004; 32(1): 278–281.
21. Gemmell C, Peterson P, Schmeling D. Potentiation of opsonization and phagocytosis of Streptococcus Pyogenes following growth in the presence of clindamycin. *J ClinInvest* 1981; 67(5): 1249–1256.
22. Stevens D, Meier K, Mitten J. Effect of antibiotics on toxin production and viability of Clostridium perfringens. *Antimicrob Agents Chemother* 1987; 31(2): 213–218.
23. Stevens D, Bryant A, Hackett S. Antiobiotic effects on bacterial viability, toxin production, and host response. *Clin Infect Dis* 1995; 20(2): S154–S157.
24. Tang WM, Ho PL, Fung KK, *et al.* Necrotizing fasciitis of a limb. *J Bone Joint Surg* (Br) 2001; 83(B): 709–714.
25. Norrby-Teglund A, Basma H, Andersson J, *et al.* Varying titers of neutralizing antibodies to streptococcal superantigens in different preparations of normal polyspecific immunoglobulin G: Implications for therapeutic efficacy. *Clin Infect Dis* 1998; 26: 631.
26. Norrby-Teglund A, Muller MP, Mcgeer A, *et al.* Successful management of severe group A streptococcal soft tissue infections using an aggressive medical regimen including intravenous polyspecific immunoglobulin together with a conservative surgical approach. *Scand J Infect Dis* 2005; 37: 166.
27. Kaide CG, Khandelwal S. Hyperbaric oxygen: Applications in infectious disease. *Emerg Med Clin North Am* 2008; 26: 571–595.

Chapter 35

The Pediatric Surgical ICU Patient

Arthur Cooper, Pamela Feuer, Logeswary Rajagopalan, Ranjith Kamity and Mary Joan Marron-Corwin

Overview

The aim of this chapter is to arm the acute care surgeon/surgical critical care specialist who rarely cares for children with a fundamental understanding of the key differences between adult and pediatric surgical critical care, so such care can be provided in the absence of a pediatric surgical critical care specialist. The most common condition for which this specialist will be consulted is major pediatric trauma. Less common conditions include respiratory and circulatory failure, neonatal surgical emergencies and postoperative surgical emergencies. Thus, while emphasizing the care of the major trauma patient, the chapter will focus on important differences between neonates, children, and adults with respect to:

1. Bedside skills necessary to determine when a pediatric patient is critically ill.
2. Respiratory structure and function, and how they may affect ventilatory management.
3. Circulatory structure and function, and how they may affect hemodynamic support.
4. Basic neurologic assessment and determination of brain death.
5. Basic fluid, electrolyte, and nutritional management, including renal replacement therapy.
6. Critical management of respiratory and circulatory failure, as well as common life-threatening pediatric surgical conditions such as major

pediatric trauma, neonatal surgical emergencies, postoperative surgical emergencies, and the use and misuse of analgesic and sedative agents.

It is important to note that pediatric critical care is provided in the multidisciplinary environment of a pediatric intensive care unit (PICU) or neonatal intensive care unit (NICU) where specialists in pediatric critical care medicine or neonatology are typically available to collaborate in the management of critically ill and injured children. In such an environment, the acute care surgeon/surgical critical care specialist will be welcomed as a collaborating partner with special expertise in the intensive care of patients with surgical conditions who, instead of acting independently, will work as a member of a team of critical care specialists. Such collaboration fits well with the patient- and family-centered approach to critical care applied in the PICU and NICU.[1] However, to optimally prepare for the moment when such collaboration is requested, the acute care surgeon/ surgical critical care specialist who rarely cares for critically ill and injured children is strongly advised to participate in educational offerings such as the *Pediatric Advanced Life Support* Course of the American Heart Association and American Academy of Pediatrics, the *Pediatric Fundamental Critical Care Support* Course of the Society of Critical Care Medicine, and the standing course in *Current Concepts in Pediatric Critical Care* offered by the same organization at its annual meeting, and to take advantage of their associated textbooks as well as resources such as the *Handbook of Pediatric Surgical Critical Care* of the American Pediatric Surgical Association recently made accessible in the public domain as the February 2015 number of *Seminars in Pediatric Surgery.*

Introduction

The goals of pediatric and adult surgical critical care are fundamentally the same; in both instances, the aims of therapy are to support vital functions until the disease process responsible for their deterioration is treated or resolved. However, the spectrum of illness confronting specialists in pediatric surgical critical care is somewhat different from that confronting their adult counterparts; this is because a major proportion of the problems confronting the specialist in pediatric surgical critical care are diseases of immaturity or prematurity which can be expected to improve with the passage of time, in contrast to the degenerative diseases which are chiefly responsible for critical illness in the adult surgical patient.

Even so, while there are a number of acquired diseases unique to the pediatric population which will also confront the specialist in pediatric surgical critical care, e.g., hemolytic-uremic syndrome (HUS) in the child, bronchopulmonary dysplasia (BPD) in the infant, there are far more which are not unique to childhood, e.g., major trauma, severe sepsis/septic shock, and multiple organ system failure (MOSF), including acute respiratory distress syndrome (ARDS). Fortunately, since the recuperative powers of the child are great, partly because most vital organs have not fully completed their growth, there is much to be gained by heroic effort: If the intervention is successful, the child may lead a normal life; yet, there is also a downside to such an aggressive approach: Precisely because of their remarkable recuperative powers, children who are saved but do not recover fully may be forced to live with severe disabilities.

While the differences between infants (particularly neonates), children, and adults may seem overwhelming to the surgical critical care specialist who cares for children infrequently, it is important to remember that there are far more similarities than there are differences. Doses of fluids and drugs must, of course, be calculated carefully on the basis of body mass, using either body weight or body surface area as a first approximation, but the effects of such interventions are generally quite similar. However, due to problems of size and scale, these doses must be determined precisely, for even small errors may have large effects when the doses are small to begin with. Use of a length-based, color-coded resuscitation tape (Broselow Pediatric Emergency Tape) or a hybrid age- and length-based, hand-aided memory aid (Handtevy Pediatric Resuscitation System) for estimation of drug dosages will minimize the chances for such error in emergencies, but it is now recognized that the tape-based and hand-based systems may underestimate drug dosages in morbidly obese children by as much as 20%, so reliance on measurement of body mass together with wall charts or published formularies, and a portable calculator, is preferred.

Nevertheless, while the "ABCs" may be the same for children and adults, marked differences in anatomy can result in sharp differences in physiology. For example, due to the small size of the infant's heart, cardiac output is more dependent upon heart rate than on stroke volume, while the decreased compliance of an infant's lungs previously mandated the use of a pressure-controlled rather than a volume-controlled ventilator, to minimize the complications of barotrauma and volutrauma (although this practice may be changing as newer ventilators have become available). Even so, whether the patient is a child or an adult, optimal perfusion is achieved when both heart rate and filling pressures are appropriate for the patient's size and condition, while adequate ventilation requires that an adequate volume of gas be exchanged even if supranormal pressures are required to achieve this. It is therefore not surprising that most treatment strategies used by specialists in pediatric surgical critical care are borrowed from their adult counterparts, although they may be adjusted to meet the particular anatomic and physiologic needs of the child.

Yet, the most important difference between infants, children, and adults is also perhaps the most obvious one: They are smaller. It is therefore crucial that physicians for caring critically ill children have at their disposal an array of cannulas, catheters, and tubes of many different sizes (which must be carefully secured to prevent dislodgement by the child's wandering hands), as well as different types and sizes of ventilators (with the smallest amount of tubing possible to minimize dead space), to allow proper monitoring as well as treatment to be performed. Of necessity, most such tools represent scaled-down versions of adult technology. Unfortunately, this sometimes leads to the erroneous conclusion that the child is nothing more than a small adult: For better, or for worse, this is most definitely not the case.

Bedside Assessment

While the late signs of physiologic distress in the neonate and infant are similar to those observed in older children and adults, the early signs may be subtle or absent. For example, the fever, lethargy, and irritability so characteristic of sepsis in the older infant and child are rarely, if ever, present in the neonate, especially if premature; instead, intolerance of feedings, clusters of apnea and bradycardia, episodes of oxygen desaturation, hypotonia, hypothermia, and hyperglycemia (or in particularly severe cases, hypoglycemia, the first indication of which, especially in the premature infant, may be a seizure), will be the earliest presenting signs. Unfortunately, ominous changes in vital signs, such as hypotension, may not occur until much later. Thus, even the slightest suspicion of sepsis, a major killer in both the PICU and the NICU, warrants an aggressive search for a source, and prophylactic treatment with antibiotics appropriate to the local epidemiology of bacterial organisms, until culture results become available.

In contrast to the neonate, the clinical signs of physiologic distress in the infant are usually not so subtle. However, they are still not very specific, and, early on, may be apparent only to the child's parents or nurse, who often may not be able to pinpoint exactly what is amiss, but know that something is wrong. Nevertheless, level of activity, particularly social activity, feeding behavior, degree of comfort, and skin color are useful parameters to follow.

Thus, children who are irritable, lethargic, have lost interest in their surroundings, do not interact with their parents, do not react to invasive procedures, who feed poorly, who assume unnatural positions, or who are pale or mottled, are usually in some sort of trouble; careful physical examination will typically lead to recognition of the precise causes of their distress.

One useful tool for rapid identification of the critically ill or injured child is the Pediatric Assessment Triangle, or PAT (Fig. 1).[2] This tool provides adult oriented clinicians with a simple method to suspect that an infant or child is ill, seriously ill, or critically ill, based on rapid visual assessment at the bedside of Appearance, work of Breathing, and Circulation to skin: If one limb of the PAT is abnormal, the infant or child is ill; if two limbs, seriously ill; if three limbs, critically ill. Moreover, the limb of the PAT that seems most deranged usually indicates which vital system is the source of the problem: respiratory, circulatory, or metabolic/neurologic; primary assessment of the "ABCDEs" is then applied to confirm the clinician's initial impression and guide initial resuscitation. Of note, the utility and accuracy of the PAT has been recently validated for use in triage by pediatric emergency nurses as well as paramedics.

Measurement of vital signs is also a key step in determining an infant's or child's level of distress. However, it must be remembered that anxiety or

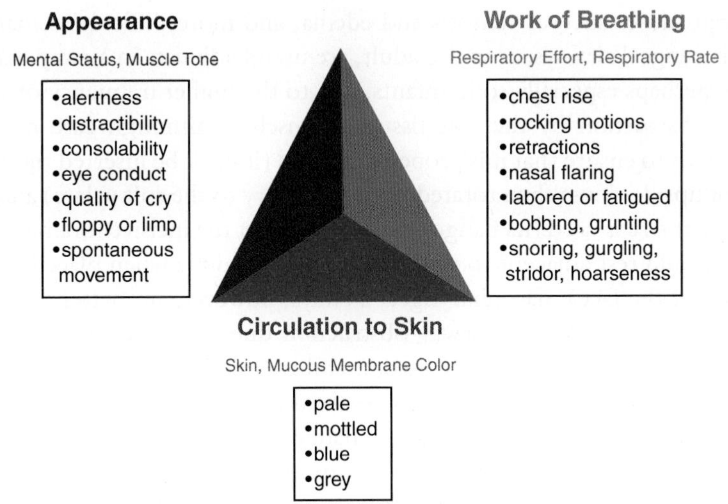

Fig. 1. The pediatric assessment triangle.

(Adapted from Horeczko T, Enriquez B, McGrath NE, Gausche-Hill M, Lewis RJ. The Pediatric Assessment Triangle: Accuracy of its application by nurses in the triage of children. *J Emerg Nurs.* 2013; 39:182–189.)

stimulation can markedly affect vital signs; it is therefore important that the rapid "primary assessment" referred to above be completed before vital signs are actually measured. The ranges of normal for vital signs vary with age and size (Table 1). Again, it must be remembered that "normal" vital signs are not always appropriate for a specific patient, and that the blood pressure measurement, in particular, will not be accurate unless obtained with the proper-sized cuff, i.e., one which is two-thirds as wide as the distance from the axilla to the antecubital fossa, or in the lower extremity of infants and small children, from the groin to the knee, or the knee to the ankle.

Airway, Lungs, and Ventilation

The tongue of the infant is larger than that of the adult, while the jaw is smaller; for this reason, and because of the need to breathe while nursing at the breast, the infant remains an obligate nasal breather until approximately six months of age. Moreover, the funnel-shaped larynx of the infant is more superior and anterior, while the trachea is shorter, narrower, and more membranous than that of the adult; as a result, the infant airway is both more susceptible to episodes of obstruction due to congenital causes such as laryngomalacia and tracheomalacia, and glottic and subglottic webs, and acquired causes such as stenosis and edema, and more difficult to manage. Oropharyngeal airways, as in the adult, are useful adjuncts in airway maintenance, perhaps especially so in infants, due to the higher frequency of upper airway obstruction by the soft tissues themselves, although care must be taken both to ensure that it is properly inserted (it must be inserted right-side up, not upside-down then rotated, to avoid injury to the soft palate) and that the proper size is used (its flange should lie against the incisive foramen while its tip should rest adjacent to the angle of the mandible when placed against the side of the face); nasopharyngeal airways, however, are better tolerated, can improve extrathoracic airway obstruction due to hypotonic pharyngeal musculature or edematous soft tissues, and may facilitate posterior pharyngeal suctioning, but they, too, must be sized correctly (the diameter should not exceed that of the naris, while the flange should lie upon the naris as its tip rests adjacent to the tragus). Indications for placement of an endotracheal tube, of course, are no different in infants and children than in adults; however, it is important to remember that the short length of the trachea in the infant (approximately 5 cm) and the small child (approximately 7 cm) makes positioning and fixation of the tube extremely crucial, while the narrow diameter of the tube predisposes to obstruction, both by kinking, and

Table 1. Normal vital signs in pediatric patients

Normal respiratory rates by age.

Age	Breaths/min
Infant (<1 year)	30–60
Toddler (1 to 3 years)	24–40
Preschooler (4 to 5 years)	22–34
School age (6 to 12 years)	18–30
Adolescent (13 to 18 years)	12–16

Normal heart rates (per minute) by age.

Age	Awake Rate	Mean	Sleeping Rate
Newborn to 3 months	85–205	140	80–160
3 months to 2 years	100–190	130	75–160
2 years to 10 years	60–140	80	60–90
>10 years	60–100	75	50–90

Normal blood pressures in children by age.

Age	Systolic blood pressure (mm Hg)		Diastolic blood pressure (mm Hg)	
	Female	Male	Female	Male
Neonate (1 day)	60–76	60–74	31–45	30–44
Neonate (4 days)	67–83	68–84	37–53	35–53
Infant (1 month)	73–91	74–94	36–56	37–55
Infant (3 months)	78–100	81–103	44–64	45–65
Infant (6 months)	82–102	87–105	46–66	48–68
Infant (1 year)	68–104	67–103	22–60	20–58
Child (2 years)	71–105	70–106	27–65	25–63
Child (7 years)	79–113	79–115	39–77	38–78
Adolescent (15 years)	93–127	95–131	47–85	45–85

(Adapted from Pediatric Subcommittee and Special Contributors, Emergency Cardiovascular Care Committee, American Heart Association, Chameides L, Samson RA, Schexnayder SM, Hazinski MF, *eds. Pediatric Advanced Life Support Provider Manual*, Professional Edition. Dallas, TX, American Heart Association, 2011.)

inspissated mucoid or secretions, thus requiring aggressive pulmonary toilet to avoid this potentially lethal complication.

Although cuffed tubes are now routinely used for the intensive management of children of all ages, as they are in adults, the tubes which are used for infants and small children may be uncuffed to allow them to fit through the subglottic area which, in contrast to the adult, is the narrowest portion of the airway; both types of tubes are most easily inserted via the oral route with the neck only slightly extended (called the "sniffing" position) using a straight (Miller)-bladed laryngoscope with its tip positioned under the vallecula, although gentle cricoid pressure may be required if the larynx is especially far anterior. While a snug fit is desirable for optimal airway protection whether using a cuffed or uncuffed tube, it is essential that the tube should fit loosely enough that a leak should be apparent when 20 cm H_2O of pressure are applied to the airway, to avoid excessive pressure (either by cuff or tube) on the subglottic tracheal mucosa and the subsequent development of subglottic stenosis; selection of the proper-sized tube (which is inserted to a depth in cm that is approximately three times the external diameter of the tube) is therefore crucial, and can be estimated by matching the size of the tube with that of the patient's naris, or using the formula: [age (yr)/4] + 3.5 (for a cuffed tube) or 4 (for an uncuffed tube)] for infants and children, reserving a 3.0 or 2.5 uncuffed tube for preterm infants. Nasotracheal intubation, although somewhat more difficult than oral intubation, as pituitary (or Rovenstein) forceps are usually required to guide the tip of the tube through the vocal cords, is preferable in term and preterm infants (except in emergencies) because the position of the tube can be more securely maintained; inadvertent extubations are therefore far less frequent, although care must be taken to avoid the risk of nasal skin breakdown that can occur with excessive pressure from a tightly fitting tube. Cricothyroidotomy is rarely indicated in the infant, yet if necessary, should not be performed surgically, but using an over-the-needle catheter attached to the barrel of a 3 mL syringe into which an adapter from an 8.0 gauge endotracheal tube has been inserted, providing oxygen via a self-inflating bag-valve, or jet insufflation, device attached to the adapter; tracheostomy is not indicated, unless the actual duration of the ventilator-dependent state has exceeded two months, unless the illness or injury warrants earlier intervention, reversal of sedation, and/or rehabilitation.

There are also significant differences in the anatomy of the chest which have important effects on the mechanics of breathing. The increased pliability of the chest wall, which results from the cartilaginous nature of the infant skeleton and the rudimentary development of the intercostal muscles, results in a relatively elastic thoracic bellows which is exquisitely sensitive to the extremes of positive and negative intrathoracic pressure and positive intra-abdominal pressure, while the more horizontal alignment of the ribs increases the overall contribution of the diaphragm to the movement of gas; the net effect of these anatomic peculiarities, when the infant is nursed supine, is that the diaphragm tends to pull the costal margins inward, rather than pull itself downward, as is the case in a more upright position. For this reason, infants who are breathing spontaneously should be nursed in a semi-erect position whenever this is feasible; moreover, because the infant is chiefly a diaphragmatic breather, anything that compromises diaphragmatic excursion, e.g., major abdominal surgery, diaphragmatic paralysis, gastric distention, or increased abdominal pressure of any other cause, will significantly affect alveolar ventilation. The presence of breath sounds, unfortunately, does not guarantee that air entry is adequate, for they are easily transmitted through the thin chest wall of the child, even if the lung directly beneath the chestpiece of the stethoscope is atelectatic; this problem may be compounded if a pediatric- or adult-sized stethoscope is used instead of an infant-sized model, but may be avoided to some extent by listening for breath sounds just below the axillae, and by always checking to be sure that breath sounds are bilaterally symmetric.

The lungs themselves are not fully mature at the time of birth; while branching is largely complete, alveoli continue to increase in number until well into childhood years. The lungs of the neonate are therefore far less compliant than those of older children and adults; unfortunately, the decreased compliance of the lungs may result in the generation of extremely high transthoracic pressures. This can lead, especially in the presence of edema and/or obstruction of the terminal airways, to "shearing" injuries which can result, in turn, in the development of barotraumatic complications such as pneumothorax, pneumomediastinum, pneumopericardium, and/or the air block syndrome, which, in its severe form, may also result in the development of pulmonary interstitial emphysema (PIE), and so-called "acquired lobar emphysema" (ALE). These problems are obviously compounded when positive pressure is required to maintain effective ventilation; of the two, high mean airway pressure, which is chiefly a function of peak inspiratory pressure, appears to be a more important etiologic factor than high end expiratory pressure. The signs of respiratory failure in the infant, of whatever cause, are tachypnea, flaring, retracting, and grunting, and in its terminal stages, cyanosis and apnea, followed if uncorrected by hypoxia, bradycardia, and death. If due to acute obstruction, severe rocking chest motions may be apparent, indicative of the infant's violent struggle for life, although neurologic or peripheral muscle disease causing hypotonia may preclude this increased work of breathing. Infants will, however, often without apparent effort or distress, tolerate much greater levels of chronic hypoxia and/or hypercarbia than older children or adults. Finally, the presenting signs of ARDS, which occurs in infants and children as it does in adults, either independently following acute lung injury (ALI) or infection, or in tandem with MOSF resulting from sepsis or trauma, are similar to those observed in the adult, although the disease may progress somewhat more rapidly; as in the adult, ARDS is defined using criteria established at the 2012 Berlin Consensus Conference: Respiratory failure not explained by cardiac failure or fluid overload occurring within one week of a known clinical insult or new respiratory symptoms; characterized by bilateral opacities on chest imaging not explained by effusions, lobar or lung collapse or nodules; and manifested by an oxygen deficit, categorized by the P_aO_2/F_iO_2 as mild (200–300), moderate (100–200), or severe (<100).

Critical Care of Life Threatening Respiratory Compromise

Indications for tracheal intubation and mechanical ventilation (hypoxemic or hypercarbic respiratory failure that cannot be successfully treated by less invasive means), and criteria for weaning (resolution of the disease process, improving pulmonary function, progressive withdrawal of support), are similar in children and adults (Table 2); the techniques are equally straightforward. Enough airway pressure must be generated to assure adequate gas insufflation, as judged not only by auscultation, but also by direct observation of the chest wall such that it is seen just to begin to rise; enough tidal volume must be generated to assure adequate minute ventilation, so as to avoid both alveolar hypoventilation and hyperventilation, recognizing that in infants, small airways close at higher lung volumes than they do in children (a process that may be mitigated by surfactant preparations in preterm infants, for rescue in those <34 weeks gestational age, for prophylaxis in those <27 weeks gestational age), such that higher than usual inflating pressures may be required to maintain adequate lung expansion. In large infants and children, synchronized intermittent mandatory ventilation (SIMV) combined with pressure support (PS) has been most frequently used in recent years; however, pressure-regulated, volume-controlled (PRVC) ventilation is increasingly commonly employed, particularly for long term mechanical

Table 2. Indications for mechanical ventilatory support in pediatric patients.

Ventilation abnormalities	Respiratory muscle dysfunction
	1. Respiratory muscle fatigue
	2. Chest wall abnormalities
	3. Neuromuscular disease
	4. Decreased ventilatory drive
	5. Increased airway resistance and/or obstruction
Oxygenation abnormalities	1. Refractory hypoxemia
	2. Need for positive end expiratory pressure
	3. Excessive work of breathing

(Adapted from Pediatric Fundamental Critical Care Support Planning Committee, Society of Critical Care Medicine, Madden MA, *ed. Pediatric Fundamental Critical Care Support*, 2 *ed.* Mount Prospect, IL: Society of Critical Care Medicine, 2013.)

ventilation, either in controlled ventilation (CV) or SIMV mode, so as to minimize the development of ALI and forestall its progression to ARDS by limiting both barotrauma and volutrauma. By contrast, while recent studies indicate that PRVC ventilation may also achieve excellent results even in neonates and small infants, due to the availability of state-of-the-art ventilators that are designed to facilitate accurate delivery even of very small breaths to these tiny patients, time-cycled, pressure-limited (TCPL) ventilation in SIMV mode combined with PS is still most often used; ventilatory strategies that seek to limit both airway pressure and tidal volume are most likely to forestall the progression to chronic lung disease, chiefly BPD.

The goal in all patients is to achieve tidal volumes that are very slightly above normal (6–8 mL/kg) so as to compensate for the mismatch in ventilation and perfusion which results from the redirection of blood flow to the posterior aspects of the lung (by gravity) and air flow to the anterior aspects of the lung (by abnormal diaphragmatic motion) when the patient is nursed supine; higher volumes (10–12 mL/kg) may be needed in patients with neuromuscular disease, lower volumes (4–6 mL/kg) in patients with ARDS. Frequency (f) and inspiratory time (TI) are matched to the patient's size, but may be increased or decreased as necessary to optimize alveolar ventilation; inspiratory:expiratory (I:E) ratios (normally 1:2), adjusted by increasing or decreasing TI above or below normal values for children (0.8–1 sec) and neonates (0.3–0.5 sec) may need to be higher (1:1) in patients with difficulty oxygenating such as ARDS, lower (1:3–1:4) in patients with outflow obstruction such as asthma or BPD. The fraction of inspired oxygen (F_iO_2) and positive end expiratory pressure (PEEP), starting respectively at 1.0 and 5 cm H_2O, should be quickly adjusted to achieve oxygen saturations (S_PO_2) of 94–99%, i.e., oxygen tensions (P_aO_2) of 90 –100 Torr, in the child, first by lowering the former; oxygen tensions in the newborn infant should be no more than the normal 70–80 Torr, as higher levels may predispose to the development of retinopathy of prematurity (ROP), chronic lung injury (BPD), and MOSF, especially in the premature infant. Use of inspired oxygen fractions greater than 0.4–0.6, peak inspiratory pressures (PIPs) that exceed 25–30 cm H_2O, and end expiratory pressures more than 8–10 cm H_2O, is discouraged, but may occasionally be required to achieve adequate oxygen saturation, recognizing that airway pressure release ventilation (APRV) or high frequency oscillatory ventilation (HFOV) should be considered to achieve adequate alveolar ventilation and oxygenation and minimize barotrauma and volutrauma whenever PIPs approach 25 cm H_2O; in select circumstances, however, it may be preferable to accept slightly lower than ideal oxygen saturations and slightly higher than ideal carbon dioxide concentrations (permissive hypercapnia) to avoid development and perpetuation of ALI, and ultimately its progression to ARDS. Obviously, whether using a volume-controlled or pressure-controlled ventilator, attempts should be made to use the minimal settings needed to obtain the desired results; weaning should be accomplished as soon as feasible, most often via SIMV, and concluding with a spontaneous breathing trial (SBT), the likely failure of which is best predicted by a rapid shallow breathing index (RSBI) of >105 breaths/min/L.

Non-invasive positive pressure ventilation (NPPV) methods are increasingly being used in the pediatric population; bilevel positive airway pressure (BiPAP) ventilation may avoid the need for intubation in cooperative older children with mild to moderate acute respiratory failure due to asthma, neuromuscular conditions, obstructive sleep apnea, and end stage cystic fibrosis, among others. In neonates, both term and preterm, use of continuous positive airway pressure (CPAP), both at bedside and during transport, most commonly in the former via an underwater seal apparatus (using an acetic acid solution to retard the growth of Pseudomonas aeruginosa and reduce the risk of ventilator-associated infections) to generate end expiratory pressure ("bubble" CPAP), using specially-designed, large-bore, low-flow nasal prongs (Hudson RCI cannula, Teleflex, Wayne, PA), less commonly in the latter via a hand-held, T-piece resuscitator (NeoPuff, Fisher & Paykel

Healthcare, Irvine, CA; Neo-Tee, Mercury Medical, Clearwater, FL), has revolutionized the management of mild to moderate forms of respiratory distress syndrome (RDS) in this patient population, as bubbling is known to have an oscillatory effect that promotes alveolarization, hence lung development; in selected cases in which bubble CPAP (or its alternative, ventilator driven CPAP, which is still being utilized in many NICUs) is insufficient to support oxygenation upon weaning from mechanical ventilation, nasal intermittent mandatory ventilation (NIMV) in a TCPL mode, using a different specially-designed nasal cannula (NeoTech RAM cannula, Valencia, CA), may be considered. Advanced modes of ventilatory assistance, such as neurally-adjusted ventilatory assistance (NAVA), in which a transesophageal detector device recognizes and transmits electromyographic evidence of diaphragmatic motion to a specially augmented ventilator, allowing earlier initiation, hence improved synchrony, of a mechanically delivered breath, are being explored, but as yet are insufficiently studied for routine use; detailed discussions of HFOV and inhaled nitric oxide (iNO) use are beyond the scope of this chapter, as patients requiring such support should be treated in tertiary, ideally extracorporeal membrane oxygenation (ECMO) capable, pediatric or neonatal centers, but are most often considered for severe (persistent or worsening) hypoxemic respiratory failure (P_aO_2 <60 Torr on F_iO_2 >0.6), such as intractable ARDS in the child, or the "pulmonary injury sequence (PIS) of prematurity" in the preterm infant (RDS which progresses to PIE or pulmonary air leak syndrome), persistent pulmonary hypertension (PPHN), and lung hypoplasia deemed compatible with life. Finally, while a detailed discussion of ECMO itself is also beyond the scope of this chapter, it too is increasingly being employed with encouraging results in selected cases of severe, intractable (unresponsive to HFOV and iNO) acute respiratory failure; consensus criteria for initiation of ECMO in neonates (most often for PPHN associated with congenital diaphragmatic hernia) are (1) gestational age >34 week, (2) weight >2.2 kg, (3) no lethal or major cardiac malformation, (4) no significant coagulopathy or uncontrollable bleeding, (5) no major intracranial hemorrhage, (6) potentially reversible lung injury, (7) duration of mechanical ventilation <10–14 da, and (8) severe, intractable respiratory failure manifested by an oxygenation index (OI) >25 (which corresponds to a mortality rate of 50%), and in children (most often for ARDS), although still in evolution, respiratory failure despite optimal therapy as manifested by (1) a P_aO_2 <60 Torr on F_iO_2 1.0 or an alveolar-arterial oxygen difference (A-aDO_2) >500 Torr, (2) persistent respiratory acidosis (pH <7.25), (3) plateau pressure (P_{plat}) >30 cm H_2O, and (4) a physiologic shunt fraction >30%.

So far as monitoring is concerned, there is no substitute for frequent arterial blood gas determinations obtained from an indwelling arterial cannula, but the complications associated therewith militate against routine use of the latter, so pulse oximetry and waveform capnography are now preferred. If invasive monitoring is needed, however, virtually any post-ductal site may be used safely for arterial cannulation, with the exception of the temporal artery, due to the possibility of cerebrovascular accidents when the catheter is flushed, although the use of end arteries should also be discouraged; the radial artery is therefore most commonly employed for intra-arterial pressure monitoring. That said, it must always be remembered, whether one is following the S_PO_2 or the P_aO_2, that what one is attempting indirectly to measure is the oxygen content of the blood; demonstrably, this depends far less upon the oxygen saturation or partial pressure of oxygen than upon hemoglobin concentration, which, in newborn infants, should be maintained above 14 g/dL to compensate for the higher level of hemoglobin F in neonatal blood. As a result, the physician must be aware that the pulse oximeter may fail to warn of inadequate oxygen saturation, hence tissue delivery, if there remains a high percentage of circulating hemoglobin F, if old or outdated blood low in 2,3-DPG has been given in significant quantity as during exchange transfusion, or if hypothermia and alkalosis, two other factors known to shift the oxyhemoglobin dissociation curve to the left, are present; additionally, it may give misleadingly high, or low, readings, if the sensor is placed at a preductal site, or is attached to an area of skin which is poorly perfused. It must also be realized that, while continuous waveform capnography is an excellent measure of exhaled CO_2, it is often lower than the actual alveolar CO_2 in severe lung disease, due to dead space ventilation; even so, it is an extremely important waveform to follow for acute ventilatory changes, obstructive airway disease, mucus plugging of the endotracheal tube, accidental extubations, and in situations of cardiac arrest.

Heart, Vessels, and Circulation

While the actual cardiac outputs of the infant and child differ significantly from those of the adult, their cardiac indices are roughly the same. However, both because the neonatal myocardium is less compliant, and because the relatively small myocardial mass precludes significant increases in stroke volume with volume loading, heart rate is far and away the most important determinant of cardiac output. Thus, with the exception of the rare supraventricular or ventricular tachycardia so rapid that it precludes adequate ventricular filling, bradycardia, of which the most common cause in the infant or child is hypoxia, is the most immediate threat to the integrity of the circulation. Unfortunately, the immaturity of the autonomic nervous system in the neonate results in exquisite sensitivity to vagal stimulation such as tracheal suctioning or gastric dilatation, dampening the effectiveness of the tachycardia response to hypoxia.

The immaturity of the autonomic nervous system is also such that incomplete myocardial innervation may make it more difficult for the neonate to respond appropriately to situations which demand sustained increases in cardiac output. Fortunately, the neonate does respond well to exogenously administered catecholamines, in doses which are generally similar, per kilogram, to those used in adults. The neonate also seems to respond better to afterload reduction than the adult. However, the reverse is also true: Increases in systemic or pulmonary vascular resistance may result in significant myocardial dysfunction.

The signs of circulatory failure in the infant, fortunately, are fairly similar to those seen in the adult. Even so, the remarkable ability of the child to vasoconstrict peripheral, and in end stages, splanchnic vascular beds is such that mean arterial pressure and core organ perfusion, but not peripheral or splanchnic organ perfusion, are preserved until late in the downward spiral, thus predisposing to earlier development of metabolic acidosis, with its deleterious effects upon myocardial function. Biventricular failure is also more common in infants and small children than in adults. However, while signs of left heart failure are usually obvious, classic signs of right heart failure, such as jugular venous distention, hepatojugular reflux, peripheral edema, or ascites, are usually absent; indeed, tiring during feeds, forehead diaphoresis, and hepatomegaly may be the only physical signs of right heart failure in infants or small children.

In part for this reason, and because the more easily obtained hemodynamic variables, e.g., pulse, blood pressure, and urine output, are often not specific enough to allow therapy to be targeted at reversal of the particular mechanism which is deranged, there is continuous emphasis upon the selective use of invasive monitoring techniques. The child who is in cardiogenic, septic, or neurogenic shock may therefore benefit from central venous pressure monitoring; so does the child in hemorrhagic or hypovolemic shock who does not respond appropriately to volume resuscitation. In highly select circumstances, measurement of pulmonary artery occlusion pressure may also be obtained; however, as placement of flow-directed balloon catheters, i.e., Swan–Ganz catheters, in infants and small children carries a greater degree of risk that in adults, it behooves the critical care specialist to use this device only when necessary, and then to obtain as much information as possible from the intervention. Models equipped with thermistors for determination of cardiac output are preferred, as measurement of this variable using the thermal dilution technique is probably the least operator-dependent of the available methods, provided reasonable precautions are taken to assure the saline tracer is maintained at the correct temperature (0°C) until the moment of infusion; with this device, one can generate an entire hemodynamic profile, i.e., oxygen consumption, systemic and pulmonary vascular resistance, by measuring mixed venous oxygen tension and saturation simultaneously with arterial values, cardiac output, and the blood hemoglobin concentration. Development of less invasive methods of cardiac output monitoring in infants, children, and adults continues to be explored; pulse contour-based, Doppler-based, and lithium dilution-based techniques have all been applied in the clinical arena, and while all have been tested in adults, results have been inconsistent to date, and little if any data are yet available in pediatric populations; fortunately, bedside echocardiography can be a highly useful tool for the evaluation of cardiac anatomy, myocardial contractility, signs of pulmonary hypertension, and/or pericardial effusion or cardiac tamponade.

Critical Care of Life Threatening Circulatory Compromise

As always, proper management of circulatory failure, of whatever cause, depends upon an understanding of the basic pathophysiology as well as careful interpretation of available data; hypovolemic shock, and to a lesser extent septic shock, are far and away the most common forms of shock encountered in the pediatric patient, and as in adults, both are treated initially with volume resuscitation. Cardiogenic shock, common in pediatric cardiac surgical patients, is uncommon in pediatric general surgical patients; regardless, by using the hemodynamic profile as a guide to therapy, it is possible to "optimize" filling pressures, cardiac work, and systemic vascular resistance in such a way as to achieve the most reasonable cardiac index for the lowest possible oxygen consumption, hence the least additional stress for an already overburdened system. Fortunately, normal values are similar for adults and children; in general, one should attempt to keep oxygen consumption at approximately 160 mL/m^2, as this value has been associated with the greatest survival. Regardless of the type of shock that may be encountered, however, its prevention by rapid recognition and treatment of the underlying cause remains the most effective therapy; it is therefore vital that the critical care specialist never forget that the presentation of circulatory failure in the child is deceptive, as the physical signs may not become manifest until late in the course of the disease, by which time shock may be irreversible, unless proper treatment has been instituted.

The circulating blood volume of the preterm infant is approximately 90–105 mL/kg, of the term infant approximately 80–85 mL/kg, and of the child approximately 70 mL/kg. While these values represent a larger proportion of circulating blood volume than in the adult, in absolute numbers these volumes are quite small; volume resuscitation should therefore proceed in small but rapidly infused aliquots ("boluses" or "pushes") of no more than 20 mL/kg (to avoid the development of acute fluid overload), repeated as necessary to restore tissue perfusion, supported in septic and neurogenic shock (once central venous pressure has been normalized) by a vasopressor agent (norepinephrine in the child, dopamine in the infant) if the patient remains hypotensive. Of course, given the relatively smaller absolute blood volume of the child, every attempt should be made to minimize the amount of blood which is drawn for laboratory tests, while the volume of each specimen obtained should be accurately recorded. Finally, because of the high concentration of hemoglobin F, which unloads oxygen suboptimally under extrauterine conditions, it is usually necessary to maintain the hematocrit of the neonate above 40%.

The treatment of severe sepsis and septic shock in pediatric patients has undergone profound change in recent years; in the pediatric surgical patient, these conditions will most likely be encountered in patients with uncontrolled intrathoracic or intra-abdominal infection from an incompletely drained empyema or complicated perforative appendicitis associated with generalized peritonitis and multiple interloop and subdiaphragmatic abscesses for which source control, if possible, is the key element of treatment. Even so, the international Surviving Sepsis Campaign, sponsored in part by the Society of Critical Care Medicine, has resulted in substantial reductions in mortality from severe sepsis and septic shock; the case fatality rate for these conditions, which once approximated 50%, has been halved in most centers, due to the introduction of what has been termed "early goal-directed therapy" (EGDT), consisting of early and aggressive fluid administration, timely antibiotic therapy, administration of a vasopressor agent for refractory shock, and reliance on diagnostic tests and prognostic indicators including blood cultures and serum lactate measurements. While the adult algorithm calls for intravenous fluids, blood cultures, and serum lactate within three hours of emergency department (ED) triage, and additional fluids, pressor agents (if needed), and repeat lactate within six hours, for adult patients with severe sepsis or septic shock, the pediatric algorithm mandates that intravenous fluids and intravenous antibiotics be given within one hour of ED triage for pediatric patients with these conditions; of note, the definitions of severe sepsis and septic shock are age-specific (Table 3).[3] The recent publication of two prospective, randomized adult trials of EGDT (ProCESS and ARISE) has dampened enthusiasm for these algorithms somewhat[4,5]; however, it is important to recognize that the enrollment criteria for both of these trials incorporated certain key elements of EGDT, while their "standard therapy" arms were provided by adult intensivists in academic centers, suggesting that EGDT was being provided informally rather than by protocol, leading the Society of Critical Care Medicine to reaffirm the Surviving Sepsis Guidelines.[6]

Cardiac arrest, fortunately, is rarely a primary event in the infant and child, and is most often due to the severe hypoxia produced by respiratory arrest, preceded and heralded by progressive "symptomatic" sinus bradycardia (less than 60 beats per minute, or bpm); reestablishing airway patency and restoring effective ventilation are therefore of paramount importance in resuscitating the infant and child. Once these have been accomplished, 100% oxygen is immediately administered, and circulation is maintained by means of chest compressions, using the two-thumb chest-encirclement or two-finger technique in the infant, or the one- or two-hand technique in the older child and adolescent, if the heart rate is less than 60 bpm; a peripheral intravenous (IV) line or tibial intraosseous (IO) needle is placed for access to the bloodstream, usually at a distal site so as not to interrupt cardiopulmonary resuscitation (CPR). In the absence of a reliable IV line or sited IO needle, all drugs except dextrose and

Table 3. Definitions of severe sepsis and septic shock in pediatric patients.

Severe sepsis
SIRS associated with a suspected or proven infection plus one of the following:
1. Cardiovascular organ dysfunction
OR
2. ARDS
OR
3. Two or more organ dysfunctions (respiratory, renal, neurologic, hematologic, or hepatic)
Septic shock
Severe sepsis with cardiovascular dysfunction

(Adapted from[3])

Table 4. Selected cardiac arrest resuscitation agents and dosages in pediatric patients.

Amiodarone	5 mg/kg bolus (maximum dose 300 mg)
Calcium chloride	20 mg/kg bolus (0.2 mL/kg)
Defibrillation	2–4 J/ kg (initial dose), 4–10 J/kg (subsequent doses)
Dobutamine	2 to 20 mcg/kg/min infusion (following ROSC)
Dopamine	2 to 20 mcg/kg/min infusion (following ROSC)
Epinephrine	0.01 mg/kg bolus (0.1 mL/kg of 1:10,000 solution)
	0.1 to 1 mcg/kg/min infusion (following ROSC)

(Adapted from Pediatric Subcommittee and Special Contributors, Emergency Cardiovascular Care Committee, American Heart Association, Chameides L, Samson RA, Schexnayder SM, Hazinski MF, eds. *Pediatric Advanced Life Support Provider Manual*, Professional Edition. Dallas, TX: American Heart Association, 2011.)

sodium bicarbonate can be given intratracheally; however, the associated metabolic acidosis is treated not with sodium bicarbonate, but rather by restoration (or return) of spontaneous circulation (ROSC), utilizing epinephrine for slow (less than 60 bpm), absent, or ineffective heart action, reserving external defibrillation and amiodarone for ventricular tachydysrhythmias (rare in infants and small children, uncommon in older children and adolescents), calcium for documented hypocalcemia or calcium channel blocker overdose, yet avoiding etomidate in cases of presumed sepsis to preclude adrenal suppression (Table 4). As in adults, cooling following pediatric cardiac arrest continues to be studied; avoidance of hyperthermia is paramount.

Fluids, Electrolytes, and Nutrition

While it is probably shorter in duration and somewhat of lesser magnitude, the best available evidence suggests that the metabolic response of the infant and child to trauma and to elective surgery parallels that of the adult. In the case of the newborn infant, this response may be superimposed upon the metabolic response to birth, which, depending upon the length and difficulty of delivery, may itself be quite significant. For example, the kidney of the newborn infant, especially if premature, has limited concentrating ability, although relatively normal diluting capacity, for the first few weeks of life. Fortunately, this does not mean that the surgical neonate, term or preterm, cannot effectively excrete a large perioperative salt load, although he or she may not do so as efficiently as the older child or adult.

However, while the response to trauma and surgery do not differ fundamentally from those of the adult, the acute changes in hydration status which accompany these insults must be interpreted in light of the markedly different anatomy of the body fluid spaces. Indeed, in contrast to the adult, water may account for some 75–80% of total body mass in the neonate, more if premature (versus 65–70% in the child and 55–60% in the adult), slightly more than half of which may be found in the extracellular compartment. Half of this extracellular water, on average, turns over every day, a fact which accounts in part for the greater susceptibility of the infant to dehydration. However, the signs of dehydration obviously depend to some extent on whether the disturbance is associated with hyper- or hypotonicity: an infant or small child with hypotonic dehydration will appear better hydrated but be less well perfused than the patient with isotonic dehydration, while the reverse is true for the patient with hypertonic dehydration.

As evaluation of fluid balance is therefore even more critical in the infant and child than it is in the adult, intake and output must be strictly and accurately recorded. Urine volume may be determined by direct measurement if an indwelling catheter or urine bag is present, or by weighing the diaper before and after use. A normally hydrated infant will excrete no less than 1.5–2.0 mL/kg/hr, and an adequately hydrated infant, or a normally hydrated child, at least 1.0 mL/kg/hr. Oliguria is present when the urine output falls below 1.0 mL/kg/ hr in an infant (as this is the minimum amount of free water necessary to excrete the average daily renal solute load, given the poor concentrating ability of the neonatal kidney), or 0.5mL/kg/ hr in a child; renal failure is present when the ratio of urinary sodium clearance to creatinine clearance, called the fractional excretion of sodium (FE_{Na}), exceeds 1.0% in the term infant or child, and 2.5–3.0% in the preterm infant. Weight should be measured daily, at the same time, and on the same scale, and should take into account the weight of arm boards and large dressings before they are applied; weight change is significant when it exceeds 50 g/d in an infant, or 100–200 g/d in a child.

The requirements for fluid roughly parallel the resting metabolic expenditure. Indeed, if one provides for "insensible" losses via lung and skin (which may be dramatically increased in the premature infant due to the effects of phototherapy, radiant warmers, and excessive transepithelial water loss, which results from thinness of the premature infant's skin) and for "sensible" losses via the urinary and gastrointestinal tracts (sweat losses are minimal in the full term infant, and virtually nil in the premature infant), each of which accounts for approximately half of the daily fluid losses (assuming that

Table 5. Holliday–Segar formula for maintenance water in pediatric patients.

0–10 kg — 100 mL/kg
10–20 kg — 1000 mL/kg + 50 mL/kg for each kg over 10 kg
20 kg and up — 1500 mL/kg + 20 mL/kg for each kg over 20 kg

(Adapted from Holliday MA, Segar WE. The maintenance need for water in parenteral fluid therapy. *Pediatrics* 1957; 19: 823–832.)

enough water is cleared by the kidney to allow an average renal solute load to be excreted at an isosthenuric specific gravity), one can readily estimate the daily maintenance fluid needs. The Holliday–Segar formula, which was derived according to these principles, is probably the most widely used method for estimating daily maintenance fluid needs, and is also probably the easiest to remember (Table 5)[7]; individual prescriptions, of course, may differ considerably, because actual maintenance requirements may vary slightly from patient to patient. However, while fluid infusions are not usually given at rates lower than "maintenance" (unless there is evidence of congestive heart failure), high rates, i.e., more than two times "maintenance" in the term infant or child, or one and one half times "maintenance" in the preterm infant, are poorly tolerated, and may predispose the infant, especially if preterm, to fluid overload and/or reopening of the ductus arteriosus, and both infant and child to the subsequent development of congestive heart failure; there is also a significant risk of iatrogenic hyponatremia in hospitalized patients receiving hypotonic fluids.

The metabolic rate itself is primarily a function of size: the smaller the size, the larger the surface area of the body and the lungs in relation to body mass, the larger the evaporative water loss, and the larger the heat loss (note that a 1°C decrease in core temperature in a preterm infant is associated with as much as a 28% increase in case fatality rate); care should therefore be taken to avoid radiant, conductive, and convective together with evaporative heat losses (increased in premature infants due to transepithelial water loss, or TEWL) by (1) maintaining room temperature at 22–26°C, surface (skin) temperature at 36.0–37.0°C, and core (rectal) temperature at 36.5–37.5°C using a radiant warmer in infants and warm standard blankets in children, (2) nursing the infant or child on a warm surface, (3) minimizing the effect of air currents (and TEWL) by nursing the infant (a) in a humidified isolette kept within the "thermoneutral range" (36.5–37.5°C), (b) on a radiant warmer as described above, taking care to cover the premature infant with a

NeoWrap (Fisher & Paykel Healthcare, Irvine, CA) or similar plastic blanket, or (c) in a combination humidified isolette and radiant warmer (Ohmeda Giraffe OmniBed, GE Healthcare Worldwide, Ho-Ho-Kus, NJ) that can decrease the total fluid requirement by as much as 100 mL/kg/d, and/or (4) wrapping the term infant or covering the child with warm standard blankets. Although there is a "thermoregulatory range" slightly below the lower limit of the thermoneutral range within which the infant can compensate for excessive heat loss, the need to generate extra energy (indicated by a surface temperature >0.5°C lower than core temperature), by means of "non-shivering thermogenesis" (metabolism of brown fat) in the preterm infant, shivering in the term infant and older child, will be minimized if surface and core temperature do not differ significantly, and are both maintained within the thermoneutral range. In general, the basal metabolic rate of the newborn infant is some two to three times that of the adult, and approximates some 45 kcal/kg/d; however, to this must be added some 10 kcal/kg/d each to account for normal heat loss, diet-induced thermogenesis, physical activity, and excessive loss of ingested nutrients in the stool. Thus, the infant's maintenance requirements for energy are approximately 75 kcal/kg/d, to which must be added some 50 kcal/kg/d (125 kcal/kg/d overall) to meet the energy costs of growth; these requirements decrease proportionally as the child grows older and larger (to approximately 100 kcal/kg/d by one year, 90 kcal/ kg/ d by five years, 70 kcal/kg/d by 10 years).

The requirements for energy intake may be met with either glucose or fat, as there is no convincing evidence that one is superior to the other as a caloric source. Of course, enough glucose must be provided to prevent the development of ketosis (>5 g/kg/d) and enough fat to prevent the development of essential fatty acid deficiency (>0.5g/kg/d), and avoid the increased work of breathing associated with carbohydrate-based, fat-free or fat-limited diets. In actual practice, these concerns are moot, since a greater reliance on diets which contain a larger proportion of fat (with its greater caloric density), whether delivered enterally or parenterally, is mandated by the infant's higher metabolic rate. However, care must also be taken to be sure the proportion of energy which is supplied by fat does not exceed some 50–55% of total caloric intake, so as to avoid metabolic derangements associated with fat deposition in the liver.

So far as requirements for protein in infants are concerned, the amount required depends chiefly upon the quality of the protein, i.e., how closely it resembles the amino acid profile of human milk. The protein content of human milk is approximately 1.1 g/dL; as the newborn infant may ingest as much as

180–200 mL/kg/d, protein intake usually ranges from 2.0–2.2 g/kg/d. Artificial cow milk-based and methionine-supplemented soy protein-based formulas closely resemble human milk in terms of protein quantity, as well as quality, as they contain approximately 1.5 g/dL of bovine or supplemented soy protein, and are designed to deliver approximately 2.25 g/kg/d of protein in a total volume of approximately 150 mL/kg/d. However, the amino acid profiles of these formulas are substantively different: human milk consists of 60% whey proteins and 40% casein, while the ratio for unmodified cow milk is 18:82; special formulas have lately been developed that more closely resemble the former.

On regimens such as these, normal infants can expect to gain some 10–15 g/kg/d after the first week of life, prior to which most infants experience approximately a 5% drop in weight before birth weight is regained, usually by the end of the first week of life; however, the premature infant may lose as much as 10–15% of birth weight in the first week of life, and, assuming oral intake is tolerated, may require as long as two weeks to regain birth weight. The premature infant also requires more calcium and phosphorus than the full term infant, approximately 2–3 mEq and 1–2 mEq/kg/d, respectively, to grow at the intrauterine rate of approximately 20 g/kg/d. Breast milk, while lower in calcium, has higher bioavailability and absorption of calcium than commercial formulas, and is also rich in lactoferrin and immunoglobulins; human milk fortifier can be added to breast milk to increase protein, calcium, and phosphorus content. For infants without access to breast milk, commercial formulas specifically tailored to the needs of the premature infant are now available, as described elsewhere in considerable detail.

Parenteral nitrogen requirements are no less dependent upon protein quality. The early amino acid solutions produced plasma amino acid profiles that tended to mimic the content of the infusate rather than the more appropriate post-prandial plasma amino acid profile of the normal breastfed infant; not surprisingly, as much as 3.5–4.0 g/kg/d of crystalline amino acids were required with these formulations to achieve consistently positive nitrogen balance. However, the current generation of solutions can achieve this with as little as 2.3–2.7 g/kg/d. Moreover, there is evidence to suggest that solutions, e.g., Trophamine® (B. Braun Medical, Irvine, CA), that were specifically designed, when infused, to reproduce the post-prandial plasma amino acid profile of a normal breastfed baby, may do so with even less.

The need for extra protein to avoid breakdown of muscle mass and its untoward effects on respiratory, cardiac, and immunologic function has been reasonably well established for surgical operations and bacterial sepsis, based on measured increases of protein degradation and urinary nitrogen excretion of 25% and 100%, respectively; unfortunately, the same is not true of the need for extra energy. Standard formulas for predicting caloric needs, such as the Harris-Benedict equation, are frequently inaccurate; moreover, the stress response to illness and injury has not been found to be so consistent or pronounced as was previously believed.[8] By contrast, the protein and energy needs of pediatric burn victims have been extensively studied over many years, and have been definitively established: protein intakes of 1.5 g/kg/day and energy intakes of 1.2 times REE are currently recommended, since greater amounts, although better able to maintain body weight, do not appear to result in preservation of lean body mass; as such, higher amounts of protein and energy are no longer routinely prescribed.[9] Moreover, overfeeding of critically ill and injured children is increasingly recognized as a serious if silent problem in the PICU; it leads to respiratory compromise through excess production and subsequent elimination of carbon dioxide, as well as hyperglycemia, hyperlipidemia, and liver dysfunction.

Critical Care of Fluids, Electrolytes, and Nutrition

Consensus recommendations for macronutrient provision to critically ill and injured pediatric patients from the American Society of Parenteral and Enteral Nutrition currently suggest:[10] (1) a protein intake of 2–3 g/kg/day for infants and toddlers, 1.5–2 g/kg/day for preschoolers and school-age children, and 1.5 g/kg/day for adolescents; and (2) an energy intake, based on resting energy expenditure (REE) as measured by indirect calorimetry, that is high in fat and low in carbohydrate, owing to the primacy of fat as an energy source in critical pediatric illness, its role in preventing EFA deficiency, and the absence of adverse effects on ventilation. If indirect calorimetry is unavailable, it may be necessary to use a standard formula, such as the Harris-Benedict equation, recognizing its tendency to overpredict REE, particularly in obese children, and modifying the calculations accordingly.[8] Every attempt should be made to avoid interruptions in feeding due to diagnostic procedures and therapeutic interventions. Ongoing consultation with a dedicated pediatric nutrition support team, if available, can assist in facilitating these aims.

Maintenance requirements for electrolytes are approximately 2–3 mEq/kg/d for sodium and chloride and 1–2 mEq/kg/d for potassium; calcium, in a dose of 1–2 mEq/kg/d (100–200 mg/kg/d as 10% gluconate), will also be required for the newborn infant, more if preterm. Other elements are probably not needed unless the patient is receiving total parenteral nutrition; fortunately, in this instance, only phosphorous (as KH_2PO_4) and magnesium (as $MgSO_4$), in doses of 1.5 mEq/kg/d and 0.25 mEq/kg/d, respectively, need to be added separately, since specific pediatric trace element supplements are available, as is also the case for vitamins. In practice, the sodium and chloride content of maintenance fluid should rarely exceed 0.22 N (taking care to avoid iatrogenic hyponatremia by minimizing excessive free water administration); even so, the post injury or postoperative patient may require sodium and chloride contents as high as 0.45 N at rates as high as 1.5 times "maintenance" for several hours following surgery or trauma (initial management of burn injury in children is discussed below) to account for third space fluid losses (especially if peritoneal inflammation is present, as in necrotizing enterocolitis or gastroschisis). Gastric drainage is generally replaced ml for ml with 0.45 N saline solution with added potassium, as this approximates the usual chloride content of gastric juice (50–60 mEq/L); similarly, chest, wound, and/or intestinal stoma drainage is replaced ml for ml with 0.9 N saline solution or lactated Ringer's solution, as these both approximate the typical electrolyte content of isotonic body fluids.

Five g/dL of dextrose are generally added to all intravenous infusions in children (10 g/dL in infants to prevent hypoglycemia) so as to normalize tonicity, avoid lysis of red cells, and spare protein, although there is data to suggest that the latter effect may not be so great in the infant as it is in the adult. All fluids should be given via an infusion pump, in aliquots which should comprise no more than 25% of the total daily fluid allotment, so as to minimize the chance for errors in administration, and to prevent inadvertent fluid overload. Intake and output must be closely monitored, and double checked, by measuring not only the amount actually infused by the infusion pump, but also how much fluid has gone from the fluid reservoir. Again, daily weights should also be measured, at the same time each day, on the same scale.

Total parenteral nutrition (TPN) should be considered if oral intake will not be resumed within five to seven days; as there appears to be no significant difference between the peripheral and central routes so far as the per diem complication rate is concerned, the choice of one or the other will depend upon other factors, i.e., desired caloric intake, anticipated duration of therapy, and accessibility of veins. Peripheral TPN can deliver up to 80–90 non-protein kcal/kg/d in the preterm infant, slightly more in the term infant, provided generally recognized dextrose (12.5%), lipid (3 g/kg/d), and fluid (150 mL/kg/d) limits are adhered to, and is most useful when nutrient needs are not exceptional, the anticipated duration of therapy is short, and there are an adequate number of veins to allow frequent changing of peripheral access sites, while central TPN can deliver up to 150–160 kcal/kg/d when using concentrations of dextrose (30%) and crystalline amino acids (3.5–4 gm/kg/d), which are usually well tolerated by all but the most premature infants, provided concentrations are advanced slowly in a stepwise fashion; while there is no particular physiologic reason to proscribe the use of adjunctive insulin, this is not recommended, both because it is rarely necessary, and because of the increased risks associated with both hyperglycemia (>200 mg/dL) and hypoglycemia (<50 mg/dL) in the infant, especially if preterm. Due to their increased caloric density, the use of "balanced" regimens which rely heavily upon the use of intravenous fat emulsions as an energy source, in addition to their role in preventing essential fatty acid deficiency syndromes and avoiding respiratory embarrassment due to carbohydrate loading, are preferred; current recommendations now allow use of the 20% emulsion, even in preterm infants, although the infusion rate of the fat emulsion should not exceed 3 g/kg/d (1g/kg/d if the infant develops cholestasis), to preclude development of cholestasis as well as fat overload syndrome (which can usually be avoided by keeping serum triglyceride levels <200 mg/dL in the term infant, <150 mg/dL in the preterm infant), recognizing that reduced lipid doses may also be needed in infants with RDS, PPHN, sepsis, and hyperglycemia. However, whether one is using parenteral or enteral nutritional support, plasma electrolytes, and blood and urine sugar, due to the lower renal threshold of the infant and child to glycosuria, must be closely monitored; if the child is parenterally fed, liver function tests must also be followed closely. Moreover, the concept that one form of artificial feeding, be it enteral or parenteral, is easier, safer, or more efficacious than another, is fallacious; close attention to the details of proper feeding are required, regardless of the method used. Adequacy of nutritional therapy in the neonate is most reliably indicated by the presence of steady weight gain in the absence of significant edema; this should approximate 10–15 g/kg/d in the term infant, but should approach the intrauterine growth rate of 20 g/kg/d in the preterm infant. Fortunately, the safety and efficacy of artificial nutritional support are now well established, such that there appears to be no valid reason to withhold such vital support unless there exists a specific contraindication to its use.

Even so, complications can and do occur. The most common complication of peripheral TPN is infiltration, and in severe infiltration, skin slough, while the most common complication of central TPN is sepsis; both types of complications are largely preventable, by rotation of access sites in the former instance, and strict adherence to catheter protocols in the latter. Percutaneously inserted central catheters (PICC lines) are now preferred for long term infusion of central TPN, especially in infants, while central venous catheters inserted via the subclavian route remain an acceptable alternative in older children; in both cases, meticulous attention to antisepsis must be maintained through rigorous adherence to catheter care "bundles", so as to avoid the possibility of central line-associated bloodstream infection (CLABSI). All infiltrated or infected peripheral catheters must, of course, be removed and replaced, but there is now good evidence that CLABSIs, particularly those caused by Gram-positive organisms, may respond to antibiotic therapy, if such therapy is given for a period of not less than two weeks via the catheter itself, recognizing that failure to clear the infection within 48 hours may constitute grounds for earlier removal.

"Metabolic" emergencies related to the use of total parenteral nutrition, fortunately, are now exceedingly rare. Obviously, the first, and often the only, step necessary in any such treatment is to discontinue the infusion. Otherwise, metabolic emergencies in patients who are not receiving artificial nutritional support are treated utilizing standard measures designed to correct the abnormality identified (Table 6). However, to avoid the disastrous complication of intraventricular hemorrhage in the neonate, due to rupture of the immature choroid plexuses following rapid infusion of a hypertonic solution, emergency infusions of glucose, electrolytes, and/or bicarbonate should be no more hypertonic than some two to three times the normal plasma osmolality of 280–300 mOsm/L, e.g., 10% dextrose, half-strength sodium bicarbonate, and should be administered by slow intravenous infusion rather than rapid intravenous push.

Acute kidney injury (AKI) resulting in acute renal failure (ARF) is uncommonly encountered in pediatric surgical critical care, prerenal causes of azotemia being more common than renal or postrenal causes; however, when present, the etiologies of AKI are similar to those observed in adults, although the RIFLE criteria for ARF, now commonly applied to adult patients, have not consistently been associated with morbidity and mortality outcomes in children with this condition. As previously noted, the diagnosis is suspected based on concomitant increases in blood urea nitrogen (BUN) and serum creatinine; it is confirmed by calculation of FE_{Na} as described above. Renal replacement therapy (RRT), in the form of ultrafiltration, hemodialysis, or peritoneal dialysis, short of renal transplantation, is available for infants and children; continuous RRT (CRRT), in the form of continuous ultrafiltration (CUF), continuous venovenous hemofiltration (CVVH), and continuous venovenous hemodialysis (CVVHD), all require insertion and maintenance of large bore central venous catheters, ideally hemodialysis

Table 6. Treatment of selected metabolic emergencies in pediatric patients

Hypocalcemia	Calcium gluconate 100mg/kg *1 (max 2 g per run)
Hypoglycemia	Dextrose 10% 0.5 g/kg
Hypomagnesemia	Magnesium sulfate 25mg/kg * 1 (max 2g per run)
Hypermagnesemia	Calcium chloride 20 mg/kg slow IV infusion
Hypokalemia	Potassium chloride 0.5–1mEq/kg (max 20 mEq per run)
Hyperkalemia (K^+ 6.0–7.0 mEq/L)	Potassium exchange resin 1 g/kg
Hyperkalemia (K^+ >7.0 mEq/L)	Regular insulin 0.1 U/ kg (2 mL/kg in D25 @ 2 mL/ min)
	AND/OR
	Sodium bicarbonate 1–2 mEq/kg slow IV push
Hyperkalemia (ECG changes)	Calcium gluconate 100 mg/kg slow IV push (max 2 g)
	Consider continuous albuterol, furosemide 1–2 mg/kg
Hyponatremia (Na^+ 120–130 mEq/L)	0.9% NaCl solution @ 1.5–2 * maintenance rate
Hyponatremia (Na^+ <120 mEq/L, seizures)	3% NaCl solution 1.2 mL/kg * Na^+ deficit slow IV push
	Na^+ deficit = 120 — serum Na^+ concerntration
Hypernatremia	0.225% NaCl solution @ 1.5–2 * maintenance rate

(Adapted from Pediatric Subcommittee and Special Contributors, Emergency Cardiovascular Care Committee, American Heart Association, Chameides L, Samson RA, Schexnayder SM, Hazinski MF, eds. *Pediatric Advanced Life Support Provider Manual*, Professional Edition. Dallas, TX: American Heart Association, 2011, and Pediatric Fundamental Critical Care Support Planning Committee, Society of Critical Care Medicine, Madden MA, *ed. Pediatric Fundamental Critical Care Support*, 2 *ed.* Mount Prospect, IL: Society of Critical Care Medicine, 2013.)

catheters, in large bore central veins, usually the internal jugular vein to minimize the risks of thrombosis and stenosis associated with use of the subclavian and femoral veins. There currently exist no studies addressing flow rates in pediatric CRRT; they should certainly not exceed the optimal adult rate of 20–25 mL/kg/hr.

Neurological Assessment and Brain Death

Although a detailed discussion of the neurologic evaluation of the critically ill infant and child is beyond the scope of this chapter, neurological assessment of the child is similar to that utilized in the adult; however, it should be noted that the incomplete development of the central and autonomic nervous systems in neonates is such that primitive postural and autonomic reflexes, e.g., the Moro and diving reflexes, are incompletely suppressed. Moreover, as spontaneous motions of the infant's extremities are directed by the basal ganglia rather than higher cortical levels, the expression of asymmetric or focal signs is extremely rare; evaluation of the infant's neurologic status will therefore be based primarily upon level of alertness, response to environmental stimuli, general level of activity, and overall muscle tone. Signs of increased intracranial pressure (ICP), fortunately, are similar in infants and adults, except to note that a bulging anterior fontanelle may be the only sign of increased ICP in an infant; it is important to realize, however, that due to incomplete closure of the cranial sutures, slight cranial enlargement, as determined by serial measurement of head circumference, may allow accommodation to increasing intracranial volume without a concomitant increase in ICP, especially when this enlargement is gradual. Finally, it must be remembered that aberrations in ventilation, oxygenation, and perfusion, as well as hypoglycemia, should always be excluded as a basis for altered mental status (AMS) before other causes are considered, while a weak, thin, high-pitched, scratchy cry is often associated with neurological disease in infants.

Criteria for determination of brain death in infants and children, excluding preterm infants for whom insufficient data are available, have recently been updated.[11] Such determination is based on (1) absence of neurological function with a known irreversible cause of coma, (2) correction of hypotension, hypothermia, and metabolic disturbances, (3) discontinuance of medications that could interfere with apnea testing, (4) two examinations including apnea testing by different attending physicians separated by an appropriate observation period (12 hour in infants and childrens, 24 hours in neonates), (5) apnea testing that documents $P_aCO_2 \geq 20$ Torr above baseline and ≥60 Torr with absence of respiratory effort during the testing period, and (6) reliance on ancillary studies (electroencephalogram and radionuclide scan) if an apnea test cannot be completed safely, or uncertainty remains about the diagnosis. This approach is in contrast to that now taken in adults, which no longer requires a second examination and apnea test. Both lack of data, and the fraught nature of declaring brain death in a child, warrant such an approach.

Life Threatening Pediatric Traumatic Emergencies

Pediatric trauma remains the leading cause of morbidity and mortality in childhood. The basic principles governing the primary survey and resuscitation of the child trauma victim are similar to those in the adult trauma patient. The need for emergency operation is indicated by the presence of hypovolemia that does not respond promptly to volume resuscitation, i.e., after two to three 20 mL/kg aliquots ("boluses" or "pushes") administered by rapid intravenous infusion over 15–20 minutes) of lactated Ringer's solution. With few exceptions, the presence of hypotensive shock itself mandates operative intervention, since the presence of this condition, given the remarkable capacity of the child to vasoconstrict in response to hypovolemia, indicates that major life-threatening hemorrhage has occurred and is likely ongoing; in such circumstances, the rapid administration of blood products, type-specific whole blood if available, O negative whole blood if not, or if only components are available, packed red blood cells (PRBCs), fresh frozen plasma (FFP), and single-donor platelet concentrates in a 1:1:1 or 2:1:1 ratio, each at 10 mL/kg, may be life-saving, recognizing that administration of PRBCs otherwise is not generally advised unless the hemoglobin concentration falls below 7 g/dL, owing to the deleterious effects of blood transfusions on immune function, and the development of transfusion-associated acute lung injury (TRALI).

Shock is present in a child when there is tachycardia, tachypnea, and impaired perfusion of body tissues sufficient to deprive them of an adequate supply of oxygen to meet their metabolic needs; it is usually caused by internal hemorrhage involving the abdomen, pelvis, and/or femora, seldom the chest, rarely if ever the head. In general, the normal systolic blood pressure in a child in mm Hg is 90 plus twice the age in years, while the diastolic pressure should be approximately two-thirds of this number; the lower limit of normal for the systolic blood pressure in mm Hg is 70 plus twice the age in years. As in the adult, rules governing the relationship between vital signs and blood loss, and the 3:1 rule for crystalloid replacement of blood loss, apply; as there is now evidence that overzealous correction of lactic acidosis due to hypoperfusion is counterproductive, acidemia should be pharmacologically treated only when the pH falls below 7.2 despite adequate volume replacement, using the formula: body weight (kg) × 0.3 × base deficit = total $NaHCO_3$, and then only until such time as adequate ventilation, oxygenation, and perfusion can be restored. Finally, as in the adult, volume resuscitation is best carried out by means of short, large bore peripheral intravenous lines; central venous catheters, except perhaps in rare cases where myocardial dysfunction and/or moderate to severe ARDS are present, will not be needed even for the monitoring of volume status, as measurement of urine output and examination of distal pulses will generally suffice for this purpose.

Blunt injuries are far more common in children than penetrating injuries: Child abuse must be suspected whenever the history proffered does not seem compatible with the type or seriousness of injury. The chest wall is extremely compliant, and major vascular injuries are rare; however, major pulmonary and myocardial contusions which can and do occur, and may be life-threatening. As the management of certain abdominal injuries, e.g., lacerations of the spleen and/or liver, is nonoperative, the presence of blood in the abdominal cavity does not constitute an automatic indication for operation; thus, peritoneal lavage, which in any case has been largely supplanted by Focused Assessment by Sonography in Trauma (FAST), is rarely utilized in children. Marked gastric distention, of course, is a concomitant of most serious childhood trauma, due to the aerophagia associated with crying; indeed, it may be so severe as to mimic abdominal injury, and mandates immediate treatment by means of gastric tube decompression.

Because the child is top-heavy, head injuries occur more frequently among children than adults; fortunately, management of head injury in the child is similar to that in the adult, although brain swelling is a far more common cause of increased ICP than mass lesions, a fact which may account for the somewhat better outcome following head injury in the child. As stated, the presence of shock is rarely, if ever, due to the head injury itself, and mandates a careful search for a source of blood loss outside the cranial vault, although it should be noted that children can lose enormous quantities of blood from scalp wounds. Also, as hypoxia represents one major cause of secondary brain injury, any child who is bradycardic due to increased ICP, or who shows other signs of hypoxia such as cyanosis, should be immediately intubated with the proper-sized endotracheal tube, and ventilated with 100% oxygen until an arterial blood gas determination can be made; adequate volume resuscitation must also be assured, as cerebral perfusion pressure depends upon the difference between mean arterial pressure, which may be decreased owing to blood loss or the presence of spinal cord injury, and ICP, which may be increased owing to brain swelling or the presence of an intracranial hematoma. Management of spine and extremity trauma is similar to that in the adult, except to note that cervical spine injuries are fortunately much less common than in adults, and that fractures through epiphyseal growth plates require special management, while vascular compromise associated with supracondylar fractures is far more common.

Critical Care of Life Threatening Pediatric Traumatic Injuries

Critical care of major pediatric trauma begins with the primary survey and resuscitation phase, which are conducted concurrently. Critical care is the responsibility of not a single individual or specialty but of a multidisciplinary team specializing in pediatric care, led by a surgeon with experience in the care of both trauma and children. It continues with the secondary survey and re-evaluation of vital functions, progresses through the tertiary survey (a scrupulous repetition of the primary and secondary surveys conducted by the admitting team once the patient is transferred to definitive care) to ensure no injuries were missed, and persists throughout the duration of hospitalization, including rehabilitation, fully encompassing the emergency, operative, critical, acute, and convalescent phases of care. Avoidance of secondary injury (injury due to persistent or recurrent hypoxia or hypoperfusion) is a major goal of critical care, and mandates continuous monitoring of vital signs, GCS score, oxygen saturation, urinary output, and, when necessary, arterial and central venous pressure, in addition to frequent re-examination.

Critical care of major pediatric trauma also depends on the type, extent, and severity of the injuries sustained. Any child requiring resuscitation should be admitted to the hospital under the care of a surgeon experienced in the management of childhood injuries. Such a child should initially not receive oral intake (because of the temporary paralytic ileus that often accompanies major blunt abdominal trauma and because general anesthesia may later be required) but intravenous fluid at a maintenance rate (assuming both normal hydration at the time of the injury and normalization of both vital signs and perfusion status after resuscitation). Soft tissue injuries also should receive proper attention (wound irrigation, debridement, cleansing, and closure, tetanus prophylaxis). Peripheral intravenous catheters inserted under substerile circumstances should be replaced to prevent the development of thrombophlebitis, while central venous lines, when needed, must be skillfully inserted and scrupulously maintained by trained providers using critical care "bundles" incorporating sterile barrier technique and chlorhexidine skin prep to avoid the development of CLABSI. Both deep venous thrombosis and venous thromboembolic complications are rare in childhood trauma, patients at greatest risk being older children with high injury severity, major vascular injury, craniotomy, or central venous catheters.[12] Prophylaxis, therefore, is seldom necessary, while a role for vena cava filters is unproven.[13,14] Urinary (Foley) catheters need not be routinely inserted, unless there is suggestive evidence of hemodynamic instability, or they are deemed necessary to the performance of FAST; they should be removed at the earliest opportunity to avoid the development of catheter associated urinary tract infection (CAUTI).

Brain

The overall mortality and morbidity of major pediatric trauma are closely linked with the functional outcome of the traumatic brain injury (TBI) that typically occurs after significant blunt impact. The results of treatment TBI are somewhat better in children 3–12 years of age than in adults with similar Glasgow Coma Scale (GCS) scores, an advantage ablated in the presence of hypotension. Conversely, outcomes are worse in children younger than 3 years of age. Although the general principles of definitive management of TBI are similar in children and adults, nonoperative management predominates because diffuse brain injuries are more common than focal injuries in pediatric patients. Surgically remediable causes of intracranial hypertension must be treated if found, but medically remediable causes are addressed aggressively. The goal of treatment is to normalize cerebral blood flow (CBF), which may decrease to half its normal value in severe TBI, through maintenance of cerebral perfusion pressure (CPP), calculated as the difference between mean arterial pressure (MAP) and ICP, and avoidance of moderate or severe hyperventilation (P_aCO_2 <30 Torr), which is known to promote cerebral ischemia.

Current management of TBI in children should adhere to evidence-based guidelines.[15] Conservative treatment, including discharge to home care under the supervision of responsible adult caretakers who have been instructed to return if signs of increased intracranial pressure (nausea, vomiting, increasing lethargy) develop, suffices for management of mild head injury (GCS score 13–15), among whom post concussive symptoms are common, but most often resolve within a few days. Neurologically intact children with isolated skull fracture may also be discharged after brief observation. Non contrast CT is indicated for all patients who sustain loss of consciousness or are amnestic, in accordance with current evidence- and population-based guidelines. Expectant management, including hospital admission, CT, and continuous neurologic observation, is employed for all patients with moderate head injury (GCS score 9–12). Repeat CT 12–24 hours following injury, previously advocated as a routine investigation to exclude injury progression, is no longer recommended absent signs of neurological deterioration.

Controlled ventilation is initiated after endotracheal intubation utilizing rapid-sequence technique (preoxygenation, followed by atropine 0.02 mg/kg [minimum 0.1 mg/kg, maximum 1.0 mg/kg], followed by judiciously applied cricoid pressure, followed by etomidate 0.3 mg/kg [0.1 mg/kg if hypovolemic] or midazolam 0.3 mg/kg [0.1 mg/kg if hypovolemic], followed by succinylcholine 1 mg/kg or rocuronium 0.6 mg/kg [if spinal cord injury or pre-existing neuromuscular disease is present or suspected]) for all patients with severe TBI (GCS score 3–8, or a sudden deterioration in GCS score of ≥2 points). Mild hyperventilation (P_aCO_2 30–35 Torr) and boluses of hypertonic saline (3%, 6.5–10 mL/kg) in preference to mannitol (0.5 mg/kg), for which scant pediatric evidence exists despite its common usage in pediatric head injury, are reserved for patients with acute evidence of intracranial hypertension (ICP >20 Torr) to prevent transtentorial (pupillary asymmetry, neurologic posturing) or cerebellar (ataxic breathing) herniation, while an infusion of hypertonic saline (3%, 0.1–1 mL/kg/hr) is used for persistent evidence of intracranial hypertension, taking care to maintain serum osmolality at a level <360 mOsm/L.[15–17] Intracranial hypertension uncontrolled by such measures may require moderate therapeutic hypothermia (32–33°C) for up to 48 hours following injury, or as a potential last resort, decompressive craniectomy.[18]

The role of ICP monitoring remains controversial. Increased ICP and inadequate CPP have both been associated with decreased survival.[19,20] As such, current evidence-based guidelines cite maintenance of a minimum CPP of 40 Torr as an option, for which the insertion of an ICP monitoring device is obviously needed.[15] The numerous studies on which these guidelines were based collectively suggest that ICP monitoring confers a probable survival benefit, corroborating historical data from the National Pediatric Trauma Registry that it improves case fatality rate in severe traumatic brain injury (GCS score 3–4) independent of the potential confounding effects of internal organ injury or systolic hypotension. However, two recently conducted prospective studies are split on the value of ICP monitoring as an adjunct to management of severe TBI.[21,22] Further research is needed before this dilemma can be resolved with certainty. Even so, it is self-evident that, short of decompressive craniectomy (the outcomes of which are uniformly disappointing despite its salutary effect in reducing ICP[18]), only ventriculostomy (short of craniectomy) offers means for physical reduction of ICP (via external drainage of excess cerebrospinal fluid), with the added benefit that it can also be used for ICP monitoring. The role of brain tissue oxygen monitoring in children with severe TBI remains uncertain, but there is no doubt that cerebral tissue hypoxia is associated with poor outcome, an outcome that is significantly worsened when cerebral tissue hypoxia is complicated by systemic hypotension. If used, the partial pressure of brain tissue oxygen ($P_{bt}O_2$) should be maintained at levels ≥10 mm Hg.[15]

Immediate operation is necessary for all acute collections of intracranial (epidural, subdural, intracerebral) blood of sufficient size to cause a mass effect (>5 mm away from the apparent midline as visualized on CT), for all open skull fractures, and for all depressed skull fractures that invade the intracranial vault by more than the thickness of the adjacent skull. Intravenous antibiotics are used only for patients with open skull fractures. Anticonvulsants (phenytoin preceded by lorazepam, as needed) are indicated for all patients with active seizures, impact seizures, or moderate or severe brain injury but should be discontinued after 2 weeks of therapy because no benefit accrues after this interval. Corticosteroid therapy is contraindicated for treatment of TBI. Moreover, nitrogen losses may be accelerated.

Acute complications of severe TBI include hyperglycemia, diabetes insipidus (DI), the syndrome of inappropriate antidiuretic hormone secretion (SIADH), and brain death. The first three are managed, respectively, through the use of insulin, desmopressin, and water restriction, while the first is associated with poor neurologic outcome for reasons not yet fully elucidated. Brain death most often results from uncontrolled intracranial hypertension. Due consideration should be given to organ preservation and donation under such circumstances, although conversations with families should be initiated by regional organ donor network personnel rather than the PICU team, to avoid the appearance of conflict of interest.

Spine

While the cervical region is often injured, the spinal cord is not. High-dose methylprednisolone, previously thought to be efficacious in mitigating the effects of spinal cord injury, is now known to add little, if any, benefit to the management of patients with such injury. Early care should therefore focus on the recognition and management of neurogenic shock (volume resuscitation followed by vasopressor agents as needed) as well as immobilization of associated fractures (extrication collar and backboard followed by skeletal traction with Gardner-Wells tongs), realizing that spinal cord injury without radiographic abnormality (SCIWORA) is far more common in children than in adults, especially those who present in traumatic coma (GCS score ≤8) or hypotensive shock. Later care addresses repair of associated vertebral fractures through the use of halo traction with or without surgical fusion.

The critical care of patients with spinal cord injury is chiefly supportive. Alternating-pressure or air-fluidizing mattresses should be used whenever available to prevent the development of decubitus ulcers. Indwelling urinary catheterization, followed by intermittent clean catheterization, should be used to prevent the development of urinary stasis and subsequent infection. Aggressive pulmonary toilet, including bronchoscopy, should be used to prevent the development of pulmonary infections, especially in patients with intercostal or diaphragmatic muscle paralysis, in whom the ability to clear respiratory secretions through spontaneous or induced coughing is most often severely compromised.

Chest

Most life-threatening chest injuries can be managed expectantly, or by tube thoracostomy inserted via the fifth intercostal space in the midaxillary line. Indications for resuscitative thoracotomy are limited to patients with physical or electrocardiographic signs of life in the field or emergency department after penetrating chest trauma. The universally dismal results preclude its use in blunt chest or abdominal trauma, even though cardiopulmonary resuscitation by itself is associated with a 23.5% survival rate, unless begun in the field and ongoing at the time of trauma center arrival, when it is zero. Emergency thoracotomy is reserved for injured patients with massive hemothorax (20 mL/kg) and ongoing hemorrhage (2–4 mL/kg/hr), massive air leak, and food or salivary drainage from the chest tube. Severe pulmonary contusions, if complicated by aspiration, overhydration, or infection, can predispose the patient to development of ARDS, which was initially described as post-traumatic pulmonary insufficiency (PTPI), or "shock lung". These complications require aggressive ventilatory support and, occasionally, ECMO. Neither isolated first rib fractures, nor isolated sternal fractures, nor isolated pneumomediastinum, nor occult pneumothorax are typically associated with serious injury in otherwise normal patients, and the latter can be safely observed, and managed without tube thoracotomy, when < 16 mm on chest imaging. Traumatic asphyxia, characterized by facial and conjunctival petechiae, requires no specific treatment, but serves to indicate the considerable severity of the impacting force.

Critical care of the respiratory insufficiency that accompanies severe chest injury is chiefly supportive, as few pulmonary contusions progress to ARDS. That said, to avoid both oxygen toxicity and resorption atelectasis, it is best to use the least amount of artificial respiratory support necessary to maintain the P_aO_2 at 70–99 Torr (hence the S_PO_2 at 94–99%) and the P_aCO_2 (or the $P_{ET}CO_2$) at 35–40 Torr. Continuous positive airway pressure (CPAP) or positive end-expiratory pressure (PEEP) should be used for maintenance of functional residual capacity whenever the F_iO_2 exceeds 0.4, but adverse effects on the circulation should be avoided. Peak inspiratory pressure should be kept below 20–25 cm H_2O whenever positive-pressure ventilation is required, especially if pneumothoraces, or fresh bronchial or pulmonary suture lines, are present. Pulmonary contusions uncomplicated by aspiration, overhydration, or infection can be expected to resolve in 7–10 days. Thus, the judicious use of pulmonary toilet, crystalloid fluid, loop diuretics, and therapeutic (not prophylactic) antibiotics to preclude the development of ARDS from pulmonary contusions or PTPI, and measures to avoid the development of ventilator-associated pneumonia (VAP) such as avoidance of both narcotics and enteral feedings use of head-of-bed elevation and sedation holidays, as well as peptic ulcer disease and deep venous thrombosis prophylaxis as indicated, are required, although nosocomial pneumonia may not affect fatality rate in afflicted children.[23]

Abdomen

Immediate management of intra-abdominal and genitourinary injuries in children is chiefly nonoperative, although not necessarily nonsurgical, as mature surgical judgment is needed to determine whether, or when, operation is needed. Nonoperative management of splenic injury is particularly advocated, to avoid the development of overwhelming post-splenectomy infection, pneumococcal vaccine being indicated for spleen-injured children if splenectomy is entertained or required. Fortunately, bleeding from renal, splenic, and hepatic injuries is mostly self-limited, and will resolve spontaneously in most cases, unless the patient is in hypotensive shock, in which case emergent operation is required (using damage control methods for patients in extremis and/or staged closure for patients with abdominal compartment syndrome) or the transfusion requirement exceeds 40 mL/kg of body weight (half the circulating blood volume) within 12–24 hours of injury, in which case urgent operation is considered.[24] Laparotomy for repair of blunt renal, pancreatic, gastrointestinal, and genitourinary injuries is infrequently required, but performed as necessary, although failure to recognize and treat blunt intestinal injuries in a timely manner may not adversely affect patient outcome. A pancreatic pseudocyst is heralded by the development of a tender epigastric mass 3–5 days after upper abdominal trauma and is likely to respond to nonoperative management composed of 4–6 weeks of bowel rest and TPN, although an internal drainage procedure is occasionally required. However, the presence of a high-grade pancreatic injury on CT of the abdomen suggests that nonoperative management may fail, and that either distal pancreatic resection with external drainage, or, in selected cases, endoscopic retrograde cholangiopancreatography (ERCP) with pancreatic ductal stenting, may ultimately be required. While abdominal compartment syndrome is uncommon in children, invasive postoperative mechanical ventilation may be needed if marked abdominal enlargement impinges on the thoracic pump, and for pain control to prevent splinting and hypoventilation. Of note, NPPV is usually not an option in an infant or child with severe ileus, as it may produce significantly increased gastric distension despite seemingly adequate gastric decompression.

Critical care of hemodynamically stable children with blunt solid visceral injuries should follow evidence-based guidelines for observation in a PICU for a minimum of 24 hours, since failure of nonoperative management (1) is uncommon, (2) is unlikely, although possible, even in the presence of a contrast blush on CT of the abdomen, (3) usually occurs within 12–24 hours, (4) does not appear to affect outcome, and (5) can be managed without resort to operation in selected cases through use of angiographic embolization or recombinant factor VIIa, while long-term complications of nonoperative management are minimal.[25,26] If respiratory care is required, incentive spirometry is preferred, as clots that are organizing may be disturbed by vigorous chest physiotherapy. The stomach should be kept decompressed following splenic injury to prevent reactivation of bleeding due to stretching of the short gastric vessels that can accompany gastric dilatation. Serial hematocrit determinations should be obtained regularly until stable. Elevated serum enzyme determinations should be repeated at intervals until normal, as should urinalyses that are positive for blood or myoglobin. Dilutional coagulopathies should be anticipated when the transfusion requirement exceeds 80 mL/kg (the entire circulating blood volume), and may require administration of fresh frozen plasma, platelet concentrates, and, potentially, intravenous calcium.

Skeleton

Because fractures of the long bones are rarely life-threatening unless associated with major bleeding (unstable pelvic fractures, and rarely, bilateral femur fractures), the general care of the injured patient takes precedence over orthopaedic care. At the same time, early stabilization will serve both to decrease patient discomfort and to limit the amount of hemorrhage. Closed treatment predominates for fractures of the clavicle, upper extremity, tibia, and femur (infants and preschoolers), although fractures of the femur increasingly involve the use of external fixation and intramedullary rods (school-age children and adolescents). Operative treatment is required for open fractures (for irrigation and debridement), displaced supracondylar fractures (because of their association with ischemic vascular injury), and major or displaced physeal fractures (which must be reduced anatomically). Owing to the ability of most long-bone fractures to remodel, reductions need not be perfectly anatomic. However, remodeling is limited in torus and greenstick fractures, as the hyperemia typical of complete fractures is unlikely to occur.

Critical care of skeletal injuries consists of careful immobilization, with emphasis on the avoidance of immobilization-related complications (friction burns and bed sores) through the use of supportive and assistive devices (egg-crate or similar mattresses and a trapeze to permit limited freedom of movement). Fracture-associated arterial insufficiency is recognized by the presence of a pulse deficit on serial observation. Detection of compartment syndrome may require measurement of compartment pressure, which mandates fasciotomy when greater than 40 cm H_2O. Traumatic fat embolism, after long-bone fracture, and rhabdomyolysis, after severe crush injury, are rare but require aggressive respiratory support and crystalloid diuresis. Early rehabilitation is vital to optimal recovery and mandates physiatric consultation on admission. Unstable pelvic fractures require special consideration. Angioembolization, initially proposed as the optimal treatment, although technically challenging in infants and small children, is still frequently employed, especially in older children and adolescents, but external fixation remains a viable alternative, using military antishock trousers (MAST) or temporary pelvic packing (potentially complicated by lower limb compartment syndrome) as temporizing measures when needed.[27]

Physical support

The care of children with major traumatic injury also involves assessment and treatment of somatic pain, for quantification of which two scales have now been validated, although neither correlates with injury severity. Since nonsteroidal anti-inflammatory drugs (NSAIDs) are contraindicated in the early postinjury or postoperative period due to their deleterious effects on platelet function, pain control typically requires narcotic use. Delivery of such agents is best accomplished in weight based increments, with appropriate monitoring for side effects and complications, and is often best done in collaboration with a pediatric pain specialist. In patients who are not eating, nutritional support and anti-acid therapies with both topical and systemic agents to avoid gastric stress ulcer bleeding are recommended. In children with hematomas of the liver, spleen, or pelvis, low-grade fever may develop as these are resorbed, but high spiking fevers should prompt investigation for a source such as infected hematomas, effusions, or pelvic osteomyelitis. In children with large retroperitoneal hematomas, hypertension may develop on rare occasions, presumably owing to pressure on the renal vessels. The temporary use of antihypertensive agents may occasionally be required, but the hematomas usually resolve without the need for surgical decompression. Children with chest tubes or long-term indwelling urinary catheters are at risk for infection and should receive prophylactic or suppressive antibiotics as long as the tube is required, recognizing that all such devices should be removed at the earliest possible opportunity.

Emotional support

Efforts must be made to attend to the emotional needs of the child and family, especially for those families facing the death of a child or a sibling. In addition to the loss of control over their child's destiny, parents of seriously injured children also may feel enormous guilt, whether or not these feelings are warranted. The responsible critical care specialist should attempt to create as normal an environment as possible for the child and allow the parents to participate meaningfully in postinjury care, as acute stress disorder (ASD) symptoms in children and parents are common after injury, and necessitate attentive follow up and supportive care by the surgeon and primary care provider; in doing so, treatment interventions will be facilitated as the child perceives that parents and staff are working together to ensure an optimal recovery, with the added benefit that long-term psychological effects such as post-traumatic stress disorder (PTSD) may be averted.[28] Even so, depression is increasingly recognized as a serious complication in adolescents after major trauma; risk factors for depression include high injury severity, other family members injured, low socio-economic status, and suicidal ideation or attempt prior to the current event, such that psychosocial evaluation is warranted.

Burns

So far as treatment of the burned child is concerned, one must remember that whatever formula is applied during initial resuscitation must take into account the higher maintenance needs of the child. The modified Parkland (O'Neill) formula is most often used, adding 2–3 mL/kg of lactated Ringer's solution for each percentage point of total body surface area (TBSA) burned to the child's normal maintenance requirements for the first 24 hours of resuscitation.[119] One must also remember that the "rule of nines" does not strictly apply to the child owing to the relatively larger size of the head and torso; instead, the Lund and Browder chart or hand area should be used in assessing the TBSA burned. Finally, as is also the case in major trauma, particularly if there is a history of previous unexplained injury, child abuse must be suspected whenever the history proffered is not compatible with the type or severity of the burn.

Disasters

The need for PICU care is known to triple in traumatic disasters involving pediatric patients. It is therefore vital that all PICUs develop, and drill, surge plans that facilitate rapid discharge of stable patients, and double PICU bed capacity, through innovative use of available space, e.g., use of narrower beds or gurneys to make room for more patients in the PICU itself, and mobilization of additional space, e.g., post anesthesia care units (PACUs) and endoscopy units to augment the total complement of critical care-capable beds, and training of additional personnel, e.g., hospitalists, to assist with pediatric critical care management. Certain aspects of pediatric critical care, e.g., intensive wound management, can be accomplished outside the PICU; such efforts, for which consensus standards have been published, will contribute to meeting the PICU's goal of trebling pediatric critical care capacity. The provision of mass critical care (MCC) to pediatric populations is an extraordinarily complex undertaking; comprehensive recommendations are available from the Task Force for Pediatric Emergency Mass Critical Care.

Life Threatening Neonatal Surgical Emergencies

Surgical conditions in the newborn infant which constitute immediate threats to life include congenital diaphragmatic hernia associated with respiratory distress, intestinal malrotation with midgut volvulus, omphalocele and gastroschisis, esophageal atresia with tracheoesophageal fistula, necrotizing enterocolitis, and tension pneumothorax or hydrops requiring timely evacuation of pleural air or fluid. The latter two respond to simple chest drainage, usually by the neonatologist, while the former two are far and away the most urgent, diaphragmatic hernia owing to progressive deterioration of ventilation and oxygenation, midgut volvulus owing to compromise of intestinal perfusion and consequent loss of the entire small bowel. Abdominal wall defects are also major threats to life, primarily because evaporative water loses can result in rapid cooling, acidosis, and death if measures are not taken early to prevent these losses. In contrast, esophageal atresia with tracheoesophageal fistula, and necrotizing enterocolitis, become immediate threats to life only when aspiration, or perforation, respectively supervene.

Critical Care of Life Threatening Neonatal Surgical Emergencies

Congenital diaphragmatic hernia

The most important point in the critical preoperative management of the infant with a congenital diaphragmatic hernia, which is readily diagnosed by simple chest roentgenography, is to avoid the injection of air into the gastrointestinal tract. Failing to do so will result in the development of what might most accurately be called a "tension pneumoenterothorax", as the bowel loops contained within the chest become filled with air; this complication can be prevented by placement of a nasogastric tube as soon as the diagnosis is suspected, and by strict avoidance of bag-mask ventilation. Instead, supplemental oxygen should be administered via an endotracheal tube; however, beware that overzealous manual compression of the bag may result in leakage of air around the endotracheal tube with subsequent air swallowing or, worse, the development of a pneumothorax in the contralateral hemithorax. Expeditious transport to a neonatal center capable of ECMO should be effected in any infant requiring intubation.

Delayed repair of the diaphragmatic defect is the rule in ECMO centers; in the absence of ECMO, repair is performed emergently. In such circumstances, critical postoperative management requires scrupulous avoidance of either overhydration or underhydration and treatment of the associated PPHN that may develop in as many as one half of these patients some 6–12 hours following operative repair of the hernia, which typically necessitates the use of pharmacologic agents such as fentanyl, prostacyclin, and sildenafil, either singly or in combination, occasionally dopamine, and, rarely, pancuronium, in an attempt to reverse or diminish the effects of PPHN, chiefly hypoxia, due to the recurrence of right to left shunts at the ductal and atrial levels; hyperventilation and induced alkalosis, formerly the mainstays of treatment, are now generally avoided, given the associated increased risks of ALI, pneumothoraces, and further worsening of PPHN. The goal of these therapies is to support life until PPHN resolves spontaneously, usually within several days. As noted, ECMO has been demonstrated to be useful in decreasing mortality when conventional methods have failed in salvageable infants (those in whom the total pulmonary mass is judged ultimately to be sufficient to maintain life, as indicated by a preductal P_aO_2 greater than 100 Torr on 100% oxygen and a P_aCO_2 less than 60 Torr at some point in the perioperative period).

Malrotation/midgut volvulus

The key element of critical management of intestinal malrotation with midgut volvulus is the earliest possible recognition of this condition. The diagnosis must be suspected whenever frank bilious emesis or gastric aspirate is noted, absent a compelling alternative explanation; it is confirmed by emergent upper gastrointestinal contrast fluoroscopy that shows the ligament of Treitz to be abnormally located in the right upper quadrant, often in association with a "corkscrew" appearance of proximal intestinal loops which are also abnormally located in the right upper quadrant. Frank midgut volvulus is often heralded by a prodrome of intermittent bilious emeses, providing the astute clinician with an opportunity to intervene before irreversible small bowel ischemia develops. Operative treatment consists of emergent laparotomy, immediate detorsion, resection of any necrotic intestinal segments, division of peritoneal

("Ladd's") bands that fix the intestine in a volvulus prone position, and incidental appendectomy; critical treatment consists of management of the septic complications of midgut volvulus, if present, followed by long term management of short bowel syndrome, if massive small bowel resection is necessitated.

Abdominal wall defects

As previously mentioned, the critical aspect of the preoperative treatment of abdominal wall defects is the avoidance of evaporative water loss. This is best accomplished by placing gauze sponges moistened with normal saline solution warmed to body temperature over the defect, then placing the baby in a large plastic bag from the neck down, thus avoiding all but radiant and conductive heat losses. Critical postoperative management consists primarily of avoiding so excessive an increase in intra-abdominal pressure that it interferes with mechanical ventilation and/or venous return. This may require that primary repair be delayed until successive shortening of a Dacron-reinforced Silastic pouch applied to the defect over exposed viscera has achieved restoration of "eminent domain" (sufficient intracavitary volume to permit intraperitoneal replacement of extruded viscera and abdominal wall closure), although immediate primary repair remains the goal if it can be accomplished without respiratory compromise.

Esophageal atresia with distal tracheoesophageal fistula

The chief danger of esophageal atresia with a distal tracheoesophageal fistula, the most common variety of this anomaly, and one that is readily diagnosed via chest roentgenography that shows coiling of a gastric tube in the proximal esophageal pouch, is that reflux of gastric acid via the fistula, once the stomach becomes distended with air, will lead to aspiration pneumonia, a serious complication which, in the past, accounted for significant mortality. Decompressive gastrostomy must therefore be performed urgently, unless primary repair is undertaken immediately. However, one must be aware that in the premature infant with very stiff lungs due to RDS, and a large tracheoesophageal fistula, a sudden loss of back pressure immediately following insertion of the gastrostomy tube may make it nearly impossible to ventilate the infant's lungs. In such situations, emergent ligation of the fistula may be lifesaving; alternatively, the fistula may be occluded by means of an endoscopically-placed Fogarty catheter.

Necrotizing enterocolitis

Necrotizing enterocolitis remains the leading cause of neonatal surgical morbidity and mortality. It is also the most common indication for abdominal operation in the newborn infant, although the need for such procedures is decreasing, likely due to advances in neonatal care, including use of breast milk, slow advancement of feedings, avoidance of feedings during blood transfusions, and administration of enteral probiotics. It occurs most commonly in the premature infant with RDS and/or episodes of apnea and bradycardia due to the immaturity of the cardiorespiratory control centers, although term infants with congenital heart disease and/or umbilical artery catheters, especially if they receive exchange transfusions, are also at significant risk. The pathogenesis of the disease appears to rest upon the triad of mucosal ischemia due to vasospastic or thrombotic events, formula feedings, and the presence of bacteria within the intestinal lumen, although immunologic and nutritional factors may also play a role.

Initial treatment consists of nasogastric decompression, intravenous antibiotics, and fluid and nutritional support; frequent examination and re-examination, serial abdominal X-ray films (supine and left lateral decubitus), and interval blood counts, platelet counts, and arterial blood gases are also performed, usually every 6–8 hours. The condition is typically heralded by abdominal distention, bilious emesis, and bloody stools; a "sentinel" intestinal loop, pneumatosis intestinalis, and, in severe cases, portal venous gas, are the classic roentgen signs. If pneumoperitoneum and/or signs of overwhelming sepsis, i.e., irreversible acidosis, severe thrombocytopenia, or disseminated intravascular coagulation, develop, laparotomy is indicated, although peritoneal drainage may be substituted in infants deemed too unstable to withstand such intervention; necrotic segments of intestine are obviously resected, but no attempt is made to perform primary anastomosis, except in rare instances. Critical postoperative management is directed toward control of the associated sepsis and its sequelae; reoperation (including planned second look reoperation in selected cases) may be indicated if sepsis cannot be adequately controlled by other means.

Life Threatening Postoperative Surgical Emergencies

A wide variety of potentially life threatening postoperative sequelae, chiefly cardiorespiratory in nature, may occur in pediatric surgical patients; a detailed preoperative history focused on preexisting conditions, associated comorbidities, current medications, allergic reactions, and risk stratification, utilizing the American Society of Anesthesiologists physical status classification system, together with a careful review of the intraoperative course, including surgical procedures, anesthetic agents, intraoperative airway size and ease of insertion, blood and fluid losses and administration, vital signs, and urinary output, will be invaluable in identifying the offending complication. Postextubation stridor is treated with oxygen, nebulized racemic epinephrine, and/or dexamethasone, while postobstructive pulmonary edema usually responds to relief of the upper airway obstruction, although rarely a single dose of furosemide may be needed; bronchospasm is treated with oxygen and nebulized β_2 agonists, while postoperative apnea, respiratory depression, or hypoventilation due to poor mechanical lung excursion may require assisted ventilation. Hemodynamic consequences of pediatric surgical procedures may include both hypovolemia and shock, or conversely, hypervolemia and congestive heart failure, due respectively to under- or over-corrected blood and/or fluid loss; hypovolemia is by far the more common problem, and is most frequently due either to under-recognition of external losses (gastrointestinal, evaporative, third space), failure to account for maintenance fluid needs in addition to replacement of operative losses, or both. Pain, which in infants and small children is manifested chiefly by tachycardia unexplained by other, more serious, respiratory or hemodynamic phenomena, should be treated with intravenous opioids (morphine or fentanyl) or non-steroidal anti-inflammatory agents (ketorolac), in accordance with validated age-appropriate pain scales, allowing for patient-controlled analgesia in older children and adolescents (demand-dosed rather than continuously-dosed), but avoiding proxy-dosing by others (especially parents); postoperative nausea and vomiting, especially common following use of inhalational anesthetics and opioid agents, is now best treated with ondansetron, while its severity will be diminished if adequate hydration and glucose supplementation have been provided preoperatively.

Use and Misuse of Analgesic and Sedative Agents

Preplanning — including consideration of non-systemic analgesic use, such as nerve blocks or epidural catheters to provide local anesthesia, when appropriate — is essential to the successful use of analgesic and sedative agents; in addition to the detailed preoperative history described above — obtained to anticipate, and avoid, any pitfalls that may accompany their use — their depth and length must be closely matched to the goals the physician wishes to achieve, so as to minimize the dosage of these potent agents, hence their depressive cardiorespiratory side effects. With respect to the former, the chief goal is to balance amelioration of patient discomfort against their known adverse reactions; with respect to the latter, the chief goals are anxiolysis, airway protection, and cardiorespiratory maintenance, which for moderate and deep sedation, necessitate an empty stomach, continuous monitoring — both

Table 7. Analgesic and sedative agents commonly used in pediatric practice

Analgesics	
Morphine[a,b]	0.05 (0.025 in neonates)-0.1 mg/kg IV q 2–4 hr
Fentanyl[c]	1–2 μg/kg IV q 1–2 hr
Ketorolac[d]	0.5 mg/kg IV q 6 hr (max 30 mg)
Sedatives	
Midazolam (bolus)	0.1 mg/kg IV q 2–4 hr (max 5 mg)
Midazolam (infusion)[b]	0.05–0.1 mg/kg/hr IV
Lorazepam[b,e]	0.05–0.1 mg/kg IV q 20 min
Propofol (bolus)[f]	1–2 mg/kg IV
Propofol (infusion)[g]	50–150 μg/kg/min IV
Etomidate[h]	0.3 mg/kg IV
Ketamine[i]	1–2 mg/kg IV; 3–4 mg/kg IM
Dexmedetomidine (bolus)[j]	1 μg/kg IV over 10 min
Dexmedetomidine (infusion)	0.2–0.75 μg/kg/hr IV

[a]Use cautiously in infants (prolonged half life) and asthma patients (IgE mediated anaphylaxis)
[b]Use cautiously in renal and hepatic failure (increased half life)
[c]Avoid rapid bolus dosing (rigid chest phenomenon)
[d]Avoid in renal insufficiency; beware gastrointestinal bleeding (decreased platelet aggregation)
[e]Avoid prolonged use, especially via infusion (lactic acidosis 2° propylene glycol vehicle)
[f]Monitor closely for apnea and hypotension
[g]Avoid in young children (propofol infusion syndrome)
[h]Use cautiously in sepsis (potential adrenal insufficiency may cause hypotension)
[i]Ideal for asthma, sepsis; increases airway secretions, intracranial and intraocular pressures; although a sympathomimetic, may produce hypotension with heart failure or catecholamine depletion
[j]Avoid rapid bolus dosing (hypotension, bradycardia)

(Adapted from Pediatric Fundamental Critical Care Support Planning Committee, Society of Critical Care Medicine, Madden MA, *ed. Pediatric Fundamental Critical Care Support*, 2 *ed.* Mount Prospect, IL: Society of Critical Care Medicine, 2013.)

electronic and visual — and the immediate availability of backup cardiorespiratory support. Pre-evaluation must include careful inspection of the airway, including both the Mallampati, and Cormack and Lehane, classifications, as numerous pathologic conditions — especially micrognathia (Pierre-Robin syndrome) and macroglossia (most often seen in infants of diabetic mothers, and Beckwith–Wiedemann syndrome), among others — are known to compromise its already narrow diameter, for which a preplanned rescue algorithm is critical; in addition, adequate time for preoxygenation, and premedication when indicated, must always be ensured. Appropriate dosage and titration of all analgesic and sedative agents is essential, and must be both weight based, and precisely calculated (Table 7); in general, the pharmacologic effects of the most commonly used analgesic and sedative agents are similar in adults and children, except to note that 1) propofol infusion syndrome is far more common in children than in adults, such that high dose and long term use of this agent should be avoided, and continuous infusion limited to precisely defined short term procedural sedation, and 2) simultaneous use of opioids and benzodiazepines in children can result in profound cardiorespiratory depression, mandating careful titration of these agents in small increments so as to avoid significant cumulative effects (including development of tolerance, resulting in increasing dosage, hence significant risk of abstinence syndromes once discontinued), as well as careful weaning of these agents (which may oblige replacement with a less problematic agent, such as dexmedetomidine, or conversion to lower dose and longer acting intravenous or enteral formulations, before weaning).

References

1. American Academy of Pediatrics Committee on Hospital Care and Institute for Patient- and Family-Centered Care. Patient- and family-centered care and the pediatrician's role. *Pediatrics* 2012; 129(2): 394–404.
2. Dieckmann RA, Brownstein D, Gausche-Hill M. The pediatric assessment triangle: A novel approach for the evaluation of children. *Pediatr Emerg Care* 2010; 26: 312–315.
3. Goldstein B, Giroir B, Randolph A, and the Members of the International Consensus Conference on Pediatric Sepsis. International Pediatric Sepsis Consensus Conference: Definitions for sepsis and organ dysfunction in pediatrics. *Pediatr Crit Care Med* 2005: 6: 2–8.
4. The Process Investigators. A randomized trial of protocol-based care for early septic shock. *N Engl J Med* 2014; 370:1683–1993.

5. The ARISE Investigators and the ANZICS Clinical Trials Group. Goal-directed resuscitation for patients with early septic shock. *N Engl J Med* 2014; 371: 1496–1506.
6. Surviving Sepsis Campaign Executive Committee. Surviving Sepsis Campaign statement regarding hemodynamic and oximetric monitoring in response to ProCESS and ARISE trials, October 1, 2014. Available at http://www.survivingsepsis.org/SiteCollectionDocuments/ProCESS-ARISE.pdf.
7. Holliday MA, Segar WE. The maintenance need for water in parenteral fluid therapy. *Pediatrics* 1957; 19: 823–832.
8. White MS, Shepherd RW, McEnierny JA. Energy expenditure in 100 ventilated, critically ill children: Improving the accuracy of predictive equations. *Crit Care Med* 2000: 28: 2307–2312.
9. Hart DW, Wolf SE, Herndon DN, *et al.* Energy expenditure and caloric balance after burn: Increased feeding leads to fat rather than lean mass accretion. *Ann Surg* 2002; 235: 152–161.
10. Mehta NM, Compher C, A.S.P.E.N. Board of Directors. A.S.P.E.N. clinical guidelines: Nutrition support of the critically ill child. *JPEN J Parenter Enteral Nutr* 2009; 33: 260–276.
11. Nakagawa TA, Ashwal S, Mathur M, Mysore M, and the Society of Critical Care Medicine, Section on Critical Care and Section on Neurology of the American Academy of Pediatrics, and the Child Neurology Society. Clinical report — guidelines for the determination of brain death in infants and children: An update of the 1987 task force recommendations. *Pediatrics* 2011: 128: e720–e740.
12. Vavilala MS, Nathens A, Jurkovich GJ, *et al.* Risk factors for venous thromboembolism in pediatric trauma. *J Trauma* 2002; 52: 922–927.
13. Azu MC, McCormack JE, Scriven RJ, *et al.* Venous thromboembolic events in pediatric trauma patients: Is prophylaxis necessary? *J Trauma* 2005; 59: 1345–1349.
14. Cook A, Shackford S, Osler T, *et al.* Use of vena cava filters in pediatric trauma patients: Data from the National Trauma Data Bank. *J Trauma* 2005; 59: 1114–1120.
15. Kochanek PM, Carney NA, Adelson PD, *et al.* Guidelines for the acute medical management of severe traumatic brain injury in infants, children, and adolescents, 2 ed. *Pediatr Crit Care Med* 2012; 13: S1–S82.
16. Fisher B, Thomas D, Peterson B. Hypertonic saline lowers raised intracranial pressure in children after head trauma. *J Neurosurg Anesthesiol* 1992; 4: 4–10.
17. Simma B, Burger R, Falk M, *et al.* A prospective, randomized, and controlled study of fluid management in children with severe head injury: Lactated Ringer's solution versus hypertonic saline. *Crit Care Med* 1998; 26: 1265–1270.
18. Rutigliano D, Egnor MR, Priebe CJ, *et al.* Decompressive craniectomy in pediatric patients with traumatic brain injury with intractable elevated intracranial pressure. *J Pediatr Surg* 2006; 41: 83–87.

19. Downard C, Hulka F, Mullins RJ, *et al.* Relationship of cerebral perfusion pressure and survival in pediatric brain-injured patients. *J Trauma* 2000; 49: 654–659.
20. Jagannathan J, Okonkwo DO, Yeoh HK, *et al.* Long-term outcomes and prognostic factors in pediatric patients with severe traumatic brain injury and elevated intracranial pressure. *J Neurosurg Pediatrics* 2008; 2: 240–249.
21. Farahvar A, Gerber LM, Chiu Y-L, *et al.* Increased mortality in patient with severe traumatic brain injury treated without intracranial pressure monitoring. *J Neurosurg* 2012; 117: 729–734.
22. Chesnut RM, Temkin N, Carney N, *et al.* A trial of intracranial-pressure monitoring in traumatic brain injury. *N Eng J Med* 2012; 367: 2471–2481.
23. Bigham MT, Amato R, Bondurrant P, *et al.* Ventilator-associated pneumonia in the pediatric intensive care unit: Characterizing the problem and implementing a sustainable solution. *J Pediatr* 2009; 154: 582–587.
24. Nance ML, Holmes JH, Wiebe DJ. Timeline to operative intervention for solid organ injuries in children. *J Trauma* 2006; 61: 1389–1392.
25. Lutz N, Mahboubi S, Nance ML, *et al.* The significance of contrast blush on computed tomography in children with splenic injuries. *J Pediatr Surg* 2004; 39: 491–494.
26. Kiankhooy A, Sartorelli KH, Vane DW, *et al.* Angiographic embolization is a safe and effective therapy for blunt abdominal solid organ injury in children. *J Trauma.* 2010; 68: 526–531.
27. Cothren CC, Moore EE, Smith WR, *et al.* Preperitoneal pelvic packing in the child with an unstable pelvis: A novel approach. *J Pediatr Surg* 2006; 41(4): e17–e19.
28. Schreier H, Ladakokos C, Morabito D, *et al.* Post trauma stress symptoms in children after mild to moderate pediatric trauma: A longitudinal examination of symptom prevalence, correlates, and parent-child symptom reporting. *J Trauma* 2005; 58: 353–363.

Index

N

O